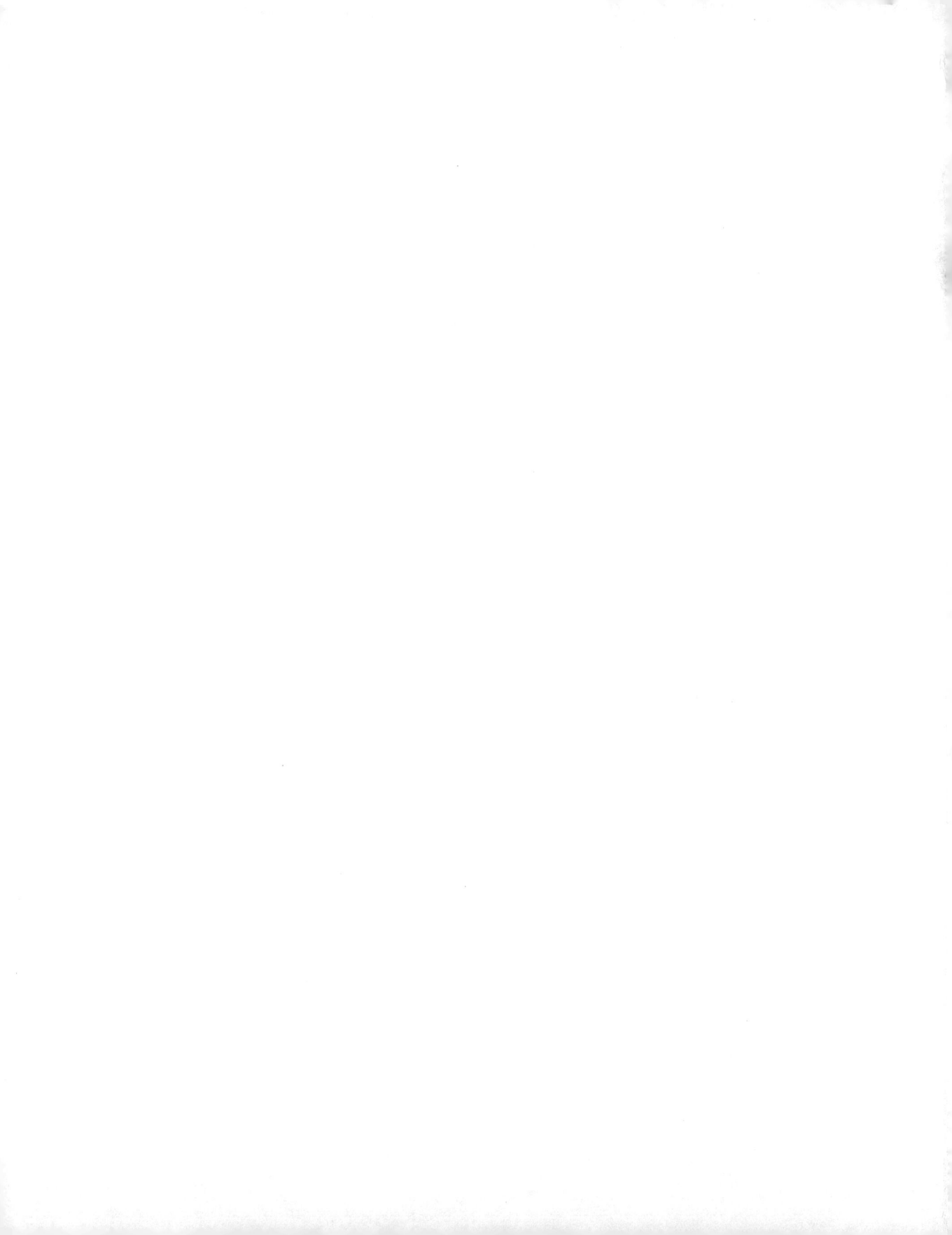

Multiple Organ Dysfunction & Failure

PATHOPHYSIOLOGY AND CLINICAL IMPLICATIONS

Multiple Organ Dysfunction & Failure

Pathophysiology and Clinical Implications

SECOND EDITION

VIRGINIA HUDDLESTON SECOR, RN, MSN

Faculty, Department of Adult Health,
Nell Hodgson Woodruff School of Nursing,
Emory University,
Atlanta, Georgia

With **109** illustrations

Mosby

St. Louis Baltimore Boston Carlsbad Chicago Naples New York Philadelphia Portland
London Madrid Mexico City Singapore Sydney Tokyo Toronto Wiesbaden

M Mosby
Dedicated to Publishing Excellence

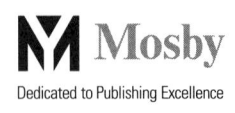

▼▶ A Times Mirror
M Company

Vice President and Publisher: Nancy Coon
Editor: Barry Bowlus
Senior Developmental Editor: Nancy Baker
Project Manager: Dana Peick
Production Editor: Dottie Martin
Manuscript Editor: Meher Dustoor
Designer: Gail Hudson
Manufacturing Manager: J.A. McAllister
Cover Art: Gail Hudson, Amy Buxton

SECOND EDITION

Copyright © 1996 by Mosby–Year Book, Inc.

Previous edition copyrighted 1992

All rights reserved. No part of this publication may be reproduced, stored in a retrieval system, or transmitted, in any form or by any means, electronic, mechanical, photocopying, recording, or otherwise, without written permission of the publisher.

Permission to photocopy or reproduce solely for internal or personal use is permitted for libraries or other users registered with the Copyright Clearance Center, provided that the base fee of $4.00 per chapter plus $.10 per page is paid directly to the Copyright Clearance Center, 27 Congress Street, Salem, MA 01970. This consent does not extend to other kinds of copying, such as copying for general distribution, for advertising or promotional purposes, for creating new collected works, or for resale.

Printed in the United States of America
Composition by Top Graphics
Printing/binding by Maple-Vail Book MFG Group

Mosby–Year Book, Inc.
11830 Westline Industrial Drive
St. Louis, Missouri 63146

Library of Congress Cataloging-in-Publication Data
Multiple organ dysfunction and failure: pathophysiology and clinical
  implications/[edited by] Virginia Huddleston Secor—2nd ed.
       p.   cm.
   Rev. ed. of: Multisystem organ failure/[edited by] Virginia Byrn
Huddleston. c1992
   Includes bibliographic references and index.
   ISBN 0-8151-4325-7
   1. Multiple organ failure—Pathophysiology. 2. Multiple organ
failure—Nursing.   I. Secor, Virginia Huddleston. II. Multisystem
organ failure.
   [DNLM: 1. Multiple Organ Failure—physiopathology—nurses'
instruction.   2. Multiple Organ Failure—complications—nurses'
instruction.   3. Multiple Organ Failure—nursing. QZ 140 M96158
1996]
RB150.M84M88   1996
616.07—dc20
DNLM/DLC
for Library of Congress   96-12507
                                                            CIP

96 97 98 99 00 / 9 8 7 6 5 4 3 2 1

Contributors

TALLY N. BELL, RN, MN, CCRN
Manager, Education,
Department of Education,
Wesley Medical Center;
Adjunct Clinical Coordinator,
Wichita State University,
Wichita, Kansas

TESS L. BRIONES, RN, PhD(c), CCRN
Research Assistant, Neurobehavior Laboratory,
The University of Michigan School of Nursing,
Ann Arbor, Michigan

SANDRA J. CZERWINSKI, RN, MS, CCRN
Director of Education,
All Children's Hospital,
St. Petersburg, Florida

C. MICHAEL DUNHAM, MD, FACS, FCCM
Associate Professor of Surgery,
Northeastern Ohio Universities, College of Medicine;
Assistant Director, Trauma/Critical Care Services,
St. Elizabeth Hospital Medical Center,
Youngstown, Ohio

DORIS M. GATES, RN, MS
Director, Cardiac Services,
Sharp HealthCare,
San Diego, California

MARGUERITE LITTLETON KEARNEY, DNSc, RN
Associate Professor,
Department of Acute and Long-Term Care,
School of Nursing,
University of Maryland at Baltimore,
Baltimore, Maryland

JOY DAVIS KIMBRELL, RN, MSN, CCRN
Faculty,
Belmont University;
Adjunct Faculty,
Vanderbilt University,
Nashville, Tennessee

JO-ELL LOHRMAN, RN, MSN, CCRN
Staff Nurse,
Surgical/Cardiovascular ICU,
Parkland Memorial Hospital,
Dallas, Texas

PATRICIA A. MOLONEY-HARMON, RN, MS, CCRN
Clinical Nurse Specialist, Children's Services,
Sinai Hospital of Baltimore,
Baltimore, Maryland

MARGARET T. MORRIS, RN, MSN, CFRN, CCRN, CEN, EMT
Program Director,
Kentucky State Trauma Systems Planning Project;
Flight Nurse,
University of Kentucky Air Medical Program;
Educational Consultant,
Lexington, Kentucky

PAMELA LASH O'NEILL, RN, BSN, CCRN
Staff Nurse, Neurosurgical Intensive Care Unit,
Harborview Medical Center,
Seattle, Washington

CAROL A. RAUEN, RN, MS, CCRN
Nursing Coordinator and Critical Care Clinical Nurse Specialist,
Cardiothoracic ICU and Stepdown Unit,
Georgetown University Medical Center,
Washington, D.C.

ELAINE V. ROBINS, RN, MS, CCRN

Staff Education Instructor,
Burn/Trauma Unit,
Emergency Services,
Ambulatory Practices,
Brigham and Women's Hospital,
Boston, Massachusetts

VIRGINIA HUDDLESTON SECOR, RN, MSN

Faculty, Department of Adult Health,
Nell Hodgson Woodruff School of Nursing,
Emory University,
Atlanta, Georgia

JANICE McMILLAN SENSING, RN, MSN, CCRN

Clinical Nurse Specialist, The Heart Group;
Adjunct Faculty,
Vanderbilt University,
Nashville, Tennessee

CHRISTINE A. STAMATOS, RN, MS, CCRN

Clinical Nurse Specialist, Cardiothoracic Surgery,
Hackensack Medical Center,
Hackensack, New Jersey

KATHLEEN H. TOTO, RN, MSN, CCRN

Coordinator, Critical Care and Trauma Nurse Internship,
Parkland Memorial Hospital,
Dallas, Texas;
Consultant, Barbara Clark Mims Associates,
Lewisville, Texas;
Adjunct Faculty, School of Nursing,
University of Texas at Arlington,
Arlington, Texas

KATHRYN T. VON RUEDEN, RN, MS, CCRN, FCCM

Clinical Nurse Specialist,
Multitrauma Critical Care Unit,
R Adams Cowley Shock Trauma Center,
Baltimore, Maryland

Reviewers

I would like to extend my appreciation to all the reviewers of the first and second editions for contributing their time and expertise to this text.

JILL ADAMS, RN, MS
Nurse Manager, Emergency Department,
University Hospital,
Augusta, Georgia

ROBERT BARKER, MD
Medical Director, Medical Intensive Care Unit,
Kettering Medical Center,
Kettering, Ohio

GORDON R. BERNARD, MD
Associate Professor of Medicine,
Vanderbilt University Medical School;
Director, Medical Intensive Care Unit,
Vanderbilt University Medical Center,
Nashville, Tennessee

JUDY L. BEZANSON, RN, MN, CCRN
Instructor of Nursing,
Nell Hodgson Woodruff School of Nursing,
Emory University,
Atlanta, Georgia

MARTHA McDANIEL BUCKNER, RN, MSN
Faculty, Belmont University School of Nursing,
Nashville, Tennessee

MARK G. CLEMENS, PhD
Robert Garrett Scholar and Associate Professor,
Pediatric Surgery and Physiology,
Johns Hopkins School of Medicine,
Johns Hopkins University,
Baltimore, Maryland

ANNE DALEIDEN, RN, MS
Assistant Trauma Coordinator/Trauma Case Manager,
Trauma Services,
Sharp Memorial Hospital,
San Diego, California

NANCY GILLIUM, RN, MS
Education Coordinator,
Tampa General Hospital,
Tampa, Florida

BETTY K. GREEN, RD, CNSD, MEd
Clinical Dietitian, Nutrition Support Team,
Summit Medical Center,
Hermitage, Tennessee

MARGUERITE LITTLETON KEARNEY, DNSc, RN
Associate Professor,
Department of Acute and Long-Term Care,
School of Nursing,
University of Maryland at Baltimore
Baltimore, Maryland

CHERYL LALONDE, BS
Senior Research Associate,
Longwood Area Trauma Center,
Boston, Massachusetts

LARRY E. LANCASTER, RN, MSN, EdD
Associate Professor,
Vanderbilt University School of Nursing,
Nashville, Tennessee

TERRY LENNIE, RN, PhD
Assistant Professor, School of Nursing,
Ohio State University,
Columbus, Ohio

ANNE R. MELTON, RN, MSN

Clinical Nurse Specialist, Telemetry,
St. Thomas Hospital,
Nashville, Tennessee

SUZANNE PREVOST, RN, PhD, CCRN

Director of Outcome Evaluation,
Associate Professor,
University of Texas Medical Branch at Galveston,
Galveston, Texas

W. EVAN SECOR, PhD

Research Microbiologist,
Immunology Branch, Division of Parasitic Diseases,
National Center for Infectious Disease,
Centers for Disease Control and Prevention,
Atlanta, Georgia

GREGORY G. STANFORD, MD

Assistant Professor of Surgery,
Department of Surgery,
University of Texas Southwestern Medical Center
   at Dallas,
Dallas, Texas

BARBARA THERRIEN, RN, PhD, FAAN

Associate Professor,
Director, Center of Excellence in Cognitive
   Neuroscience,
The University of Michigan School of Nursing,
Ann Arbor, Michigan

ROBERT D. TOTO, MD

Professor, Department of Internal Medicine,
Clinical Director, Renal Division,
The University of Texas Southwestern Medical School,
Dallas, Texas

PENNY VAUGHAN, RN, MSN

Associate Director,
Critical Care Program,
University of Tennessee,
Nashville, Tennessee

JOHN A. WEIGELT, MD, FACS

Chairman, Department of Surgery,
St. Paul-Ramsey Medical Center,
St. Paul, Minnesota;
Professor and Vice Chairman,
Department of Surgery,
University of Minnesota Medical School,
Minneapolis, Minnesota

This book is dedicated to my parents

Mr. and Mrs. Robert Alvis Huddleston, Jr.

for their constant and generous support of all my endeavors,
for the example they set, and for their love.

V.H.S.

Foreword

"To act is easy, to think is hard"
JOHANN WOLFGANG VON GOETHE

In 1996 critical care nurses not only must be able to act, they also must be able to think. Competent actions are a primary component of nursing practice. Yet, actions must be based on critical thinking—the ability to apply information from a broad knowledge base to complex patient care situations to effect a positive patient outcome. Careful reading of this comprehensive text on multiple organ dysfunction and failure is one way that critical care nurses can broaden their knowledge base and acquire a better understanding of the syndrome that has been called "the final common pathway to death."

I would suggest that the nurse who reads this book do so carefully. The subject is not a simple one, and the material presented is advanced. Topics are not covered superficially, but with completeness and sophisticated integration.

Multiple Organ Dysfunction and Failure: Pathophysiology and Clinical Implications thoroughly addresses the subject of multiple organ dysfunction syndrome. In doing so, the book also addresses many aspects of general critical care. Information presented in the text is applicable to a variety of patients, including those with shock, trauma, coagulopathies, respiratory failure, cardiac failure, liver failure, gastrointestinal dysfunction, and sepsis. In the decade ahead, this book will serve as a valuable resource to advanced practitioners, educators, and other health team members involved in the care of critically ill patients, especially those with multiple organ dysfunction and failure.

Twenty-five years ago, when critical care nursing was in its infancy, complex pathophysiologic concepts, as described in this text, would not have been found in nursing literature; rather, such information would have appeared only in medical writings. To have the subject of multiple organ dysfunction and failure described in such a thorough, well-documented work written solely by nurses is a major step forward in nursing literature and an advancement for the nursing profession. I applaud the advanced practitioners who have combined their personal clinical experiences with well-documented medical and nursing research to produce this compehensive text.

Vee Rice, RN, PhD
Critical Care Coordinator,
Critical Care Program,
The University of Tennessee,
Nashville, Tennessee

Preface

While awaiting publication of a major work, particularly one in press for months, every author and editor fears that a "major" finding or change in theory will occur *promptly* after publication. In the case of this text's first edition, it took only 1 month. In June of 1992, the recommendations of the American College of Chest Physicians and the Society of Critical Care Medicine Consensus Conference* were published, changing the very names of the syndromes to which we had just devoted an entire text! I guess I should not complain too loudly because I also changed *my* name as well, marrying 3 months after the first edition was published. So this second edition brings not only new science but also new nomenclature, which is immediately obvious by the change in title.

In this second edition, we have attempted to bring the reader up-to-date on the state of the art and science of multiple organ dysfunction syndrome (MODS). The term *dysfunction* emphasizes the dynamic nature of the process that is the leading cause of death in the noncoronary intensive care unit. Since the first edition, a wealth of research and information has been published concerning MODS, with an even heavier emphasis on the role of inflammation and the endothelium than 4 years ago. This shift in approach is reflected by the use of terms such as the *systemic inflammatory response syndrome* (SIRS) to describe the clinical presentation and pathophysiology associated with severe clinical insults such as multiple trauma, sepsis, burns, and acute pancreatitis. As we become more aware of the interplay between organs in both their physiologic and pathophysiologic states, it has become apparent that organ-organ interaction is also a major facet of MODS pathophysiology and progression; therefore it is also highlighted in this edition.

As was the goal of the first edition, the purpose of this text is to provide the experienced critical care nurse and other critical care providers with the pathophysiologic background and understanding of MODS necessary to develop an effective plan of care and anticipate events associated with this syndrome. The text not only presents *what* you see but *why* you see it. The information presented assumes that the reader possesses a working knowledge of basic critical care assessment parameters, hemodynamic monitoring, and routine standards of care for the critically ill population; therefore basic nursing care is not included. The focus is on integration of clinical assessment into a pathophysiologic knowledge base so that decision-making is based on a foundation of science and research rather than tradition.

Section I provides an overview of the syndrome, along with a complete chapter on the inflammatory/immune response (IIR) and its impact on the critically ill patient. The development of SIRS and the inflammatory mediators playing a principal role in sepsis and MODS are presented in Chapter 3. Because coagulation and the endothelium are closely related to the IIR, the role of disseminated intravascular coagulation (DIC) in the potentiation of MODS has been given individual attention in Chapter 4.

Section II presents the major pathophysiologic derangements occurring in sepsis, SIRS, and MODS. As major etiologic factors in MODS, sepsis and SIRS are common threads running through the text. Many of the pathophysiologic changes present in sepsis parallel the development and progression of MODS. Detail is given about the source of these changes, as well as the clinical presentation accompanying each change. Section III then presents each organ as a piece of the entire puzzle of MODS.

---

*American College of Chest Physicians/Society of Critical Care Medicine Consensus Conference Committee. Definitions for sepsis and organ failure and guidelines for the use of innovative therapies in sepsis. Crit Care Med 1992;20:864-874.

Damage sustained, clinical evidence of failure, and the ensuing impact that each particular organ's dysfunction produces are discussed. While individual organ support continues to be a major element of the therapeutic regimen, it is no longer the primary focus of research and management.

Section IV provides an overview of MODS and associated therapeutic interventions. Special concerns for the pediatric patient and a new chapter on geriatric patients are presented separately. The evaluation and management of oxygen supply and demand has become a burgeoning area of research and controversy in critical care; therefore in this second edition, a new chapter has been added that addresses this particular aspect of therapeutic management. As a leading cause of morbidity and late mortality in the critical care unit, MODS presents a tremendous challenge to the health care team caring for the critically ill patient. A collaborative approach to management serves as the foundation for discussion of assessment and intervention in this text. As case management moves to the forefront of health care delivery and the one set of goals/one plan of care approach (critical pathways) becomes more common, patient goal attainment will depend on our ability to collaborate and work together rather than in isolation.* In a unique study, Knaus and associates† reported a decrease in expected mortality rates in those intensive care units that demonstrated a high degree of nurse-physician collaboration. Because nurses are at the bedside 24 hours a day, they play a key role in early intervention and successful management of the patient with MODS, including coordination of the numerous disciplines involved. Nursing care of the patient with MODS requires a great degree of knowledge, independent judgment, and skill. Accurate monitoring, astute assessment, and genuine compassion all combine to enhance the care and comfort of the critically ill patient.

Section IV also provides an overview of current investigational therapies. The study of MODS is an explosive area of research both in pathogenic mechanisms and therapeutic modalities. New data become available almost daily concerning the numerous mediators that have been implicated in the pathogenesis of this complex phenomenon. Present investigational therapies are aimed at inhibiting the IIR and maximizing regional tissue perfusion and oxygen extraction.

Because MODS can strike any patient in any type of critical care area, knowledge of MODS and its associated clinical conditions is imperative to the critical care nurse. It is beyond the scope and purpose of this text to comprehensively cover all areas of critical care. However, much of the information presented here can be applied to almost any patient in the unit. Most of the secondary complications occurring in critical care are related to infection, inflammation, or ischemia, which are covered in greath depth in the following chapters. Remember that every aspect of the patient's condition and treatment, from tube feedings, wound care, and pain control to mechanical ventilation, pulmonary artery catheterization, and hemodialysis, has the potential to impact the MODS process. By understanding the etiologic factors and pathophysiologic mechanisms operating in MODS, the nurse can more effectively assess the patient, implement an individualized plan of care, and evaluate the patient's response to the therapeutic regimen.

How to use this text

This text is one of a rare number of books in the nursing literature that focuses on a single clinical syndrome and its pathophysiologic background. Although written at an advanced level and primarily intended for an experienced audience, the format of this text does allow for use by the less experienced practitioner.

Level of reader

For the experienced reader with a strong background in basic anatomy, physiology, and pathophysiology, Sections I and II provide an in-depth pathophysiologic discussion on prevailing systemic alterations that actually set the stage for damage in the individual organs. For the reader without a strong background in pathophysiologic mechanisms or enough time to cover the entire text, the organ chapters (Section III) provide an overview of normal physiology and then proceed to a discussion on pathophysiology, significant assessment parameters, and management strategies for each major organ

---
*Zander K, McGill R. Critical and anticipated recovery paths: only the beginning. Nurs Manage 1994;24:34-7, 40.
†Knaus WA, Draper EA, Wagner DP, Zimmerman JE. An evaluation of outcome from intensive care in major medical centers. Ann Intern Med 1986;104:410-418.

system. The organ chapters are the clinical "meat" of the text.

For the reader newer to the critical care arena, reading the introduction (Chapter 1) and overview (Chapter 18) will expose you to a baseline understanding of MODS and its management. Reading the text in reverse order (Section IV to Section I) may actually enhance understanding of the more difficult material. Begin with the overview, then delve a little deeper into normal anatomy and physiology and pathophysiology in the various organs, applying it to clinical assessment and management. When a grasp of the material is acquired, move to the in-depth pathophysiologic derangements in Section II. Keep in mind that these pathophysiologic changes actually incite the organ damage discussed in Section III.

Points of notice

Because Chapter 3 extensively examines the physiologic role and the pathophysiologic impact of the principal inflammatory mediators thought to be involved in the organ dysfunction observed in MODS, each chapter author focuses only on the mediators' role within his or her topic. The reader is referred to Chapter 3 for additional background information, such as the mediators' source, activation, and biologic activity. Appendix A also provides a quick reference to the major mediators.

Many charts and flow diagrams have been included in the text to give the reader an overall view of the cascade of events occurring in the various systems. In material of this depth, it is easy to get lost in the details and lose sight of the overall process as it affects the patient. The charts and diagrams assist the reader in integrating complex physiologic concepts into clinical practice and decision-making, often showing the sequence of events that lead up to a particular clinical presentation. An extensive reference list at the end of each chapter provides bibliographic support for that chapter's presentation, but it is also developed to furnish further source material for those who choose to research a particular area in more depth.

Acknowledgments

Once again, my deepest appreciation goes to the contributing authors of this text. Their attention to detail, knowledge of the subject matter, and interest in providing the most state-of-the-art information have produced a text that is both physiologically based and clinically relevant. I also value their willingness to contribute to this project a second time. I would like to extend my gratitude to the expert reviewers for sharing their expertise, valuable time, and helpful suggestions to ensure the accuracy of this text. Finally, thank you to the staff at Mosby for their support and assistance in the preparation of this manuscript.

On a more personal note, I would like to extend my deepest gratitude to Barbara Clark Mims, RN, MSN, CCRN, for her invaluable support of my nursing career and professional development from the time I was a new graduate. My decision to become an educator was primarily inspired by listening to her take complex physiologic material and make it both understandable *and* clinically applicable. She has provided me most of the major opportunities I have pursued in both speaking and publishing, including the opportunity to edit and publish the first edition of this text in the beginning. Barbara is a gifted educator and an accomplished role model, and I am forever indebted to her. I would also like to thank the faculty in the Department of Adult Health at Emory University's Nell Hodgson Woodruff School of Nursing for their support and patience with me in my attempt to get this manuscript out by deadline. They have been a tremendous source of inspiration for me and my academic career during the last year.

Finally, I would like to thank you, the reader. The feedback from the first edition has been very rewarding as many experienced nurses have expressed enthusiasm at having complex material presented in such an advanced but clinically applicable fashion. To those and other critical care nurses interested in an increased understanding of both physiology and pathophysiology and its application at the bedside, this text is for you.

The study of MODS has advanced since the publication of the first edition of this text more than four years ago. We are continually seeking to understand the syndrome in all its sophisticated detail and devastating results. I hope this second edition will provide you with a new appreciation for the complexity of the syndrome, challenge you to an increased awareness of the role of inflammation in critical illness, and enhance your understanding of the assessment and interventions required to care for the patient with MODS.

Virginia Huddleston Secor

Contents

SECTION ONE
Primary Events and Mediator Release

1 Multiple Organ Dysfunction Syndrome: Background, Etiology, and Sequence of Events, 1

Virginia Huddleston Secor

History and Background, 3
New Theory versus Old Theory, 4
Classification, 7
Primary Events, 8
Sequelae, 14
Conclusion, 16

2 The Inflammatory/Immune Response: Implications for the Critically Ill, 19

Virginia Huddleston Secor

Components of the Inflammatory/Immune Response, 20
Inflammatory/Immune Response: Levels of Host Defense, 23
Immune Response Abnormalities and Clinical Implications, 31
Assessment and Laboratory Findings, 36
Conclusion, 41

3 The Systemic Inflammatory Response Syndrome: Role of Inflammatory Mediators in Multiple Organ Dysfunction Syndrome, 46

Virginia Huddleston Secor

Systemic Inflammatory Response Syndrome, 46
Endothelium, 49

Nitric Oxide, 52
Endothelin, 53
Plasma Enzyme Cascades: Complement, 53
Plasma Enzyme Cascades: Coagulation and Fibrinolysis, 56
Plasma Enzyme Cascades: Kallikrein/Kinin System, 57
Neutrophils, 57
Toxic Oxygen Metabolites, 58
Proteolytic Enzymes, 59
Mononuclear Phagocytic System and the Macrophage, 60
Tumor Necrosis Factor, 61
Interleukin-1, 62
Interleukin-6, 64
Arachidonic Acid Metabolites, 64
Platelet Activating Factor, 66
Platelets, 66
Transforming Growth Factor-beta, 66
Mast Cells, 67
Summary: Intrinsic Control: Function and Failure, 67

4 Coagulation and Disseminated Intravascular Coagulation, 73

Tally N. Bell

Normal Hemostatic Mechanisms, 74
Etiology of DIC, 82
Pathophysiologic Alterations in DIC, 84
Relationship of DIC and MODS, 87
Clinical Presentation and Assessment Parameters, 91
Diagnosis and Laboratory Data, 92
Therapeutic Management, 95
Conclusion, 100

SECTION TWO

Pathophysiologic Changes

5 Maldistribution of Circulating Volume, 107
Elaine V. Robins

Pathophysiology, 107
Failure of Compensatory Mechanisms, 113
Regional Blood Flow, 113
Postischemic Reperfusion Injury, 119
Clinical Presentation and Assessment, 123
Therapeutic Management, 125
Investigational Therapies, 131
Conclusion, 132

6 Imbalance of Oxygen Supply and Demand, 135
Marguerite Littleton Kearney

Cellular Bioenergetics, 135
Oxygen Transport and Utilization, 138
Oxygen Supply-Demand Relationships, 141
Pathophysiology of Oxygen Supply-Demand Imbalance in MODS, 142
Conclusion, 145

7 Alterations in Metabolism, 148
Joy Davis Kimbrell

Pathophysiology of the Metabolic Response, 148
Metabolic Support, 152
Investigational Therapies, 160
Conclusion, 160

SECTION THREE

Organ Involvement and Clinical Presentation

8 Adult Respiratory Distress Syndrome, 167
Margaret T. Morris

Definition and Diagnosis, 168
Pulmonary Physiology, 169
Pathophysiology, 174
Clinical Presentation and Assessment, 178
Therapeutic Management, 180
Investigational Therapies, 185
Recommendations for Management with Investigational Therapies, 186
Research and Management in the Future Health Care Environment, 187
Conclusion, 188

9 Hepatic Dysfunction, Hypermetabolism, and Multiple Organ Dysfunction Syndrome, 196
Jo-ell Lohrman

Anatomy of the Liver, 196
Liver Function and Physiology, 197
Secretory Function, 201
Hypermetabolism, Liver Function, and the Progression to MODS, 201
Mechanism of Liver Damage Sustained in the MODS Process, 203
Clinical Presentation and Assessment, 206
Impact of Liver Failure on the MODS Process, 207
Therapeutic Management, 208
Conclusion, 211

10 Gastrointestinal System: Target Organ and Source of Multiple Organ Dysfunction Syndrome, 215
Pamela Lash O'Neill

Anatomy and Physiology, 215
Gut Defenses, 221
Pathophysiology, 223
Clinical Presentation and Assessment, 227
Therapeutic Management, 231
Conclusion, 234

11 Acute Pancreatitis and Multiple Organ Dysfunction Syndrome, 238
Janice McMillan Sensing

Anatomy and Physiology, 238
Etiology, 240
Pathophysiology Hypotheses, 242
Clinical Presentation and Assessment, 243
Complications, 248
Multisystem Involvement, 248
Therapeutic Management, 249
Conclusion, 250

12 Myocardial Dysfunction in Sepsis and Multiple Organ Dysfunction Syndrome, 252

Doris M. Gates

Historical Perspective, 252
Pathophysiology and Clinical Presentation, 253
Etiology of Myocardial Dysfunction, 265
Role of Monitoring, 267
Therapeutic Management, 268
Conclusion, 273

13 The Kidney in Multiple Organ Dysfunction Syndrome, 276

Kathleen H. Toto

Basic Physiologic Concepts, 276
Definition and Classification of Acute Renal Failure, 280
Acute Renal Failure—Sepsis—MODS, 285
Prevention and Treatment of Acute Renal Failure, 294
Future Trends in Management and Prevention of Acute Tubular Necrosis, 298
Conclusion, 301

14 Central Nervous System Dysfunction in Multiple Organ Dysfunction Syndrome, 304

Tess L. Briones

Etiology and Pathophysiology, 304
Clinical Manifestations, 312
Therapeutic Management, 314
Future Directions, 321
Conclusion, 322

SECTION FOUR

Management and Special Considerations

15 The Pediatric Patient with Multiple Organ Dysfunction Syndrome, 327

Patricia A. Moloney-Harmon
Sandra J. Czerwinski

Pathophysiology, 329
Respiratory System Dysfunction, 330
Cardiovascular System Dysfunction, 333
Central Nervous System Dysfunction, 338
Hematologic System Dysfunction, 340
Renal System Dysfunction, 342
Hepatic Dysfunction, 345
Nutritional Support, 347
Infection, 348
Skin Integrity, 349
Pain Management, 349
Growth and Development, 352
Family Support, 353
Conclusion, 354

16 The Geriatric Patient with Multiple Organ Dysfunction Syndrome, 357

Carol A. Rauen
Christine A. Stamatos

Physiology of Aging, 361
Effects of Aging on Organ Structure and Function, 366
Therapeutic Management, 375
Conclusion, 381

17 Evaluation and Management of Oxygen Delivery and Consumption in Multiple Organ Dysfunction Syndrome, 384

Kathryn T. Von Rueden
C. Michael Dunham

Clinical Evaluation of Oxygen Delivery, Consumption, and Debt, 385
Relationship of Oxygen Delivery, Consumption, and Debt, 390
Management Targets Related to Oxygen Delivery and Consumption, 392
Therapeutic Interventions, 394
Practical Considerations and Conclusions, 397

18 Multiple Organ Dysfunction Syndrome: Overview and Conclusions, 402

Virginia Huddleston Secor

Summary of Pathophysiology, 402
Assessment, 408
Overview of Therapeutic Management, 408
Investigational Therapies, 412
Ethical and Psychosocial Considerations, 418
Conclusion, 418

Appendices

A Inflammatory Mediators, 427
B Abbreviations, 436
C Glossary, 438

Section 1

PRIMARY EVENTS AND MEDIATOR RELEASE

The multiple organ dysfunction syndrome ultimately results from the body's response to physiologic insult such as trauma, shock, sepsis, and ischemia. Following insult, the body triggers two major responses to protect itself, limit the extent of injury, and promote rapid healing. These two responses are neuroendocrine activation and the inflammatory/immune response, both of which involve the production and release of numerous biologically active mediators. Localized to the site of injury, these mediators elicit changes in the organ systems, macrocirculation, microcirculation, and white blood cell activity necessary for tissue repair and organ protection. However, overwhelming activation and loss of regulatory control of these same systems shift activity from the local site to the systemic circulation and distant tissue. In addition to neuroendocrine activation and the inflammatory/immune response, other primary events associated with the injury and resuscitation occur, including endothelial damage and ischemia/reperfusion injury, that also trigger the release of mediators into the tissue and circulation. Consequently, the systemic inflammatory response rages out of control and initiates pathophysiologic changes throughout the body. The patients most at risk for developing the syndrome are those experiencing a significant amount of infection, inflammation, or ischemia, which are all potent triggers of the early primary events.

1. Multiple Organ Dysfunction Syndrome: Background, Etiology, and Sequence of Events
2. The Inflammatory/Immune Response: Implications for the Critically Ill
3. The Systemic Inflammatory Response Syndrome: Role of Inflammatory Mediators in Multiple Organ Dysfunction Syndrome
4. Coagulation and Disseminated Intravascular Coagulation

CHAPTER *1*

Multiple Organ Dysfunction Syndrome: Background, Etiology, and Sequence of Events

Virginia Huddleston Secor

Despite the tremendous advances made in both the understanding and management of critical illness and injury over the last 50 years, mortality from secondary complications remains appallingly high[1,2] and, in some syndromes, virtually unchanged or even increased from the time of their initial description.[3] Multiple organ dysfunction syndrome (MODS) has emerged as the pivotal syndrome of critical care in the 1990s, with its presence or absence often determining survival. MODS is the major cause of death following septic, burn, and traumatic insults, with reported mortality rates of 40% to 100%.[4-10] A high correlation exists between number of organs involved, length of time organ dysfunction continues, and percent mortality.[1,6,11] The first chapter of this text on MODS presents a brief history and overview of the syndrome with an emphasis on inflammatory stimuli as a major etiologic event in the development and progression of the syndrome (see the box on p. 4).

HISTORY AND BACKGROUND

In the 1950s and 1960s, single organ failure was the leading cause of death following major traumatic and surgical insults. Renal failure and, more predominantly, respiratory failure had mortality rates greater than 70%.[10,12] With the advent of sophisticated modes of resuscitation and invasive monitoring, more patients survived previously lethal insults. With this increase in survival, new patterns of morbidity and mortality emerged in the ICU. Although respiratory failure, namely the adult respiratory distress syndrome (ARDS), still presents early in the process, the cause of death today is not usually failure of gas exchange as seen in the 1960s and early 1970s, but instead is due to sepsis-related complications, systemic inflammation, and multiple organ dysfunction.[12] As therapies and understanding of disease processes such as sepsis and shock improve, the appearance of "new" complications and syndromes has kept pace.[13] Today patients rarely die from their initial insult, but from complications related to it. MODS, which has been dubbed "the disease of intensive care units," may be considered the final common pathway to death in the 20th century ICU, often following severe trauma, major surgery, intraabdominal sepsis, and other forms of critical illness.

Our understanding of MODS pathophysiology and management has evolved over the past 20 years.[11,14-17] Several early reports described an association between impaired function of multiple organs and gram-negative sepsis or shock.[4,18,19] In 1973, Tilney et al[5] described a syndrome of sequential organ failure occurring in patients following hemorrhage from abdominal aortic aneurysms. The concept of failure in *multiple* organs remote from the injured site was formalized by Baue[20] in his 1975 editorial. In that classic editorial, Baue also asserted that the emergence of the syndrome was, in part, related to ICU technology and the increased survival of patients following insults from which

> **TRIGGERS OF THE INFLAMMATORY/IMMUNE RESPONSE**
>
> **Mechanical tissue damage**
> Burns
> Crush injuries
> Surgical procedures
>
> **Global perfusion deficits**
> Shock states
> Cardiopulmonary arrest
>
> **Regional perfusion deficits**
> Vascular injury
> Vascular repair procedures
> Thromboembolic events
>
> **Ischemic/necrotic tissue**
> Myocardial infarction
> Pancreatitis
> DIC
>
> **Microbial invasion**
> Immunosuppressed states
> Surgery/trauma
> Community exposure
> Nosocomial exposure
>
> **Endotoxin release**
> Gram-negative sepsis
> Translocation of bacterial products from the gut
>
> **Abscesses**
> Intraabdominal
> Intracranial
> Other

they previously would have died. Over the next several years, Eiseman et al[8] and Fry et al[6] coined the terms multiple organ failure (MOF) and multiple system organ failure (MSOF), respectively. Other names also found in the literature include remote organ failure,[21] sequential organ failure,[20] or hypermetabolism organ failure complex.[22]

Although initially these terms were used only to label the patient at end-stage experiencing failure of multiple organ systems, the entity they describe has come into its own as a distinct clinical syndrome. However, much confusion and inconsistency arose concerning definitions, diagnostic criteria, and the actual etiology of MODS; therefore, in 1991, the American College of Chest Physicians and the Society of Critical Care Medicine met at a consensus conference to clarify terminology related to sepsis and organ failure and set forth guidelines for the use of innovative therapies in sepsis.[23,24] Their definitions are reported in the box on p. 5. At this conference, the interrelationship between systemic inflammation, sepsis, and infection was conceptually formulated, as depicted in Figure 3-1. A major conceptual outcome of this conference was the identification of inflammation (with or without infection) as a major pathogenic factor in the development of sepsis and organ failure. Two new terms were developed to address this shift in thinking: systemic inflammatory response syndrome (SIRS) and multiple organ dysfunction syndrome (MODS).[25]

The term *multiple organ failure* implies an all-or-none phenomenon that is usually irreversible. However, in the clinical progression, the organs become dysfunctional before they irreversibly fail. In contrast, the term *multiple organ dysfunction* emphasizes the dynamic nature of the clinical continuum through which many of these patients progress.[1] MODS is a nonspecific expression of critical illness involving progressive dysfunction of two or more organ systems, which is driven by the presence of numerous circulating mediators and clinical conditions, most notably the systemic inflammatory response syndrome (see the box at left).[1,23,24]

NEW THEORY VERSUS OLD THEORY

On autopsy, many organs remote from the injury or septic source display similar patterns of tissue damage in the MODS patient.[9,26] If the organs are suffering similar injury, could their damage be related, and could it be caused by systemic alterations rather than *isolated* derangements in each organ? The search for a "final common pathway" to the development of MODS has been the primary goal of recent research; therefore newer theories concerning the pathophysiologic mechanisms involved in MODS have focused on common pathways and interactions between the organ systems rather than on isolated processes. The availability of more advanced biochemical instrumentation and techniques in recent years has provided the foundation for more extensive research into the processes associated with the MODS complex.

DEFINITIONS

Infection
Microbial phenomenon characterized by an inflammatory response to the presence of microorganisms or the invasion of normally sterile host tissue by those organisms

Bacteremia
The presence of viable bacteria in the blood

Systemic inflammatory response syndrome
The systemic inflammatory response to a variety of severe clinical insults. The response is manifested by two or more of the following conditions:
Temperature >38°C or <36°C
Heart rate >90 beats/min
Respiratory rate >20 breaths/min or $PaCO_2$ <32 torr (<4.3 kPa)
WBC >12,000 cells/mm^3, <4000 cells/mm^3, or >10% immature (band) forms

Sepsis
The systemic response to infection. This systemic response is manifested by two or more of the following conditions as a result of infection:
Temperature >38°C or <36°C
Heart rate >90 beats/min
Respiratory rate >20 breaths/min or $PaCO_2$ <32 torr (<4.3 kPa)
WBC >12,000 cells/mm^3, <4000 cells/mm^3, or >10% immature (band) forms

Severe sepsis
Sepsis associated with organ dysfunction, hypoperfusion, or hypotension. Hypoperfusion and perfusion abnormalities may include, but are not limited to, lactic acidosis, oliguria, or an acute alteration in mental status

Septic shock
Sepsis with hypotension, despite adequate fluid resuscitation, along with the presence of perfusion abnormalities that may include, but are not limited to, lactic acidosis, oliguria, or an acute alteration in mental status. Patients who are on inotropic or vasopressor agents may not be hypotensive at the time that perfusion abnormalities are measured

Hypotension
A systolic BP of <90 mm Hg or a reduction of >40 mm Hg from baseline in the absence of other causes for hypotension

Multiple organ dysfunction syndrome
Presence of altered organ function in an acutely ill patient such that homeostasis cannot be maintained without intervention

From American College of Chest Physicians/Society of Critical Care Medicine Consensus Conference Committee. Definitions for sepsis and organ failure and guidelines for the use of innovative therapies in sepsis. Crit Care Med 1992;20:866.

Initially the common pathway among patients with MODS was thought to be infection. Early studies on the epidemiology of the syndrome identified sepsis as the etiologic and pathophysiologic mechanism causing much of the organ dysfunction and cardiopulmonary deterioration in critical illness[6,8]; therefore in the late 1970s and early 1980s a major focus of basic and clinical research was on the role of infection in the development of MODS. However, during this period, research and management continued to focus on organ-specific dysfunction and therapies rather than organ interactions and systemic processes triggered immediately postinsult. The realization in the late 1980s and early 1990s that MODS was a systemic process related not to the actions of invading bacteria but instead to the effects of an uncontrolled host response has led to a shift in research. Identification of early pathogenic mechanisms related to the insult, and the body's response to that insult, is a major goal of clinical and basic investigation (Fig. 1-1).[2,23,24,27-31] Although clinical evidence of organ dysfunction may not be readily apparent in the immediate postinsult period, damage to the ultrastructure may already be occurring, which is actually similar from organ to organ.[26,32] While infection can play a role in many patients, it may be more of a secondary event, with many patients dying "with" rather than "of" infection.[33]

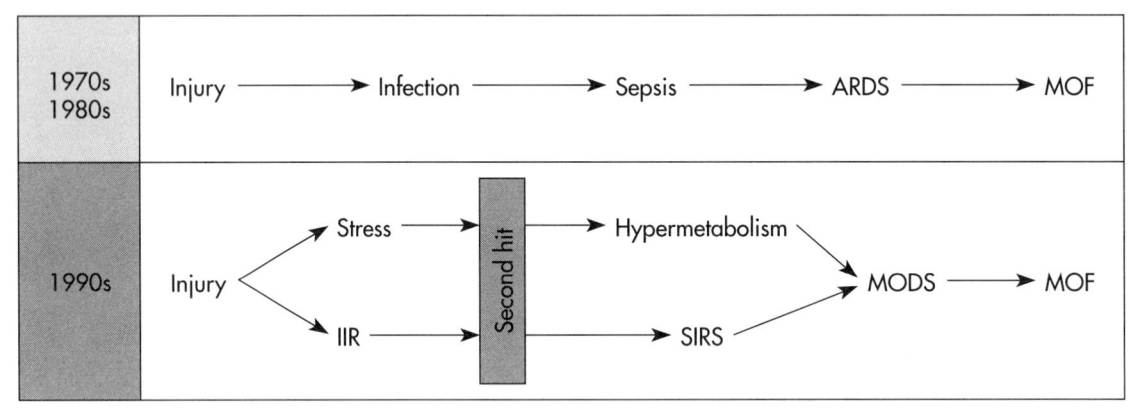

Fig. 1-1 Current and past theories of the etiology and clinical progression of MODS. *ARDS*, Adult respiratory distress syndrome; *MOF*, multiple organ failure; *IIR*, inflammatory/immune response; *SIRS*, systemic inflammatory response syndrome; *MODS*, multiple organ dysfunction syndrome.

Inflammation versus infection

As numerous investigators have described the syndrome over the last two decades, an interesting finding is becoming increasingly evident: clinical infection is not needed to initiate the MODS process. While septicemia and septic shock remain the most common single etiologic factor in the development of MODS, 25% to 50% of MODS patients do not have positive blood cultures or another focus of infection.[1,2,9,26,33] Other major conditions including perfusion deficits and persistent inflammatory foci are also associated with the development of MODS and the liberation of inflammatory mediators (see the box at right).

The common pathway in all these clinical conditions is triggering of the inflammatory/immune response (IIR) and release of inflammatory mediators, even in classically "noninfectious" states such as hypovolemic shock,[34,35] myocardial infarction,[36] congestive heart failure,[37] or coronary artery bypass grafting.[38,39] As tissue perfusion decreases, cellular oxygen metabolism is altered and by-products of anaerobic metabolism and numerous mediators are released, including lactic acid, proteases, toxic oxygen metabolites, catabolic hormones (epinephrine, glucagon, glucocorticoids), opioids, arachidonic acid metabolites, and cytokines.

Nonbacteremic sepsis and *malignant intravascular inflammation* were two terms commonly used in reference to the patients who demonstrated a classic "septic" presentation yet had no source of infection that could be found.[12,40] The newer term, SIRS, re-

---

MEDIATORS PRODUCED IN INFECTION, INFLAMMATION, AND ISCHEMIA

Cytokines
Chemokines
Colony-stimulating factors
Interleukins
Interferons
Tumor necrosis factor

Plasma enzyme cascades
Complement
Coagulation factors
Fibrinolytic factors
Kallikrein/kinins

Lipid mediators
Arachidonic acid metabolites (eicosanoids)
　Leukotrienes
　Prostaglandins
　Thromboxanes
Platelet activating factor

Toxic oxygen metabolites (oxygen-derived free radicals)
Hydrogen peroxide
Hydroxyl radical
Superoxide anion

Other
Endothelin
Nitric oxide
Proteases

places these older terms and is supported by the autopsy findings of Nuytinck et al[26] and Goris et al[9] and clinical findings of Rangel-Frausto et al[1] showing that inflammation was present, often without infection or a septic focus. These patients, with or without positive cultures, present in a hyperdynamic, hypermetabolic state.[41] Elevated cardiac output, decreased systemic vascular resistance (SVR), leukocytosis, tachycardia, and fever are prominent. Major alterations in tissue perfusion, metabolism, and oxygen utilization occur. The major danger of this syndrome appears to be its self-propagating nature. Once the inflammatory process reaches a certain level of activation, minimal stimulus is necessary to keep it going.[12] This makes prevention and early identification crucial in this patient population. Special attention must be given to identification of early markers of infection, inflammation, and ischemia. Whether systemic inflammation causes the ischemia or the ischemia causes the inflammation, the outcome is often the same: organ system dysfunction and failure.

Interaction versus isolation

A consequence of this shift in thinking (from invasion of the patient and late infection to early changes involving the body's response to insult) is the change in the view of MODS from individual problems in individual organs to an emphasis on organ-organ interaction.[10,42-45] The systemic nature of SIRS has the potential to incite damage in the individual organs, but the organs themselves also have the ability to interact with each other, particularly as they become dysfunctional. The most noted examples in MODS appear to be liver-lung interactions[46]; the effects of intestinal ischemia/reperfusion injury on the lungs and other organs[45]; and other systems and pathways not classically considered organs, i.e., the interrelationship between coagulation and inflammation.[47-49]

Organ interactions occur via neural, hormonal, inflammatory/immune, hemodynamic, biochemical, and metabolic pathways.[50] As more is understood about these pathways, it has become increasingly apparent that they are intricately related to each other and do not operate in isolation. Deviations in one have an impact on the other pathways, as well as numerous organ systems; therefore dysfunction of any particular organ cannot be attributed to intraorgan processes alone.[17,42]

A major link between the organ and pathway interactions is the endothelium. In his editorial, Wetzel[51] describes the endothelium as a distinctive organ system linking and modulating organ interaction. The role of the endothelium in health and disease appears almost boundless. Its role in vasoregulation and anticoagulation, as well as its anatomic distribution throughout the body, place it in a key position to affect almost every body process both physiologically and pathophysiologically.[52] All circulating substances come in contact with the endothelium, including those moving into the extravascular tissues.[51] Although the lungs are sensitive to endothelial damage and are often the first organ to clinically manifest dysfunction, endothelial injury occurs in many organs simultaneously with the lung injury; therefore, other organs suffer damage concurrently with the lungs.[44,46]

CLASSIFICATION

In keeping with the change in terminology and new conceptual framework, newer classification schemes have been developed to describe different forms or stages of MODS.[16,17,53,54] Although there are minor differences in the classification schemes, most are developed around a "hit" model. In the single-hit scenario, the insult itself, along with resuscitative measures, contributes directly to the development of rapid respiratory failure followed by renal and cardiovascular failure. Infection may or may not be present, and death ensues within two to four days of admission. Direct pulmonary trauma (hemothorax/pneumothorax, pulmonary contusion, aspiration), severe head injury, and delayed or inadequate resuscitative measures greatly contribute to the single-hit or primary MODS.[16,17,53,54]

In secondary MODS (also know as double-hit), secondary complications (sepsis, shock, myocardial infarction) and persistent inflammation and ischemia contribute to activation of host defense systems,[12,27,35,55] hypermetabolism,[22,54,56] overwhelming inflammation,[9,26,27,57] and loss of gut barrier function.[53,58-60] The initial insult is thought to prime the inflammatory response.[61,62] Even a minor secondary insult may then be able to reactivate the inflammatory response at an exaggerated level.[16,27] SIRS and MODS are the ultimate sequelae (Fig. 1-1). Pulmonary dysfunction usually occurs first, followed by liver/GI dysfunction, cardiovascular instability, and renal failure. The central nervous system and hematologic system may also be involved. Late mortality (defined as 14 to 21 days postinsult) is often the final outcome.

PRIMARY EVENTS

Many investigators believe the presence and activity of numerous mediators provide the common pathway to the development of MODS, with or without septicemia and shock.* But from where do these mediators come and why are they released? Following bodily insult, whether it be multisystem trauma, microbial invasion, or myocardial infarction, the body triggers two major responses to protect itself, limit the extent of injury, and promote rapid healing. These two responses are neuroendocrine activation and the inflammatory/immune response. Along with these two physiologic responses, other primary events associated with the injury and resuscitation occur that also trigger the release of mediators into the tissue and circulation, including endothelial damage and ischemia/reperfusion injury.

Neuroendocrine activation

One of the most rapid responses to injury is neuroendocrine activation, commonly known as the stress response. The nervous and endocrine systems are intimately linked in their control of tissue function. The nervous system generates biochemical agents that act as hormones, and the endocrine system produces substances that mediate activity within the central nervous system. The two systems therefore are often referred to as one functional unit and given the name *neuroendocrine* (neurohumoral, neurohormonal). Neuroendocrine activation involves the acute phase response, endocrine activation, sympathetic nervous system activity (SNS), renin-angiotensin activity, and metabolic alterations.

Acute phase response. Following injury, an acute phase response (APR) is triggered in the body with the liver as its focal point. Plasma protein synthesis by the hepatocytes shifts to an increased synthesis of proteins known as acute phase proteins and a decreased synthesis of other plasma proteins, such as albumin. The acute phase proteins include α_1-acid glycoprotein, alpha$_1$-proteinase inhibitor (alpha$_1$-antitrypsin), C-reactive protein (CRP), ceruloplasmin, clotting factors, complement components, ferritin, fibrinogen, fibrinolytic proteins, haptoglobin, kininogen, and serum amyloid.[65] The acute phase proteins participate in a wide variety of functions, including coagulation, inflammation, and metabolism. The catabolism of skeletal muscle is initiated during the APR to meet the increased amino acid need by the liver. Also, changes in lipogenic enzymes lead to increased lipolysis, increased serum lipoproteins, and cachexia.

The APR is self-limiting and the homeostatic balance returns to normal if the initial stimulus (trauma, infection, infarction) responds to the body's own healing processes or interventional therapies. Conversely, if the initial stimulus is unresponsive to therapy and continues unabated, the APR (and the accompanying physiologic changes that it induces) becomes persistent and can actually precipitate pathophysiologic events. Inflammatory mediators such as IL-1 and IL-6 are thought to be responsible for triggering the APR.[65,66]

Endocrine activation. The hypothalamus is the monitoring system of neuroendocrine activity (Fig. 1-2).[67] Following an insult, activation of the neuroendocrine system stimulates the hypothalamus to secrete its releasing hormones, which in turn trigger the pituitary to release its hormones, such as adrenocorticotropin hormone (ACTH) from the anterior pituitary and antidiuretic hormone (ADH) from the posterior pituitary. ACTH triggers the release of glucocorticoids (cortisol) and mineralocorticoids (aldosterone) from the adrenal cortex. Endorphins, growth hormone, and prolactin levels are also increased following exposure to stressful stimuli. Numerous nervous, endocrine, and metabolic actions are triggered (Table 1-1).

Sympathetic nervous system activation. Sympathetic nervous system (SNS) activity is another major component of neuroendocrine activation. Norepinephrine and epinephrine from sympathetic nerves and the adrenal medulla mediate many of the effects of SNS activity, which functions to rapidly manage blood flow and preferentially perfuse vital organs such as the heart and brain.

The "mass discharge" of the sympathetic nervous system occurs almost instantaneously, with the autonomic centers of the brain stimulating almost all the sympathetic nerves at once.[68] The sympathetic nervous system can effect change in target organs with extreme rapidity and intensity. Heart rate can double in 3 to 5 seconds, blood pressure can double in 10 to 15 seconds, and cardiac output can increase fourfold. Sweating and involuntary bladder emptying can also occur within seconds.[68]

---

*References 9, 12, 26, 27, 33, 40, 57, 63, 64.

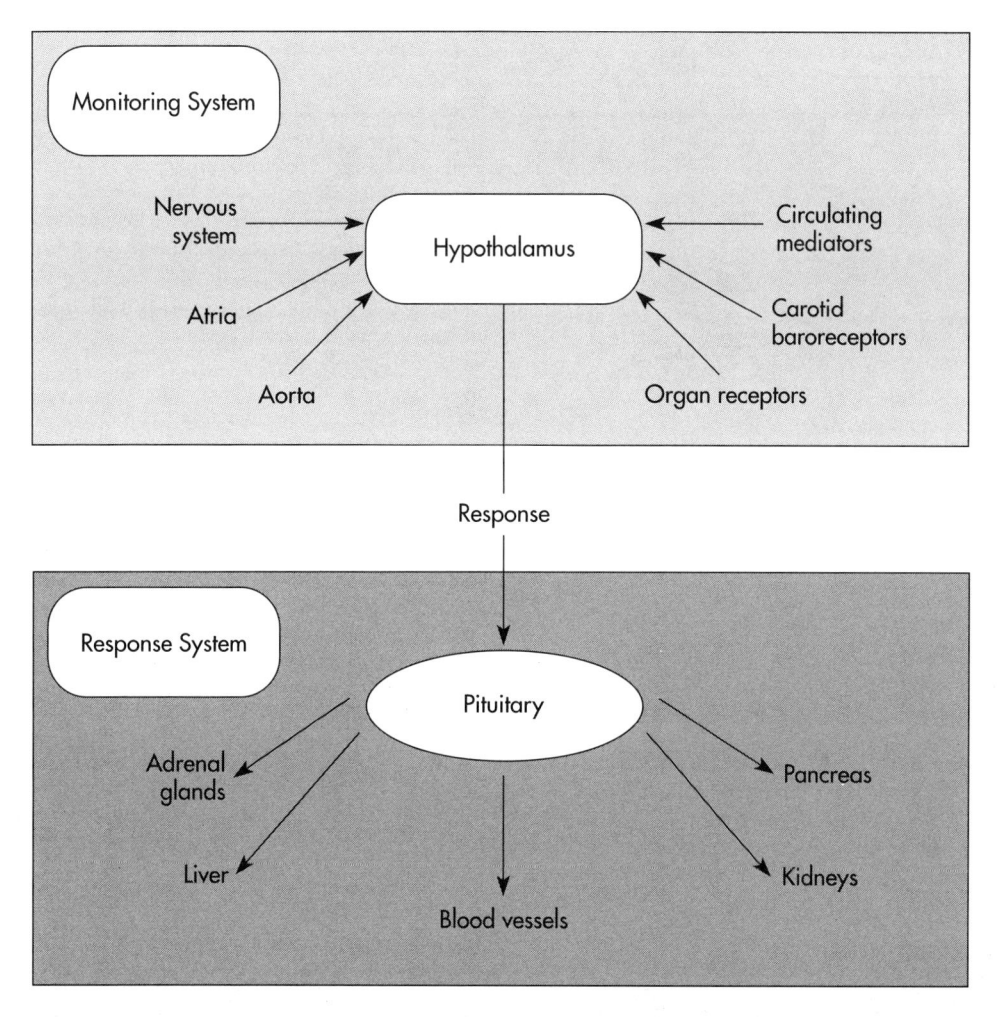

Fig. 1-2 Hypothalamic control of the neuroendocrine response. The hypothalamus monitors signals from sensors located throughout the body and processes these signals to determine if a threat is present and then initiates the appropriate response to the threat. (From Stanford GG. The stress response to trauma and critical illness. Crit Care Nurs Clin North Am 1994;6:695.)

The secretion of catecholamines and "stress hormones" and these metabolic alterations prepare the body for fight or flight from the insult, as well as for ultimate healing of the injured tissue. The hormones also allow the body to compensate for complications occurring secondary to the insult, such as fluid losses, hypotension, and microbial invasion. Other changes, including increased blood flow, increased capillary permeability, and increased blood glucose, provide an environment necessary for adequate repair and healing. In the face of hemorrhage and massive third-spacing, other mediators responsible for maintaining circulating volume will also be released, such as aldosterone and renin.

Inflammatory/immune response

Activation of the IIR represents a major physiologic event in the body. Following an insult, multiple IIR mechanisms are activated to protect the host from invading microorganisms, limit the extent of

Table 1-1 Neuroendocrine Hormone Activity in the Stress State

Hormone	Secretory source	Activity
ACTH	Anterior pituitary	Stimulated release of cortisol and aldosterone from adrenal cortex Increased lipolysis Increased amino acid and glucose uptake in muscle Increased beta-cell release of insulin
Cortisol	Adrenal cortex	Increased gluconeogenesis Decreased extrahepatic cellular protein synthesis Increased hepatic protein synthesis Mobilization of fatty acids Stabilized lysosomal membrane Decreased capillary permeability Depressed WBC activity and mediator release Lymphocyte suppression
Catecholamines (epinephrine and norepinephrine)	Adrenal medulla and sympathetic nerve endings	Increased sweat production Increased heart rate and contractility Increased blood pressure Increased respiratory rate Bronchodilatation Decreased peristalsis Increased gluconeogenesis and glycogenolysis Increased basal metabolic rate Increased lipolysis
Growth hormone	Anterior pituitary	Increased protein synthesis Increased fatty acid mobilization Decreased glucose utilization rate (conservation of carbohydrates)
Endorphins	Hypothalamus, anterior pituitary, pancreas, and GI tract	Enhanced ACTH secretion Suppressed cortisol levels Induced analgesia Euphoria
Glucagon	Alpha cells of pancreas	Increased liver breakdown of glycogen stores leading to increased blood glucose Increased gluconeogenesis
Aldosterone	Adrenal cortex	Increased renal tubular reabsorption of Na^+ and H_2O Increased secretion of K^+ and H^+
Antidiuretic hormone (ADH)	Posterior pituitary	Increased H_2O reabsorption at the renal collecting duct and distal tubule Concentrated urine

injury, and promote rapid healing of involved tissues. A series of complex interactions occur with numerous activating and inhibiting feedback loops and redundant pathways. These interactions occur via humoral, cellular, and biochemical mediators (Appendix A). While the process is initiated to protect the host, lack of appropriate regulation can lead to a malignant (uncontrolled) systemic inflammation that ultimately harms the host.[13,27,33,40,57] Inflammatory mediators produced by white blood cells and other cells, such as tumor necrosis factor (TNF),[69-71] interleukin-1 (IL-1),[72,73] toxic oxygen metabolites,[74] proteases, and arachidonic acid metabolites,[75,76] are very damaging to tissues and vessels and are associated with many signs and symptoms seen in MODS.[77,78] A vicious self-activating cycle may occur and previously protective mechanisms actually contribute to the three pathophysiologic disturbances in MODS: maldistribution of volume, imbalance of oxygen supply and demand, and alterations in metabolism (Fig. 1-3).[56,79-82] If these pathophysiologic changes can-

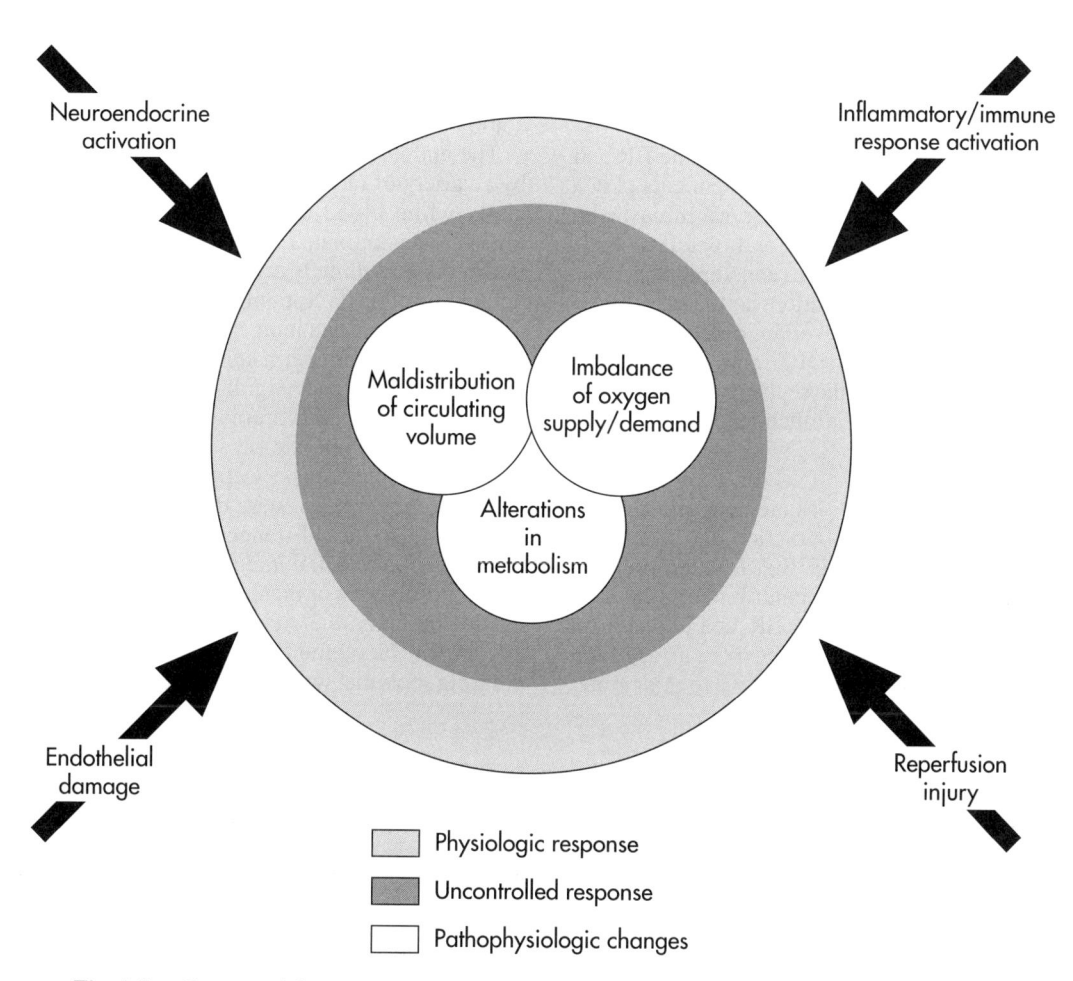

Fig. 1-3 Conceptual framework depicting relationship between primary events and pathophysiologic changes. Once insulted, primary events such as neuroendocrine activation, IIR activation, endothelial damage, and ischemia/reperfusion injury trigger the release of numerous mediators. Under proper regulation (outer circle), many effects are local and specific. If control is lost (dark circle), the cycle becomes self-propagating, and the mediators initially released to protect the host actually provoke the three major pathophysiologic changes (inner white circles). (From Huddleston VB. Multisystem organ failure: A pathophysiologic approach. Boston, 1991;5.)

not be reversed or slowed, organ dysfunction and failure ensue (Table 1-2).[83] See Chapters 2 and 3 for further information on the exquisite and complicated mechanism of IIR activity.

The wound's role in the systemic response has also become a focus of investigation.[84,85] The wound produces extensive inflammation by activating large numbers of neutrophils and macrophages, which in turn produce inflammatory mediators such as TNF, toxic oxygen metabolites, and proteases.[86] These mediators can be systemically absorbed and target distant organs. The wound also makes oxygen and metabolic demands on an already stressed system.[84]

An extensive overlap exists between the IIR and coagulation. Several circulating components play a role in both processes: kallikrein/kinin cascade, complement, Hageman factor, and platelets. Activation of the IIR often leads to concomitant activation of coagulation or alterations in the hemostatic balance. Because of this overlap, disseminated intravascular coagulation (DIC) and other coagulopathies are common in the septic patient or the patient experiencing a major inflammatory insult.

Endothelial damage

Coagulation abnormalities are also prevalent in the critically ill patient population due to the extensive endothelial damage that is often present. The endothelium is a major contributor to the activation and potentiation of the IIR, coagulopathies, and MODS because of its extensive surface area (throughout the body), susceptibility to injury, and metabolic functions. Once thought to be an inert barrier between the flowing blood and the substructure of the blood vessels and tissue, the endothelium is now recognized as an active metabolic organ (see Chapter 3).[51] Two of the major functions of the endothelium are anticoagulation and vasoregulation, particularly in the microcirculation.[52,87] When damaged, the endothelium loses many of its anticoagulant properties and may even generate and release procoagulant substances, such as tissue factor.[88-90] If the vasoregulatory properties of the endothelium are lost, autoregulation in the tissue beds may not occur and oxygen delivery could be compromised.[87]

The endothelium is very susceptible to damage by a variety of factors (see the box on p. 13), especially white blood cell–endothelial cell interactions.[91-93] Endotoxin, TNF, and other inflammatory mediators also directly or indirectly damage the endothelium.[69,73,94-97] Not only does endothelial damage potentiate coagulation abnormalities, but it may also affect capillary permeability. Direct damage or mediator activity may significantly increase capillary permeability, thus promoting edema formation and changes in oncotic pressure gradients.[94,98,99] Whether the patient is a victim of a fresh myocardial infarction, multisystem trauma, or pneumonia, potentially toxic substances are circulating that could alter endothelial integrity and incite coagulation abnormalities or increased vascular permeability. In summary, the endothelium not only aids in keeping the blood fluid but also in retaining the circulating volume within the vascular space and

Table 1-2 Definition of Pathophysiologic Changes

Maldistribution of circulating volume	Imbalance of oxygen supply and demand	Alterations in metabolism
Capillary permeability	V/Q mismatching	Hypermetabolism
Vasodilatation	Intrapulmonary shunting	Inadequate substrate metabolism
Selective vasoconstriction	Maldistribution of volume	Protein catabolism
Loss of autoregulation	Microcirculatory abnormalities	Liver dysfunction
Microvascular thrombi	Oxygen extraction defects	Peripheral cell dysfunction
Vascular obstruction	Increased demand	Resistance to exogenous administration
Tissue edema	Pain	
Cellular aggregation	Fever	
Microthrombi	Tachycardia	
Myocardial dysfunction	Restlessness	
Fluid imbalances	Increased work of breathing	

FACTORS IMPAIRING ENDOTHELIAL INTEGRITY AND FUNCTION

Mechanical disruption
Microorganisms and their toxins
Immune complexes
Shock
Hypoxemia
Acidosis
Platelet aggregation leading to microthrombi, mechanical obstruction, and decreased nutrition
Neutrophil aggregation and adhesion leading to mechanical obstruction, free radical formation, and protease release and damage
Coagulation on the endothelial surface
Direct action of mediators such as TNF and IL-1

TNF, tumor necrosis factor; *IL-1*, interleukin-1.

maintaining oxygen delivery to the tissues. Both activation of the IIR and endothelial damage contribute to the coagulopathies seen in sepsis and MODS.[47,49,94,100]

Ischemia/reperfusion injury

Ischemia/reperfusion injury has also been shown to play a role in remote organ damage and MODS and is thought to be primarily mediated by toxic oxygen metabolites (free radicals) and neutrophils.[101,102] It is especially prevalent following low-flow or ischemic events, such as shock states, cardiopulmonary arrest, myocardial infarctions, and aortic cross-clamping.[85,103,104] During ischemia, specific enzymes and substances in the tissue undergo transformations. An enzyme, xanthine dehydrogenase, is converted to another enzyme, xanthine oxidase. Concurrently, ATP is broken down to hypoxanthine and xanthine. When blood and oxygen are returned to the tissue during reperfusion, the molecular oxygen (O_2) reacts with these "new" enzymes and substances to produce the superoxide radical (Fig. 1-4). The formation of hydrogen peroxide follows, and in the presence of iron, hydroxyl radical production can occur. In myocardial reperfusion, the formation of free radicals irritates the myocardium, potentially causing the increased ectopy often seen postreperfusion during thrombolytic therapy.

The free radicals, along with the lactic acid, potassium, and other substances released from reperfused tissues, are very toxic to tissues and the endothelium and may perpetuate damage that has already occurred secondary to ischemia. Increased capillary permeability, tissue edema, and microcirculatory compression may occur and cause further damage to already compromised limbs or organs. The "stunned" myocardium seen after the patient comes off bypass may also be related to production of free radicals in the revascularized myocardium.[103]

Damage in ischemia/reperfusion is not limited to the organ that was initially ischemic. Following reperfusion of a previously ischemic bowel, a systemic inflammatory response[105] is noted, highlighted by neutrophil sequestration in several organs,[106] most notably the lungs and liver. These neutrophils also demonstrate heightened superoxide radical and protease generation.[45] Consequent to these actions, lung microvascular permeability increases and evidence of endothelial damage is noted. An ARDS-type presentation can occur. Activated complement, cytokines, and adhesion molecules most likely play a role in the pathogenesis of pulmonary microvascular injury following intestinal ischemia/reperfusion injury, but the mechanisms are not fully defined.[45]

Summary of primary events

The body suffering an insult is exposed not only to direct damage by the insult but also to the effects of many activated mediators. Substances and systems initially primed and activated to protect and defend the host actually cause severe tissue damage, shock, and death secondary to MODS.* The mediators released during the two primary events of IIR activation and neuroendocrine activation initially serve a physiologic function in host defense and repair, but the loss of regulation and overwhelming of clearance mechanisms lead to a pathologic "build-up" of many mediators. Previously localized responses become systemic derangements exacerbated by endothelial damage and ischemia/reperfusion in-

---

*References 1, 13, 27, 33, 57, 86.

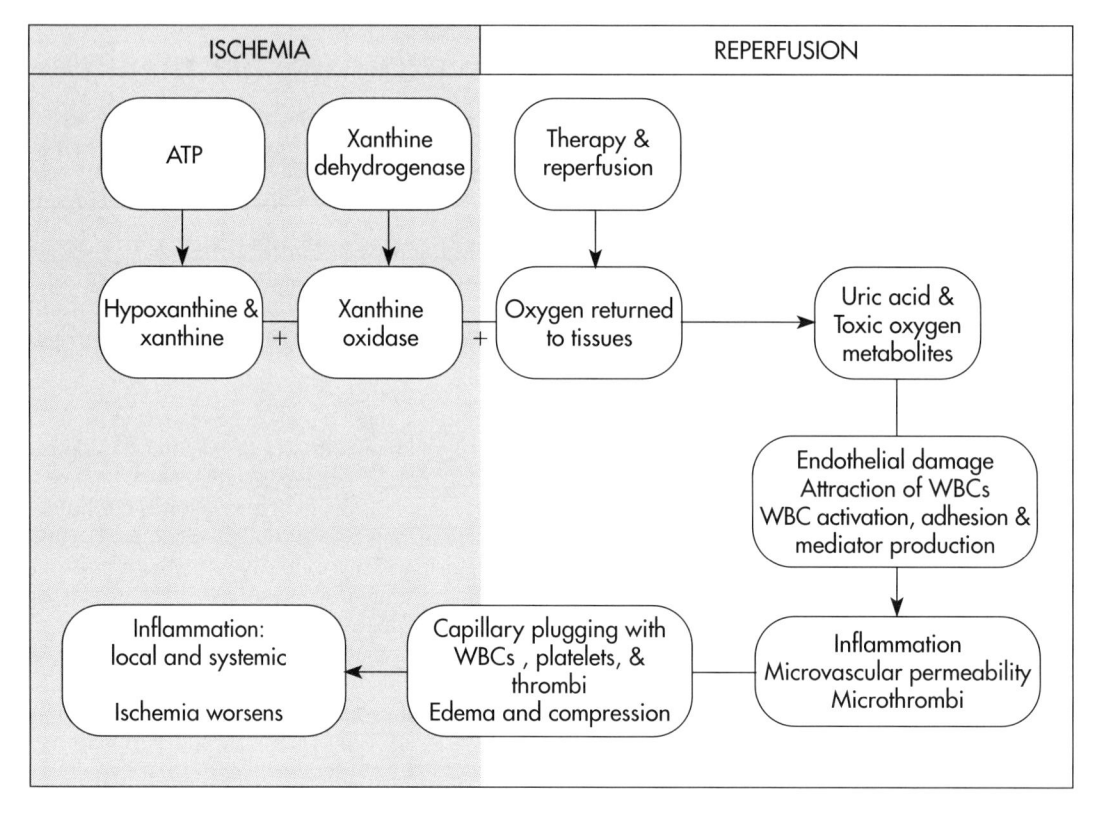

Fig. 1-4 Toxic oxygen metabolite (TOM) formation in ischemia and reperfusion injury. The TOMs produced during reperfusion injury attract and activate WBCs, which can produce more TOMs and other inflammatory mediators such as proteases. (From Huddleston VB. Multisystem organ failure: A pathophysiologic approach. Boston, 1991;35.)

jury. For example, vasodilatation occurring at the site of injury secondary to kinin and complement activity may occur systemically, if the mediator levels increase above a threshold value. Severe decreases in SVR and BP then ensue.

The numerous mediators released provoke three pathophysiologic derangements: (1) maldistribution of circulating volume, (2) imbalance of oxygen supply/demand, and (3) alterations in metabolism. These pathophysiologic derangements are discussed in Chapters 5, 6, and 7, respectively. Figure 1-5 diagrams the relationship between the primary events, pathophysiologic derangements, and the ensuing clinical presentation that progresses to MODS and, ultimately, organ failure. Due to the autoactivating nature of the stimulated IIR, the IIR becomes malignant and perpetuates itself in a vicious cycle requiring minimal additional stimulus. In other words, once the system becomes activated, it may keep itself going despite the removal of initial stimuli such as abscesses, microbes, or necrotic tissue (Fig. 1-5).[12,40]

SEQUELAE
Determining factors

Organ dysfunction and failure occurring secondary to the pathophysiologic changes are not predictable on admission. Why does the patient in bed 1 develop fulminant MODS and the patient in bed 2 overcome the obstacles and recover? The progression into organ dysfunction and failure following insult and pathophysiologic derangements is determined by the severity of insult, host-related factors, therapeutic interventions, and other undefined mechanisms. Numerous scoring systems and diag-

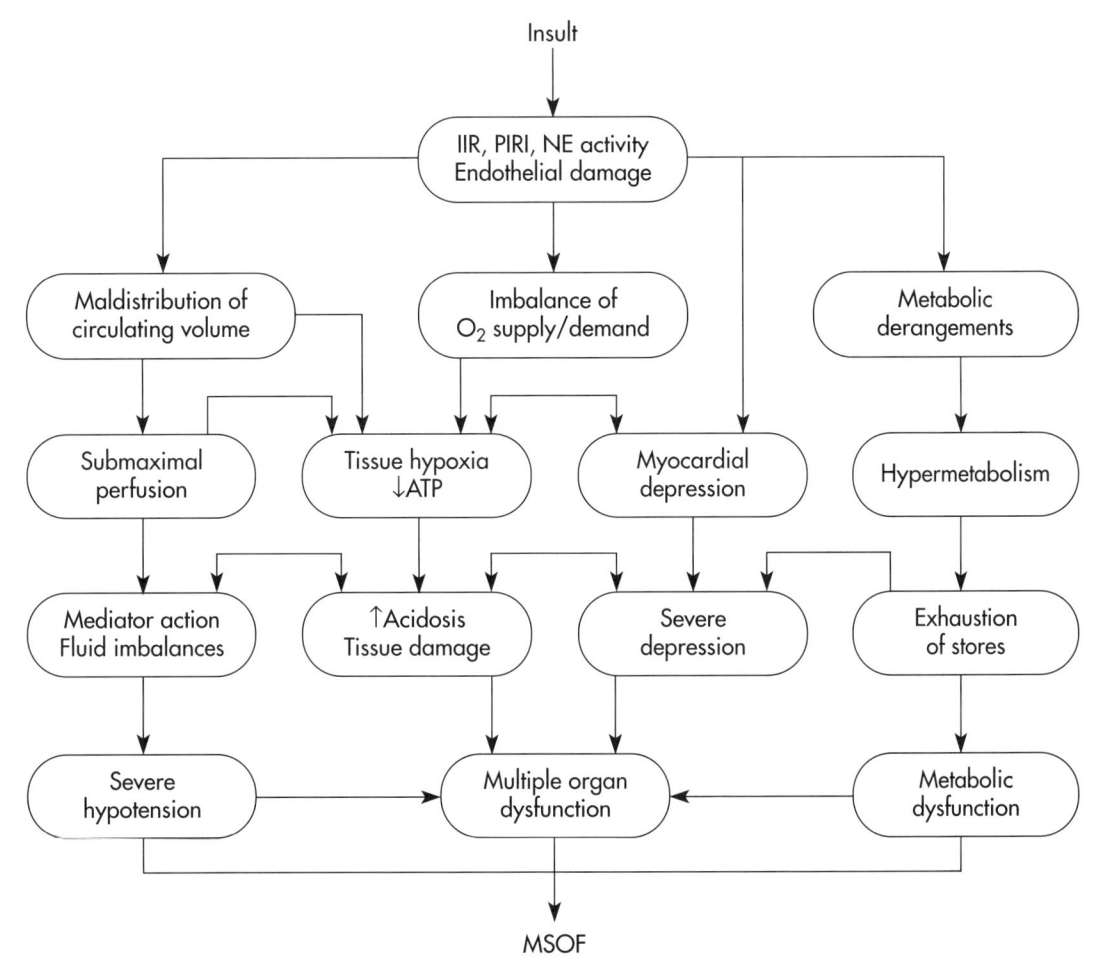

Fig. 1-5 Pathophysiologic cascade mechanism of multiple organ dysfunction and failure. *IIR,* Inflammatory/immune response; *NE,* neuroendocrine; *PIRI,* postischemic reperfusion injury; *ATP,* adenosine triphosphate; *MSOF,* multisystem organ failure. (From Huddleston VB. Multisystem organ failure: A pathophysiologic approach. Boston, 1991;24.)

nostic criteria based on initial clinical presentation and other factors have been developed with varying levels of success in an attempt to prospectively identify those patients most likely to develop MODS.[17,23,107-111]

Obviously, the more severe the insult, the more likely the patient will develop complications. Host-related factors, including age, chronic disease states, and immunosuppression, may increase the risk of MODS. Genetic predisposition may also play a role.[16,112,113] In the patient with altered defense mechanisms or increased severity of insult, normal regulatory and clearance mechanisms are more likely to be overwhelmed. The body cannot clear the elevated levels of potentially toxic mediators, and the mediators begin to inflict damage on vessels and tissue. Iatrogenic factors such as invasive lines and catheters, immunosuppressant therapy, surgical procedures, and antibiotic therapy predispose the patient to the development of sepsis and thus MODS.[114] See Chapter 2 for further discussion on contributing factors and immunosuppression.

Organ involvement

Although the heart, lung, liver, and kidney are most often addressed in discussions of MODS, every organ has the potential to suffer damage. Even peripheral neuropathies are now associated with critical illness and MODS.[115] Every organ is at risk because every organ receives a blood supply that may contain many of the inflammatory mediators. Not all organs have equal susceptibility to injury, nor does each organ's failure affect patient survival with the same magnitude. Factors affecting organ system involvement include (1) sensitivity of the organ's vascular bed to mediators and hypoperfusion, (2) regional degree of inflammation and proximity to the primary site of trauma or infection, and (3) responsiveness to the therapeutic regimen; i.e., what may help one organ may harm another.[40,84,116]

The damage suffered by an individual organ may be a contributing factor to the development of MODS or a direct result of the ongoing inflammatory process. In other words, the organ may be the source of the problem or a victim of the process. For example, ARDS may potentiate the development of MODS, or ARDS may develop secondary to mediators and toxins circulating in the blood during SIRS and MODS. As previously described, present emphasis is not on isolated failures but on systemic processes and organ-organ interaction.*

CONCLUSION

The complex phenomenon of MODS, once thought to be a clinical presentation stemming solely from sepsis and cardiovascular instability, is now recognized as a systemic disturbance mediated by a sustained inflammatory response, hypermetabolism, hypoperfusion, and ultimately dysfunctional cellular activity and oxygen extraction/utilization defects. No longer viewed as a series of isolated failures, MODS represents a complex interaction of organ systems in both functioning and pathophysiologic states and may represent the failure of the body to maintain a balance between protective and destructive actions of the inflammatory/immune response. Future therapies focus on inhibition of this uncontrolled, systemic response.

---

*References 10, 43, 44, 46, 47, 93.

REFERENCES

1. Rangel-Frausto M et al. The natural history of the systemic inflammatory response syndrome (SIRS). JAMA 1995;273:117-123.
2. Bone RC. Toward an epidemiology and natural history of SIRS (systemic inflammatory response syndrome). JAMA 1992;268:3452-3455.
3. Deitch EA. Multiple organ failure: Pathophysiology and potential future therapy. Ann Surg 1992;216:117-134.
4. Skillman JJ et al. Respiratory failure, hypotension, sepsis, and jaundice. Am J Surg 1969;117:523-530.
5. Tilney NL, Bailey GL, Morgan AP. Sequential system failure after rupture of abdominal aortic aneurysms: An unsolved problem in postoperative care. Ann Surg 1973;178:117-122.
6. Fry DE et al. Multiple system organ failure: The role of uncontrolled infection. Arch Surg 1980;115:136-140.
7. Sweet SJ et al. Synergistic effect of acute renal failure and respiratory failure in the surgical intensive care unit. Am J Surg 1981;141:492-496.
8. Eiseman B, Beart R, Norton L. Multiple organ failure. Surg Gynecol Obstet 1977;144:323-326.
9. Goris RJ et al. Multiple organ failure: Generalized autodestructive inflammation. Arch Surg 1985;120:1109-1115.
10. Bone RC et al. Adult respiratory distress syndrome: Sequence and importance of development of multiple organ failure. Chest 1992;101:320-326.
11. Deitch EA. Multiple organ failure. Adv Surg 1993;26:333-356.
12. DeCamp MM, Demling RH. Posttraumatic multisystem organ failure. JAMA 1988;260:530-534.
13. Pinsky MR. Multiple systems organ failure: Malignant intravascular inflammation. Crit Care Clin 1989;5:195-198.
14. Cipolle MD, Pasquale MD, Cerra FB. Secondary organ dysfunction: From clinical perspectives to molecular mediators. Crit Care Clin 1993;9:261-298.
15. Beal AL, Cerra FB. Multiple organ failure syndrome in the 1990s: Systemic inflammatory response and organ dysfunction. JAMA 1994;271:226-233.
16. Demling R et al. Multiple organ dysfunction in the surgical patient: Pathophysiology, prevention, and treatment. Curr Probl Surg 1993;30:348-414.
17. Moore FA, Moore EE. Evolving concepts in the pathogenesis of postinjury multiple organ failure. Surg Clin North Am 1995;75:257-277.
18. Burke JF, Pontopiddan H, Welch CE. High output respiratory failure: An important cause of death ascribed to peritonitis or ileus. Ann Surg 1963;158:581-595.
19. Clowes GHA et al. Observations on the pathogenesis of the pneumonitis associated with severe infections in other parts of the body. Ann Surg 1968;167:630-650.
20. Baue AE. Multiple, progressive, or sequential systems failure: A syndrome of the 1970s. Arch Surg 1975;110:779-781.
21. Polk HC, Shields CL. Remote organ failure: A valid sign of occult intraabdominal infection. Surgery 1977;81:310-313.
22. Cerra FB. Hypermetabolism, organ failure, and metabolic support. Surgery 1987;101:1-14.
23. American College of Chest Physicians/Society of Critical Care Medicine Consensus Conference Committee. Definitions for sepsis and organ failure and guidelines for the use of innovative therapies in sepsis. Crit Care Med 1992;20:864-874.

24. Bone RC et al. Definitions for sepsis and organ failure and guidelines for the use of innovative therapies in sepsis. The ACCP/SCCM Consensus Conference Committee. Chest 1992;101:1644-1655.
25. Ackerman MH. The systemic inflammatory response, sepsis, and multiple organ dysfunction: New definitions for an old problem. Crit Care Nurs Clin North Am 1994;6:243-250.
26. Nuytinck HKS et al. Whole-body inflammation in trauma patients. Arch Surg 1988;123:1519-1524.
27. Anderson BO, Harken AH. Multiple organ failure: inflammatory priming and activation sequences promote autologous tissue injury. J Trauma 1990;30:S44-S49.
28. Dinarello CA, Gelfand JA, Wolff SM. Anticytokine strategies in the treatment of the systemic inflammatory response syndrome. JAMA 1993;269:1829-1835.
29. Lowry SF. Anticytokine therapies in sepsis. New Horiz 1993;1:120-126.
30. Giroir BP. Mediators of septic shock: New approaches for interrupting the endogenous inflammatory cascade. Crit Care Med 1993;21:780-789.
31. Christman JW, Holden EP, Blackwell TS. Strategies for blocking the systemic effects of cytokines in the sepsis syndrome. Crit Care Med 1995;23:955-963.
32. Schlag G, Redl H. Introduction: "Organ in shock," "Early organ failure," "Late organ failure." In: Schlag G, Redl H, eds. Pathophysiology of shock, sepsis, and organ failure. Berlin: Springer-Verlag, 1993:1-3.
33. Waydas C et al. Inflammatory mediators, infection, sepsis, and multiple organ failure after severe trauma. Arch Surg 1992;127:460-467.
34. Roumen RMH et al. Cytokine patterns in patients after major vascular surgery, hemorrhagic shock, and severe blunt trauma. Ann Surg 1993;218:769-776.
35. Svoboda P, Kantorova I, Ochmann J. Dynamics of interleukin 1, 2, and 6 and tumor necrosis factor alpha in multiple trauma patients. J Trauma 1994;36:336-340.
36. Kilgore KS, Lucchesi BR. Reperfusion injury after myocardial infarction: The role of free radicals and the inflammatory response. Clin Biochem 1993;26:359-370.
37. Mann DL, Young JB. Basic mechanisms of congestive heart failure: Recognizing the role of proinflammatory cytokines. Chest 1994;105:897-904.
38. Casey LC. Role of cytokines in the pathogenesis of cardiopulmonary-induced multisystem organ failure. Ann Thorac Surg 1993;56:S92-S96.
39. Butler J, Rocker GM, Westaby S. Inflammatory response to cardiopulmonary bypass. Ann Thorac Surg 1993;55:552-559.
40. Pinsky MR, Matuschak GM. Multiple systems organ failure: Failure of host defense homeostasis. Crit Care Clin 1989;5:199-220.
41. Ronco JJ et al. No differences in hemodynamics, ventricular function, and oxygen delivery in septic and nonseptic patients with the adult respiratory distress syndrome. Crit Care Med 1994;22:777-782.
42. Matuschak GM, ed. Organ interactions in critical illness [entire issue]. New Horiz 1994;2:413-581.
43. Matuschak GM. Organ interactions in critical illness: Paradigms and mechanisms. New Horiz 1994;2:413-414.
44. Crouser ED, Dorinsky PM. Gastrointestinal tract dysfunction in critical illness: Pathophysiology and interaction with acute lung injury in adult respiratory distress syndrome/multiple organ dysfunction syndrome. New Horiz 1994;2:476-487.
45. Turnage RH, Guice KS, Oldham KT. Pulmonary microvascular injury following intestinal reperfusion. New Horiz 1994;2:463-475.
46. Matuschak GM. Liver-lung interactions in critical illness. New Horiz 1994;2:488-504.
47. Taylor FB. The inflammatory-coagulant axis in the host response to Gram-negative sepsis: Regulatory roles of proteins and inhibitors of tissue factor. New Horiz 1994;2:555-565.
48. Bone RC. Modulators of coagulation: A critical appraisal of their role in sepsis. Arch Intern Med 1992;152:1381-1389.
49. Secor VH. Mediators of coagulation and inflammation: Relationship and clinical significance. Crit Care Nurs Clin North Am 1993;5:411-433.
50. Buchman TG, Zahnbauer BA. Molecular biology in the intensive care unit: A framework for interpretation. New Horiz 1995;3:139-145.
51. Wetzel RC. The intensivist's system. Crit Care Med 1993;21(9 suppl):S341-S344.
52. Schiffrin EL. The endothelium and control of blood vessel function in health and disease. Clin Invest Med 1994;17:602-620.
53. Meakins JL. Etiology of multiple organ failure. J Trauma 1990;30:S165-S168.
54. Lekander BJ, Cerra FB. The syndrome of multiple organ failure. Crit Care Nurs Clin North Am 1990;2:331-342.
55. Border JR. Hypothesis: Sepsis, multiple systems organ failure, and the macrophage [editorial]. Arch Surg 1988;123:285-286.
56. Barton R, Cerra FB. The hypermetabolism, multiple organ failure syndrome. Chest 1989;96:1153-1160.
57. Goris RJ. Multiple organ failure: Whole body inflammation? Schweiz Med Wochenschr 1989;119:347-353.
58. Deitch EA. The role of intestinal barrier failure and bacterial translocation in the development of systemic infection and multiple organ failure. Arch Surg 1990;125:403-404.
59. Ryan CM et al. Increased gut permeability early after burns correlates with the extent of burn injury. Crit Care Med 1992;20:1508-1512.
60. Fiddian-Green RG. Associations between intramucosal acidosis in the gut and organ failure. Crit Care Med 1993;21(suppl):S103-S107.
61. Vercellotti GM et al. Platelet-activating factor primes neutrophil responses to agonists: Role in promoting neutrophil-mediated endothelial damage. Blood 1988;71:1100-1107.
62. Worthen GS et al. The priming of neutrophils by lipopolysaccharide for production of intracellular platelet-activating factor: Potential role in mediation of enhanced superoxide secretion. J Immunol 1988;140:3553-3559.
63. Roumen RMH et al. Inflammatory mediators in relation to the development of multiple organ failure in patients after severe blunt trauma. Crit Care Med 1995;23:474-480.
64. Donnelly TJ et al. Cytokine, complement, and endotoxin profiles associated with the development of the adult respiratory distress syndrome after severe injury. Crit Care Med 1994;22:768-776.
65. Pannen BHJ, Robotham JL. The acute-phase response. New Horiz 1995;3:183-197.
66. Kushner I. Postmodernism, the acute phase response, and interpretation of data. Ann NY Acad Sci 1989;557:240-242.
67. Stanford GG. The stress response to trauma and critical illness. Crit Care Nurs Clin North Am 1994;6:693-702.
68. Guyton AC. Textbook of medical physiology. 8th ed. Philadelphia: WB Saunders, 1991.

69. Beutler B. Endotoxin, tumor necrosis factor, and related mediators: New approaches to shock. New Horiz 1993;1:3-12.
70. Beutler B, Milsark IW, Cerami AC. Passive immunization against cachectin/tumor necrosis factor protects mice from lethal effect of endotoxin. Science 1985;229:869-871.
71. Tracey KJ, Cerami A. Tumor necrosis factor: An updated review of its biology. Crit Care Med 1993;21:S415-S422.
72. Dinarello CA, Wolff SM. The role of interleukin-1 in disease. N Engl J Med 1993;328:106-113.
73. Yi ES, Ulich TR. Endotoxin, interleukin-1, and tumor necrosis factor cause neutrophil-dependent microvascular leakage in postcapillary venules. Am J Pathol 1992;140:659-663.
74. Goode HF, Webster NR. Free radicals and antioxidants in sepsis. Crit Care Med 1993;21:1770-1776.
75. Fink MP. Phospholipases A2: Potential mediators of the systemic inflammatory response syndrome and the multiple organ dysfunction syndrome [editorial]. Crit Care Med 1993;21:957-959.
76. Fletcher JR. Eicosanoids: Critical agents in the physiological process and cellular injury. Arch Surg 1993;128:1192-1196.
77. Parrillo JE. Pathogenetic mechanisms of septic shock. N Engl J Med 1993;328:1471-1477.
78. Bone RC. The pathogenesis of sepsis. Ann Intern Med 1991;115:457-469.
79. Dantzker D. Oxygen delivery and utilization in sepsis. Crit Care Clin 1989;5:81-98.
80. Gutierrez G, Lund N, Bryan-Brown CW. Cellular oxygen utilization during multiple organ failure. Crit Care Clin 1989;5:271-288.
81. Bersten A, Sibbald WJ. Circulatory disturbances in multiple systems organ failure. Crit Care Clin 1989;5:233-254.
82. Cunnion RE, Parrillo JE. Myocardial dysfunction in sepsis. Crit Care Clin 1989;5:99-118.
83. Brass N, ed. Multiple systems organ failure [entire issue]. Crit Care Nurs Q 1994;16(4):1-105.
84. Baue AE. Multiple organ failure: Patient care and prevention. St. Louis: Mosby, 1990.
85. Baxter CR. Future prospectives in trauma and burn care. J Trauma 1990;30(Suppl 12):S208-S209.
86. Demling RH. Wound inflammatory mediators and multisystem organ failure. Prog Clin Biol Res 1987;236A:525-537.
87. Beerthuizen GIJM. Response of the microcirculation: Tissue oxygenation. In: Schlag G, Redl H, eds. Pathophysiology of shock, sepsis, and organ failure. Berlin: Springer-Verlag, 1993:230-241.
88. Müller-Berghaus G. Pathophysiologic and biochemical events in disseminated intravascular coagulation: Dysregulation of procoagulant and anticoagulant pathways. Semin Thromb Hemost 1989;15:58-87.
89. Müller-Berghaus G. Septicemia and the vessel wall. In: Verstraete M, Vermylen J, Lijnen R, Arnout J, eds. Thrombosis and haemostasis. Leuven, Belgium: Leuven University Press, 1987:619-671.
90. Morrissey JH, Drake TA. Procoagulant response of the endothelium and monocytes. In: Schlag G, Redl H, eds. Pathophysiology of shock, sepsis, and organ failure. Berlin: Springer-Verlag, 1993:564-574.
91. Weiss SJ. Tissue destruction by neutrophils. N Engl J Med 1989;320:365-376.
92. Brigham KL, Meyrick B. Interactions of granulocytes with lungs. Circ Res 1984;54:623-635.
93. Talbott GA et al. Leukocyte-endothelial interactions and organ injury: The role of adhesion molecules. New Horiz 1994;2:545-554.
94. Meyrick B, Johnson JE, Brigham KL. Endotoxin-induced pulmonary endothelial injury. Prog Clin Biol Res: Second Vienna Shock Forum 1989;308:91-100.
95. Tracey KJ et al. Shock and tissue injury induced by recombinant human cachectin. Science 1986;234:470-474.
96. Ghosh S et al. Endotoxin-induced organ injury. Crit Care Med 1993;21(suppl):S19-S24.
97. Zivot JB, Hoffman WD. Pathogenic effects of endotoxin. New Horiz 1995;3:267-275.
98. Freudenberg N. Reaction of the vascular intima to endotoxin shock. Prog Clin Biol Res: Second Vienna Shock Forum 1989;308:77-89.
99. Del Vecchio PJ, Malik AB. Thrombin-induced neutrophil adhesion. Prog Clin Biol Res: Second Vienna Shock Forum 1989;308:101-112.
100. Bell TN. Disseminated intravascular coagulation: Clinical complexities of aberrant coagulation. Crit Care Nurs Clin North Am 1993;5:389-410.
101. Nelson K, Herndon B, Reisz G. Pulmonary effects of ischemic limb reperfusion: Evidence for a role of oxygen-derived radicals. Crit Care Med 1991;19:360-363.
102. Welbourn CRB et al. Pathophysiology of ischaemia reperfusion injury: Central role of the neutrophil. Br J Surg 1991;78:651-655.
103. Kloner RA, Przyklenk K, Patel B. Altered myocardial states: The stunned and hibernating myocardium. Am J Med 1989;86(suppl 1A):14-22.
104. Black L, Coombs VJ, Townsend SN. Reperfusion and reperfusion injury in acute myocardial infarction. Heart Lung 1990;19:274-284.
105. Oldham KT et al. The systemic consequences of intestinal ischemia-reperfusion injury. J Vasc Surg 1993;1:1136-1137.
106. Hechtman HB. Mediators of local and remote injury following gut ischemia. J Vasc Surg 1993;18:134-135.
107. Barie PS, Hydo LJ, Fischer E. A prospective comparison of two multiple organ dysfunction/failure scoring systems for prediction of mortality in critical surgical illness. J Trauma 1994;37:660-666.
108. Knaus WA, Wagner DP. Multiple systems organ failure: Epidemiology and prognosis. Crit Care Clin 1989;5:221-232.
109. Fry DE. Multiple system organ failure. St. Louis: Mosby, 1992.
110. Dunham CM et al. Inflammatory markers: Superior predictors of adverse outcome in blunt trauma patients. Crit Care Med 1994;22:667-672.
111. Tran DD et al. Risk factors for multiple organ system failure and death in critically injured patients. Surgery 1993;114:21-30.
112. Gerritsen ME, Bloor CM. Endothelial cell gene expression in response to injury. FASEB J 1993;7:523-532.
113. Rauen CA. Too old to live. Too young to die. Multiple organ dysfunction syndrome in the elderly. Crit Care Nurs Clin North Am 1994;6:535-542.
114. Giraud T et al. Iatrogenic complications in adult intensive care units: A prospective two-center study. Crit Care Med 1993;21:40-51.
115. Witt NJ et al. Peripheral nerve function in sepsis and multiple organ failure. Chest 1991;99:176-184.
116. Goodwin CW. Multiple organ failure: clinical overview of the syndrome. J Trauma 1990;30:S163-S165.

CHAPTER 2

The Inflammatory/Immune Response: Implications for the Critically Ill

Virginia Huddleston Secor

The inflammatory/immune response (IIR) represents one of the most exquisite and complicated homeostatic mechanisms of the body. IIR activity spans all levels of physiologic interaction—from the molecular to the systemic—via numerous humoral, cellular, and biochemical pathways. When the body receives an insult, whether it be mechanical (surgery, crush injury), ischemic (shock, myocardial infarction), chemical (ingestion of toxic substances, drug abuse), or microbial (bacterial, viral, fungal, parasitic), multiple systems are activated to protect the host from invading pathogens, limit the extent of injury, and promote rapid healing of involved tissues.[1] A series of complex interactions occurs along numerous activating and inhibiting feedback loops and redundant pathways.

The identification of the signs and symptoms of IIR activity dates back to 3000 B.C., when the Mesopotamian culture recognized fever in association with disease. By 200 B.C., the Chinese and Egyptians recognized the importance of acquired immunity by performing rudimentary vaccination (variolation) against smallpox. In the first century, Celsus identified the four cardinal signs of inflammation: tumor, rubor, dolor, calor.[2] The 1950s heralded the era of modern immunology with the recognition of histocompatibility antigens, the delineation of antibody structure, and increased understanding of immunopathologic conditions.[2] On the forefront of immunologic research today are mechanisms of cellular activation and regulation, the role of genetic coding in specific immune recognition, and the nature of soluble messengers and cell surface receptors.

But what does this mean for the critical care patient today? For the team caring for that patient? Why is knowledge of the IIR not only helpful but necessary in caring for the critically ill patient? The IIR plays a role not only in multiple organ dysfunction syndrome (MODS) but in many other areas of critical care as well. A major emphasis of research into the pathogenesis and treatment of many pathologic conditions involves the function of the IIR. Cancer, acquired immunodeficiency syndrome (AIDS), organ transplantation, diabetes, traumatic injury, and reperfusion injury are common examples. Even myocardial infarction is now seen as both an inflammatory event and an ischemic event. In addition to the pathology of many disease states, most patients in critical care areas have many risk factors for immunosuppression or dysfunction: trauma, stress, and malnutrition (see the box on p. 20). Because the endothelium and the process of coagulation are intimately involved in the IIR, individual attention has also been given to their activity and role in the potentiation of MODS.

Knowledge of the IIR is vital not only in understanding the pathophysiology of disease states, but in understanding drug therapy and assessment findings as well.[3] How does one safely administer interleukin-2 (IL-2) in cancer patients if one does not know what IL-2 is, what it does, or what the com-

RISK FACTORS FOR IMMUNE DYSFUNCTION	
Host-related	**Treatment-related**
Age	Invasive lines, catheters, devices
Malnutrition	Malnutrition
Chronic diseases	Antibiotic therapy
Debilitated states	Immunosuppressant therapy
Stress	Stress
Trauma/burns	Trauma/surgery/anesthesia
Hemorrhage	Blood transfusions
Perfusion deficit	Perfusion deficit
Sepsis	Sepsis
Inflammatory foci	Inflammatory foci

mon side-effects are? Why do we give some patients nitric oxide, and yet attempt to block its activity in other patients? What do we monitor to assess the effectiveness of these therapeutic regimens? Confusing these pharmacologic agents and their effects could gravely injure patients or expedite their demise.

It is beyond the scope and purpose of this text to give a comprehensive presentation of the entire IIR and associated immunopathologies in disease states. The discussion in this chapter presents a brief overview and background of the major components of the IIR and describes how these components contribute to host defense through nonspecific inflammatory responses and specific immune activity. A discussion on clinical conditions associated with immune dysfunction and common assessment parameters also follows. Chapter 3 presents a comprehensive discussion of the major cells and mediators of the inflammatory response and their role in the development and progression of MODS. Sepsis, inflammation, and dysfunction of immunoregulatory mechanisms play a key role in the development and potentiation of MODS, with inflammatory changes present in most patients dying of MODS.[4-8] The final common pathway of organ system dysfunction and failure has not been fully described; however, the IIR certainly plays a role. The extent of that role is yet to be defined.[4,8-10]

COMPONENTS OF THE INFLAMMATORY/IMMUNE RESPONSE

The IIR is not a function of white blood cells alone, but instead, the response is governed by the integrated activity of various immune and nonimmune cells and the soluble mediators they generate and secrete.[11] Although very beneficial as a local response, appropriate regulation of inflammation is necessary to keep the cells and mediators sequestered in the region of injury and prevent their spread to the systemic circulation and remote sites. These cells and mediators can be grouped into three major categories: plasma enzyme cascades, cellular components, and other intercellular mediators.

Plasma enzyme cascades

The four interlocking enzymatic cascades in plasma produce a rapid, highly amplified response to numerous stimuli, such as ischemia, tissue debris, and endotoxin. Also known as humoral mediators because of their presence in the plasma, the enzymatic cascades quickly become amplified, because the product of one reaction is the enzymatic catalyst for the next reaction. The four primary enzymatic cascades play major roles in injury and in the nonspecific immune response and include the complement, coagulation, fibrinolysis, and kallikrein/kinin cascades (Table 2-1).

Cellular components

Cellular components play a major role in host protection through their activity and production of the numerous mediators necessary to carry out an IIR[10,12] (Table 2-2). The primary cellular components of the IIR are the white blood cells (WBCs). The inflammatory WBCs (neutrophils and monocytes/macrophages) are primarily phagocytic cells that aid in the clearance of microorganisms and

Table 2-1 Activity of Plasma Enzyme Cascades

Cascade	Activity	Role in injury
Complement	Induction of inflammation Opsonization Activation of phagocytic cells Direct target cell lysis	Excessive inflammation Excessive cellular activation with mediator release
Coagulation	Hemostasis	Excessive intravascular coagulation leading to vascular obstruction, endothelial damage, and tissue ischemia
Fibrinolysis	Degradation of fibrin clot Prevention of extensive clot formation	Hemorrhage leading to decreased oxygen delivery and tissue ischemia
Kallikrein/Kinin (Bradykinin)	Enhanced IIR activity Enhanced fibrinolytic cascade Possible role in renal blood flow regulation	Massive vasodilatation Increased microvascular permeability Bronchoconstriction Excessive inflammation Excessive cellular activation

other debris. The immune WBCs (T and B lymphocytes) carry out immunoregulatory functions and antibody production. Other immune and non-immune cells operating in the IIR include endothelial cells, platelets, mast cells, basophils, eosinophils, fibroblasts, dendritic cells, and Langerhans cells.

The endothelial cell, although not a primary immunologic cell, has more recently been shown to play a significant role in IIR activities and sepsis.[13-15] The endothelium, once thought to be an inert lining of the vasculature with little biologic activity, is now known to possess numerous metabolic, anticoagulant, and inflammatory functions. In inflammation, the endothelium is not only a target of numerous mediators that affect its function, but it also produces many mediators, including inhibitors and activators of coagulation, inflammatory substances, and adhesion molecules.[13-15] The endothelium may thus engineer many pathophysiologic processes, particularly if it has been perturbed.

Cytokines and other intercellular mediators

Cytokines and other inflammatory mediators are produced and secreted primarily by WBCs, but they can also be generated by stimulated or damaged endothelium and cells in the wound. Cytokines are proteins that serve as the physiologic messengers of the IIR and include tumor necrosis factor (TNF), interleukins (IL), interferons (IFN), transforming growth factor-beta (TGF-β), and colony-stimulating factors (CSFs). Cytokines trigger various activities in the IIR (see the box below). In general, they direct cell activation, differentiation, and further release of mediators. Other inflammatory mediators produced by WBCs, endothelial cells, fibroblasts, mast cells, and platelets include arachidonic acid metabolites (prostaglandins, thromboxane, leukotrienes, and lipoxins), platelet activating factor, toxic oxygen metabolites (free radicals), nitric oxide, and proteases.

Like the cellular components, the mediators are necessary in the function of the physiologic protective IIR; their uncontrolled activation can, however,

---

CYTOKINES: DEFINITION AND ACTIVITY[34]

Cytokines
Soluble protein molecules that serve as intercellular messengers in the IIR

Regulatory activities
Cell growth
Cell activation
Inflammation
Immunity
Tissue repair
Fibrosis
Morphogenesis
Chemotaxis

Table 2-2 Cellular Mediators of the Inflammatory/Immune Response

Cell	Mediators
Neutrophil	Arachidonic acid metabolites Interleukins Lysozyme Myeloperoxidase Platelet activating factor Proteases Tissue factor (tissue thromboplastin) Toxic oxygen metabolites (oxygen-derived free radicals)
Macrophages	Arachidonic acid metabolites Colony-stimulating factors Complement proteins Coagulation factors Growth factors Interferons Interleukins Lysozyme Nitric oxide Plasminogen activators Platelet activating factor Proteases Toxic oxygen metabolites (oxygen-derived free radicals) Tumor necrosis factor-alpha
Lymphocytes	Antibodies Arachidonic acid metabolites Colony-stimulating factors Growth factors Interleukins Interferons Tumor necrosis factor-beta
Mast cells	Arachidonic acid metabolites Heparin Histamine Interleukins Platelet activating factor Proteases
Platelets	Arachidonic acid metabolites Chemotactants Growth factors Histamine Platelet activating factor Serotonin
Endothelial cells	Arachidonic acid metabolites Endothelins Interleukins Nitric oxide Platelet activating factor Tissue factor (tissue thromboplastin)

lead to pathologic levels of these mediators. Excessive cellular activation and mediator production cause detrimental changes in circulating volume, oxygen supply/demand balance, and metabolism.[10,16-23] Chapter 3 and Appendix A provide further information on the major cells and mediators of the IIR and MODS.

INFLAMMATORY/IMMUNE RESPONSE: LEVELS OF HOST DEFENSE

The host defense operates at three levels: external barriers against invasion; nonspecific systems against injury and invasion; and antigen-specific responses to foreign pathogens. These three levels work in concert by integrating the major components of the IIR described above to prevent invasion by foreign pathogens and to promote healing of damaged tissue.[11]

External barriers

The host defense system makes a valiant attempt to prevent invasion rather than fight it. The body is equipped with various natural defenses or external barriers to prevent microbial invasion[11,24] (Table 2-3). These mechanisms of defense include: (1) the mechanical barrier provided by intact skin and epithelium, (2) flushing or mechanical removal, (3) cilia and activity of mucus, (4) pH changes, (5) secretions containing enzymes and IgA, and (6) the presence of normal flora (commensal organisms) that compete with pathogenic species for nutrients and attachment sites and produce inhibitory substances.

Unfortunately for the patient in the intensive care unit (ICU), many therapeutic interventions alter the natural defenses. Antibiotics destroy the balance of normal flora; antacids and H_2-blockers raise gastric pH; sedatives depress respiratory depth and secretion removal and also potentiate intestinal ileus; and endotracheal tubes bypass the protective mechanisms of the respiratory system. Invasive devices and procedures that breach the external barrier of the skin provide added portals of entry for opportunistic and pathogenic organisms.

Nonspecific response and mechanisms of inflammation

Although in theory the nonspecific and specific immune responses can be viewed separately, their activities are intricately interwoven, with each pro-

Table 2-3 Natural Defenses and External Barriers[11,28]

Defense/barrier	System
Intact epithelium	Integument
	Respiratory
	Gastrointestinal
	Genitourinary
Acidic pH	Gastrointestinal
	Genitourinary
	Integument
Resident flora	Integument
	Respiratory
	Gastrointestinal
	Genitourinary
Mechanical removal/ flushing	Respiratory: cough, sneeze
	Gastrointestinal: peristalsis, defecation
	Genitourinary: urination
Cilia activity and mucus production	Respiratory
	Gastrointestinal
	Genitourinary
Bactericidal secretions	Gastric juices: acid, enzymes
	Milk: lactoperoxidase
	Tears, saliva, perspiration: lysozyme
	Sebum: fatty acids
	Semen: spermine
Secretory IgA	Respiratory
	Gastrointestinal
	Genitourinary

moting the effectiveness of the other. Classically, the nonspecific immune response involves inflammation and phagocytosis. Inflammation is the initial response of the body to insult or invasion and involves a nonspecific response to tissue injury triggered by mechanical, chemical, or microbial stimuli.[11] The goal of inflammation is to enhance the movement of nutrients and IIR cells and mediators to the site of injury, thus preventing foreign invasion and extension of the injury.

The four major physiologic mechanisms of the inflammatory response are vasodilatation, increased microvascular permeability, cellular activation and adhesion, and coagulation (Fig. 2-1). Following injury, the plasma enzyme cascades and phagocytic cells, such as neutrophils (in the circulation) and macrophages (in the tissue), are activated by microorganisms, cell debris, and endothelial damage. These components, acting in concert with other in-

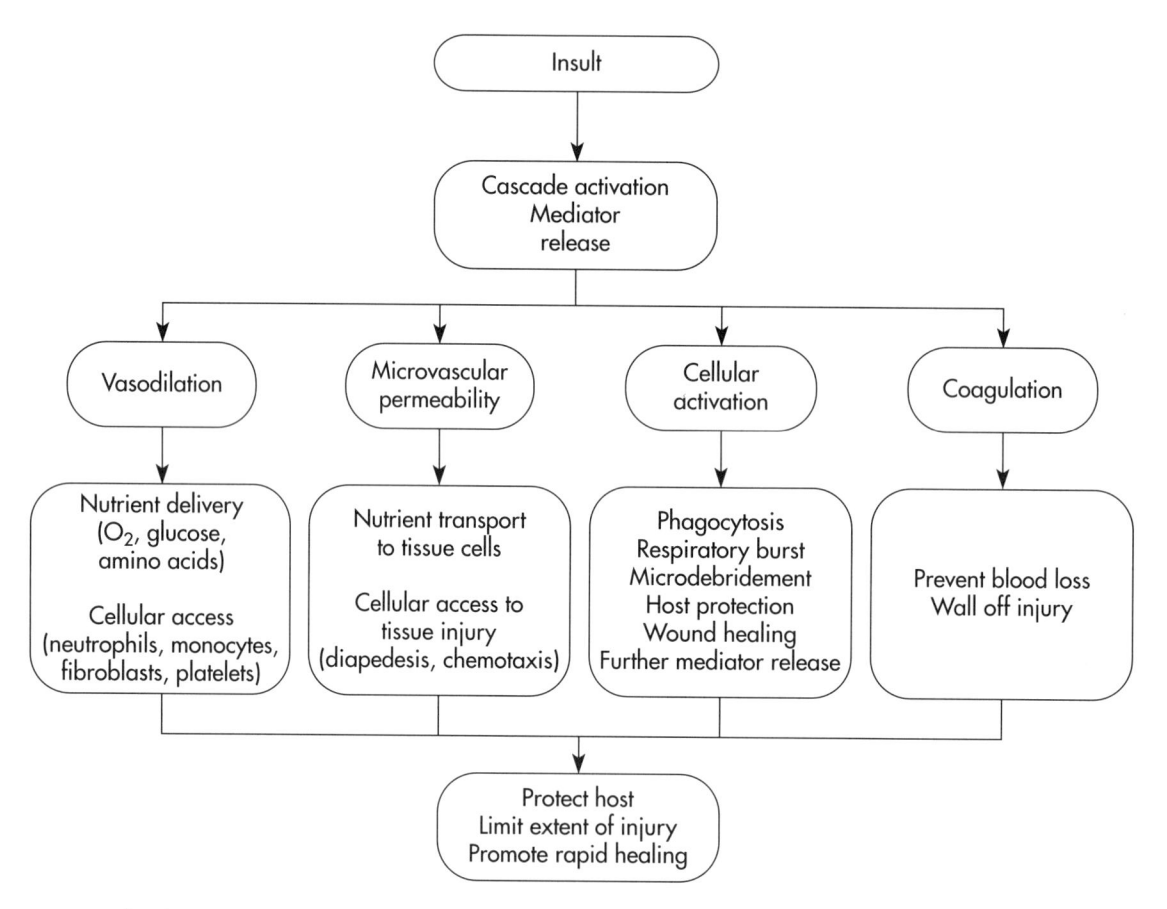

Fig. 2-1 Cascade of inflammation (From Huddleston VB. Multisystem organ failure: A pathophysiologic approach. Boston, 1991;6.)

flammatory mediators and WBCs, cause the vasodilatation and increased vascular permeability that are responsible for the classic signs and symptoms commonly associated with inflammation: rubor (erythema), tumor (edema), calor (heat), and dolor (pain).

Vasodilatation at the local site of injury increases nutrient (e.g., oxygen and glucose) delivery to the injured area, and the increased microvascular permeability allows these nutrients and other large proteins and factors, such as antibodies, complement, and kinins, to mobilize more quickly from the vasculature into the tissue. The plasma enzyme cascades also activate WBCs and attract them into the area of injury.

WBC activation, adhesion, and transmigration into the tissue promote phagocytosis of foreign debris and microdebridement of the wound. Only recently have researchers and clinicians begun to understand the mechanics of WBC adhesion to the vascular endothelium and its clinical implications. For a WBC, such as a neutrophil, to migrate into injured or infected tissue, it must stop flowing in the blood stream and adhere to the endothelial lining of a vessel, usually the postcapillary venule. Initially the WBC rolls along the surface of the vessel and then eventually tightly adheres to the endothelium (a process known as margination or pavementing) if the appropriate adhesion molecules are present on both the WBC and the endothelium.[14,25-27] Numerous adhesion molecules have been identified. The selectins are a group of adhesion molecules that mediate the initial rolling of the WBCs on the endothelium and include P-selectin and E-selectin.

The integrins on the WBC and other adhesion molecules (from the immunoglobulin gene superfamily, e.g., intercellular adhesion molecule-1 [ICAM-1]) on the endothelium institute tight binding between the WBC and the endothelium[27] (Fig. 2-2). The differential expression of adhesion molecules on cells and endothelium dictates which cell types enter which tissues.

After adhesion, the WBC squeezes through the vessel wall (diapedesis, transmigration) and moves into the area of injured tissue where it can phagocytize invading pathogens and necrotic tissue (Fig. 2-3). The neutrophil and monocyte must use this migration process to enter the injured tissue. In contrast, the macrophage, which resides in the tissue, is already present in many organ beds. Phagocytes have nonspecific receptors for binding foreign pathogens and do not require previous exposure to the pathogen to be effective; however, phagocytosis is enhanced if the microorganism is opsonized (coated) by antibodies or complement. Opsonization of the pathogen enhances phagocytosis because the phagocytes have receptors specific for antibody and complement. Therefore the phagocyte attaches to the pathogen by binding the antibody or complement coating the pathogen[11,28,29] (Fig. 2-4). Once engulfed, the WBC kills the pathogen and isolates the area with highly toxic substances, such as toxic oxygen metabolites and proteases.[30]

The fourth aspect of inflammation is the triggering of coagulation. Coagulation minimizes blood loss and walls off the injury. Inflammation and coagulation are intricately interwoven, particularly at the blood-endothelial interface through the activity of numerous cells and mediators common to both tissues, such as platelets, complement, Hageman factor (clotting factor XII), the kallikrein/kinin system, TNF, IL-1, toxic oxygen metabolites, pro-

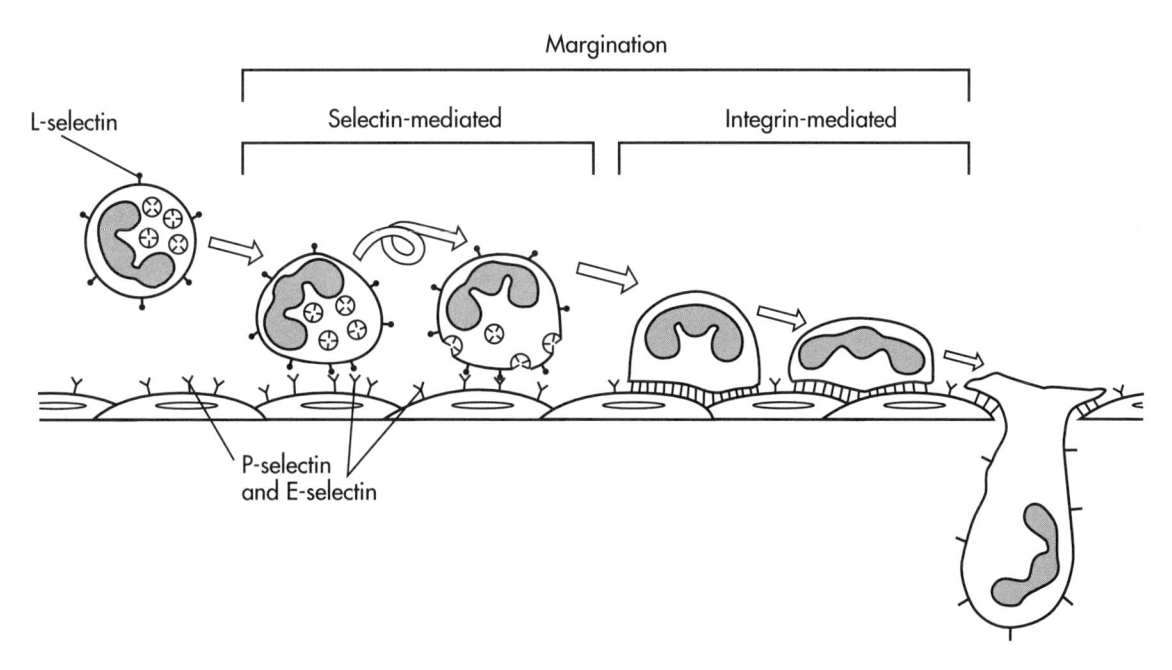

Fig. 2-2 Neutrophil margination and transmigration. The initial weak binding is mediated by adhesion molecules (known as selectins) on the neutrophil and on activated endothelial cells. On contact with the endothelium, L-selectin is rapidly shed from the neutrophil surface, and presynthesized adhesion molecules (known as integrins) move from storage granules onto the surface of the neutrophil. The integrins mediate tight binding to the endothelial surface and later facilitate emigration and migration through the tissue. The emigrating neutrophil passes between endothelial cells, with their active collaboration. (From Parslow TG. The phagocytic neutrophils and macrophages. In: Stites DP, Terr AI, Parslow TG, eds. Basic and clinical immunology. 8th ed. Norwalk, CT: Appleton & Lange;1994:13.)

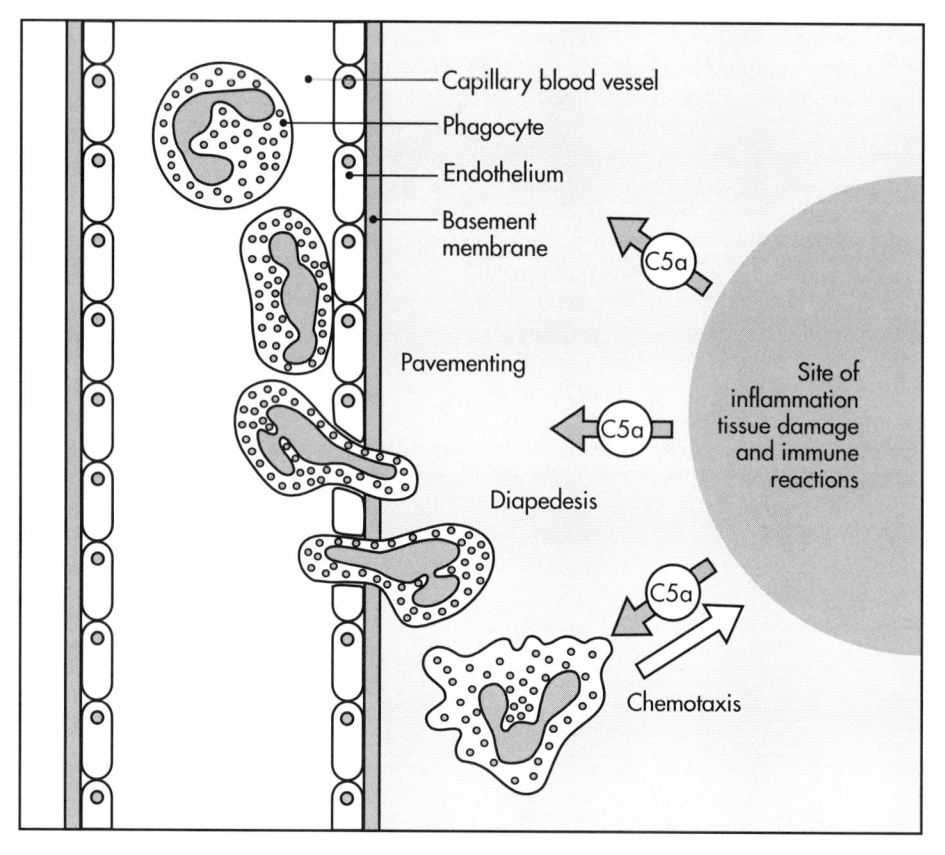

Fig. 2-3 Chemotaxis and migration of phagocytes from the blood to the tissue. (From Male D, Roitt I. Introduction to the immune system. In: Roitt I, Brostoff J, Male D, eds. Immunology. 3rd ed. London:Mosby;1993: 1.10.)

teases, platelet activating factor, and arachidonic acid metabolites.[31-33] Activation of either coagulation or inflammation in turn activates the other system, thus providing the body with dual protection in a controlled response.[31-33]

The inflammatory response does not conclude with these four mechanisms. After phagocytosis or contact with a foreign pathogen, macrophages and other antigen-presenting cells (APCs) (Table 3-2) process the antigen, return it to the surface of the APC, and present it to T cells residing in the peripheral lymphoid tissue. This antigen processing and presentation is a vital aspect of macrophage–T cell interaction and links the nonspecific to the specific immune response.[11,34]

Specific response and lymphoid tissue

The specific response is mediated by T lymphocytes and B lymphocytes, whose activation primarily takes place in the lymphoid tissue. Lymphocyte activity is classically divided into cell-mediated immunity (CMI) and humoral immunity (HI). CMI and HI are distinguished from other levels of host defense by two important characteristics: specificity and memory. Each T or B cell reacts only with the specific antigen that it recognizes. Genetically, the body has the potential to produce over 10^9 different specificities through specific antibodies or antigen receptors on T cells.[35] Antibodies produced by plasma cells that arise from a single B lymphocyte all recognize the same antigen and are known as

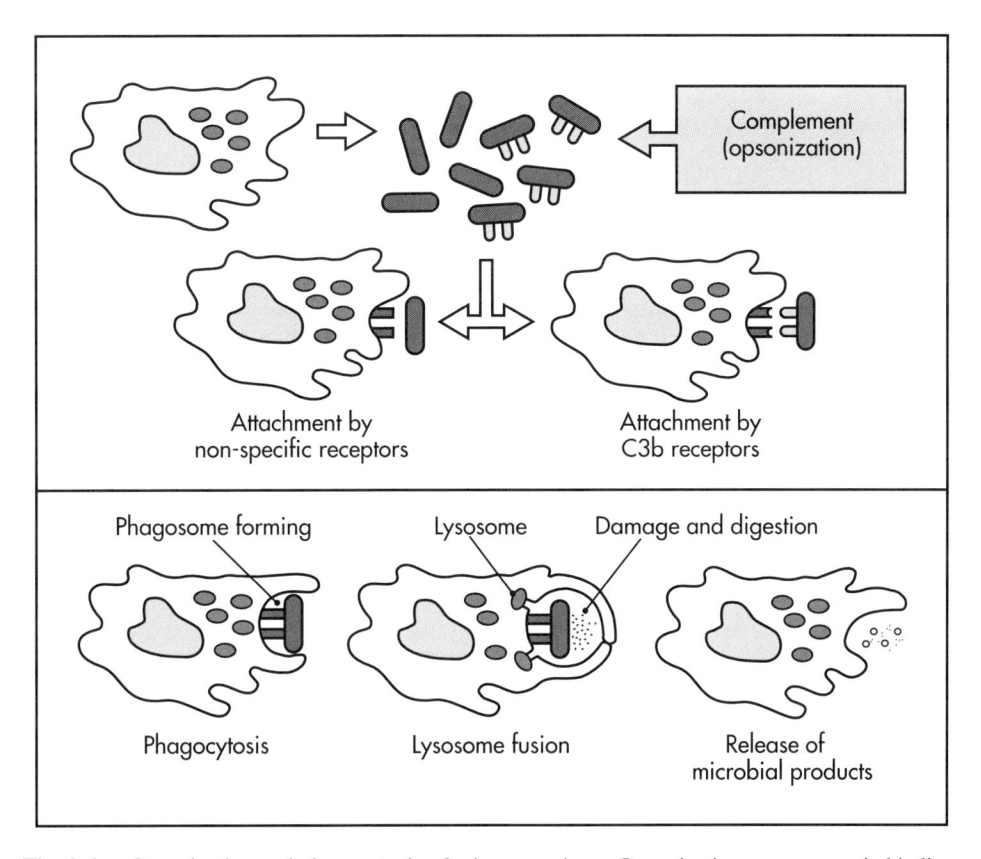

Fig. 2-4 Opsonization and phagocytosis of microorganisms. Opsonization may occur via binding with complement and/or antibody. (From Male D, Roitt I. Introduction to the immune system. In: Roitt I, Brostoff J, Male D, eds. Immunology. 3rd ed. London: Mosby;1993: 1.9.)

monoclonal antibodies.[11] This concept of specificity, coupled with the ability of investigators to produce monoclonal antibodies, has become important in generating new immunomodulation techniques and treatment regimens for the MODS patient.[36-38] See Chapter 18 for additional discussion on immunomodulation.

The second important characteristic of lymphocytes and the specific immune response is memory. After exposure to antigen, most T cells and B cells carry out specific immune functions while a small percentage of lymphocytes return to the secondary lymphoid tissue and reside there as memory cells. The memory cells enable the host to mount a more rapid and vigorous response with repeated exposures to the same antigen.[11,39]

Cell-mediated immunity. In CMI, different T-lymphocyte subsets orchestrate the IIR and regulate its function. The subsets are distinguished from each other by the presence of specific markers or receptors on their cell surfaces, known as clusters of determination (CD). The most common division of T cells used clinically is the $CD4^+$ T cells (also known as helper T cells [TH]) and $CD8^+$ T cells (also known as cytotoxic T cells [TC]). The $CD4^+$ cells, upon recognition by the T-cell receptor of the antigen presented by APCs, proliferate and produce cytokines that (1) enhance B-cell proliferation, differentiation, and antibody production, (2) activate macrophages, or (3) stimulate additional T-cell activity.[34,40] Without $CD4^+$ cell activity, the entire IIR becomes severely dysfunctional.

The $CD8^+$ cells participate in cytotoxic activities against intracellular infections, tumor cells, and foreign donor tissue, and possibly in other regulatory activity, such as down regulation of the IIR (suppressor activity).[41] Previously referred to as "suppressor T cells," these cells were (are?) thought to prevent the IIR from turning into an uncontrolled response to a given antigen; however, this terminology has come into question, because a subset of CD8+ cells distinct from the cytotoxic CD8+ cells has not been cloned and demonstrated to perform this function in vitro.[42,43]

The ratio of CD4+ cells to CD8+ cells reflects the balance between activation and suppression of the immune response and is approximately 2:1 in healthy individuals. Changes in both the absolute count, as well as in the CD4+:CD8+ ratio, occur in both healthy immune responses and dysfunction of the immune system.[44] In infection, the ratio is increased because of an increase in CD4+ cells; the ratio is decreased in AIDS secondary to destruction of CD4+ cells by the virus and possibly increased multiplication of CD8+ cells.

Another cell considered to be of lymphoid lineage that has many of the same cytolytic properties as the Tc cell is the natural killer (NK) cell. Although maturation of NK cells can occur in the absence of a functional thymus, NK precursor cells have been found in the thymus.[45] Like Tc cells, NK cells produce cytokines, such as IFN-γ. Unlike Tc cells, NK cells can kill tumor cells and virus-infected cells without previous sensitization and without classical antigenic stimulation or major histocompatibility complex (MHC) restriction. Detailed features of NK cell maturation, interaction with other lymphocytes, and mechanisms of target cell killing require further study.

Humoral immunity. In humoral immunity (HI), specific B cells recognize the antigen as it is bound by their surface immunoglobulins (Fig. 2-5), which are large glycoproteins (proteins with carbohydrate moieties attached). Once the antigen is bound, it triggers the B cell to proliferate and differentiate into antibody-producing plasma cells. When the secreted antibodies (which are identical to the surface immunoglobulins that recognized the antigen initially) find their specific antigen, they bind the antigen to form antigen-antibody immune complexes. This complex is engulfed by phagocytic cells, particularly in the mononuclear phagocytic system (previously known as the reticuloendothelial system).[39,46] Recognition of antigen by B cells and activation of B cells are highly complex events and require precise cell-cell and cytokine-TH cell inter-

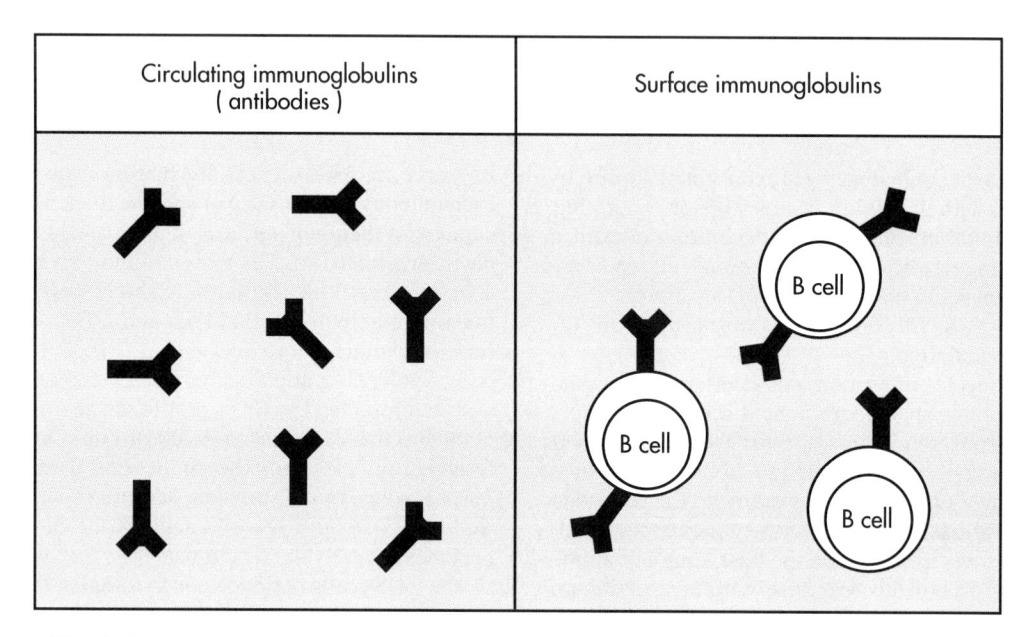

Fig. 2-5 Circulating immunoglobulins (antibodies) and B cell surface immunoglobulins. The B cell recognizes and binds specific antigen via its surface immunoglobulins. It then differentiates into a plasma cell that produces circulating antibodies.

actions through mechanisms that are just being described.[30,34,47,48]

Primary lymphoid tissue. Lymphoid organs are classified as either primary (central) or secondary (peripheral) organs. Lymphopoiesis (the differentiation and maturation of functional lymphocytes) occurs in the primary lymphoid organs—the thymus (for T cells) and bone marrow (for B cells). During the fetal and the neonatal periods, the lymphocytes develop and acquire the ability to recognize antigens. Those B or T cells that recognize the "self" antigens of the body as foreign are eliminated. T lymphocytes learn to differentiate between self and nonself in the thymus, a process know as thymic education. This education is conducted in the context of specific molecules that reside in the thymus, as well as on the surface of most body cells. These molecules (also known as surface antigens) are genetically coded by the MHC, which plays an important role in regulating APC–T cell interactions.[49] In humans, MHC genes, which are located on the short arm of chromosome 6, encode for surface molecules known as human leukocyte antigens (HLA).

Because the major role of the MHC is the regulation of immune responsiveness and the distinction of self from nonself, HLA typing is important in organ transplantation. MHC gene products are classified as Class I or Class II antigens. Class I antigens are found on the cell membrane of all nucleated cells and function as surface recognition molecules for CD8+ T cells. Class II antigens are not as widely distributed and are primarily expressed on APCs. Under certain conditions, lymphocytes and endothelial cells can be induced to express Class II antigens; however, they do not express Class II antigens constitutively.[41]

CD4+ cells only recognize antigen presented on the surface of APCs in the context of specific Class II molecules; therefore, MHC Class II surface antigens must be present on the cell surface of APCs, such as macrophages, for the CD4+ cell to recognize and respond to foreign antigen (Fig. 2-6). This macrophage–T cell interaction is termed "MHC-restricted" because MHC surface antigens must be present for the interaction to take place. Other immune interactions that can be MHC-restricted include T cell-T cell, T cell-B cell, and cytotoxic T cell-target cell activity.[41]

These cellular interactions and MHC restriction have clinical implications because much of the immunosuppression of trauma, stress, hemorrhage, surgery, and blood transfusions discussed in the following pages is related to macrophage–T cell interaction. Decreased MHC Class II surface molecule expression may be partially responsible for this poor interaction. Ertel and co-workers[50] have shown that the elevated intracellular calcium level seen postischemia induces a decrease in MHC Class II expression, an effect that can be attenuated with calcium channel blockers. In summary, for effective lymphocyte activity, the lymphocytes must be able to differentiate self from nonself and must be able to interact with the antigen presented by the APC. The presence of MHC Class II molecules facilitates both of these activities.

Secondary lymphoid tissue. Secondary lymphoid tissue is organized into either discretely encapsulated organs (spleen, lymph nodes) or nonencapsulated accumulations of lymphoid tissue in the periphery. Approximately 95% of the total lymphocytes in the body are in the lymphoid tissue at any given time, with only 5% actually circulating in the blood. Lymphocytes interact with each other, with APCs, and with antigens they encounter in the secondary lymphoid tissue. The white pulp of the spleen contains large numbers of lymphocytes, macrophages, and other APCs. As blood flows through the spleen, microorganisms are trapped by the splenic macrophages, processed, and presented to the surrounding T lymphocytes. The T lymphocytes are activated and begin proliferating. The active T cells produce cytokines that stimulate other immune cells, including B cells, which differentiate into antibody-producing plasma cells.[49]

Similar activity occurs in the lymph nodes, which frequently are located at branches of lymphatic vessels. Many APCs with large amounts of MHC antigen on their surfaces are present within these nodes. As lymph passes through the nodes, the APCs phagocytize, process, and present any antigen in the lymph fluid to the resident lymphocytes, and activation occurs again. When presented antigen stimulates lymphocyte proliferation, the secondary lymphoid tissue, particularly the lymph nodes, enlarge because of the lymphocyte expansion.[49]

The nonencapsulated tissue of the lymphoid system, known as mucosa-associated lymphoid tissue (MALT), is commonly associated with the mucosal surfaces of the gut, respiratory tract, and genital tract, which are common access sites for microorganisms to enter the body. Tonsils in the upper re-

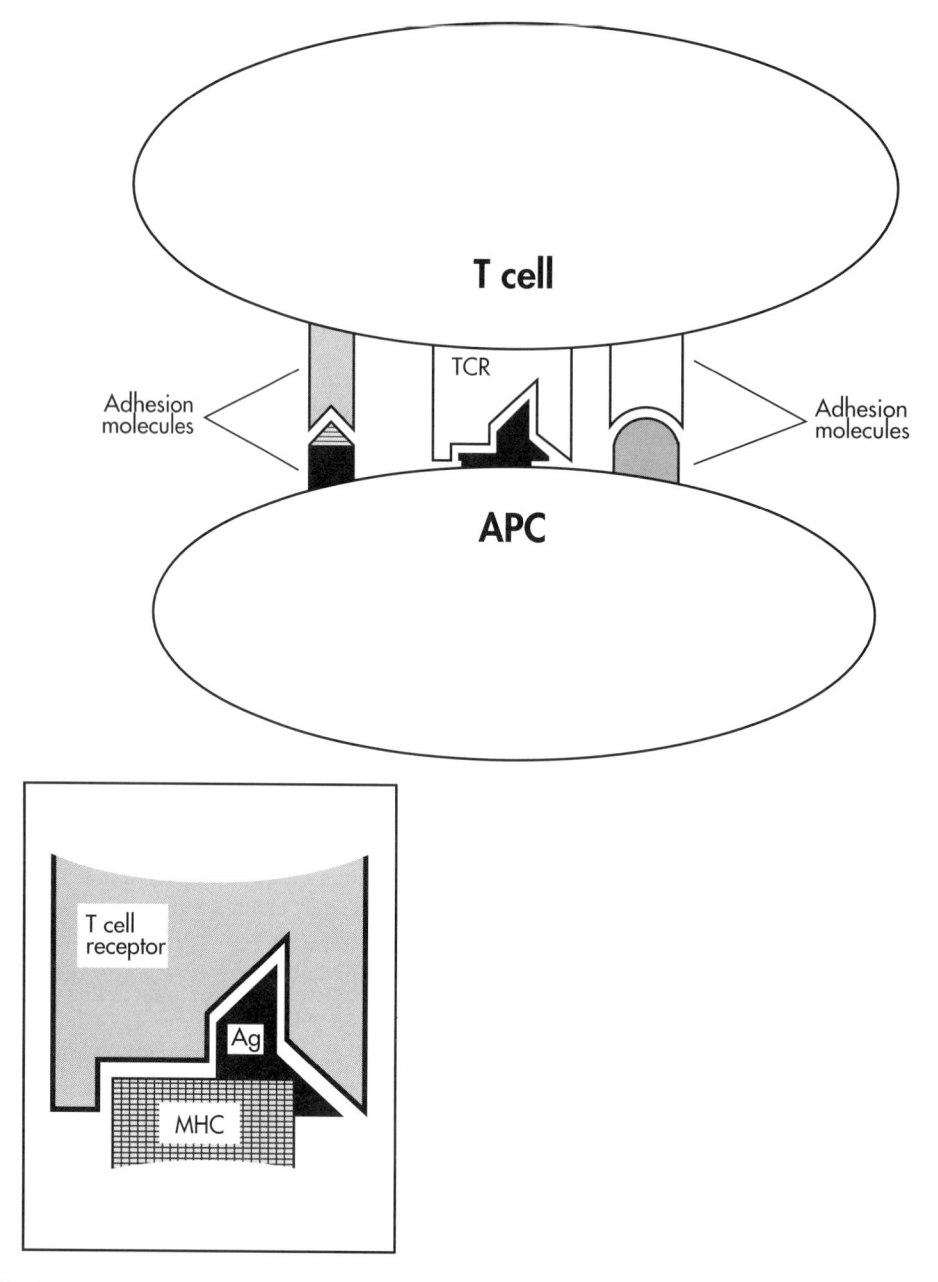

Fig. 2-6 Macrophage/T cell interaction requiring the presence of MHC Class II surface antigen on the macrophage. The macrophage is an antigen presenting cell. *TCR*, T cell receptor; *APC*, antigen presenting cell; *MHC*, major histocompatibility complex; *Ag*, presented antigen.

spiratory tract and the Peyer's patches in the gut are examples of MALT.

The lymphocytes not only migrate from the primary to the secondary lymphoid tissue after maturation but also, during their life span, constantly recirculate between the blood, the lymph, and other secondary organs. Interestingly, recent studies have shown that this circulation is not random. Lymphocytes have a tendency to "home" to particular lymphoid organs, particularly those lymphocytes with previous antigenic exposure and activation.[51,52] The circulation of a lymphocyte ceases after its entry into a node in which its specific antigen is present. Antigen-specific lymphocytes are retained in the nodes that drain the area of antigen invasion or accumulation for a period ranging from hours to days.[49,52]

Summary

The response of the body to injury involves inflammation, immunologic activity, and repair. Depending on the agent (bacterial, viral, fungal, parasitic) and the site of infection (intracellular, tissues, body fluids), one mode of response plays a more dominant role than another. CMI plays a major role in viral and parasitic infections, while HI and phagocytosis are the chief mechanisms used to combat bacterial infection.[30,53] In an uncomplicated scenario, the response is rapid, localized, and results in healing. Unfortunately, in the critical care environment, a myriad of complications is common. Immunosuppression, dysregulation, and uncontrolled inflammatory activity often occur, resulting in tissue damage and organ dysfunction that can ultimately lead to MODS.[4-10,15,16,33]

IMMUNE RESPONSE ABNORMALITIES AND CLINICAL IMPLICATIONS

The term *immunosuppression* is commonly used in the ICU. Patients can become immunosuppressed because they are stressed, malnourished, or suffering from a traumatic insult. But what exactly does the term mean? What impact does it have on the patient? On care and assessment? Is one patient's immunosuppression the same as another's? Probably not, at least not exactly. There are actually three areas of immune dysfunction: (1) immunosuppression—ineffective or hindered response, (2) hypersensitivity—overactive response, and (3) autoimmunity—mistaken recognition of self as antigen.[11]

Immunosuppression is the primary focus of this next section; the overactive response (systemic inflammatory response syndrome) is the focus of Chapter 3; autoimmunity is beyond the scope of this text.

The intricacy of the IIR is overwhelming in its complexity, components, and interrelationships. Alterations can occur anywhere among the numerous pathways, cells, and mediators. Global interventions to prevent infection or stimulation of inflammation, such as handwashing, aseptic technique, and nutrition, are crucial but may not be enough to protect the critically ill patient exposed to alterations in the IIR, resistant environmental pathogens, and breakdown of natural defense barriers. As knowledge of immune mechanisms increases, future therapies can be targeted more precisely to specific dysfunctions in the IIR.[37,38] Numerous risk factors have been implicated in the development and progression of immune dysfunction in critical illness, including stress, trauma, hemorrhage, blood transfusions, surgery, anesthesia, and malnutrition (Table 2-4).

Stress

As our understanding of the IIR expands, evidence increasingly links the nervous system, the endocrine system, and the immune system into a complex, integrated response, with an overlap of many of their regulatory molecules, such as corticosteroids, cytokines, and neurotransmitters.[54] Nowhere does the interaction of these three systems appear more evident than in the stress state. A wealth of literature has been published in recent years and new fields, such as neuroendocrinimmunology, neuroimmunomodulation, and psychoneuroimmunology have arisen. The reader is referred to several recent reviews.[54,55]

Stress is a "physical, chemical, or emotional factor to which an individual fails to make a satisfactory adaptation, and which causes physiologic tensions that may be a contributory cause of disease."[56] Observations that stressful conditions contribute to immunosuppression have been in the literature for decades.[57-59] In the last 10 years, stressful conditions have been shown to affect many aspects of the IIR, including phagocytosis, lymphocyte cytotoxicity, and antibody production.[59-61]

Steroids have long been associated with the immunosuppressive effects of stress.[62,63] Circulating steroids, both endogenous (cortisol) and exogenous

Table 2-4 Clinical Conditions with Hypothesized Immune Alterations/Dysfunction

Condition	Alteration in immune activity
Stress*	↑ neutrophil counts ↑ IL-1, ? ↑ TNF, IL-6 ↓ lymphocyte, monocyte, basophil counts ↓ chemotaxis ↓ phagocytosis ↓ mediator release ↓ IL-2 ↓ antibody production ↓ IL-2 receptors on T-cells ↓ NK activity
Trauma[74-77]	↓ macrophage–T cell interaction ↓ antigen processing and presentation ↓ T$_H$ cell proliferation and activity ↑ PGE$_2$ (inhibitory) production by macrophages ↓ antibody production ↑ T-cell suppressor activity ↓ neutrophil phagocytic activity ↓ IL-2 ↑ IL-1, ↑ TNF
Hemorrhage†	↓ macrophage–T cell interaction ↓ antigen processing and presentation ↓ T-cell proliferation and cytokine production ↓ antibody production ↓ phagocytic activity ↓ NK cell activity ↓ MHC Class II expression ↓ Kupffer cell phagocytic capability but ↑ cytokine production ↑ TGF-β and PGE$_2$
Blood transfusion‡	↓ antigen processing and presentation ↓ T-cell proliferation ↓ CD4$^+$:CD8$^+$ ratio ↓ NK cell activity ↑ PGE$_2$
Surgery/anesthesia§	↓ macrophage–T cell interaction ↓ antigen processing and presentation ↓ T$_H$ cell proliferation and activity ↑ PGE$_2$ production by macrophages ↑ T-cell suppressor activity ↓ lymphocyte traffic out of lymph nodes ↓ phagocytosis ↓ antibody production
Malnutrition[113,114]	↓ cell-mediated immunity ↓ lymphocyte counts ↓ CD4$^+$:CD8$^+$ ratio ↓ NK activity ↓ humoral immunity Impaired macrophage respiratory burst

IL, Interleukin; *MHC*, major histocompatibility complex; *NK*, natural killer; *PG*, prostaglandin; *TNF*, tumor necrosis factor; *TGF-β*, transforming growth factor-beta.
*References 59, 61, 62, 65, 70-73.
†References 50, 78, 83, 85, 86, 88, 89.
‡References 82, 84, 96-98, 100, 103.
§References 74, 98, 100, 105-109.

(prednisone, methylprednisolone) have antiinflammatory and antilymphocyte effects (Fig. 2-7). Steroids decrease lymphocyte, monocyte, and basophil counts.[62] This effect may partly be caused by the redistribution of lymphocytes from the circulating pool to the peripheral lymphoid tissue.[63,64]

Monocyte/macrophage activity is also hindered by the corticosteroids; therefore, chemotaxis, phagocytosis, and mediator release necessary for the inflammatory process may be inhibited. Although neutrophil counts increase, the cells have a decreased ability to adhere to the vessel wall and to move through it to a site of injury. Other effects seen with large doses of corticosteroids include decreased IL-1, IL-2, and IgG levels, T$_H$ cell proliferation, and arachidonic acid metabolism.[65]

While the antiinflammatory effects of corticosteroids would seem to be helpful in patients with sepsis and MODS who are suffering from overwhelming inflammation and "loss of control," the potent immunosuppressant effects of steroids can be devastating to an immunocompromised patient exposed to numerous pathogenic organisms. Large-scale clinical trials have shown that high-dose corticosteroid therapy does not decrease mortality associated with sepsis and MODS.[66-69]

Although circulating corticosteroids can have profound effects on immune activity, studies have shown that even when the release of circulating steroids is inhibited, immunosuppression still occurs in the stress state. Along with glucocorticoid receptors, many immune cells (especially lymphocytes) have receptors on their surfaces for catecholamines, acetylcholine, insulin, and other neuroendocrine hormonal substances that are released during the stress state and that have the potential to affect specific aspects of the IIR.[59] In addition, the lymphoid organs are innervated by the autonomic nervous system, and their function may be affected by autonomic nervous system activity.[59,60]

Several mechanisms have been proposed for the steroid-independent immunosuppression seen in stress. IL-2, which is necessary for T-cell proliferation, is decreased after stress. Investigators have shown that T cells also have fewer IL-2 receptors to bind the IL-2 that is present.[61] Without T$_H$ cell proliferation and cytokine production, other aspects of the IIR that depend on T$_H$ cell assistance are not as effective. Weiss and co-workers hypothesize that a circulating protein factor is present during the stress state that suppresses the immune response.[61]

Not only does the neuroendocrine system affect the immune response but the immune response affects the neuroendocrine system. Some cytokines released during the IIR act as neurotransmitters. IL-1 has been shown to be linked to the activation

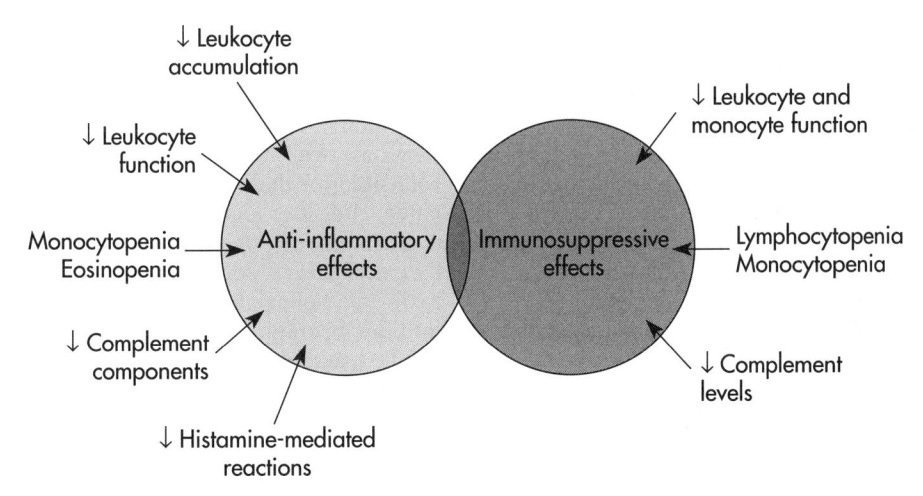

Fig. 2-7 The antiinflammatory and immunosuppressive effects of corticosteroids. (From Hooks MA. Immunosuppressive agents used in transplantation. In: Smith SL, ed. Tissue and organ transplantation: Implications for professional nursing practice. St. Louis: Mosby, 1990;57.)

of the hypothalamic-pituitary-adrenal (HPA) axis through the triggering of corticotropin-releasing factor (CRF).[70] CRF may cause immunosuppression directly by altering the functions of various immune components or indirectly through its activation of the HPA axis leading to the production of glucocorticoids. Cortisol release may be a protective mechanism to limit destructive activity, such as overwhelming inflammation.[54,71] The ability of IL-1 to induce fever is another example of its effects as a neurotransmitter.

Stress disturbs the homeostasis of the major regulatory systems: nervous, endocrine, and immune. IL-1, released in many stress states such as trauma, is thought to be a major messenger within and between these three body systems.[70,72] The intricate balance between the various hormones required for the body to maintain equilibrium is lost during the stress state and multiple derangements are clinically observable.[59,73]

Trauma

Research on the "immunosuppression of trauma" is expanding as advances in immune techniques and trauma care allow more advanced study of the phenomenon. Clinically, trauma-related immunosuppression leads to an increase in both opportunistic and pathogenic infections in this population of patients. Progression into fulminant septic shock and MODS can ensue. Therefore the critical care team should make all attempts to prevent infection, identify and treat it early when it does occur, and enhance the ability of the body to respond to invasion. This enhancement requires knowledge of the immune alterations occurring posttrauma and is currently an area of much interest and research.

Alterations in cytokine production, as well as in cell number and activity, have been noted after traumatic injury, particularly severe burns.[74-76] The mediators most often implicated in posttraumatic immunosuppression are the prostaglandins and the cytokines produced by activated immune cells.[77,78] The major problem occurring posttrauma appears to be a depression of macrophage–T cell interaction caused by increased production of the inhibitory prostaglandin PGE_2, decreased MHC Class II expression by macrophages, and decreased production of IL-2 by T cells.[50,78-80] Both IL-1 and IL-2 facilitate T_H cell activity. Without proper antigen processing, presentation, and macrophage–T cell interaction, T_H cell stimulation does not occur; therefore, further activation of macrophages and stimulation of antibody production by B cells is lost. Ingestion of alcohol has been shown to exacerbate the immunosuppression of trauma.[81] T-cell suppressor activity is also increased.[77]

Hemorrhage

Not only does the trauma victim experience direct injury, but the patient is also exposed to stress, hemorrhage, surgery, anesthesia, and blood transfusions, all of which have immunosuppressive effects.[59,82-84] Hemorrhage causes major disturbances in organ systems and the immune response, even in the absence of massive tissue trauma.[83,85] Alterations in the immune response include decreases in T-cell proliferation, cytokine production, and NK activity.[50] In addition, macrophage activity, including antigen processing, presentation, and MHC Class II expression, is also depressed.[86]

Hepatocellular dysfunction has been shown to occur early after hemorrhage and to persist despite aggressive fluid resuscitation.[87] Because the liver plays a key role in overall immune activity and because macrophage–T cell interaction is so crucial in activating the antigen-specific component of the IIR, increased susceptibility to infection is a major concern for trauma patients and others experiencing a hemorrhagic event. Although production of the cytokines, IL-2 and IFN-γ, is decreased in trauma, recent evidence has shown that Kupffer cell production of TNF, IL-1, and TGF-β are increased following trauma or hemorrhage.[85,88,89] TNF and IL-1 are proinflammatory cytokines that could trigger the inflammatory cascade, systemic inflammatory response syndrome (SIRS), and septic shock.

Although the changes that occur in trauma patients are well-documented, the mechanisms responsible for these changes have yet to be elucidated. Because calcium channel blockers can augment antigen presentation and IL-1 production by macrophages, some investigators believe that a toxic influx of calcium from the extracellular space into the macrophage may be partially responsible for the macrophage dysfunction[50] and concomitant T-cell depression seen in hemorrhage and ischemia (Fig. 2-8).[90] An interesting point is that this calcium influx is thought to occur during resuscitation at the time of reperfusion, not during the ischemic period.[91] This may be of clinical benefit because damage occurs not in the field but at the time of resuscitation; therefore, preventive measures may be

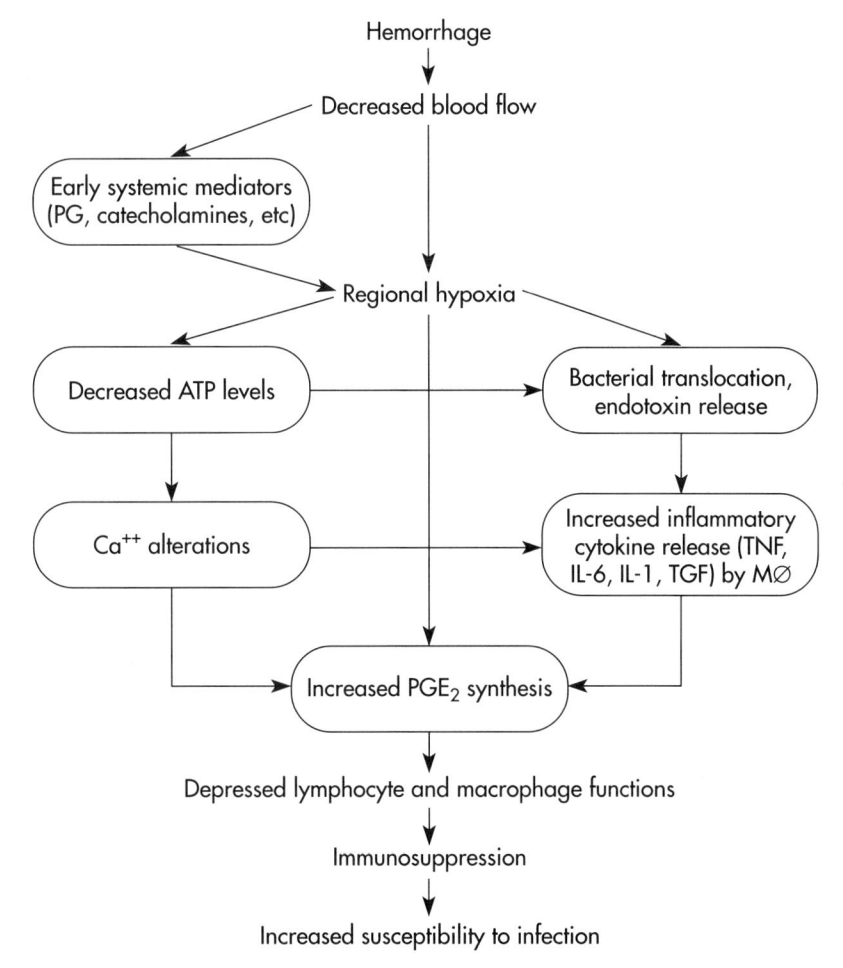

```
                        Hemorrhage
                            │
                            ▼
                  ┌── Decreased blood flow
                  │         │
                  ▼         │
        ┌──────────────────┐│
        │ Early systemic   ││
        │ mediators        ││
        │ (PG,             ││
        │ catecholamines,  ││
        │ etc)             ││
        └──────────────────┘│
                  │         │
                  ▼         ▼
                → Regional hypoxia ←
```

Fig. 2-8 Hypothesis of the cascade of events following hemorrhage leading to immunosuppression and increased susceptibility to infection. *PG*, Prostaglandins; *ATP*, adenosine triphosphate; *TNF*, tumor necrosis factor; *IL*, interleukin; *TGF*-β, transforming growth factor-beta; *MØ*, macrophage. (From Chaudry IH, Ayala A. Mechanism of increased susceptibility to infection following hemorrhage. Am J Surg 1993;165(2A suppl):59S-67S.)

taken during the resuscitation. Investigators postulate that lipid peroxidation—caused by oxygen-derived free radicals formed via the xanthine oxidase pathway during reperfusion—alters membrane permeability and integrity and allows large amounts of calcium to enter the cell.[50]

In addition to the direct immunosuppression of trauma, the patient is also at increased risk for septic complications because hemorrhagic shock greatly affects gut integrity. Ischemia and loss of gut barrier function contribute to increased permeability of the gut wall and the possible movement of bacteria, bacterial products, or other inflammatory stimuli into the lymph and portal circulation.[92,93]

Blood transfusions

Blood transfusions are often used in trauma patients and others to combat hemorrhage which adds further insult to the compromised patient. Numerous studies have implicated blood transfusions in immunosuppression. This was initially observed when donor graft survival was lengthened in transplant patients who had received transfusions before the transplantation. The point was raised that if blood transfusions suppressed immune rejection of the graft, they were perhaps also suppressing the IIR against other foreign agents, thus increasing the risk of infection or even malignancies.[94,95]

Changes seen after blood transfusion include decreased helper cell/cytotoxic cell (CD4+:CD8+) ratios, decreased NK activity, decreased antigen processing and presentation, and decreased T-cell proliferation.[96-99] Decreased production of IL-2 ("good" cytokine) and increased production of PGE_2 ("bad" prostaglandin) after blood transfusion may partially mediate this dysfunction; there are other studies, however, that have shown that the PGE_2 may be responsible for the signs or symptoms of sepsis but not the immune dysfunction of trauma or transfusion.[100,101] IL-2 is necessary for effective TH activity, and PGE_2 depresses macrophage–T cell interaction. The question remains whether blood transfusion alone causes immunosuppression or whether the other factors (i.e., hemorrhage) involved in a traumatic or septic insult work together to produce immunosuppression.[102] The IIR alterations seen in graft survival, which are specific responses, may be different from the alterations seen after trauma or sepsis, which are associated with both specific and nonspecific responses.[84,103]

Surgery and anesthesia

Patients undergoing surgical procedures have long been known to have impaired immunologic reactivity.[104,105] Because the surgical procedure is accompanied by anesthesia, trauma to the body, possible blood transfusion, and an overall stress response, it is difficult to isolate which events cause which alterations in the IIR. Most likely, these events operate synergistically to mediate overall host immunosuppression, resulting in increased susceptibility to infection.[82,106,107] Alterations noted in surgical patients include ineffective CD4+ cell proliferation, increased suppressor activity of CD8+ cells, and dysfunctional monocytes and macrophages.[108] These effects lead to other alterations including a decrease in IL-2 synthesis and decreased antibody production.[109,110]

Malnutrition and substance abuse

Malnutrition, both starvation and protein deficiency, impairs a variety of systemic functions: the most profoundly affected are immunologic functions and wound healing, although the exact mechanisms are unclear. Immunocompetence and wound healing are closely related because effective immune system function is necessary for wound microdébridement and protection. Malnutrition deprives the patient of protein, glucose, oxygen, and other nutrients needed for stable tissue formation and wound repair. T-cell proliferation and helper ability are impaired in the malnourished patient but can often be restored following adequate protein and calorie supplementation.[111]

Malnutrition is often associated with, and may be secondary to, chronic drug and alcohol abuse. Alcohol affects neutrophil production and other immune functions.[112] Excessive substance abuse leads to decreased food intake and alters nutrient digestion, absorption, storage, and utilization. All aspects of metabolism are affected and gut integrity is compromised.[112,113] Alcohol may also increase the breakdown and turnover of many vitamins and minerals, thus further increasing the demand on an already decreased supply.[114]

Summary

Although more patients are surviving their initial injury, secondary complications remain a major source of morbidity and mortality in critical care units. There are six strikes against trauma patients—trauma, stress, hemorrhage, blood transfusions, surgery, and anesthesia—even before they arrive in the unit, where they will then be bombarded with antibiotics (which can select for resistant organisms), invasive procedures, and often iatrogenic malnutrition. Surgical patients and other critically ill individuals also have several of these risk factors. The risk, therefore, is great for septic complications and MODS in the critically ill patient. This is confirmed in the literature, which continues to report major morbidity and mortality in the trauma patient secondary to septic and inflammatory complications and MODS.[6-8,10,16,19] Destruction of surface barriers, overload of tissue debris, and activation of coagulation all contribute to the already complicated clinical scenario.

ASSESSMENT AND LABORATORY FINDINGS

With the advent of newer laboratory equipment and more sophisticated techniques, the clinician is no longer solely dependent on the simple WBC count with differential to assess the immune response. In addition to total cell counts, mediator levels and activity, effectiveness of both humoral and cell-mediated immune responses, and counts of specific cellular subsets can be determined.[115] While some of these advanced techniques are only available to investigators for research purposes, many are now being utilized in clinical diagnosis and prognostication.

For intelligent interpretation of laboratory data and assessment of therapeutic effectiveness, knowledge of the significance and implications of a test is vital to the clinician's ability to provide thorough, rationale-based care. Although sophisticated laboratory techniques are very helpful, the general status of the immune system and defense capabilities of the patient is also apparent from data obtained during a routine physical assessment.

Natural defenses

Assessing the status of natural defenses or external barriers to invasion is the initial step in assessment of host defense.[116] Is the skin intact? Is it fragile? Is it edematous? Are there numerous invasive lines and devices in place that would permit the invasion of microorganisms? Table 2-5 details organ-specific assessment parameters and their effect on immune function.[24,116]

Cells and tissues of the immune system

The complete blood count (CBC) and CBC with differential are two of the most commonly ordered laboratory tests in the ICU. Not only do they provide information concerning absolute cell counts, such as those of neutrophils, monocytes, and lymphocytes, but the percentage of each relative to the total is also reported, providing the clinician with information necessary to assess the status and activity of the IIR (Table 2-6).[24] The ability of other organs, such as the bone marrow and lymphoid organs, to meet the peripheral demand is also reflected in the cell counts.

Neutrophils. In bacterial infection the neutrophil count is increased, and in viral infections the lymphocyte count is increased. It must be remembered that cell counts measure only those cells actually circulating in the blood. Neutrophils marginated along vessel walls and lymphocytes sequestered in the lymph nodes and the lymphatic circulation are not reflected in the count. As mentioned previously, 90% to 95% of the lymphocytes in the body reside in the secondary lymphoid tissue of the spleen, lymph nodes, and mucosa-associated lymphoid tissue. In addition to inflammation or infection, other factors can also increase WBC counts. By increasing cardiac output and blood flow, exercise and catecholamine release can increase the neutrophil count (neutrophilia, leukocytosis) because marginated cells are flushed off the vessel wall and into the circulation.

If inflammation and infection continue, more immature neutrophils (known as bands) are released by the bone marrow as it attempts to meet the increased demand in the periphery. The appearance of circulating bands and other immature cells is referred to as a "shift to the left" because the immature cells are traditionally drawn on the left side of the page in maturation diagrams (Fig. 2-9). The bone marrow eventually becomes exhausted and can no longer match the demands in the periphery. Low neutrophil counts (neutropenia) are not uncommon at the end stage of sepsis and MODS, and infection can still be present even when the WBC count decreases. Chemotherapy, radiation therapy, and hematologic malignancies also contribute to neutropenia. Because neutrophils are necessary for the development of pus, a severely neutropenic patient can have an infection without the presence of purulent drainage. The loss of neutrophils also contributes to the inability of the body to remove bacteria and other foreign debris.

The presence of neutrophil adhesion molecules can also be assayed. In a recent study by Goya and co-workers[117] neutrophils from septic patients were found to exhibit enhanced endothelial cell adhesion, chemotaxis, free radical generation, and enzyme release in association with complement activation. The authors concluded that neutrophil activity is central to the pathogenesis of septic MODS.[117]

Lymphocytes. In assessing humoral immunity, both B-cell counts and specific antibody assays can be performed. In cell-mediated immunity, absolute T-cell counts, as well as subset ratios, are examined. A low CD4+:CD8+ ratio reflects a decrease in CD4+ cells or an increase in the CD8+ cells; therefore, the ratios must be interpreted concurrently with absolute cell counts and the patient's clinical picture.[44] The low ratio could signify an imbalance of immune regulation toward down-regulation of the spe-

Table 2-5 Systems Assessment with Potential IIR Impact and Complications[24,116]

System	Risk factors	Impact on IIR	Potential complications	Assessment
Central nervous system	Invasive drains ICP monitoring Incision line Cranial nerve impairment Spinal cord injury	Increased microbial access IIR activation Impaired natural defenses (gag, cough, blink)	Inflammation/infection Aspiration Corneal abrasions Immobility → skin breakdown	↓ LOC, ↓ CPP, inflammation at wound site, respiratory depression, ↑↓ temperature, ↑↓ BP, ↑↓ heart rate, ↓ Glasgow Coma Score, ↑↓ respiratory rate, ↑↓ tidal volume, skin breakdown
Pulmonary	Artificial airway Mechanical ventilation Barotrauma High FiO$_2$ levels	Bypass of natural defenses (humidity, mucociliary escalator) Increased microbial access (ETT, oral secretions) Activation of alveolar macrophages with toxic mediator release Altered surfactant production	Aspiration Atelectasis Pneumonia ARDS Oxygen toxicity and alveolocapillary damage	↑↓ respiratory rate, ↓ depth, ↑ SOB, dyspnea, diaphoresis, use of accessory muscles, ↓ SEC, ↑ PIP, thick and greenish-yellow sputum, ↑ V/Q mismatching, intrapulmonary shunt >20%, wheezes, crackles, infiltrates on CXR, ventilatory dependence, ↓ pH, ↓ SaO$_2$, ↓ SvO$_2$, ↓ PaO$_2$, ↑ PaCO$_2$, ↑ lactate
Cardiovascular	Invasive monitoring Poor perfusion	Increased microbial access Tissue ischemia → IIR activation with third spacing and edema Cellular activation and mediator release	Reperfusion injury Cellulitis Bacteremia/septicemia Endothelial damage and clotting abnormalities	↑↓ CO, ↓↑ SVR, ↑↓ heart rate, ↓ BP, ↓ ejection fraction, ↑ PAP, ↓↑ PCWP, ↓↑ CVP, cold and pale skin, inflammation at access sites, weak pulses, narrow pulse pressure, ectopy, MI, ↑ isoenzymes, ↑ lactate

Gastrointestinal	Nasogastric tube Antacid therapy H₂-blocker therapy Stress ulceration Antibiotics Ileus	↑ pH → ↑ bacterial colonization IIR activation Inhibition of normal flora's protective functions Inability to clear bacterial load	Colonization of esophagus and tracheobronchial tree Pneumonia Overgrowth of pathogenic organisms in the GI tract Translocation of bacteria to the lymph and blood	↓ bowel sounds, upper/lower GI bleeding, abdominal distention, diarrhea, impaction, ileus, stress ulceration/erosion, mucosal atrophy, guaiac+ stool, enteric organisms on blood culture, jaundice, ascites, ↓ drug clearance, bleeding, ↑ liver function tests, ↓ plasma proteins, ↑ ammonia, ↓ clotting factors, hepatomegaly, splenomegaly
Genitourinary	Bladder catheter Antibiotics Hyperglycemia	Increased microbial access Altered normal flora in vagina Promotion of yeast growth	Urinary tract infection Septicemia *Candida* infections	↑↓ urine output, malodorous discharge, ↑ PCWP, ↑ CVP, ↑ weight, peripheral edema, ↑ BUN, ↑ creatinine, ↑ potassium, ↑ magnesium, ↓ pH, ↓ bicarbonate

ARDS, Adult respiratory distress syndrome; *BP*, blood pressure; *BUN*, blood urea nitrogen; *CO*, cardiac output; *CPP*, cerebral perfusion pressure; *CVP*, central venous pressure; *ETT*, endotracheal tube; *Fio₂*, fraction of inspired oxygen; *GI*, gastrointestinal; *H₂*, histamine type 2 receptor; *ICP*, intracranial pressure; *IIR*, inflammatory/immune response; *LOC*, level of consciousness; *MI*, myocardial infarction; *Paco₂*, partial pressure of carbon dioxide in arterial blood; *Pao₂*, partial pressure of oxygen in arterial blood; *PAP*, pulmonary artery pressure; *PCWP*, pulmonary capillary wedge pressure; *PIP*, peak inspiratory pressure; *Sao₂*, arterial oxygen saturation; *SEC*, static effective compliance; *SOB*, shortness of breath; *Svo₂*, venous oxygen saturation; *SVR*, systemic vascular resistance; *V/Q*, ventilation/perfusion ratio.

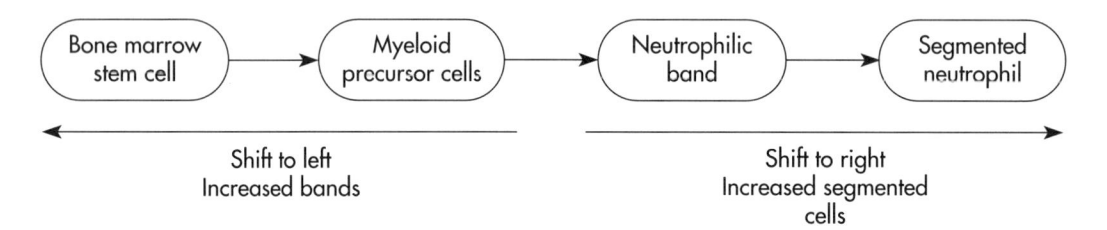

Fig. 2-9 Maturational diagram of the neutrophil.

Table 2-6 Normal White Blood Cell Values

Cell type	Absolute number (mm³)	Differential (%)	Function/change
Granulocytes			
Neutrophils	3000-7000	60-70	↑ with inflammation or infection ↓ with bone marrow suppression or exhaustion
Segmented	2800-5600	56	↑ value-right shift
Bands (immature)	150-600	3-6	↑ value-left shift
Eosinophils	50-500	1-4	↑ in allergy and parasitic infections
Basophils	25-100	0.5-1	Involved in Type I hypersensitivity reactions (anaphylactoid) ? role in infection
Mononuclear cells			
Monocytes	100-800	2-8	↑ with chronic infection, TB, malaria, some viral infections
Lymphocytes (total)	1000-4000	20-45	↑ in viral infections ↓ in HIV disease
T cells	800-3200	80% of TLC	
B cells	100-600	10%-15% of TLC	
NK cells	50-400	5%-10% of TLC	

Modified from Tribett D. Immune system function: Implications for critical care nursing practice. Crit Care Nurs Clin North Am 1989;1:727.
HIV, Human immunodeficiency virus; *NK*, natural killer; *TB*, tuberculosis; *TLC*, total lymphocyte count; *WBC*, white blood count.

cific immune response. The CD4+:CD8+ ratio has been shown to be generally decreased in sepsis[118] and AIDS.[119] Conversely, a high ratio signifies an increase in CD4+ cell activity or a decrease in CD8+ cell activity. CD4+ cell activity is greatly increased as a normal response to bacterial invasion, and the ratio may increase to 20:1 in *Staphylococcus* and *Klebsiella* infections.[44] A decrease in the CD8+ cell count is often present in autoimmune diseases, reflecting a lack of immunoregulation. In a study by Dahn and co-workers,[118] one interesting subset of nonsurvivors of sepsis demonstrated a high CD4+:CD8+ ratio secondary to decreased numbers of CD8+ cells. Without the regulatory, controlling action of the CD8+ cells, the IIR is not limited and an exaggerated immune and metabolic response could overwhelm the host.[118] These data provide further support for the hypothesis that MODS may be a result of overwhelming inflammation and activation of the IIR. The use of the CD4+:CD8+ ratio has become controversial as the functional lines between CD4+ cells and CD8+ cells have become blurred. Some CD4+ cells may have suppressor activity and some CD8+ cells may have helper activity. Although the use of the ratio is under question, the measurement of T-cell subsets continues to be used clinically.[44]

Lymphoid tissue. Because the liver, spleen, and lymph nodes play a major role in host defense, knowledge of previous alterations in these organs aids in assessment of immune function. If the patient has a history of cirrhosis or other hepatic disease, the Kupffer cells (liver macrophages) may not adequately clear foreign matter in the circulation or debris leaking from the gut.[4,120] Congestive heart failure accompanied by hepatic congestion may also decrease the phagocytic capabilities of the liver.

A previous splenectomy can predispose the patient to infectious complications, especially in children and young adults. Research has shown that this increased incidence of infection, when it does occur, is more likely to occur months to years after the splenectomy and not in the perioperative period.[99] An increased incidence of sepsis and thromboembolic complications has been observed 10 to 15 years postsplenectomy.[121-123] The spleen is a major lymphoid organ with a large population of T and B cells. Following the removal of the spleen, the other lymphoid organs usually "make up the difference," but this compensatory activity may be stressed in times of overwhelming infection.[121-123]

Enlarged lymph nodes signify the proliferation of T and B cells in the nodal tissue following antigen exposure. Although their enlargement indicates the presence of infection, it also demonstrates the ability of the lymphocytes to respond and proliferate.[49] Past resection of nodal tissue should be noted on the patient's chart.

Circulating mediators of the inflammatory/immune response

Because many of the mediators in sepsis and MODS are unstable or occur in only minute concentrations, the levels of specific mediators are difficult to measure directly. The presence of a mediator may have to be extrapolated from the existence of its metabolites, from levels of precursor molecules, or from the presence of activity that is attributable to the mediator in question.[115,124] Two common techniques used to measure mediator or mediator metabolite concentrations are the radioimmunoassay (RIA) and enzyme-linked immunosorbent assay (ELISA). The ELISA technique is often preferable because it does not involve the handling and disposal restrictions associated with the use of radioactive materials; however, the RIA is generally more sensitive for mediators present at low concentrations.

Several mediators that can presently be measured include activated complement proteins (split products), endotoxin, arachidonic acid metabolites, prothrombin, and cytokines, such as TNF, IL-1, IL-2, and IL-6. More attention is now being given to making these tests more clinically feasible and timely. Activated macrophages release neopterin, and increased levels have been shown to correlate with the development of sepsis and MODS.[125-128]

Immunologic responsiveness

Cell counts and mediator concentrations give the clinician clues concerning the availability of IIR components, but the assessment can be taken one step further by measuring the actual responsiveness of the cells to specific mediators. The mediator levels are insignificant if the cell has no receptor and thus no ability to respond to the mediator. Changes in receptor number and type have been noted in the septic state.[129] The ability of T and B cells to proliferate in response to antigen exposure can be measured in the laboratory, along with circulating antibody levels. The capacity of neutrophils for chemotaxis, phagocytosis, and bactericidal activity can also be determined.

The intradermal injection of antigens to which most people have been previously exposed (streptococcal products, diphtheria toxoid, tetanus toxoid, *Candida* antigens) is used to evaluate overall immune responsiveness. Skin testing involves a delayed-type hypersensitivity (DTH) reaction in which sensitized lymphocytes are drawn to the local area of injection.[130,131] On arrival, the T cells release cytokines that attract macrophages to the area, setting up a local inflammatory reaction (erythema, induration, warmth). If lymphocytes and macrophages are unresponsive to the antigen, no inflammation is seen, and the patient is considered anergic. Anergy is associated with increased incidence of sepsis and greater mortality.[132,133]

CONCLUSION

The inflammatory/immune response is designed to protect the host and limit the extent of injury. In the setting of critical illness, however, regulation of this exquisite response is often lost for reasons that remain to be elucidated. The dysregulation can occur at either end of the spectrum ("too much" or "too little"), and interestingly enough may be present at both ends of the spectrum in some patients. In other words, some patients could be experiencing immunosuppression of their specific immune response but overactivity of their inflammatory (nonspecific) response.[89] Loss of regulation combined with infection, inflammation, or ischemia often leads to the development of the systemic inflammatory response syndrome, which is frequently associated with the development of septic shock, multiple organ dysfunction and failure, and other complications of critical illness.[134-136]

With knowledge of mediator activity and immune status, patient management can focus on controlling the immune response. Known as immunotherapeutics or immunomodulation, these therapies are aimed at enhancing IIR, restoring control, and inhibiting excessive mediator activity. By monitoring the mediators of inflammation and modifying their presence and excessive activity, the health care team may have the potential to upset the fatal course that many of these patients travel.

REFERENCES

1. Roitt I, Brostoff J, Male D. Immunology. 3rd ed. London: Mosby; 1993.
2. Sell S. Immunology, immunopathology and immunity. 4th ed. New York: Elsevier; 1987.
3. Byram DA. Future expectations for critical care nurses: Competence in immunotherapy. Crit Care Nurs Clin North Am 1989;1:797-806.
4. Baue AE. Multiple organ failure: Patient care and prevention. St. Louis: Mosby; 1990.
5. Dorinsky PM, Gadek JE. Multiple organ failure. Clin Chest Med 1990;11:581-591.
6. Goris RJ. Multiple organ failure: Whole body inflammation? Schweiz Med Wochenschr 1989;119:347-353.
7. Goris RJ, Boekhorst TE, Nuytinck JK, Gimbrére JSF. Multiple organ failure: Generalized autodestructive inflammation. Arch Surg 1985;120:1109-1115.
8. Goris RJ et al. Multiple organ failure and sepsis without bacteria. Arch Surg 1986;121:897-901.
9. Pinsky MR. Multiple systems organ failure: Malignant intravascular inflammation. Crit Care Clin 1989;5:195-198.
10. Pinsky MR, Matuschak GM. Multiple systems organ failure: Failure of host defense homeostasis. Crit Care Clin 1989;5:199-220.
11. Male D, Roitt I. Introduction to the immune system. In: Roitt I, Brostoff J, Male D, eds. Immunology. 3rd ed. London: Mosby;1993:1.1-1.12.
12. Hyers TM, Gee M, Andreadis NA. Cellular interactions in the multiple organ injury syndrome. Am Rev Respir Dis 1987;135:952-953.
13. Bevilacqua MP, Gimbrone MA. Inducible endothelial functions in inflammation and coagulation. Semin Thromb Hemost 1988;13:425-433.
14. Pober JS, Cotran RS. The role of endothelial cells in inflammation. Transplantation 1990;50:537-544.
15. Vallance P, Moncada S. Role of endogenous nitric oxide in septic shock. New Horiz 1993;1:77-86.
16. DeCamp MM, Demling RH. Posttraumatic multisystem organ failure. JAMA 1988;260:530-534.
17. Cunnion RE, Parrillo JE. Myocardial dysfunction in sepsis. Crit Care Clin 1989;5:99-118.
18. Bersten A, Sibbald WJ. Circulatory disturbances in multiple systems organ failure. Crit Care Clin 1989;5:233-254.
19. Anderson BO, Harken AH. Multiple organ failure: Inflammatory priming and activation sequences promote autologous tissue injury. J Trauma 1990;30:S44-S49.
20. Dantzker D. Oxygen delivery and utilization in sepsis. Crit Care Clin 1989;5:81-98.
21. Hotter AN. The pathophysiology of multi-system organ failure in the trauma patient. AACN Clin Issues Crit Care Nurs 1990;1:465-478.
22. Gutierrez G, Lund N, Bryan-Brown CW. Cellular oxygen utilization during multiple organ failure. Crit Care Clin 1989;5:271-288.
23. Barton R, Cerra FB. The hypermetabolism multiple organ failure syndrome. Chest 1989;96:1153-1160.
24. Tribett D. Immune system function: Implications for critical care nursing practice. Crit Care Nurs Clin North Am 1989;1:725-740.
25. Mackay CR, Imhof BA. Cell adhesion in the immune system. Immunol Today 1993;14:99-102.
26. Springer TA. Adhesion receptors of the immune system. Nature 1990;346:425-434.
27. Talbott GA et al. Leukocyte-endothelial interactions and organ injury: The role of adhesion molecules. New Horiz 1994;2:545-554.
28. Walport M. Complement. In: Roitt I, Brostoff J, Male D, eds. Immunology. 3rd ed. London: Mosby;1993:12.1-12.17.
29. Hood LE, Weissman IL, Wood WB, Wilson JH. Immune effector mechanisms and the complement system. In: Hood LE, Weissman IL, Wood WB, Wilson JH, eds. Immunology. 2nd ed. Menlo Park, CA: Benjamin/Cummings Publishing Co; 1984:334-365.
30. Rook G. Immunity to viruses, bacteria and fungi. In: Roitt I, Brostoff J, Male D, eds. Immunology. 3rd ed. London: Mosby;1993:15.1-15.22.
31. Bone RC. Modulators of coagulation: A critical appraisal of their role in sepsis. Arch Intern Med 1992;152:1381-1389.
32. Taylor FB. The inflammatory-coagulant axis in the host response to Gram-negative sepsis: Regulatory roles of proteins and inhibitors of tissue factor. New Horiz 1994;2:555-565.
33. Secor VH. Mediators of coagulation and inflammation: Relationship and clinical significance. Crit Care Nurs Clin North Am 1993;5:411-433.
34. Feldmann M, Male D. Cell cooperation in the antibody response. In: Roitt I, Brostoff J, Male D, eds. Immunology. 3rd ed. London: Mosby; 1993:7.1-7.16.

35. Hay F. The generation of diversity. In: Roitt I, Brostoff J, Male D, eds. Immunology. 3rd ed. London:Mosby; 1993: 5.1-5.14.
36. Boyd JL, Stanford GG, Chernow B. The pharmacotherapy of septic shock. Crit Care Clin 1989;5:151-156.
37. Dinarello CA, Gelfand JA, Wolff SM. Anticytokine strategies in the treatment of the systemic inflammatory response syndrome. JAMA 1993;269: 1829-1835.
38. Hazinski MF. Mediator-specific therapies for the systemic inflammatory response syndrome, sepsis, severe sepsis, and septic shock: Present and future approaches. Crit Care Nurs Clin North Am 1994;6:309-319.
39. Parslow TG. The phagocytic neutrophils and macrophages. In: Stites DP, Terr AI, Parslow TG, eds. Basic and clinical immunology. 8th ed. Norwalk, CT: Appleton & Lange; 1994:9-21.
40. Rook G. Cell-mediated immune reactions. In: Roitt I, Brostoff J, Male D, eds. Immunology. 3rd ed. London: Mosby; 1993:8.1-8.16.
41. Lydyard P, Grossi C. Cells involved in immune responses. In: Roitt I, Brostoff J, Male D, eds. Immunology. 3rd ed. London:Mosby; 1993:2.1-2.20.
42. Bloom BR, Salgame P, Diamond B. Revisiting and revising suppressor T cells. Immunol Today 1992;13:131-136.
43. Green DR, Webb DR. Saying the "S" word in public. Immunol Today 1993;14:523-525.
44. Giorgi JV. Lymphocyte subset measurements: Significance in clinical medicine. In: Rose NR, Friedman H, Fahey JL, eds. Manual of clinical laboratory immunology. 3rd ed. Washington, D.C.: American Society for Microbiology;1986:236-246.
45. Moretta L et al. Ontogeny, specific functions and receptors of human natural killer cells. Immunol Lett 1994;40(2):83-88.
46. Owen M, Steward M. Antigen recognition. In: Roitt I, Brostoff J, Male D, eds. Immunology. 3rd ed. London: Mosby; 1993:6.1-6.14.
47. Cambier JC, Pleiman CM, Clark MR. Signal transduction by the B cell antigen receptor and its coreceptors. Annu Rev Immunol 1994;12:457-486.
48. Parker DC. T cell-dependent B cell activation. Annu Rev Immunol 1993;11:331-360.
49. Lydyard P, Grossi C. The lymphoid system. In: Roitt I, Brostoff J, Male D, eds. Immunology. 3rd ed. London: Mosby;1993:3.1-3.12.
50. Ertel W et al. Immunoprotective effect of a calcium channel blocker on macrophage antigen presentation function, major histocompatability class II antigen expression, and interleukin-1 synthesis after hemorrhage. Surgery 1990;108:154-160.
51. Picker LJ et al. Differential expression of homing-associated adhesion molecules by T-cell subsets in man. J Immunol 1990;145:3247-3255.
52. Picker LJ, Butcher EC. Physiological and molecular mechanisms of lymphocyte homing. Annu Rev Immunol 1992;10:561-591.
53. Taverne J. Immunity to protozoa and worms. In: Roitt I, Brostoff J, Male D, eds. Immunology. 3rd ed. London: Mosby; 1993:16.1-16.22.
54. Wilder RL. Neuroendocrine-immune system interactions and autoimmunity. Annu Rev Immunol 1995;13:307-338.
55. Michelson D, Gold PW, Sternberg EM. The stress response in critical illness. New Horiz 1994;2:426-431.
56. Webster's Third New International Dictionary. Unabridged. Springfield, MA:Merriam-Webster Inc;1986.
57. Ishigami T. The influence of psychic acts on the progress of pulmonary tuberculosis. Am Rev Tubercul 1919;2:470-484.
58. Holmes TH, Rahe RH. The social readjustment rating scale. J Psychosom Res 1967;11:213-218.
59. Khansari DN, Murgo AJ, Faith RE. Effects of stress on the immune system. Immunol Today 1990;11:170-175.
60. Dunn AJ. Nervous system–immune system interactions: An overview. J Recept Res 1988;8:589-607.
61. Weiss JM, Sundar SK, Becker KJ, Cierpial MA. Behavioral and neural influences on cellular immune responses: Effects of stress and interleukin-1. J Clin Psych 1989;50(5 suppl):43-53.
62. Cupps TR, Fauci AS. Corticosteroid-mediated immunoregulation in man. Immunol Rev 1982;65:133-155.
63. Ogawa K, Sueda K, Matsui N. The effect of cortisol, progesterone and transcortin on phytohemagglutinin-stimulated human blood mononuclear cells and their interplay. J Clin Endocrinol Metab 1983;56:121-126.
64. Fauci AS, Dale DC. Alternate-day prednisone therapy and human lymphocyte subpopulations. J Clin Invest 1975;55:22-32.
65. Hooks MA. Immunosuppressive agents used in transplantation. In: Smith SL, ed. Tissue and organ transplantation: Implications for professional nursing practice. St. Louis: Mosby; 1990:48-80.
66. Bone RC at al. A controlled clinical trial of high-dose methylprednisolone in the treatment of severe sepsis and septic shock. N Engl J Med 1987;317:653-658.
67. Veterans Administration Systemic Sepsis Cooperative Study Group. Effect of high-dose glucocorticoid therapy on mortality in patients with clinical signs of systemic sepsis. N Engl J Mcd 1987;317:659-665.
68. Bernard GR et al. High-dose corticosteroids in patients with the adult respiratory distress syndrome. N Engl J Med 1987;317:1565-1570.
69. Nicholson DP. Review of corticosteroid treatment in sepsis and septic shock: Pro or con. Crit Care Clin 1989;5:151-155.
70. Saperstein A et al. Interleukin 1 beta mediates stress-induced immunosuppression via corticotropin-releasing factor. Endocrinol 1992;130:152-158.
71. Besedovsky H, Del Rey A, Sorkin E, Dinarello CA. Immunoregulatory feedback between interleukin-1 and glucocorticoid hormones. Science 1986;233:652-654.
72. Dobbin JP et al. Cytokine production and lymphocyte transformation during stress. Brain, Behavior, and Immunity 1991;5:339-348.
73. Abraham E. Effects of stress on cytokine production. Methods and Achieve Exp Pathol 1991;14:45-62.
74. Holch MW et al. Graduation of immunosuppression after surgery or severe trauma. Prog Clin Biol Res: Second Vienna Shock Forum 1989;308:491-494.
75. Griswold JA. White blood cell response to burn injury. Semin Nephrol 1993;13:409-415.
76. Barlow Y. T lymphocytes and immunosuppression in the burned patient: A review. Burns 1994;20:487-490.
77. Faist E et al. Mediators and the trauma induced cascade of immunologic defects. Prog Clin Biol Res: Second Vienna Shock Forum 1989;308:495-506.

78. Ertel W et al. Modulation of macrophage membrane phospholipids by ω-3 polyunsaturated fatty acids increases interleukin 1 release and prevents suppression of cellular immunity following hemorrhagic shock. Arch Surg 1993;128:15-20.
79. Polk HC. Factors influencing the risk of infection after trauma. Am J Surg 1993;165:2S-7S.
80. Cheadle WG. The human leukocyte antigens and their relationship to infection. Am J Surg 1993;165:75S-81S.
81. Szabo G et al. Acute ethanol consumption synergizes with trauma to increase monocyte tumor necrosis factor alpha production late postinjury. J Clin Immunol 1994;14:340-352.
82. Waymack JP et al. Effect of blood transfusion and anesthesia on resistance to bacterial peritonitis. J Surg Res 1987;42:528-535.
83. Chaudry IH. Hemorrhage and resuscitation [editorial]. Am J Physiol 1990;259(4 Part 2):R663-R678.
84. Brunson ME, Alexander JW. Mechanisms of transfusion-induced immunosuppression. Transfusion 1990;30:651-658.
85. Ayala A et al. The release of transforming growth factor-beta following haemorrhage: Its role as a mediator of host immunosuppression. Immunology 1993;79:479-484.
86. Ertel W et al. Insights into the mechanisms of defective antigen presentation following hemorrhage. Surgery 1991; 110:440-447.
87. Wang P, Hauptman JG, Chaudry IH. Hepatocellular dysfunction occurs early after hemorrhage and persists despite fluid resuscitation. J Surg Res 1990;48:466-470.
88. Chaudry IH, Ayala A. Mechanisms of increased susceptibility to infection following hemorrhage. Am J Surg 1993;165:59S-67S.
89. Ayala A et al. Differential effects of hemorrhage on Kupffer cells: Decreased antigen presentation despite increased inflammatory cytokine (IL-1, IL-6, and TNF) release. Cytokine 1992;4:66-75.
90. Unanue ER, Allen PM. The basis of the immunoregulatory role of macrophages and other accessory cells. Science 1987;236:551-557.
91. Yano Y et al. Calcium-accented ischemic damage during reperfusion: The time course of the reperfusion injury in the isolated working rat heart model. J Surg Res 1987;42:51-55.
92. Baker JW et al. Hemorrhagic shock induces bacterial translocation from the gut. J Trauma 1988;28:896-906.
93. Ryan CM et al. Increased gut permeability early after burns correlates with the extent of burn injury. Crit Care Med 1992;20:1508-1512.
94. Gantt CL. Red blood cells for cancer patients [letter]. Lancet 1981;2:363.
95. Francis DMA, Sheaton BK. Blood transfusion and tumour growth: Evidence from laboratory animals [letter]. Lancet 1981;2:871.
96. Kaplan J et al. Diminished helper/suppressor lymphocyte ratios and natural killer activity in recipients of repeated blood transfusions. Blood 1984;64:308-310.
97. Stephan RN et al. Effect of blood transfusion on antigen presentation function and on interleukin-2 generation. Arch Surg 1988;123:235-240.
98. Maeta M et al. Perioperative allogeneic blood transfusion exacerbates surgical stress-induced postoperative immunosuppression and has negative effect on prognosis in patients with gastric cancer. J Surg Oncol 1994;55:149-153.
99. Duke BJ et al. Transfusion significantly increases the risk for infection after splenic injury. Arch Surg 1993;128:1125-1132.
100. Ross WB et al. Macrophage prostaglandin E2 and oxidative responses to endotoxin during immunosuppression associated with anaesthesia and transfusion. Prostaglandins, Leukot Essent Fatty Acids 1993;49:945-953.
101. Waymack JP et al. Effect of prostaglandin E on immune function in normal healthy volunteers. Surg Gynecol Obstet 1992;175:329-332.
102. Cue JI, Peyton JC, Malangoni MA. Does blood transfusion or hemorrhagic shock induce immunosuppression? J Trauma 1992;32:613-617.
103. Brunson ME, Ing R, Tchervenkov JI, Alexander JW. Variable infection risk following allogeneic blood transfusions. J Surg Res 1990;48:308-312.
104. Graham EA. The influence of ether and ether anesthesia on bacteriolysis, agglutination, and phagocytosis. J Infect Dis 1911;8:147-175.
105. Moore TC. Anesthesia-associated depression in lymphocyte traffic and its modulation. Am J Surg 1984;147:807-812.
106. Spruck CH, Moore TC. Anesthesia-associated depression of peripheral node lymphocyte traffic and antibody production in sheep accompanied by elevations in arachidonic acid metabolites in efferent lymph. Transplant Proc 1988;20:1169-1174.
107. Browder W, Williams D. Immunosuppression in the surgical patient. J Natl Med Assoc 1988;80:531-536.
108. Costa A et al. Endocrine, hematological and immunological changes in surgical patients undergoing general anesthesia. Ital J Surg Sci 1989;19:41-49.
109. Gebhard F, Kaffenberger W, Hartel W. Peripheral blood immune responses to surgically induced lung tissue injury. Eur Surg Res 1994;26(3):156-162.
110. Deehan DJ et al. Modulation of the cytokine and acute-phase response to major surgery by recombinant interleukin-2. Br J Surg 1995;82:86-90.
111. Pizzini RP et al. Dietary nucleotides reverse malnutrition and starvation-induced immunosuppression. Arch Surg 1990;125:86-90.
112. Watzl B, Watson RR. Role of alcohol abuse in nutritional immunosuppression. J Nutr 1991;110:311-317.
113. Leonard TK, Mohs ME, Watson RR. The cardiovascular effects of alcohol. I. In: Watson RR, ed. Nutrition and heart disease. Boca Raton:CRC Press;1987:19-47.
114. Mohs ME, Watson RR. Ethanol induced malnutrition, a potential cause of immunosuppression during AIDS. Prog Clin Biol Res 1990;325:433-444.
115. Redl H, Schlag G. Biochemical analysis in posttraumatic and postoperative organ failure. Prog Clin Biol Res: Second Vienna Shock Forum 1989;308:649-672.
116. Hoyt NJ. Host defense mechanisms and compromises in the trauma patient. Crit Care Nurs Clin North Am 1989;1:753-766.
117. Goya T, Morisaki T, Torisu M. Immunologic assessment of host defense impairment in patients with septic multiple organ failure: Relationship between complement activation and changes in neutrophil function. Surgery 1994;115:145-155.
118. Dahn MS et al. Altered T-lymphocyte subsets in severe sepsis. Am Surg 1988;54:450-455.

119. Chachoua A et al. Prognostic factors and staging classification of patients with epidemic Kaposi's sarcoma. J Clin Oncol 1989;7:774-780.
120. Tinkoff G et al. Cirrhosis in the trauma victim. Effect on mortality rates. Ann Surg 1990;211:172-177.
121. Pimpl W et al. Incidence of septic and thromboembolic-related deaths after splenectomy in adults. Br J Surg 1989;76:517-521.
122. Shaw JHF, Print CG. Postsplenectomy sepsis. Br J Surg 1989;76:1074-1081.
123. Styrt B. Infection associated with asplenia: Risks, mechanisms, and prevention. Am J Med 1990;88(5):33n-42n.
124. Steward M, Male D. Immunological techniques. In: Roitt I, Brostoff J, Male D, eds. Immunology. 3rd ed. London: Mosby; 1993:25.1-25.16.
125. Pacher R, Redl H, Woloszczuk W. Plasma levels of granulocyte elastase and neopterin in patients with MOF. Prog Clin Biol Res: Second Vienna Shock Forum 1989;308:683-688.
126. Pacher R et al. Relationship between neopterin and granulocyte elastase plasma levels and the severity of multiple organ failure. Crit Care Med 1989;17:221-226.
127. Jochum M et al. Posttraumatic plasma levels of mediators of organ failure. Prog Clin Biol Res: Second Vienna Shock Forum 1989;308:673-681.
128. Martich GD et al. Relation of serum neopterin to the hemodynamic and cytokine response following intravenous endotoxin administration to normal humans [abstract]. Crit Care Med 1991;19(4 suppl):S14.
129. Spitzer JA et al. Receptor changes in endotoxemia. Prog Clin Biol Res: Perspectives in Shock Research 1989; 299:95-106.
130. Barnetson R, Gawkrodger D. Hypersensitivity-Type IV. In: Roitt I, Brostoff J, Male D, eds. Immunology. 3rd ed. London: Mosby;1993:22.1-22.12.
131. Chapel H, Haeney M. Techniques in clinical immunology. In: Chapel H, Haeney M, eds. Essentials of clinical immunology. 3rd ed. London: Blackwell Scientific Publications; 1993:302-327.
132. Meakins JL et al. Delayed hypersensitivity and neutrophil chemotaxis. Effect of trauma. J Trauma 1978;18:240-247.
133. Christou NV et al. Estimating mortality risk in preoperative patients using immunologic, nutritional, and acute-phase response variables. Ann Surg 1989;210:69-77.
134. Nuytinck HKS et al. Whole-body inflammation in trauma patients. Arch Surg 1988;123: 1519-1524.
135. Nerlich ML. The trigger for posttraumatic multiple organ failure: Surgical sepsis or inflammation? Prog Clin Biol Res: Second Vienna Shock Forum 1989;308:413-417.
136. Parrillo JE. Pathogenetic mechanisms of septic shock. N Engl J Med 1993;328:1471-1477.

CHAPTER 3

The Systemic Inflammatory Response Syndrome: Role of Inflammatory Mediators in Multiple Organ Dysfunction Syndrome

Virginia Huddleston Secor

From the initial discussions by Baue[1] and others[2,3] in the midseventies up through more recent research on the multiple organ dysfunction syndrome (MODS), investigators in both basic science and clinical research have attempted to delineate a common thread running through patients presenting with and succumbing to MODS. While shock, hypoperfusion, endotoxemia, and sepsis are common denominators in the development of organ dysfunction, recent research increasingly points to overwhelming inflammatory activity as a primary underlying mechanism resulting in organ dysfunction and failure distant to the initial site of insult.[4-9]

The discussion in this chapter presents an overview of the systemic inflammatory response syndrome (SIRS) and the physiologic and pathophysiologic roles of the major inflammatory mediators of sepsis, SIRS, and MODS. The mediators discussed are not limited to soluble substances in the circulation, but include structures such as the endothelium, cells such as white blood cells (WBCs) and platelets, and biochemical substances such as toxic oxygen metabolites. As Baue[10] states, "The mediators of inflammatory responses are numerous, fascinating, complex, and incompletely understood. . . . The biologic purpose of these cells and activities is sound: they are necessary for mounting an inflammatory response, for healing, and for survival. However, they may also run wild, becoming toxic to other cells." Although presented here in isolation for purposes of discussion, in the critically ill patient, these mediators are continuously affected by interactions among themselves, with the physiologic environment, and with treatment regimens. Failure of host defense homeostasis is related not only to overwhelming activation but to loss of inhibitory pathways as well.[11] Appendix A provides a quick reference of the major mediators.

SYSTEMIC INFLAMMATORY RESPONSE SYNDROME
Definition

The definitions of syndromes such as septic shock, disseminated intravascular coagulation (DIC), and MODS, along with their diagnostic criteria and recommended therapies, are widely disparate in both the literature and clinical practice. To address this problem, the American College of Chest Physicians and the Society of Critical Care Medicine met at a 1991 consensus conference to standardize the terminology and diagnostic criteria used in evaluating patients with systemic responses to sepsis and trauma. The primary focus of this conference was the systemic inflammatory response.[12-14]

SIRS is defined as the systemic inflammatory response to a severe clinical insult, including tissue trauma, ischemia, infection, and shock. The response is manifested by alterations in body temperature (higher than 38° C or lower than 36° C), tachycardia (more than 90 beats/minute), tachypnea or hyperventilation (respiratory rate greater than 20 breaths/minute or partial arterial pressure of carbon dioxide [$PaCO_2$] less than 32 torr), and changes in WBC count (WBC count greater than 12,000 cells/mm³ or less than 4000 cells/mm³ or greater than 10% immature [band] forms).[12,13] In the past, the term *sepsis* was used in relation to the systemic response arising from infection. What has become apparent more recently is that this same clinical response can be seen in the *absence of infection* in such conditions as multiple trauma, shock, and pancreatitis[15,16] (Fig. 3-1). Even on autopsy, an infectious focus is often not found, although the clinical presentation before death is almost identical to that seen with sepsis and septic shock.[17,18] Because of this confusion in terminology and clinical presentation, the consensus conference also set forth standardized definitions (see the box on p. 5 in Chapter 1).

Pathophysiology of SIRS

As described in Chapter 2, localized inflammation is a physiologic, protective response involving the mechanisms of vasodilatation, increased microvascular permeability, cellular activation and adhesion, and coagulation. However, this response must be tightly controlled by the body at the local site of injury or the response becomes overly activated, leading to an exaggerated, systemic response in each of these four mechanisms.[6,15,19,20]

Exaggerated mechanisms of inflammation in SIRS. Although vasodilatation in the local area increases nutrient delivery, uncontrolled systemic vasodilatation leads to decreased systemic vascular resistance and hypotension, which is often refractory to fluid therapy. The increased microvascular per-

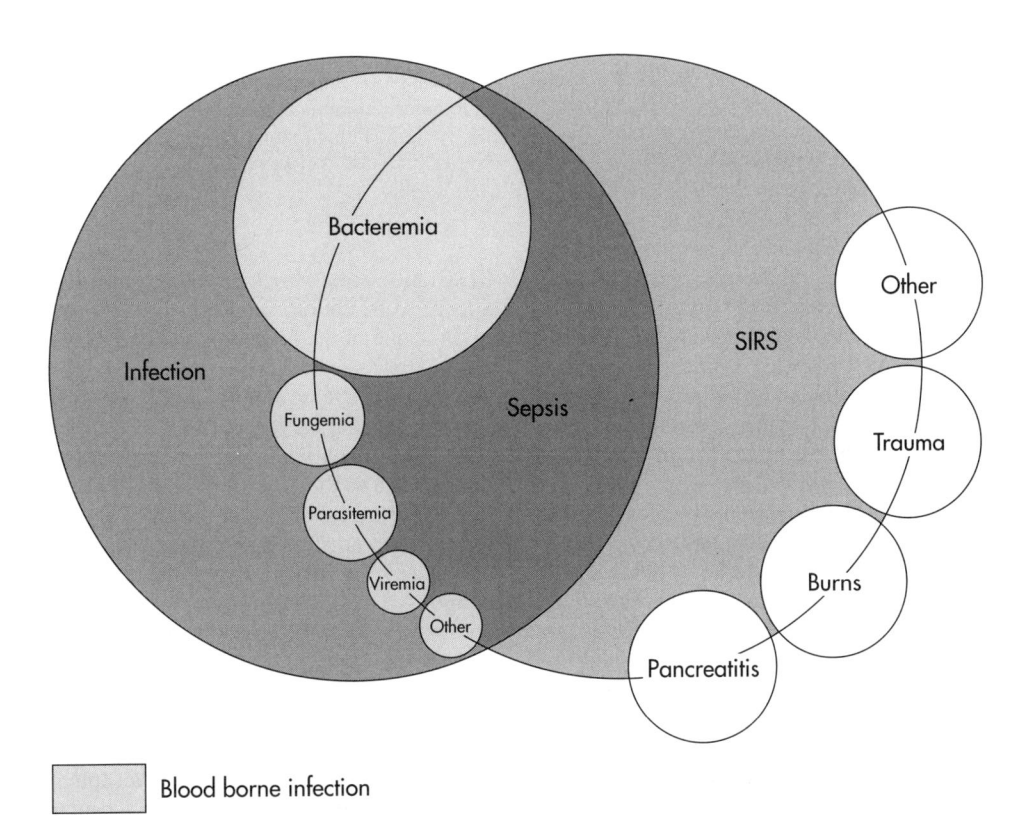

Fig. 3-1 Interrelationships among the systemic inflammatory response syndrome (SIRS), sepsis, and infection. (From American College of Chest Physicians/Society of Critical Care Medicine Consensus Conference Committee. Definitions for sepsis and organ failure and guidelines for the use of innovative therapies in sepsis. Crit Care Med 1992;20:865.)

meability can also be destructive at the systemic level. Instead of localized edema occurring only at the site of injury, generalized peripheral edema is often present. The leaky vasculature makes it difficult to volume resuscitate these patients adequately because they third-space so much of their volume into the extravascular space. Although not as clinically observable, the increased microvascular permeability also leads to edema in the organ beds, which can negatively affect organ function and hinder intraorgan blood flow.

Overwhelming cellular activation and adhesion leads to increased cellular aggregation, vascular obstruction, tissue infiltration, and excessive mediator production, all of which perpetuate the response. In disease states, such as the adult respiratory distress syndrome (ARDS) and MODS, large numbers of WBCs adhere to the vessel wall and can obstruct the microcirculation. This is thought to be at least partially related to an increase in the number of adhesion molecules present on the endothelium[21-23] (Fig. 3-2). Tumor necrosis factor (TNF), interleukin-1 (IL-1), and other mediators have been shown to trigger the endothelium to produce an increased number of adhesion molecules.[23,24] In addition to the blockage, the active WBCs are producing their toxic mediators that can then damage the surrounding tissue and vasculature, especially if the WBCs are tightly adhered to the endothelium.[25,26] The endothelium is fragile and susceptible to damage. An uncontrolled response hinders the anticoagulant properties of the endothelium and predisposes the damaged area to a procoagulant state, the development of excessive microthrombi, and further obstruction of blood flow.

Contributing to the production of excessive microthrombi is the accelerated coagulation occurring secondary to overwhelming endothelial damage and the interaction between inflammation and coagulation. Remember, as one cascade is activated, it in turn activates the other. Thus excessive inflammation usually triggers excessive coagulation because of the interplay between many of the mediators common to both pathways.[27,28] Acquired coagulopathies such as DIC often develop, further contributing to the multiple complications critically ill patients experience.[20,29]

Role of the septic triad: endotoxin, TNF, and IL-1. Although a multitude of mediators operate in

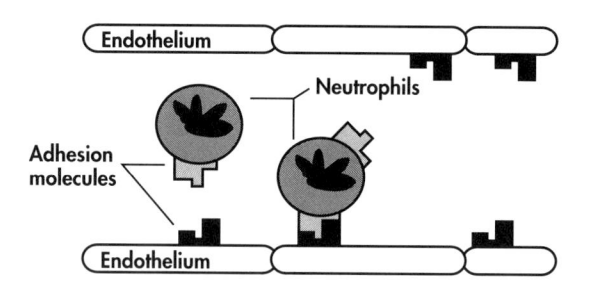

Fig. 3-2 Schematic representation of adhesion between the endothelium and neutrophils. Adhesion molecules present on both the neutrophil and endothelial cell are necessary for adhesion and emigration of the neutrophil from the blood into the tissues. (From Secor VH. The inflammatory/immune response in critical illness: Role of the systemic inflammatory response syndrome. Crit Care Nurs Clin North Am 1994;6:256.)

SIRS and septic shock, the three most influential appear to be endotoxin, TNF, and IL-1.[30-32] Endotoxin is one of the most powerful triggers of the inflammatory response, often causing the response to progress to the systemic level. Endotoxin is a lipopolysaccharide present in the outer membrane of all gram-negative organisms, and it is shed from the bacteria as they multiply or die.[33] Once thought to exert direct damage at multiple sites, much of the damage attributed to endotoxin is most likely related to its ability to trigger the plasma cascades, phagocytic cells, and inflammatory mediator production. Endotoxin is a potent activator of the complement cascade and coagulation, which further contribute to the increased microvascular permeability, vasodilatation, and microthrombi common in septic patients.[33-35] The endotoxin-activated phagocytic cells, particularly macrophages, produce potent inflammatory mediators such as TNF and IL-1 that then carry out much of the direct damage by inducing a procoagulant state, causing endothelial damage, and inciting metabolic abnormalities.[32-36] The specific roles of TNF and IL-1 are discussed later in this chapter.

Pathophysiologic sequelae of SIRS. Systemic activation of inflammation and coagulation is self-perpetuating and often extremely difficult to slow or halt once the responses become widespread. Systemic activation of these two processes can be a major contributor to the development and progression of secondary complications common in critical illness. Sir William Osler said, "Patients die not of their disease. They die of the physiological abnormalities of their disease."[37] In the last several years, it has become increasingly apparent that secondary complications are a major contributor to death in the intensive care unit (ICU) and that SIRS is a major etiologic factor in the development of DIC, ARDS, septic shock, and MODS, especially if a second insult, such as shock, infection, or ischemia follows the initial injury (Fig. 3-3).

The potentially destructive changes occurring in SIRS (increased peripheral vasodilatation, excessive microvascular permeability, and accelerated microvascular clotting) contribute to the development of profound pathophysiologic changes in the body (Table 3-1). These changes are associated with a maldistribution in circulating volume, an imbalance of oxygen supply and demand, and alterations in metabolism.[29,38] If these major pathophysiologic events are not reversed or slowed, inadequate oxygen utilization and multiple organ dysfunction and failure often ensue. Therefore knowledge of the mediators and cells involved in SIRS is necessary to more effectively assess, manage, and develop new strategies for the patients suffering from SIRS, MODS, and other complications of critical illness. The endothelium is a major site of damage and propagation of SIRS because of its interaction with these cells and mediators.

ENDOTHELIUM
Physiologic role

Once thought to function solely as an inert barrier between the fluid phase of blood and the solid phase of tissue, the endothelial layer is now recognized as a dynamic, metabolic site.[28,39] The endothelium is a unicellular layer of specialized cells that lines the entire vascular system from the aorta, arteries, and capillary beds, through the venules and veins, and back through the vena cava to the heart.

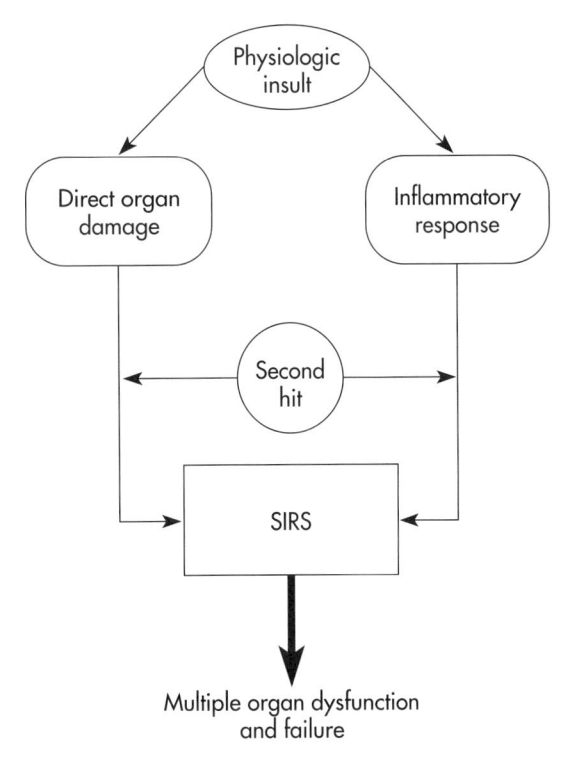

Fig. 3-3 Relationship between initial insult, second hit, and SIRS. The initial insult can cause direct organ damage and triggering of the inflammatory response. If the response is not controlled, the SIRS can occur, particularly if a second hit, such as infection or shock is present. (From Secor VH. The inflammatory/immune response in critical illness: Role of the systemic inflammatory response syndrome. Crit Care Nurs Clin North Am 1994; 6:259.)

In major vessels, the endothelium overlays the subendothelial structures of collagen, smooth muscle fibers, and elastic tissue; however, in the capillary bed, only the endothelium remains (Fig. 3-4). The endothelial cells are surrounded by a basement membrane on the tissue side of the vessel.

The endothelial cells approximate at sites known as intercellular clefts or junctions. In response to mediators such as complement, histamine, and kinin, endothelial cells retract and the junctions widen, leading to the increased capillary permeability and edema commonly seen in inflammation.[31,40] These widened junctions allow for the

Table 3-1 Pathophysiologic Derangements with Associated Mediators and Contributing Factors

Derangement	Mediators/factors	
Systemic vasodilatation	Bradykinin Complement Endorphins Histamine	Nitric oxide Prostaglandins Serotonin Tumor necrosis factor
Microvascular permeability	Arachidonic acid metabolites Bradykinin Complement Histamine	Leukotrienes Platelet activating factor Toxic oxygen metabolites Tumor necrosis factor
Coagulation/microvascular thrombi	Arachidonic acid metabolites Endothelial damage Endotoxin Hageman factor Interleukins	Platelet aggregation Tissue factor Tissue trauma Toxic oxygen metabolites Tumor necrosis factor WBC aggregation
Selective vasoconstriction	Arachidonic acid metabolites Catecholamines Endothelins	Hypoxia (lungs) Platelet activating factor Renin/angiotensin system Serotonin
Endothelial damage	Acidosis Complement Endotoxin Histamine Hypoxia Immune complexes	Interleukins Lysosomal enzymes Platelet aggregation Toxic oxygen metabolites Tumor necrosis factor WBC aggregation
Myocardial depression	Acidosis Complement Endorphins Endotoxin Impaired adrenergic responsiveness	Ischemia Myocardial depressant factor Nitric oxide Tumor necrosis factor
Excessive cellular activity	Arachidonic acid metabolites Cell debris Complement Kinins	Interleukins Platelet activating factor Platelets Proteases Tumor necrosis factor

Modified from Huddleston VB. Multisystem organ failure: A pathophysiologic approach, 1990:12.

egress of nutrients and other large proteins such as antibodies, complement factors, and kinins.

The endothelium serves many purposes in addition to its barrier function between blood and tissue (see the box on p. 51). It produces potent vasoactive substances, such as nitric oxide and endothelin, whose production is thought to be altered in sepsis, SIRS, and MODS. One of the most important functions of the endothelium is to keep the blood fluid, and thus it has many anticoagulant properties.[41] Therefore, if the function and integrity of the endothelium are disrupted, the hemostatic balance may be severely impaired. Procoagulant activity results, leading to thrombin formation and fibrin de-

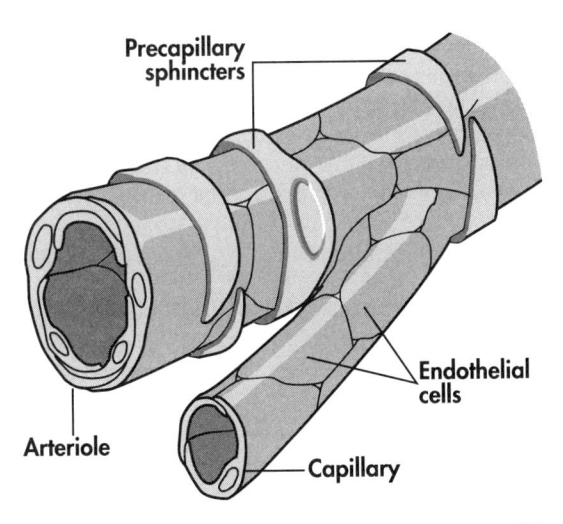

Fig. 3-4 Endothelial anatomy. (From Thibodeau GA, ed. Structure and function of the body. 9th ed. St. Louis: Mosby, 1992.)

FUNCTIONS OF THE ENDOTHELIUM

Anticoagulation via maintenance of smooth, nonadherent lining, formation of t-PA, generation of prostacyclin, and generation of other activators and inhibitors of platelet aggregation, coagulation, and fibrinolysis

Vasoregulation through its production of nitric oxide, endothelin, and other relaxing and constricting factors

Hydrolysis (inactivation) of vasoactive peptides such as bradykinin, angiotensin, and serotonin

Synthesis and release of growth factors

Endocytosis of small particles, including immune complexes, endotoxin, and bacteria

Antigen processing and presentation (uncommon)

Modulation of carbohydrate and lipid metabolism via receptors for insulin, low-density lipoproteins, very low-density lipoproteins, and lipoprotein lipase

Synthesis and release of mediators: nitric oxide, endothelins, arachidonic acid metabolites, and tissue factor (when injured)

---

t-PA, Tissue plasminogen activator.

---

position.[42,43] The role of the endothelium in the homeostasis of coagulation includes the following:

1. Maintenance of a smooth, continuous blood vessel lining to prevent adherence of platelets to subendothelial structures
2. Generation of prostacyclin (metabolite of arachidonic acid), a vasodilatory, antiplatelet aggregator
3. Synthesis and release of tissue plasminogen activator (t-PA) to promote clot breakdown
4. Synthesis and release of antithrombin III and thrombomodulin, both of which are inhibitors of the procoagulant activity of thrombin

Unfortunately, many mediators and clinical conditions commonly seen in the critically ill patient damage the endothelium (see the box on p. 52). Its extensive surface area, susceptibility to injury, and metabolic functions make it a key focus of research in sepsis, DIC, ARDS, and MODS.[43-45]

Impact on MODS process

Although the endothelium has the potential to repair itself and maintain normal function, extensive damage overwhelms the repair mechanisms of the endothelium, resulting in widespread permeability and coagulation abnormalities.[27,46,47] If the endothelial damage is severe, the increased capillary permeability can become systemic, accompanied by large fluid losses to the tissues and organs. As tissues continue to swell, vascular flow is further obstructed, and tissue ischemia worsens. Proteins and other plasma elements lost to the tissue cause tissue damage, osmotic derangements, and lymph drainage system overload. The fluid loss can precipitate hemoconcentration in the local microvasculature, leading to increased plasma viscosity and red blood cell aggregation.[48]

As the endothelium suffers damage to its anticoagulant mechanisms, coagulation becomes accelerated and large amounts of fibrin may be deposited in the vasculature, further obstructing flow and potentiating ischemia, especially in the microvasculature. Damaged endothelium has actually been shown to express tissue factor, a potent activator of the extrinsic pathway of coagulation. This may actually be the most procoagulant stimulus for the initiation of DIC.[28,42-44]

Endothelial damage also hinders other endothelial metabolic and receptor functions, leading to vasomotor abnormalities and decreased detoxification

> **FACTORS IMPAIRING ENDOTHELIAL INTEGRITY AND FUNCTION**
>
> Mechanical disruption
> Microorganisms and their toxins
> Immune complexes
> Shock, hypoxemia, and acidosis
> Platelet aggregation leading to microthrombi and decreased nutrition
> Neutrophil aggregation leading to mechanical obstruction and toxic mediator release
> Coagulation on the endothelial surface
> Direct action of mediators such as TNF and IL-1

IL-1, Interleukin-1; *TNF*, tumor necrosis factor.

of vasoactive substances, such as bradykinin, angiotensin, and serotonin.[49,50] Damage to the endothelium further stimulates the inflammatory/immune response (IIR), making it central to the self-propagation of the vicious cycle culminating in MODS.[42-44] In conclusion, the endothelium converts from an anticoagulant/antiinflammatory site to a procoagulant/proinflammatory site. This conversion results in focal microvascular thrombosis and leukocyte-mediated endothelial injury.[51]

NITRIC OXIDE
Physiologic role

Nitric oxide is a biochemical molecule synthesized from the amino acid, L-arginine, by the actions of enzymes known as nitric oxide synthases. Although it is a ubiquitous molecule that carries out more functions than virtually any other known messenger molecule,[52] its importance in physiologic and pathophysiologic processes in the body has only become apparent over the last decade. In 1992 it was named "Molecule of the Year" by the American Association for the Advancement of Science.[52,53]

Nitric oxide is produced constitutively (under resting conditions) in endothelial cells, certain neurons, endocardium, myocardium, and platelets and acts as a physiologic messenger in intercellular and intracellular communication. Its physiologic activity includes signalling in the central nervous system, maintenance of vascular tone and organ blood flow, and enhancement of inflammatory/immune activity.[53,54] Nitric oxide production can also be induced in numerous cells following their exposure to endotoxin, cytokines, and other mediators. Inducible nitric oxide production has been shown to occur in vascular endothelial and smooth muscle cells, macrophages, neutrophils, cardiac cells (myocytes and endocardium), hepatic cells (hepatocytes and Kupffer cells), and numerous other fixed tissue macrophages and organ tissues.[52,53]

In 1980 Furchgott and Zawadzki[55] demonstrated that the endothelium had to be present for certain vasodilator substances to cause vascular relaxation and reported the presence of an endothelium-derived relaxation factor (EDRF).[55] Over the next 8 to 10 years, several groups of investigators reported that EDRF was nitric oxide or a closely related molecule.[56,57] During the same time period, other studies were beginning to show that macrophage cytotoxicity also involved the conversion of arginine to nitrates or nitrites.[58] Nitric oxide has been shown to participate in the antimicrobial activities of neutrophils and macrophages, although the exact mechanisms have not been defined.[54,59] Thus a picture began to emerge of nitric oxide as a principal molecule in vascular and inflammatory functions, whose activities extended throughout the body. It has also become apparent that nitric oxide exhibits both protective and pathologic roles, particularly in shock and cardiovascular disease.[60]

Role in injury

The dual role of nitric oxide as a mediator of both inflammation and cardiovascular responses could be the link between sepsis or SIRS and the dramatic cardiovascular responses occurring in these clinical states. The cytokines TNF and IL-1 increase the production of nitric oxide and cause nitric oxide–mediated vasodilatation and decreased responsiveness to catecholamines and other vasoconstrictor agents in animal models.[60-62] Other mediators have also been shown to affect or be affected by the production of nitric oxide, including platelet-activating factor, toxic oxygen metabolites, and glucocorticoids.[54,59]

Nitric oxide is also thought to cause or amplify the following: myocardial depression; hepatic, pancreatic, and neurologic dysfunction; endothelial damage and increased vascular permeability; and the mitochondrial dysfunction and defective cellular respiration that occur in sepsis and SIRS.[39,52,53,60]

The numerous effects of nitric oxide, both protective and pathologic, and the fact that the constitutive and inducible forms may have different mechanisms of action make it difficult to isolate and treat the syndromes in which this multifaceted molecule is thought to play a role. Inhibition of nitric oxide production has shown varying results in studies of sepsis.[63] Researchers have actually taken advantage of the vasodilatory effects of nitric oxide by administering it to patients with ARDS, where it is thought to improve ventilation/perfusion matching by relaxing vasoconstricted pulmonary vessels.[64] Nitric oxide continues to be a major focus of study for researchers in many different fields, and understanding its mechanisms of action and interactions with other mediators such as endothelin holds promise for future treatment modalities.

ENDOTHELIN
Physiologic role

In many areas of physiologic activity, mediators with antagonistic actions work together to achieve a "balanced effect." The endothelium generates contracting factors, which act in opposition to the relaxation factors such as nitric oxide as discussed in the previous section. One of the most important contracting factors generated by the endothelium is endothelin-1, which was first reported by Yanagisawa and co-workers in 1988.[65] Endothelins are peptides that trigger powerful vasoconstriction and growth responses, and endothelin-1 is the main endothelin produced by the endothelium. The endothelins are released in response to hypoxia, angiotensin II, vasopressin, norepinephrine, bradykinin, and transforming growth factor-beta.[39]

Role in injury

Elevated values of endothelin have been noted in patients with sepsis, burns, and DIC.[66-70] Whether the endothelin release is triggered as part of a specific response or whether it leaks from the damaged endothelium is still under investigation.[39] The release of endothelin is thought to be partially dependent on TNF and IL-1 activity, which once again links these two inflammatory cytokines to much of the pathophysiology of sepsis and organ failure.[71] The organ beds, particularly the renal vasculature, appear to be a selective target of endothelin-1 activity.[72] Therefore endothelin could be a mediator of the selective vasoconstriction that occurs in many of the organ beds during the septic and inflammatory processes.

PLASMA CASCADES: COMPLEMENT
Physiologic role

The complement cascade is a triggered enzyme system consisting of a complex series of approximately 20 circulating proteins operating in cascade fashion and 5 regulatory membrane-bound proteins (Fig. 3-5). Although initially described over 100 years ago, the complement cascade is still being widely studied. Its primary role is to amplify the IIR, primarily in bacterial infections. The peptides splitting from the inactive "parent" molecules are biologically active, with C3a and C5a (also known as anaphylatoxins) being the best described. C3 is the major protein of the cascade.[73,74]

The major physiologic function of complement is to initiate, enhance, or "complement" the inflammatory response. Activities include (1) induction of inflammation, (2) opsonization of foreign particles, (3) cellular activation of phagocytic cells (neutrophils, monocytes/macrophages), and (4) direct lysis of target cells.[51,73]

Induction of inflammation primarily results from the action of the anaphylatoxins. Not only do anaphylatoxins increase capillary permeability and vasodilatation directly, but they cause the degranulation of mast cells and basophils, which leads to the release of histamine and other proinflammatory mediators that also increase vasodilatation, capillary permeability, and phagocytic activation.

Opsonization facilitates phagocytosis through the deposition (coating or binding) of opsonins such as antibodies or C3b onto the antigen. The presence of opsonin on the antigen enhances binding with phagocytic cells such as neutrophils, monocytes/macrophages, natural killer (NK) cells, and antigen-presenting cells, all of which have receptors for the C3b or the antibody (Fig. 3-6). Once bound, the phagocytes can engulf the microbe and kill it. Complement enhances the binding with these phagocytes.

Complement assists in the cellular activation of the phagocytic cells of the IIR. The cells must be drawn to the injury site (chemotaxis) and activated to kill (respiratory burst). A concentration gradient of complement or other chemotactic substances develops near the injury site, and WBCs move up the concentration gradient to the site of inflamma-

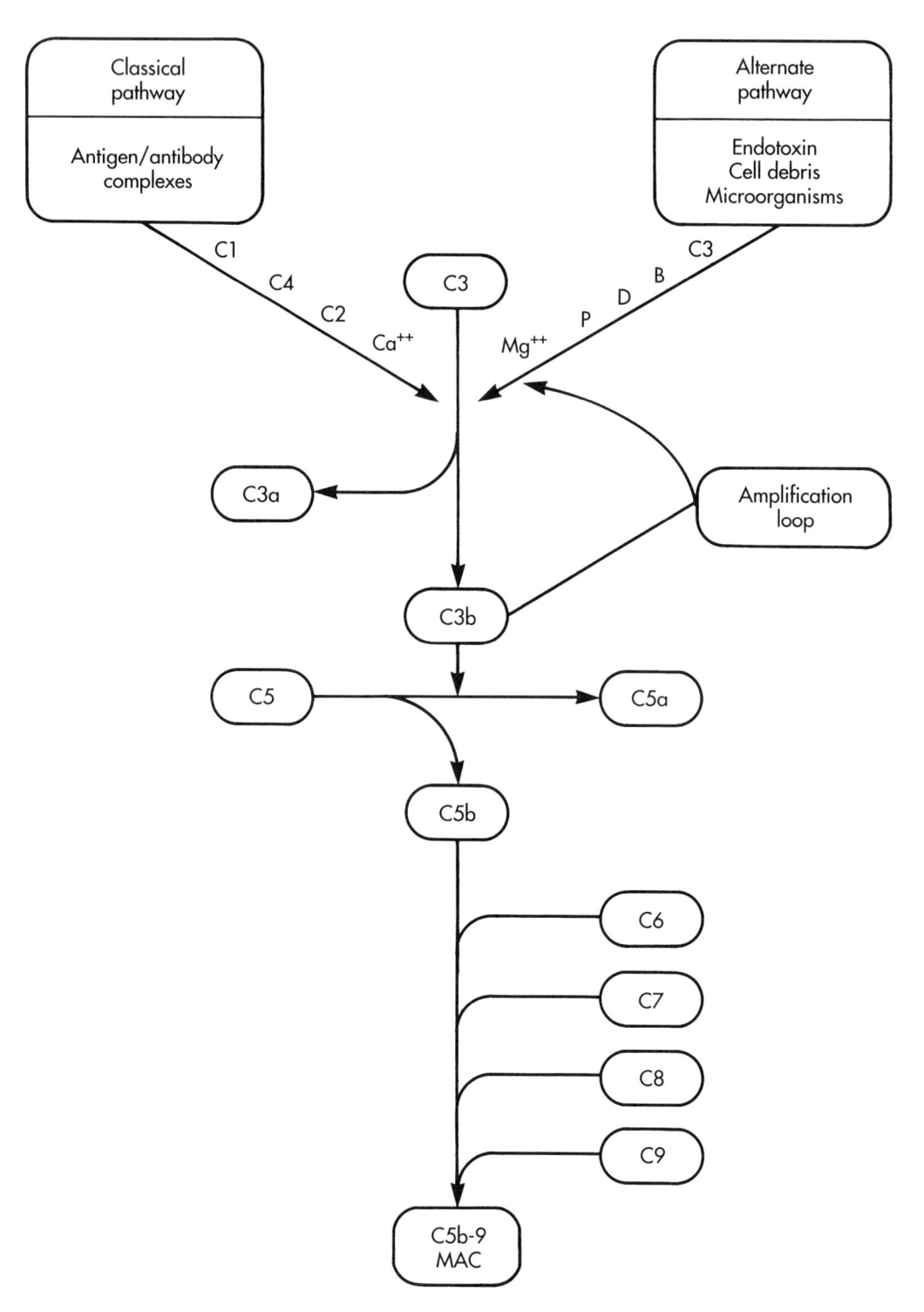

Fig. 3-5 Complement cascade. *MAC*, Membrane attack complex; *P*, properdin; *B*, Factor B; *D*, Factor D; *C*, complement. (Modified from Hood LE, Weissman IL, Wood WB, Wilson JH, eds. Immunology. 2nd edition. Menlo Park, CA: Benjamin/Cummings Publishing, 1984;343.)

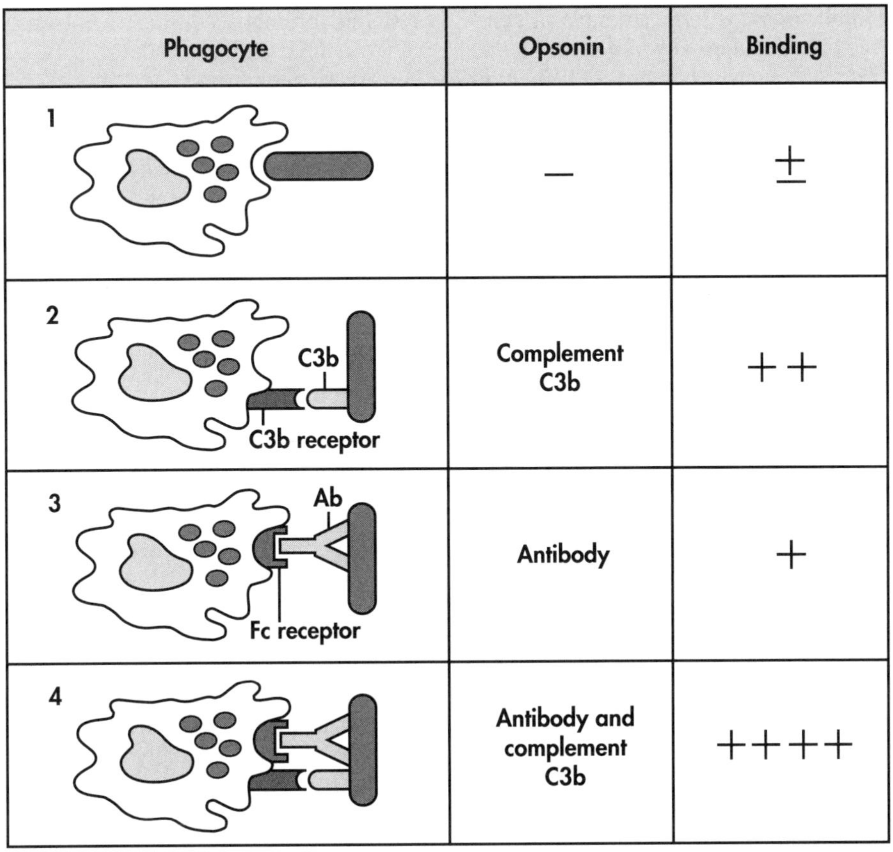

Phagocyte	Opsonin	Binding
1	—	±
2 C3b / C3b receptor	Complement C3b	++
3 Ab / Fc receptor	Antibody	+
4	Antibody and complement C3b	++++

Fig. 3-6 Opsonization of microorganisms. Opsonization may occur via binding with complement and/or antibody. (From Male D, Roitt I. Introduction to the immune system. In: Roitt I, Brostoff J, Male D, eds. Immunology. 3rd edition. London: Mosby, 1993;1.7.)

tion. Once the WBC is activated, it undergoes a respiratory burst and produces microbicidal mediators to use in combination with preformed mediators present within its granules and lysosomes to kill the invader. Degranulation of mast cells and basophils also occurs secondary to complement activation.

Target cell lysis occurs via the activity of the membrane attack complex (MAC), which is formed at the termination of the complement cascade. The MAC (C5b to C9) inserts into the membrane of the target cell leading to osmotic disequilibrium, cell lysis, and possibly increased arachidonic acid metabolism.[73] In this scenario, the pathogen is killed before phagocytosis occurs. Phagocytosis is still necessary to degrade and remove cell debris; therefore the ultimate destruction of bacteria requires synergistic action with phagocytic cells.

Although complement is a major pathway in the process of inflammation and the nonspecific immune response, its actions are enhanced by specific immune response activity. Complement has a high avidity for the immunoglobulins IgG and IgM, and the classic pathway of complement is triggered by antigen-antibody complexes formed during the specific immune response.[73]

Impact on MODS process

As with the other inflammatory mediators, the effects of complement serve a very protective function, but only if production is regulated and localized to the site of injury. If large amounts of complement are activated and escape into the systemic circulation, its action may become detrimental. Overwhelming vasodilatation, capillary permeability, and activation of phagocytic cells with their concomitant release of toxic by-products all serve to perpetuate the edema formation, cardiovascular instability, endothelial damage, clotting abnormalities, and other signs or symptoms seen in the MODS patient.[51,75-77] Elevated levels have been noted in victims of multiple trauma.[7]

Studies show that complement activation produces tissue and organ damage, especially in the lungs and vasculature.[78,79] Hemodynamic changes and perfusion abnormalities in the liver and kidneys are also related to complement activation.[80,81] The difficulty comes in trying to determine the point at which the system crosses the line of a protective response and begins to damage the host. Levels of circulating complement components can be assayed directly, or their functional capabilities can be determined.[82]

PLASMA CASCADES: COAGULATION & FIBRINOLYSIS
Physiologic role

Coagulation and fibrinolysis are dependent on numerous anticoagulant and procoagulant factors operating in dynamic equilibrium. If the exquisite balance between these two systems is disrupted, systemic thrombosis or gross hemorrhage could result, often presenting simultaneously in a patient as DIC.[83] As mentioned, activation of hemostatic mechanisms accompanies injury, localized inflammation, and damage to the endothelium. Hemostasis is necessary to prevent excessive blood loss and isolate the injured site. Like the IIR, hemostasis is protective only if it remains localized to the site of injury. When coagulation is not contained or regulated, systemic abnormalities and coagulopathies such as DIC can result. Chapter 4 presents a comprehensive discussion of DIC.

Impact on MODS process

The combined effects of stagnation of blood flow, tissue injury, and endothelial damage seen in shock, sepsis, and trauma may stimulate excessive coagulation. The close interrelationship between the IIR and coagulation potentiates the activation of both systems when either is stimulated. The enzymatic plasma cascades are tightly interwoven in their activities, both in their physiologic and pathophysiologic states. Hageman factor (factor XII) is a major link in this interdependency (Fig. 3-7). In the protective state this is very efficient because injury that requires hemostasis usually requires immune protection; however, in a poorly regulated situation, overwhelming inflammation, coagulation, and fibrinolysis can ensue and be constantly reactivated. Mediators then leave the confines of the local site of in-

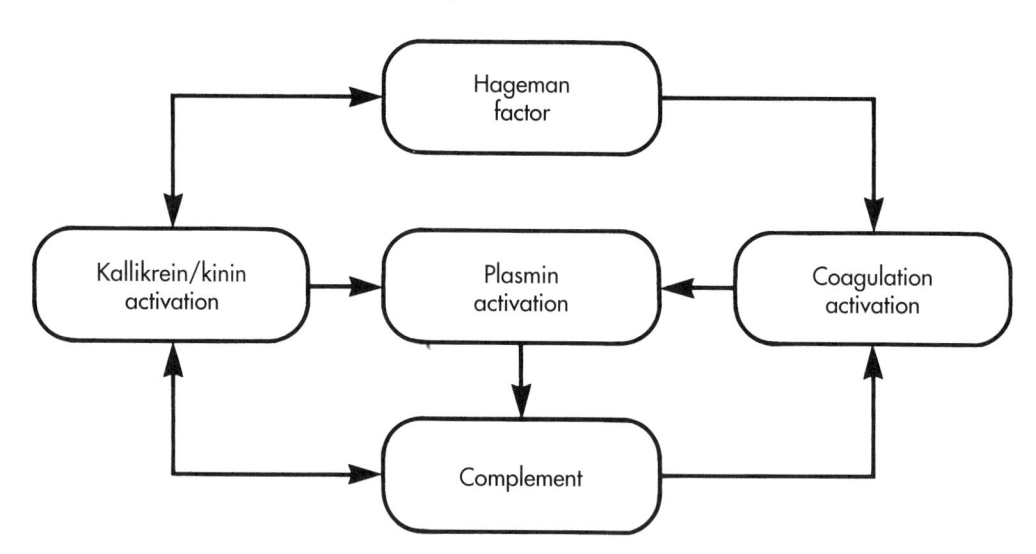

Fig. 3-7 Hageman factor as the link in the interlocking network of the plasma enzyme cascades.

jury and move to the systemic circulation, causing alterations in organs remote from the site of injury.

Clotting abnormalities greatly increase the incidence of vascular obstruction, tissue ischemia, and organ damage. While there are many stimuli that trigger the hemostatic mechanism, damage to the vascular endothelium is currently thought to be the primary mechanism that induces the intravascular procoagulant state.[27,42-44] Certain mediators (endotoxin, TNF, IL-1, immune complexes) can induce the generation of tissue factor on the cell surface of endothelial cells[42-44] and macrophages (cells not normally thrombogenic), thus providing another link between inflammation and thrombosis.[27,29,84,85]

PLASMA CASCADES: KALLIKREIN/KININ SYSTEM
Physiologic role

The kallikrein/kinin system is the fourth enzyme system of the interlocking plasma protein cascades. As mentioned above, these systems work together following an insult to initiate hemostasis, the inflammatory response, tissue repair, and host protection.[86] The role of the kallikrein/kinin system has not been fully delineated. One of the major metabolites, bradykinin, is a potent vasodilator and has been shown to increase capillary permeability in some tissue beds.[87] It is also thought to play a role in blood pressure regulation and renal blood flow.[88] The kinins have been shown to stimulate neutrophil chemotaxis, phagocytosis, and respiratory burst activity. Kinin release also increases bronchoconstriction and microvascular permeability.[89]

As mentioned earlier, Hageman factor provides the major link between the plasma enzyme cascades with its concomitant activation of the intrinsic coagulation cascade and kallikrein. Kallikrein then catalyzes the conversion of kininogen to kinin.[90] The kinins also indirectly activate complement,[86] further propagating the IIR.

Bradykinin has a very short half-life, so its presence and impact are inferred from the circulating levels of its precursors and activators. Previous research has implicated bradykinin in physiologic abnormalities seen in hemorrhagic shock, septic shock, endotoxemia, and tissue injury.[10]

Impact on MODS process

Severe infection is associated with increased activation of the kinin cascade.[91] As a potent vasodilator, bradykinin certainly potentiates problems of low systemic vascular resistance and hemodynamic instability seen in shock and MODS. Increased capillary permeability and neutrophil stimulation also exacerbate the damage that may occur in a nonspecific, uncontrolled inflammatory response. Tissue edema and leukocyte aggregation lead to vascular compression and obstruction, further tissue ischemia, and maldistribution of circulating volume. Because bradykinin plays a role in coagulation and fibrinolysis, alterations in its activity as seen in MODS have a potential impact on the development of microemboli and increased permeability.[86] Research has identified isoproterenol as a potential inhibitor of bradykinin-induced microvascular permeability.[87]

NEUTROPHILS
Physiologic role

The neutrophil is the major polymorphonuclear (PMN) granulocyte in the circulation. Along with eosinophils and basophils, the neutrophil differentiates from the hematopoietic stem cell in the bone marrow and matures through the myeloid lineage. Commonly referred to as PMNs, polymorphs, granulocytes, or polys, their primary function is surveillance and phagocytosis of debris and foreign pathogens. This may occur in the blood or after migration of the neutrophil into the tissue during the inflammatory response. Neutrophils are readily available, and have a short life-span and high phagocytic activity.[92] A significant number of neutrophils are also sequestered in the lungs, where they adhere (marginate) to the lining of the pulmonary vasculature.

Once injury has occurred, neutrophils are drawn to the site by various chemotactic factors (complement, arachidonic acid metabolites, kinins) and adhesion molecules; activated by numerous cytokines (TNF, IL-1), bacterial wall fragments, prostaglandins, and cell debris; and dedicated to phagocytize the pathogen or debris. Following activation, the neutrophil undergoes a respiratory burst and converts to oxidative metabolism. These oxygen-dependent reactions produce highly reactive oxygen species, collectively referred to as toxic oxygen metabolites (TOMs) or oxygen-derived free radicals (ODFR).[25]

These oxygen-dependent TOMs, along with the non–oxygen-dependent cytotoxic enzymes and substances (lysozyme, myeloperoxidase, lactoferrin) in the granules and lysosomes of the neutrophil, are then secreted into the phagolysosome where they carry out their microbicidal activity and breakdown of cellular debris.[93] During the process of phagocytosis and intracellular killing, the neutrophil also releases these microbicidal substances into the extracellular environment. While this increases the protective function and activity of the neutrophil, excessive activation and secretion may potentiate tissue damage and organ dysfunction.[25]

Impact on MODS process

Neutrophils are systemically activated after thermal injury and other traumatic events, and this activation is possibly mediated by complement or endotoxin.[92] Neutrophils are thought to play a pathophysiologic role in the development of systemic inflammation, and their activity has been shown to be up-regulated in SIRS.[94] Neutrophil aggregation caused by the up-regulation of adhesion molecules on the surface of the neutrophil and the endothelium can also cause direct vascular obstruction or endothelial damage and thrombosis, further contributing to tissue ischemia and inflammation.[21-24] At what point the activity of the neutrophil ceases to be protective and becomes damaging, and to what extent that damage occurs, is still a matter of great debate.[95] There is no question that mediators synthesized and released by activated neutrophils (see the box below) damage vascular endothelium and parenchymal tissue.

Much of the work done on neutrophil-related organ damage is found in the literature on ARDS.[96-100] While the neutrophil and its products are implicated in the pulmonary hypertension, abnormal lung mechanics (decreased compliance, increased resistance to air flow), and vascular permeability that are the hallmarks of ARDS, research has shown that ARDS can occur in the neutropenic patient as well.[101] However, other research has shown that the severity of damage is lessened if neutrophils are depleted.[102,103] This suggests that other factors working either independently or in concert with neutrophil activation and activity may be responsible for the pathogenesis of ARDS.[10]

Neutrophils provide a necessary element in the inflammation and protective actions of the nonspecific response, but if a persistent inflammatory focus (abscess, necrotic tissue, occult infection) or improper down-regulation is present, neutrophil aggregation, activity, and mediator release may contribute to organ damage and host demise.[7,104]

TOXIC OXYGEN METABOLITES
Physiologic role

Toxic oxygen metabolites (also known as oxygen-derived free radicals and reactive oxygen species) and their roles in homeostasis and pathogenesis of disease are presently an exciting and expanding area of both basic science and clinical research. TOMs are generated from numerous sources in the body: activated phagocytes, xanthine oxidase systems, mitochondrial respiration, and arachidonic acid pathways.[105] The primary TOMs are superoxide anion (O_2^-), hydrogen peroxide (H_2O_2), and the hydroxyl radical (OH^-). They may be formed at toxic levels during the respiratory burst of phagocytic cells and during postischemic reperfusion. The myocardial infarction (MI) patient and reperfusion injury,[106] the vascular patient and restoration of flow,[107] the coronary artery bypass graft patient post-pump,[108] mechanical ventilation and oxygen toxicity,[109] and ARDS and neutrophil activation,[25,109] all provide settings in which reactive oxygen species may develop and interact with surrounding tissue.

Two of the TOMs (superoxide anion and hydroxyl radical) are free radicals, and this is the term commonly used to identify them. A *radical* (all are "free" by definition) is an atom or group of atoms carrying an unpaired electron in the outer orbits.

SELECTED MEDIATORS GENERATED BY NEUTROPHILS

Interleukins
Leukotrienes
Lysozyme
Myeloperoxidase
Platelet activating factor
Proteases
Prostaglandins
Tissue factor (tissue thromboplastin)
Toxic oxygen metabolites (oxygen-derived free radicals)

They are normally produced during oxidative metabolism in small concentrations, and they are highly reactive and very unstable.[110,111] Although hydrogen peroxide is a TOM and is often referred to as a free radical, it is not a true free radical, because it does not have an unpaired electron in its outer orbit. Once produced, the free radicals do not travel far, and reactivity and toxicity vary with the particular species. The body has numerous enzyme systems (superoxide dismutase, catalase, and the glutathione redox system) and membrane antioxidants (vitamin E, beta-carotenes) to break them down further into nontoxic species, usually H_2O and O_2.[25,111,112]

Impact on MODS process

The increased presence of free radicals and other oxygen metabolites can cause significant damage to cell membranes of both vascular endothelial cells and tissue cells. TOMs can cause damage via three mechanisms: (1) damage to cell structure, (2) damage to cellular processes, or (3) damage to the genetic information and activity of the cell.[113] Lipid peroxidation occurs as TOMs react with polyunsaturated fatty acids in the cell membrane. This alters the fluidity, secretory function, and ionic gradients of the membrane.[10,114] Endothelial damage, increased capillary permeability, altered cell receptor function, and denaturation of protein may also occur, further stimulating the IIR.[10,112] If the endothelium is damaged, procoagulant factors may initiate the development of thrombi in the microcirculation.

The increased permeability, edema, and inflammation that accompany free radical damage may lead to vascular occlusion, either from edematous tissue compression or accelerated microthrombi formation. Tissue ischemia, extended infarcts, compartment syndrome, and loss of organ system integrity may all ensue. The "stunned" myocardium seen after the patient comes off bypass may also be related to production of TOMs in the revascularized myocardium.[108]

TOM production also increases during the respiratory burst of phagocytic cells. TOMs are useful for their bactericidal activity, but they may escape from the cell and cause damage to the surrounding tissue and vasculature. Because of the leukocytosis and margination of neutrophils and their increased production of TOMs when activated, it is highly plausible that TOMs are playing a definitive role in the organ damage that occurs in MODS.*

A patient experiencing a low-flow state (cardiopulmonary arrest, shock, cross-clamp placement) followed by resuscitation may also have increased production of TOMs, as the tissues are reperfused in the postresuscitation period. Assessment of edema, capillary refill, pulses, and skin temperature are necessary to assess adequacy of limb perfusion. Unfortunately, measuring regional perfusion in various vital organs is not possible at the bedside on a routine basis. Indirect measures such as urine output, level of consciousness, liver enzymes, and other laboratory values have to be used to assess adequacy of organ perfusion, although their sensitivity is less than desired.

PROTEOLYTIC ENZYMES
Physiologic role

Following activation, many phagocytic cells release proteolytic enzymes (proteases). The ability of the enzymes to digest bacteria and other foreign protein matter makes them a necessary part of the IIR and wound healing. Proteases also serve as enzymatic catalysts in the four enzyme cascades: complement, kallikrein/kinin, coagulation, and fibrinolysis.[25,117] Common proteases include collagenase, elastase, and cathepsins.

Impact on MODS process

Collagenase and elastase degrade the collagen and elastin found in blood vessels, leading to vascular damage and remodelling. Free radicals enhance the destructive capabilities of the proteases, because the free radicals damage enzymes, such as alpha$_1$-proteinase inhibitor, that normally inactivate the proteases.[25,117] Vascular permeability increases with resultant tissue edema.

The proteases attack not only vascular structures, but extracellular tissue matrix as well.[118,119] Direct parenchymal damage may be further inflicted on the organs (in addition to the existing ischemia and altered microvascular perfusion) by the proteases as they actually digest tissue walls.[25] Further inflammation is incited and the vicious cycle continues. One severe example of this concerns the premature activation of proteolytic enzymes in the pancreas, which are ultimately formed for digestion. Prema-

---

*References 25,109,111,115,116.

ture activation leads to extensive tissue damage in the body of the pancreas itself, setting up the intense IIR responses seen in pancreatitis (see Chapter 11).

It must be remembered that inflammation can occur without the presence of microorganisms.[120] Proteases play a significant role in this "aseptic inflammation" secondary to their tissue-damaging capabilities. Elastase also degrades and inactivates inhibitors of the clotting cascade, thereby allowing clotting to continue unabated. Increased levels of elastase have been found after trauma, surgery, and hemorrhage.[7,9,121]

MONONUCLEAR PHAGOCYTIC SYSTEM AND THE MACROPHAGE
Physiologic role

The mononuclear phagocytic system (formerly known as the reticuloendothelial system) is a network of phagocytic tissue macrophages including the resident macrophages of the liver, spleen, and bone marrow, as well as the more mobile tissue macrophages that are present in many organs and tissues throughout the body (Table 3-2). Other antigen-presenting cells (APC), such as follicular dendritic cells of the lymph nodes and spleen, Langerhans cells of the skin, and interdigitating cells of the thymus, are also included in the mononuclear phagocytic system.[93]

Many tissues are inhabited by resident macrophages that do not circulate. The different resident macrophages vary in their morphology and therefore are assigned specific names. The resident macrophages may be tissue-fixed, such as the microglia of the central nervous system (CNS); wandering, such as the alveolar macrophages of the lung; or fixed to endothelial cells such as the Kupffer cells of the liver.[122] During inflammation and infection, monocytes circulating in the blood adhere to the vascular endothelium and then migrate into injured tissues where they differentiate into the mature inflammatory macrophages, which are a major source of mediator release[123] (see the box below). Macrophages aid in ridding the injured site of foreign material, cell debris, and dying leukocytes, providing microdébridement in the wound, and also aid in wound granulation by producing locally acting growth factors.[124,125]

The major function of the monocytes and macrophages is the antigen processing and presentation that follows the nonspecific phagocytosis and removal of particulate and soluble antigen from the circulation, tissue, and body cavities. The antigens include bacteria, endotoxin, denatured protein, collagen, damaged red blood cells (RBCs), platelet aggregates, tissue debris, and other microaggregates.

Table 3-2 Tissue Macrophages and Other Antigen-Presenting Cells

Cell	Organ/anatomic site
Alveolar macrophages	Lungs
Splenic macrophages	Spleen
Monocytes	Blood
Synovial A cells	Synovia
Intraglomerular mesangial cells	Kidneys
Kupffer cells	Liver
Microglial cells	Brain
Langerhans cells	Skin
Interdigitating dendritic cells	Lymphoid tissue
Follicular dendritic cells	Lymphoid tissue
Follicular cells	Thyroid
Astrocytes	Brain
Endothelial cells	Vasculature
Fibroblasts	Connective tissue

Modified from Male D, Roitt I. Introduction to the immune system. In: Roitt I, Brostoff J, Male D, eds. Immunology, ed 3. London: Mosby; 1993:1.1-1.12.

SELECTED MEDIATORS GENERATED BY MACROPHAGES

Colony-stimulating factors
Complement proteins
Coagulation factors
Growth factors
Interferons
Interleukins
Leukotrienes
Lysozyme
Nitric oxide
Plasminogen activators
Platelet activating factor
Prostaglandins
Proteases
Toxic oxygen metabolites (oxygen-derived free radicals)
Tumor necrosis factor

The macrophage may engulf pure antigen or opsonized antigen. Phagocytosis is enhanced by opsonization because the macrophage has receptors on its cell surface for complement and antibodies.

Once the macrophage has phagocytized the antigen, the antigen is degraded (processed) into fragments that may then be presented to lymphocytes to induce their activation and proliferation. The macrophage releases IL-1, which activates T cells and surrounding macrophages. Although the macrophage can phagocytize antigen without previous T-cell activation and interaction, T-cell activation and mediator (IL-2, IFN-γ) release increase macrophage phagocytic capabilities. Thus the macrophages provide a major link between the nonspecific and specific immune responses.[93]

Macrophages are also involved in the generation and secretion of various inflammatory mediators (complement components, proteases, lysozyme) and cytokines (TNF, IL-1).[125] Each cytokine can have several functions, act on several different target tissues, or have functions that overlap with other cytokines. The cytokines are thought to play a central role in the problems associated with septic shock, DIC, and MODS, although alterations in activation or inhibition of phagocytosis and antigen processing and presentation can also have an impact on the process. Further information on the cytokines TNF and IL-1 is presented later in this chapter.

Impact on MODS process

Increased attention is being given to the macrophage and its role in the development and potentiation of MODS. Many of the mediators thought to play a central role in this syndrome are released by activated macrophages.[126,127] Although macrophage activation and phagocytic activity are necessary to prevent systemic invasion by bacteria and other foreign agents, extensive macrophage activation leads to increased release of potentially harmful mediators, such as TNF, IL-1, prostaglandins, and TOMs.[125,128]

Bacteria and their products can enter the circulation from numerous sources: wound abscesses, infection in remote organs (lungs, kidneys, bladder), or translocation from the gut. As the resident tissue macrophages (especially hepatic Kupffer cells) attempt to fight this pathogenic onslaught, they begin to release both preformed and newly synthesized mediators.[125,127,128] These mediators not only cause direct damage such as capillary permeability and vasodilatation, but also cause increased activation or degranulation of other cells. Mast cells, basophils, other macrophages, lymphocytes, and neutrophils then amplify the process with release of their own mediators.[11] A mushrooming effect occurs in which the system "feeds" off itself. Once a certain level of activation is reached, minimal stimulation is required from outside sources to keep the process active. In other words, even if the initial stimulus is treated by antibiotics, surgical débridement, or other appropriate treatment, the process may not be reversible. Accelerated coagulation, DIC, tissue ischemia, and organ damage continue unabated.[129] Like the endothelium, the macrophage can be triggered by cytokines to express tissue factor and thus promote a procoagulant state. Macrophages also decrease fibrinolytic activity, which furthers the procoagulant state.[44,127]

Macrophages play a major role in wound repair and defense, and the wound itself is a major source of macrophage accumulation, activation, and mediator release.[130] Macrophages are necessary for removal of tissue and bacterial debris, fibroblast and healing activities, and microdébridement.[125,128] Baue[10] even views the wound as an organ in itself, which calls upon the circulation, lungs, liver, and kidneys to support it. It communicates with the host and may make demands the host cannot keep, especially if the wound becomes infected. The septic wound "may initiate or activate processes that directly damage other organs,"[10] such as WBC aggregation and free radical release, complement activation, and immune complex formation. Research implicates the macrophage as a source of increased PGE_2 postinjury, which depresses antigen processing and presentation.[131]

TUMOR NECROSIS FACTOR
Physiologic role

Tumor necrosis factors are cytokines produced by macrophages, lymphocytes, and other IIR cells. Tumor necrosis factor-beta is produced by lymphocytes and is also known as lymphotoxin. Tumor necrosis factor-alpha (TNF-α) is the form produced primarily by activated macrophages, especially in response to endotoxin exposure. It is the form most dominant in sepsis, SIRS, and MODS and is the form referred to when the acronym TNF is used without an alpha or beta notation. Also known as cachectin, its isolation and characterization resulted from two distinct lines of investigation. One group of investigators was looking for the substance that caused hemorrhagic necrosis of tumors when the patient was also septic (TNF-α); the other group was looking for a substance that caused the wasting and cachexia commonly seen in patients with cancer or sepsis (cachectin). Beutler and coworkers purified the substance in 1985.[132]

While TNF-α is now considered to be the "major mediator of sepsis and MODS," it does serve physiologic functions in the normal IIR. It enhances the phagocytic and killing activity of both neutrophils and macrophages and may render tissue cells such as hepatocytes resistant to invasion, especially in parasitic infections.[30,36,133,134] TNF-α has also been shown to enhance lymphocyte activity and stimulate IL-1, platelet activating factor (PAF), and IFN-γ release from various cells involved in the immune response. Stress hormone production is also increased. TNF-α induces fever and stimulates collagenase production, which leads to the tissue remodelling necessary for growth and repair of injured tissue. Because TNF-α suppresses lipoprotein lipase activity, fat uptake and storage is decreased, and cachexia is a common result.[132]

Impact on MODS process

When the macrophage is activated by substances such as endotoxin, the macrophage releases TNF-α; TNF-α thus mediates many of the toxic effects of endotoxin.[36,133] The TNF-α not only affects local cells, but may enter the circulation and effect changes in distant organs and tissues not normally associated with a classic immune response* (Table 3-3). When isolated TNF-α is injected into noninfected laboratory animals, the animals exhibit many of the same signs and symptoms commonly found in sepsis and MODS, including hypotension, tachycardia, tachypnea, hyperglycemia, metabolic acidosis, fluid shifts, gastrointestinal (GI) ischemia, and alveolar thickening.[135-137] Therefore the endotoxin causes indirect damage by stimulating the macrophage to release TNF-α, which then causes the actual direct damage or, in turn, triggers the release of other toxic mediators. Direct activities of TNF-α that contribute to organ dysfunction include stimulation of TOM release from neutrophils, endothelial damage, decreased vascular responsiveness to catecholamines, severe anorexia, increased capillary permeability, and other signs listed above.[36,138]

The discovery of over 100 mediators in the blood of patients with MODS, many of which initially serve a protective function, makes it very difficult to understand the intricate relationship between the various factors and also to know which factors to treat and which to leave alone.[118,139,140] At this point, TNF-α appears to be one of the primary mediators in initiating organ dysfunction and damage, either alone or in concert with other mediators.[30,133,141] TNF-α is a proximal mediator that triggers the release of many other inflammatory mediators. It is one of the few mediators known to cause the entire spectrum of signs and symptoms associated with sepsis, SIRS, and MODS.[133,142] Pharmacologic agents that inhibit TNF-α synthesis or activity have been shown to attenuate some of these signs and symptoms or lower TNF-α levels in the serum.[143-146] Monoclonal antibodies to TNF-α and to TNF-α receptors are presently under investigation.[143,145,147-150]

INTERLEUKIN-1
Physiologic role

Interleukins (ILs) are another class of substances involved in signalling between (inter) cells of the immune response (leukocyte). They are numbered consecutively, and at the time of printing, 17 interleukins have been identified. IL-1β and IL-6 are the best known and documented in relation to MODS pathology and clinical presentation.[32,151,152] Like TNF, IL-1 has several forms. The dominant active form is IL-1β, which may be referred to as IL-1β or simply as IL-1. Many functions of IL-1β and TNF-α overlap. Like TNF-α, IL-1β serves many beneficial effects in the IIR, but it has also been implicated in organ damage and failure.[32,151]

Macrophages and blood monocytes are a major source of IL-1β, along with fibroblasts, NK cells, and damaged endothelium. The presence of thrombi or simple hemorrhage can also increase IL-1β release. IL-1β stimulates leukocytosis, fever, and metabolic changes. Additionally, it stimulates B-cell and T-cell activity and proliferation, activation of macrophage and NK cells, and stimulation of hematopoiesis.[153] Production of acute-phase reactants and an increase in adhesion of circulating WBCs to vascular endothelium is also seen.[32] IL-1β is necessary for fibroblast proliferation and wound

---
*References 30, 31, 36, 133, 135.

Table 3-3 Biologic Effects of Tumor Necrosis Factor (Abridged)

System	Effect
Nervous	Fever
	Hypothalamic-pituitary release of CRF and ACTH
	Anorexia
	Meningeal inflammation
Cardiovascular	Shock
	Myocardial suppression
	Capillary leakage syndrome
	Biosynthesis of nitric oxide
Pulmonary	Adult respiratory distress syndrome
	Edema
	Hypoxia
Gastrointestinal	Necrosis
	Biosynthesis of platelet activating factor
	Hepatic production of acute-phase proteins
	Diarrhea
Renal	Diuresis followed by oliguric renal failure
	Acute tubular necrosis
Hematopoietic	Suppressed erythropoiesis and increased RBC destruction
	Disseminated intravascular coagulation
	Neutrophilia or neutropenia
Endocrine	Euthyroid sick syndrome
	Lactic acidosis
	Hyperaminoacidemia
	Hyperglycemia, followed by hypoglycemia

From Tracey KJ, Cerami A. Tumor necrosis factor: An updated review of its biology. Crit Care Med 1993;21(10 suppl):S417.
ACTH, Adrenocorticotropic hormone; *CRF*, corticotropin-releasing factor; *RBC*, red blood cell.

healing and plays a key role in linking the immune response to the neuroendocrine system.[154-156]

Impact on MODS process

Increased cellular activation and release of IL-1β may lead to detrimental effects in the body. Isolated IL-1β inflicts cellular and tissue injury,[32] but more recent research focuses on its amplification of TNF-α activity and damage. Working in concert, TNF-α and IL-1β synergistically interact with numerous target cells and tissues.[153] Induction of procoagulant activity on the endothelium, decreased vascular responsiveness to catecholamines, and increased muscle proteolysis,[157,158] and negative nitrogen balance have all been associated with IL-1β activity.[32,151,152,159] Once known as endogenous pyrogen, IL-1β also induces fever, which may or may not be helpful depending on the clinical scenario. TNF-α and IL-1β may indirectly exacerbate vascular or tissue damage by causing increased adhesion of neutrophils to the endothelium.[151,152] Free radicals and proteases, which are byproducts of the respiratory burst and mediator release from the neutrophils, may then cause direct vascular or tissue damage.[25]

INTERLEUKIN-6
Physiologic role

Interleukin-6 (IL-6) is a cytokine produced by macrophages and other cells throughout the body, including those in the brain, pituitary gland, adrenal glands, ovaries, and testes. Tissue injury and the cytokines TNF-α and IL-1β are considered the most potent triggers of IL-6 production. IL-6 is thought to be a pivotal mediator in the acute-phase response. It also triggers the hypothalamic-pituitary-adrenal axis. Unlike many of the other mediators whose actions are primarily confined to the local area of release, IL-6 is thought to act in a more endocrine fashion and its activation leads to systemic effects.[142,160] Other activities of IL-6 include the promotion of B-cell and T-cell differentiation and proliferation and the inhibition of tumor growth.[161,162]

Impact on MODS process

Elevated levels of IL-6 have been noted in sepsis, trauma, and hemorrhage and have been associated with increased mortality.[8,161,163] Because the functions of IL-6 overlap those of TNF-α and IL-1β, isolating its effects in the pathophysiology of sepsis and SIRS is difficult. IL-6 interacting with these cytokines, as well as with other mediators, could potentially extend or accelerate the response and the sequelae associated with SIRS.[161] Recent research has shown that IL-6 acting synergistically with PAF primes neutrophils.[164] As described above, neutrophil activation sets into motion a cascade of events responsible for much of the pathology of sepsis, SIRS, and MODS.

ARACHIDONIC ACID METABOLITES
Physiologic role

Arachidonic acid (eicosatetraenoic acid) is a fatty acid present in the phospholipid of most cell membranes except those of RBCs. Following stimulation by cytokines, catecholamines, neuroendocrine responses, tissue injury, ischemia, hypoxia, or endotoxin, phospholipase A_2 hydrolytically cleaves or liberates arachidonic acid, which then enters the cyclooxygenase or lipoxygenase pathway within the cell[165,166] (Fig. 3-8). The resulting metabolites of these two pathways are collectively known as eicosanoids, and they participate in many biologic activities (see the box on p. 65). The major eicosanoid classes are the prostaglandins (PGs) and thromboxanes (TXs) from the cyclooxygenase pathway and the leukotrienes and lipoxins from the lipoxygenase pathway.[167-169] The eicosanoids function in provision and regulation of the inflammatory response and have also been implicated in regulation of renal blood flow, initiation of labor, fever, and shock.[170]

Many different eicosanoids are produced by the various tissues and have effects on virtually every tissue in the body.[171] Often the actions of different eicosanoids are antagonistic. PGI_2 (prostacyclin) causes vasodilatation and decreased platelet aggregation, while thromboxane causes vasoconstriction and increased platelet aggregation.[170] Their functions often overlap: PGE_1 and PGI_2 both cause vasodilatation; $PGF_{2\alpha}$ and TXA_2 both cause pulmonary hypertension. The specific eicosanoid generated is most likely determined by the cell type producing it, but other factors may lead to one or more being favored.[168,172]

Impact on MODS process

Phospholipase A_2 and eicosanoid production have been implicated in many of the signs and symptoms of the septic state, ARDS, and MODS, both systemically and in individual organs.[166,173,174] Investigations into inhibition of the cyclooxygenase and lipoxygenase pathways have shown attenuation of signs and symptoms associated with these syndromes.[167,168,175,176] The most promising agents appear to be the nonsteroidal antiinflammatory agents, such as ibuprofen and indomethacin, which inhibit the cyclooxygenase pathway.[176-179] Although the exact mechanism of action is yet to be established, improvements include decreased eicosanoid synthesis, inhibition of WBCs, and inhibition of free radical production. Some of the vasodilatory prostaglandins (PGI_2 and PGE_1) have actually been infused to counteract pulmonary hypertension.[180,181] Along with pulmonary vasodilatation, an improvement in microcirculatory flow, inhibition of platelet aggregation, and improvement of oxygen delivery (DO_2) and oxygen consumption (VO_2) also occur.[181,182] Whether these effects will decrease the overall morbidity and mortality in ARDS and MODS is yet to be seen.[183]

Eicosanoids play a role in shock, ischemia, ARDS, burn edema, reperfusion injury, and the redistribution of flow seen in the septic state.[168,174,184,185] The leukotrienes and thromboxane

```
Stimulation → Phospholipase activation
Cell membrane phospholipid → Arachidonic acid released
Phospholipase activation → Arachidonic acid released
Arachidonic acid released → Lipoxygenase pathway → Leukotrienes
Arachidonic acid released → Cyclooxygenase pathway → Prostaglandins / Thromboxanes
```

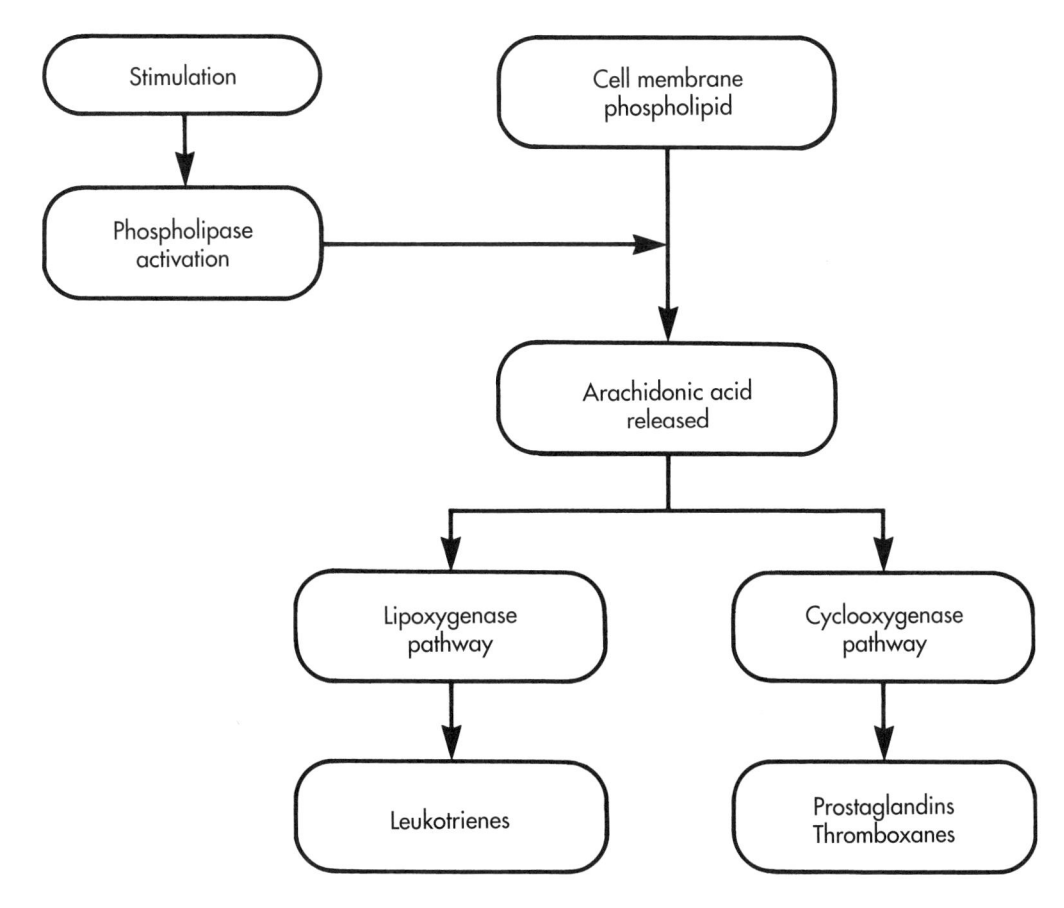

Fig. 3-8 Arachidonic acid metabolism.

BIOLOGIC TARGETS OF ARACHIDONIC ACID METABOLITES

Vasomotor tone
Microvascular permeability
Platelet aggregation
Macrophage–T cell interaction
Temperature regulation
Cellular activation and mediator release
Bronchial smooth muscle tone
GI motility, secretion, and blood flow

GI, Gastrointestinal.

have been strongly implicated in the vascular and airway changes that occur in ARDS.[167,174] Leukotrienes increase neutrophil chemotaxis and influx into the interstitium.[186] Another interesting finding in lung injury shows a shift in the ratio of the "good" eicosanoid to the "bad" eicosanoid. In ARDS, there is a decrease in prostacyclin and an increase in TX A_2, leading to vasoconstriction and platelet aggregation.[187] Eicosanoids have also been implicated in dysfunction in other organs such as the kidneys. See the chapters on specific organs in Section 3 for more specific information. Through their proplatelet activity, eicosanoids can enhance platelet aggregation, microembolization, and endothelial damage. Concomitant vasoconstriction can potentiate ischemia, further hindering blood flow to the organ beds.

PLATELET ACTIVATING FACTOR
Physiologic role

Platelet activating factor (PAF) is a lipid mediator produced from the cell membrane of many different cells of the IIR after phospholipase A_2 activation, including mast cells, basophils, monocytes/macrophages, neutrophils, platelets, and damaged endothelium.[188] Once in the circulation, PAF triggers platelet activation and morphologic changes that increase the ability of the platelets to aggregate. PAF can also promote neutrophil adhesion and stimulate their respiratory burst and degranulation (release of free radicals and digestive enzymes). Increased vascular permeability and vasomotor changes have also been associated with PAF release.[189]

Impact on MODS process

PAF triggers the release of many inflammatory mediators and is thus likely to play a pivotal role in sepsis and MODS.[190] PAF has been shown to induce the release of leukotrienes and TOMs from granulocytes. PAF, TNF-α, and endothelial damage may all contribute to the tissue destruction seen in MODS.[141,191] In animal studies, PAF has also induced hypotension, myocardial depression, decreased coronary artery flow, vascular changes, renal dysfunction, metabolic acidosis, bronchoconstriction, and thrombocytopenia.[188,192-195]

Because excessive platelet activation can lead to increased endothelial damage and clot formation, increased levels of PAF are ultimately dangerous for the host, especially if the PAF leaves the localized area of injury and circulates farther downstream. Microcirculatory abnormalities caused by platelet plugs and vasoconstriction contribute to further tissue ischemia and necrosis. PAF may exacerbate preexisting coagulopathies such as DIC.[189,191]

PLATELETS
Physiologic role

Platelets differentiate from hematopoietic stem cells in the bone marrow and mature through the myeloid lineage. Their principal activity is in the phase of primary hemostasis. After vessel injury, the platelets are activated by endothelial disruption and begin to swell and change shape. Their change in shape increases their surface area for adhesion and promotes aggregation and the formation of the platelet plug. After activation platelets produce many mediators (e.g., chemoattractants) that play a role not only in coagulation, but also in inflammation.

Impact on MODS process

Excessive platelet activity can lead to accelerated platelet aggregation, vascular obstruction, and excessive WBC activity and mediator release. Coagulation and the deposition of microthrombi are also potentially increased. The platelet provides another link between the processes of inflammation and coagulation and serves to perpetuate both responses.

Platelet dysfunction is often present in critically ill patients.[196] An adequate platelet count does not always indicate adequate platelet function. Abnormalities include both hyperreactive and hyporeactive platelets. The presence of sepsis and microorganisms has also been shown to affect platelet function.

TRANSFORMING GROWTH FACTOR-BETA
Physiologic role

The cytokine transforming growth factor-beta (TGF-β) is a peptide growth factor that is also involved in many other biologic processes, including inflammation, tissue repair, and tumorigenesis.[197-199] TGF-β is secreted primarily from platelets and also from activated macrophages and fibroblasts. It has both stimulatory and inhibitory activity. The apparent contradictory actions of TGF-β on various cells of the IIR is related to its effects on resting cells versus its effects on activated cells. In general, TGF-β triggers resting cells and plays a role in increasing adhesion molecules, enhancing chemotaxis, and triggering the release of other cytokines in the IIR. Conversely, TGF-β also inhibits inflammatory cells that were previously activated; therefore TGF-β can "convert an active inflammatory site into one dominated by resolution and repair."[197] If the delicate balance between TGF-β activities is disrupted, the potential for pathologic consequences is high, particularly in the area of host defense.

Impact on MODS process

Elevated TGF-β levels have been observed after injury and in sepsis,[200] but the exact impact of TGF-β on MODS is unknown. Because of its contradictory behavior in various settings, it is difficult to determine whether the effects of TGF-β in sepsis and MODS are primarily stimulatory or immunosuppressive.

MAST CELLS
Physiologic role

Mast cells are found in almost all tissues of the body, especially near blood vessels and the external environment. There are at least two types of morphologically distinct mast cells. One is found predominantly in the connective tissue of the peritoneal and pleural spaces and the skin. The majority of the granules of this mast cell contain heparin sulfates, histamine, and a chymotrypsin-like enzyme. The mast cells in the gastrointestinal mucosa contain chondroitin sulfates, a trypsinlike enzyme, and less histamine. The mast cell originates in the bone marrow and is very similar to the blood basophil, both in structure and function. Their relationship is not completely defined.

The mast cell plays a key role in the acute response to injury (primarily inflammation) but may affect the microenvironment in latter responses as well.[11] The mast cell releases both preformed and newly generated mediators when it is stimulated or directly injured by mechanical factors (crush, burn), endotoxin, complement, or bradykinin. Preformed substances released include histamine, proteases, heparin, and chemotactic factors. Generated substances include prostaglandins and leukotrienes. PAF and TNF may also be released.[201] Not only is the immediate environment affected (local response), but these substances may enter the circulation and cause systemic disturbances such as anaphylaxis.

Impact on MODS process

The mast cell, as a major source of mediators, may play a role in the development of MODS, although definitive documentation is not yet available. The major mediators released by mast cells are histamine, proteases, and arachidonic acid metabolites. The inflammatory effects of histamine include vasodilatation, increased capillary permeability, and chemo-kinesis (increased WBC movement, but not necessarily toward the specific site). It can also cause urticaria, bronchoconstriction, and increased gastric acid secretion, all of which are detrimental in a critically ill patient.

The arachidonic acid metabolites contribute to the bronchoconstriction, platelet aggregation, and vasodilatation already mentioned. Once again, initially protective physiologic functions in host defense are augmenting activity that is detrimental to the host. This scenario occurs repeatedly with many of the components of the IIR.

SUMMARY
Intrinsic control: function and failure

It is evident that numerous pathways are not only operating in MODS, but their activities are interdependent on each other and often synergistic in effect: vasodilatation, vasoconstriction, endothelial damage, microvascular permeability, tissue edema, fibrin deposition, leukocyte aggregation, vascular obstruction, and metabolic derangements. The pathways continually activate themselves and each other. Their synergistic effects contribute to the pathophysiology of MODS and combine to initiate and maintain maldistribution of circulating volume, imbalances in oxygen supply and demand, and metabolic abnormalities.[29,139,142,153]

Although the same cytokines are produced in a variety of clinical conditions such as trauma, hemorrhage, and surgery, the cytokine profiles (levels, timing of appearance, peaks) vary from one scenario to another.[163] There is, however, some consistency in the cytokine activity in nonsurvivors, regardless of the initial insult. Patients who die exhibit much higher levels of TNF-α, IL-1β, and IL-6 early after injury.[163] IL-6 appears to be a sensitive indicator of the severity of illness.[8]

Not only is activation overwhelming, but also inhibitory pathways may not be effective, leading to the uncontrolled, devastating responses of septic shock, tissue damage, and MODS. This failure of inhibition is just as significant as overwhelming activation.[11,25] "Malignant intravascular inflammation" was the initial term coined by Pinsky and Matuschak[129,202] to describe what is now known as SIRS and is thought by many to be the final common pathway in the journey to multiple organ dysfunction and failure.[5,9,19,129]

When does the IIR cease to be protective and move to a malignant, uncontrolled state? What is protective in one clinical situation seems to be destructive in another setting. How can there be immunosuppression leading to sepsis and overwhelming inflammation leading to septic shock and MODS in the same patient? Are they not antagonistic? Many research efforts are presently examining these questions, and a major focus of research is aimed at modulating this uncontrolled response. The difficulty comes in suppressing the uncontrolled response, yet keeping the protective response intact. One cannot help but think of the old adage: Too much of a good thing is bad. For the critically ill patient with MODS, "bad" is often fatal. Future research holds the key to keeping the good things good or, at the very least, under control.

REFERENCES

1. Baue AE. Multiple, progressive, or sequential systems failure: a syndrome of the 1970s. Arch Surg 1975;110:779-781.
2. Tilney NL, Bailey GL, Morgan AP. Sequential system failure after rupture of abdominal aortic aneurysms. Ann Surg 1973;178:117-122.
3. Eiseman B, Beart R, Norton L. Multiple organ failure. Surg Gynecol Obstet 1977;144:323-326.
4. DeCamp MM, Demling RH. Posttraumatic multisystem organ failure. JAMA 1988;260:530-534.
5. Goris RJ. Multiple organ failure: Whole body inflammation? Schweiz Med Wochenschr 1989;119:347-353.
6. Anderson BO, Harken AH. Multiple organ failure: Inflammatory priming and activation sequences promote autologous tissue injury. J Trauma 1990;30:S44-S49.
7. Roumen RMH et al. Inflammatory mediators in relation to the development of multiple organ failure in patients after severe blunt trauma. Crit Care Med 1995;23:474-480.
8. Svoboda P, Kantorova I, Ochmann J. Dynamics of interleukin 1, 2, and 6 and tumor necrosis factor alpha in multiple trauma patients. J Trauma 1994;36:336-340.
9. Waydas C et al. Inflammatory mediators, infection, sepsis, and multiple organ failure after severe trauma. Arch Surg 1992;127:460-467.
10. Baue AE. Multiple organ failure: Patient care and prevention. St. Louis: Mosby; 1990.
11. Yurt RW, Lowry SF. Role of the macrophage and endogenous mediators in multiple organ failure. In: Deitch EA, ed. Multiple organ failure: Pathophysiology and basic concepts of therapy. New York: Thieme Medical Publishers; 1990: 60-71.
12. American College of Chest Physicians/Society of Critical Care Medicine Consensus Conference Committee. Definitions for sepsis and organ failure and guidelines for the use of innovative therapies in sepsis. Crit Care Med 1992;20:864-874.
13. Bone RC et al. Definitions for sepsis and organ failure and guidelines for the use of innovative therapies in sepsis. The ACCP/SCCM Consensus Conference Committee. Chest 1992;101:1644-1655.
14. Ackerman MH. The systemic inflammatory response, sepsis, and multiple organ dysfunction: New definitions for an old problem. Crit Care Nurs Clin North Am 1994;6:243-250.
15. Bone RC. Toward an epidemiology and natural history of SIRS (systemic inflammatory response syndrome). JAMA 1992;268:3452-3455.
16. Hoch RC et al. Effects of accidental trauma on cytokine and endotoxin production. Crit Care Med 1993;21:839-845.
17. Goris RJ et al. Multiple organ failure: Generalized autodestructive inflammation. Arch Surg 1985;120:1109-1115.
18. Nuytinck HKS et al. Whole-body inflammation in trauma patients. Arch Surg 1988;123:1519-1524.
19. Abraham E, ed. Sepsis: Cellular and physiologic mechanisms. New Horiz 1993;1:1-159.
20. Secor VH. The inflammatory/immune response in critical illness: Role of the systemic inflammatory response syndrome. Crit Care Nurs Clin North Am 1994;6:251-264.
21. Osborn L. Leukocyte adhesion to endothelium in inflammation. Cell 1990;62:3-6.
22. Malik AB. Endothelial cell interactions and integrins. New Horiz 1993;1:37-51.
23. Talbott GA et al. Leukocyte-endothelial interactions and organ injury: The role of adhesion molecules. New Horiz 1994;2:545-554.
24. Bevilacqua MP et al. Identification of an inducible endothelial-leukocyte adhesion molecule. Proc Natl Acad Sci USA 1987;84:9238-9242.
25. Weiss SJ. Tissue destruction by neutrophils. N Engl J Med 1989;320:365-376.
26. Welbourn R et al. Role of neutrophil adherence receptors (CD 18) in lung permeability following lower torso ischemia. Circ Res 1992;71:82-86.
27. Bone RC. Modulators of coagulation: A critical appraisal of their role in sepsis. Arch Intern Med 1992;152:1381-1389.
28. Bevilacqua MP, Gimbrone MA. Inducible endothelial functions in inflammation and coagulation. Semin Thromb Hemost 1988;13:425-433.
29. Secor VH. Mediators of coagulation and inflammation: Relationship and clinical significance. Crit Care Nurs Clin North Am 1993;5:411-433.
30. Beutler B. Endotoxin, tumor necrosis factor, and related mediators: New Approaches to shock. New Horiz 1993;1:3-12.
31. Yi ES, Ulich TR. Endotoxin, interleukin-1, and tumor necrosis factor cause neutrophil-dependent microvascular leakage in postcapillary venules. Am J Pathol 1992;140:659-663.
32. Dinarello CA, Wolff SM. The role of interleukin-1 in disease. N Engl J Med 1993;328:106-113.
33. Rietschel ET, Brade H. Bacterial endotoxins. Scientific American 1992;August:54-61.
34. Ghosh S et al. Endotoxin-induced organ injury. Crit Care Med 1993;21(suppl):S19-S24.
35. Welbourn CRB et al. Pathophysiology of ischaemia reperfusion injury: Central role of the neutrophil. Br J Surg 1991;78:651-655.
36. Beutler B, Grau GE. Tumor necrosis factor in the pathogenesis of infectious diseases. Crit Care Med 1993;21:S423-S435.
37. Bean RB. Sir William Osler: Aphorisms. New York: Henry Shumar; 1950.
38. Demling R et al. Multiple organ dysfunction in the surgical patient: Pathophysiology, prevention, and treatment. Curr Probl Surg 1993;30:348-414.
39. Schiffrin EL. The endothelium and control of blood vessel function in health and disease. Clin Invest Med 1994;17:602-620.
40. Majno G, Shea S, Leventhal M. Endothelial contraction induced by histamine type mediators: An electron microscopic study. J Cell Biol 1969;42:647-672.

41. Gimbrone MA, ed. Vascular endothelium in hemostasis and thrombosis. New York: Churchill Livingstone; 1986.
42. Müller-Berghaus G. Septicemia and the vessel wall. In: Verstraete M, Vermylen J, Lijnen R, Arnout J, eds. Thrombosis and haemostasis. Leuven, Belgium: Leuven University Press; 1987:619-671.
43. Müller-Berghaus G. Pathophysiologic and biochemical events in disseminated intravascular coagulation: Dysregulation of procoagulant and anticoagulant pathways. Semin Thromb Hemost 1989;15:58-87.
44. Morrissey JH, Drake TA. Procoagulant response of the endothelium and monocytes. In: Schlag G, Redl H, eds. Pathophysiology of shock, sepsis, and organ failure. Berlin: Springer-Verlag; 1993:564-574.
45. Meyrick B, Johnson JE, Brigham KL. Endotoxin-induced pulmonary endothelial injury. Prog Clin Biol Res: Second Vienna Shock Forum 1989;308:91-100.
46. Freudenberg N. Reaction of the vascular intima to endotoxin shock. Prog Clin Biol Res: Second Vienna Shock Forum 1989;308:77-89.
47. Del Vecchio PJ, Malik AB. Thrombin-induced neutrophil adhesion. Prog Clin Biol Res: Second Vienna Shock Forum 1989;308:101-112.
48. Beerthuizen GIJM. Response of the microcirculation: Tissue oxygenation. In: Schlag G, Redl H, eds. Pathophysiology of shock, sepsis, and organ failure. Berlin: Springer-Verlag; 1993:230-241.
49. Gidlof A, Lewis DH. Do endotoxinemia and sepsis impair the regulatory functions of capillary endothelial cells. Prog Clin Biol Res: Second Vienna Shock Forum 1989;308:157-162.
50. Pober JS, Cotran RS. The role of endothelial cells in inflammation. Transplantation 1990;50:537-544.
51. Deitch EA, Mancini MC. Complement receptors in shock and transplantation. Arch Surg 1993;128:1222-1226.
52. Star RA. Nitric oxide: Friend and foe. Medical Grand Rounds. Dallas, TX: Parkland Memorial Hospital, 1995 Feb.
53. Vallance P, Moncada S. Role of endogenous nitric oxide in septic shock. New Horiz 1993;1:77-86.
54. Albina JE, Reichner JS. Nitric oxide in inflammation and immunity. New Horiz 1995;3:46-64.
55. Furchgott RF, Zawadzki JV. The obligatory role of endothelial cells in the relaxation of arterial smooth muscle by acetylcholine. Nature 1980;288:373-376.
56. Palmer RMJ, Ferrige AG, Moncada S. Nitric oxide release accounts for the biological activity of endothelium-derived relaxing factor. Nature 1987;325:524-526.
57. Ignarro LJ. Biological actions and properties of endothelium-derived nitric oxide formed and released from artery and vein. Circ Res 1989;65:1-21.
58. Hibbs JB, Taintor RR, Vavrin Z. Macrophage cytotoxicity: A role for L-arginine deiminase activity and imino nitrogen oxidation to nitrite. Science 1987;235:473-476.
59. Szabo C. Alterations in nitric oxide production in various forms of circulatory shock. New Horiz 1995;3:2-32.
60. Wright CE, Rees DD, Moncada S. Protective and pathological roles of nitric oxide in endotoxin shock. Cardiovasc Res 1992;26:48-57.
61. Kilbourn RG, Belloni P. Endothelial cell production of nitrogen oxides in response to interferon gamma in combination with tumor necrosis factor, interleukin-1, or endotoxin. J Natl Cancer Inst 1990;82:772-776.
62. Kosaka H et al. Synergistic stimulation of nitric oxide hemoglobin production in rats by recombinant interleukin-1 and tumor necrosis factor. Biochem Biophys 1992;189:392-397.
63. Booke M et al. Use of nitric oxide synthase inhibitors in animal models of sepsis. New Horiz 1995;3:123-138.
64. Cioffi WG, Ogura TR. Inhaled nitric oxide in acute lung disease. New Horiz 1995;3:73-85.
65. Yanagisawa M et al. A novel potent vasoconstrictor peptide produced by vascular endothelial cells. Nature 1988;332:411-415.
66. Huribal M et al. Endothelin-1 and prostaglandin E_2 levels increase in patients with burns. J Am Coll Surg 1995;180:318-322.
67. Myhre U et al. Endothelin-1 and endotoxemia. J Cardiovasc Pharmacol 1993;22(Suppl 8):S291-S294.
68. Weitzberg E, Lundberg JM, Rudehill A. Elevated plasma levels of endothelin in patients with sepsis syndrome. Circ Shock 1991;33:222-227.
69. Pittet JF et al. Elevated plasma endothelin-1 concentrations are associated with the severity of illness in patients with sepsis. Ann Surg 1991;213:261-264.
70. Voerman HJ et al. Plasma endothelin levels are increased during septic shock. Crit Care Med 1992;20:1097-1101.
71. Redl H et al. Big-endothelin release in baboon bacteremia is partially TNF-dependent. J Lab Clin Med 1994;124:796-801.
72. Kohan DE. Role of endothelin and tumour necrosis factor in the renal response to sepsis. Nephrol Dialysis Transplant 1994;9(suppl 4):73-77.
73. Walport M. Complement. In: Roitt I, Brostoff J, Male D, eds. Immunology. 3rd ed. London: Mosby; 1993:12.1-12.17.
74. Johnston RB. The complement system in host defense and inflammation: The cutting edges of a double-edged sword. Pediatr Infect Dis J 1993;12:933-941.
75. Zimmerman T et al. The role of the complement system in the pathogenesis of multiple organ failure in shock. Prog Clin Biol Res: Second Vienna Shock Forum 1989;308:291-298.
76. Roxvall L, Bengtson A, Heideman M. Anaphylatoxin generation and multisystem organ failure in acute pancreatitis. J Surg Res 1989;47:138-143.
77. Bengtsson A, Redl H, Schlag G. Complement in sepsis. In: Schlag G, Redl H, eds. Pathophysiology of shock, sepsis, and organ failure. Berlin: Springer-Verlag; 1993:447-458.
78. Bengtson A, Heideman M. Anaphylatoxin formation in sepsis. Arch Surg 1988;123:645-649.
79. Langlois PF et al. Accentuated complement activation in patient plasma during the adult respiratory distress syndrome: A potential mechanism for pulmonary inflammation. Heart Lung 1989;18:71-84.
80. Schirmer WJ et al. Complement activation in peritonitis. Association with hepatic and renal perfusion abnormalities. Am Surg 1987;53:683-687.
81. Schirmer WJ et al. Systemic complement activation produces hemodynamic changes characteristic of sepsis. Arch Surg 1988;123:316-321.
82. Steward M, Male D. Immunological techniques. In: Roitt I, Brostoff J, Male D, eds. Immunology. 3rd ed. London: Mosby; 1993:25.1-25.16.

83. Bell TN. Disseminated intravascular coagulation: Clinical complexities of aberrant coagulation. Crit Care Nurs Clin North Am 1993;5:389-410.
84. McGee MP et al. Tissue factor and factor VII messenger RNAs in human alveolar macrophages: Effects of breathing ozone. Blood 1990;75:122-127.
85. Lyberg T et al. Procoagulant (thromboplastin) activity in human bronchoalveolar lavage fluids is derived from alveolar macrophages. Eur Resp J 1990;3:61-67.
86. Aasen AO, Buo L. Activation of humoral systems: The role of coagulation, fibrinolysis, and the plasma kallikrein-kinin system. In: Schlag R, Redl H, eds. Pathophysiology of shock, sepsis, and organ failure. Berlin: Springer-Verlag; 1993:36-45.
87. Mullins RJ, Malias MA, Hudgens RW. Isoproterenol inhibits the increase in microvascular membrane permeability produced by bradykinin. J Trauma 1989;29:1053-1063.
88. Carmines PK, Fleming JT. Control of the renal microvasculature by vasoactive peptides. FASEB J 1990;4:3300-3309.
89. Ichinose M, Barnes PJ. Bradykinin-induced airway microvascular leakage and bronchoconstriction are mediated via a bradykinin B_2 receptor. Am Rev Resp Dis 1990; 142:1104-1107.
90. Kaplan AP, Silverberg M. The coagulation-kinin pathway of human plasma. Blood 1987;70:1-15.
91. Hesselvik JF et al. Coagulation, fibrinolysis, and kallikrein systems in sepsis: Relation to outcome. Crit Care Med 1989;17:724-733.
92. Cioffi WG, Burleson DG, Pruitt BA. Leukocyte responses to injury. Arch Surg 1993;128:1260-1267.
93. Parslow TG. The phagocytic neutrophils and macrophages. In: Stites DP, Terr AI, Parslow TG, eds. Basic and clinical immunology. 8th ed. Norwalk, CT: Appleton & Lange; 1994:9-21.
94. Simms HH, D'Amico R. Polymorphonuclear leukocyte dysregulation during the systemic inflammatory response syndrome. Blood 1994;83:1398-1407.
95. Vedder NB et al. Neutrophil-mediated vascular injury in shock and multiple organ failure. Prog Clin Biol Res: Perspectives in Shock Research 1989;299:181-192.
96. Brigham KL, Meyrick B. Interactions of granulocytes with lungs. Circ Res 1984;54:623-635.
97. Heflin C, Brigham KL. Granulocyte depletion prevents increased lung vascular permeability after endotoxemia in sheep. Clin Res 1979;27:399A.
98. Tate RM et al. Oxygen radical-induced pulmonary edema: A mechanism for the production of non-cardiogenic pulmonary edema by neutrophils. Chest 1982;81:57S-59S.
99. Burchardi H et al. Neutrophil stimulation by PMA increases alveolar permeability in rabbits. Prog Clin Biol Res: Second Vienna Shock Forum 1989;308:323-330.
100. Rivkind AI et al. Sequential patterns of eicosanoid, platelet, and neutrophil interactions in the evolution of the fulminant post-traumatic adult respiratory distress syndrome. Ann Surg 1989;210:355-372.
101. Ognibene FP et al. Adult respiratory distress syndrome in patients with severe neutropenia. N Engl J Med 1986; 315:547-551.
102. Mallick AA et al. Multiple organ damage caused by tumor necrosis factor and prevented by prior neutrophil depletion. Chest 1989;95:1114-1120.
103. Perkett EA, Brigham KL, Meyrick B. Granulocyte depletion attenuates sustained pulmonary hypertension and increased pulmonary vasoreactivity caused by continuous air embolization in sheep. Am Rev Resp Dis 1990;141: 456-465.
104. Bersten A, Sibbald WJ. Acute lung injury in septic shock. Crit Care Clin 1989;5:49-80.
105. Mullane KM, Salmon JA, Kraemer R. Leukocyte-derived metabolites of arachidonic acid in ischemia-induced myocardial injury. Fed Proc 1987;46:2422-2433.
106. Black L, Coombs VJ, Townsend SN. Reperfusion and reperfusion injury in acute myocardial infarction. Heart Lung 1990;19:274-286.
107. Nelson K, Herndon D, Reisz G. Pulmonary effects of ischemic limb reperfusion: Evidence for a role of oxygen-derived radicals. Crit Care Med 1991;19:360-363.
108. Kloner RA, Przyklenk K, Patel B. Altered myocardial states: The stunned and hibernating myocardium. Am J Med 1989;86(suppl 1A):14-22.
109. Brigham KL. Role of free radicals in lung injury. Chest 1986;89:859-863.
110. Dormandy TL. Free-radical pathology and medicine. J Royal Coll Physicians London 1989;23:221-227.
111. McCord JM. Oxygen-derived free radicals. New Horiz 1993;1:70-76.
112. van der Kraaij AMM et al. Lipid peroxidation and its significance for postischemic cardiovascular injury. Prog Clin Biol Res 1989;301:61-72.
113. Goode HF, Webster NR. Free radicals and antioxidants in sepsis. Crit Care Med 1993;21:1770-1776.
114. Machiedo GW et al. The incidence of decreased red blood cell deformability in sepsis and the association with oxygen free radical damage and multiple-system organ failure. Arch Surg 1989;124:1386-1389.
115. Werns SW, Lucchesi BR. Leukocytes, oxygen radicals, and myocardial injury due to ischemia and reperfusion. Free Radical Biol Med 1988;4:31-37.
116. Kloner RA, Przyklenk K, Whittaker P. Deleterious effects of oxygen radicals in ischemia/reperfusion: Resolved and unresolved issues. Circulation 1989;80:1115-1127.
117. Neuhof H et al. Proteases as mediators of pulmonary vascular permeability. Prog Clin Biol Res: Second Vienna Shock Forum 1989;308:305-314.
118. Jochum M et al. Posttraumatic plasma levels of mediators of organ failure. Prog Clin Biol Res: Second Vienna Shock Forum 1989;308:673-681.
119. Lang H, Fritz H. The role of phagocytic proteinases in the pathobiochemistry of inflammation. Adv Clin Enzymol 1986;3:168-178.
120. van Bebber IPT et al. Endotoxin does not play a key role in the pathogenesis of multiple organ failure. An experimental study. Prog Clin Biol Res: Second Vienna Shock Forum 1989;308:419-423.
121. Jochum M et al. The role of phagocyte proteinases and proteinase inhibitors in multiple organ failure. Am J Resp Crit Care Med 1994;150:S123-S130.

122. Male D, Roitt I. Introduction to the immune system. In: Roitt I, Brostoff J, Male D, eds. Immunology. 3rd ed. London: Mosby; 1993:1.1-1.12.
123. Kuijpers TW, Harlan JM. Monocyte-endothelial interactions: Insights and questions. J Lab Clin Med 1993; 122:641-651.
124. Knighton DR, Riegel VD. The macrophages: effector cell wound repair. Prog Clin Biol Res: Perspectives in Shock Research 1989;299:217-226.
125. Ford HR et al. Characterization of wound cytokines in the sponge matrix model. Arch Surg 1989;124:1422-1428.
126. Cerra FB et al. Hypermetabolism/organ failure: The role of the activated macrophage as a metabolic regulator. Prog Clin Biol Res 1988;264:27-42.
127. Border JR. Hypothesis: Sepsis, multiple systems organ failure, and the macrophage. Arch Surg 1988;123:285-286.
128. Lazarou SA et al. The wound is a possible source of posttraumatic immunosuppression. Arch Surg 1989;124:1429-1431.
129. Pinsky MR, Matuschak GM. Multiple systems organ failure: Failure of host defense homeostasis. Crit Care Clin 1989;5:199-220.
130. Demling RH. Wound inflammatory mediators and multisystem organ failure. Prog Clin Biol Res 1987;236A:525-537.
131. Faist E et al. Mediators and the trauma induced cascade of immunologic defects. Prog Clin Biol Res: Second Vienna Shock Forum: 1989;308:495-506.
132. Beutler B et al. Purification of cachectin, a lipoprotein lipase-suppressing homone secreted by endotoxin-induced RAW 264.7 cells. J Exp Med 1985;161:984-995.
133. Tracey KJ, Cerami A. Tumor necrosis factor: An updated review of its biology. Crit Care Med 1993;21:S415-S422.
134. Vassalli P. The pathophysiology of tumor necrosis factors. Annu Rev Immunol 1992;10:411-452.
135. Schirmer WJ, Schirmer JM, Fry DE. Recombinant human tumor necrosis factor produces hemodynamic changes characteristic of sepsis and endotoxemia. Arch Surg 1989;124:445-448.
136. Tracey KJ et al. Shock and tissue injury induced by recombinant human cachectin. Science 1986;234:470-474.
137. Johnson J et al. Human recombinant tumor necrosis factor alpha infusion mimics endotoxemia in awake sheep. J Appl Physiol 1989;66:1448-1454.
138. Stephens KE et al. Tumor necrosis factor causes increased pulmonary permeability and edema. Comparison to septic acute lung injury. Am Rev Resp Dis 1988;137:1364-1370.
139. Schlag G, Redl H, eds. Pathophysiologic role of mediators and mediator inhibitors in shock. Prog Clin Biol Res: First Vienna Shock Forum 1987;236A.
140. Neugebauer E et al. Mediators in septic shock: Strategies of securing them and assessment of their causal significance. Chirurg 1987;58:470-481.
141. Camussi G et al. Tumor necrosis factor/cachectin stimulates peritoneal macrophages, polymorphonuclear neutrophils, and vascular endothelial cells to synthesize and release PAF. J Exp Med 1987;166:1390-1404.
142. Lowry SF. Cytokine mediators of immunity and inflammation. Arch Surg 1993;128:1235-1241.
143. Tracey KJ et al. Anticachectin/TNF monoclonal antibodies prevent shock during lethal bacteraemia. Nature 1987;330:662-665.
144. Evans DA. The effects of tumor necrosis factor and their selective inhibition by ibuprofen. Ann Surg 1989;209:312-321.
145. Bodmer M, Fournel MA, Hinshaw LB. Preclinical review of anti-tumor necrosis factor monoclonal antibodies. Crit Care Med 1993;21:S441-S446.
146. Fisher CJ et al. Influence of an anti-tumor necrosis factor monoclonal antibody on cytokine levels in patients with sepsis. The CB0006 Sepsis Syndrome Study Group [see comments]. Crit Care Med 1993;21:318-327.
147. Hinshaw LB et al. Survival of primates in LD100 septic shock following therapy with antibody to tumor necrosis factor (TNF alpha). Circ Shock 1990;30:279-292.
148. Shalaby MR et al. Binding and regulation of cellular functions by monoclonal antibodies against human tumor necrosis factor receptors. J Exp Med 1990;172:1517-1520.
149. Espevik T et al. Characterization of binding and biological effects of monoclonal antibodies against a human tumor necrosis factor receptor. J Exp Med 1990;171:415-426.
150. Wherry JC, Pennington JE, Wenzel RP. Tumor necrosis factor and the therapeutic potential of anti-tumor necrosis factor antibodies. Crit Care Med 1993;21:S436-S440.
151. Dinarello CA. Biology of interleukin 1. FASEB J 1988; 2:108-115.
152. Kampschmidt RF. The numerous postulated biological manifestations of interleukin-1. J Leukocyte Biol 1984; 36:341-355.
153. Tracey KJ, Lowry SF. The role of cytokine mediators in septic shock. Adv Surg 1990;23:21-56.
154. Bernton EW et al. Release of multiple hormones by a direct action of interleukin-1 on pituitary cells. Science 1987;238:519-521.
155. Cunningham ET Jr, de Souza EB. Interleukin 1 receptors in the brain and endocrine tissues. Immunol Today 1993;14: 171-176.
156. Tilders FJH et al. Activation of the hypothalamus-pituitary-adrenal axis by bacterial endotoxins: Routes and intermediate signals. Psychoneuroendocrinol 1994;19:209-232.
157. Baracos V et al. Stimulation of muscle protein degradation and prostaglandin E2 release by leukocytic pyrogen (interleukin-1). N Engl J Med 1983;308:553-558.
158. Cozzolino F et al. Potential role of interleukin-1 as the trigger for diffuse intravascular coagulation in acute nonlymphoblastic leukemia. Am J Med 1988;84:240-250.
159. Dinarello CA et al. Multiple biological activities of human recombinant interleukin-1. J Clin Invest 1986;77:1734-1739.
160. Wilder RL. Neuroendocrine-immune system interactions and autoimmunity. Annu Rev Immunol 1995;13:307-338.
161. Borden EC, Chin P. Interleukin-6: A cytokine with potential diagnostic and therapeutic roles. J Lab Clin Med 1994; 123:824-829.
162. Molloy RG, Mannick JA, Rodrick ML. Cytokines, sepsis, and immunomodulation. Br J Surg 1993;80:289-297.
163. Roumen RMH et al. Cytokine patterns in patients after major vascular surgery, hemorrhagic shock, and severe blunt trauma. Ann Surg 1993;218:769-776.

164. Biffl WL et al. Interleukin-6 potentiates neutrophil priming with platelet-activating factor. Arch Surg 1994;129:1131-1136.
165. Isakson P et al. Cytokine regulation of eicosanoid generation. Ann NY Acad Sci 1994;744:181-183.
166. Fink MP. Phospholipases A2: Potential mediators of the systemic inflammatory response syndrome and the multiple organ dysfunction syndrome [editorial]. Crit Care Med 1993;21:957-959.
167. Sprague RS et al. Proposed role for leukotrienes in the pathophysiology of multiple systems organ failure. Crit Care Clin 1989;5:315-330.
168. Petrak RA, Balk RA, Bone RC. Prostaglandins, cyclo-oxygenase inhibitors, and thromboxane synthetase inhibitors in the pathogenesis of multiple systems organ failure. Crit Care Clin 1989;5:302-314.
169. Samuelsson B et al. Leukotrienes and lipoxins: Structures, biosynthesis, and biological effects. Science 1987;237:1171-1176.
170. Ogletree ML. Overview of physiological and pathophysiological effects of thromboxane A2. Fed Proc 1987;46:133-138.
171. Fletcher JR. Eicosanoids: Critical agents in the physiological process and cellular injury. Arch Surg 1993;128:1192-1196.
172. Ninnemann JL. Prostaglandins, leukotrienes, and the immune response. New York: Cambridge University Press; 1988.
173. Anderson BO, Moore EE, Banerjee A. Phospholipase A2 regulates critical inflammatory mediators of multiple organ failure. J Surg Res 1994;56:199-205.
174. Bernard GR et al. Persistent generation of peptido leukotrienes in patients with the adult respiratory distress syndrome. Am Rev Resp Dis 1991;144:263-267.
175. Brigham KL. Conference summary: Lipid mediators in the pulmonary circulation. Am Rev Resp Dis 1987;136:785-788.
176. Bernard GR et al. Prostacyclin and thromboxane A2 formation is increased in human sepsis syndrome. Effects of cyclooxygenase inhibition. Am Rev Resp Dis 1991;144:1095-1101.
177. Byrne K et al. Increased survival time after delayed histamine and prostaglandin blockade in a porcine model of severe sepsis-induced lung injury. Crit Care Med 1990;18:303-308.
178. Waymack JP. The effect of ibuprofen on postburn metabolic and immunologic function. J Surg Res 1989;46:172-176.
179. Cook JA et al. Prostaglandins, thromboxanes, leukotrienes, and cytochrome-P450 metabolites of arachidonic acid. New Horiz 1993;1:60-69.
180. Demling RH et al. The effect of prostacyclin infusion on endotoxin-induced lung injury. Surgery 1981;89:257-263.
181. Bihari DJ, Tinker J. The therapeutic value of vasodilator prostaglandins in multiple organ failure associated with sepsis. Intens Care Med 1988;15:2-7.
182. Silverman HJ et al. Effects of prostaglandin E1 on oxygen delivery and consumption in patients with the adult respiratory distress syndrome. Results from the prostaglandin E1 multicenter trial. Chest 1990;98:405-410.
183. Russell JA, Ronco JJ, Dodek PM. Physiologic effects and side-effects of prostaglandin E1 in adult respiratory distress syndrome. Chest 1990;97:684-692.
184. Mullane K et al. Myocardial salvage induced by REV-5901: An inhibitor and antagonist of the leukotrienes. J Cardiovasc Pharmacol 1987;10:398-406.
185. Brigham KL, Sheller JR. Leukotrienes and ARDS. Intens Care Med 1989;15:422-423.
186. Henderson WR. The role of leukotrienes in inflammation. Ann Intern Med 1994;121:684-697.
187. Yellin SA et al. Prostacyclin and thromboxane A2 in septic shock: Species differences. Circ Shock 1986;20:291-297.
188. Lefer AM. Induction of tissue injury and altered cardiovascular performance by platelet-activating factor: Relevance to multiple systems organ failure. Crit Care Clin 1989;5:331-352.
189. Braquet P, Hosford D. The potential role of platelet-activating factor (PAF) in shock, sepsis and adult respiratory distress syndrome (ARDS). Prog Clin Biol Res: Second Vienna Shock Forum 1989;308:425-439.
190. Koltai M, Hosford D, Braquet PG. Platelet-activating factor in septic shock. New Horiz 1993;1:87-95.
191. Bonavida B et al. The involvement of platelet-activating factor (PAF)-induced monocyte activation and tumor necrosis factor (TNF) production in shock. Prog Clin Biol Res: Second Vienna Shock Forum 1989;308:485-489.
192. Vargaftig BB et al. Platelet-activating factor induces a platelet-dependent bronchoconstriction unrelated to the formation of prostaglandin derivatives. Eur J Pharmacol 1980;65:185-192.
193. Kenzora JL, Perez JE, Bergman SR, Lange LG. Effects of acetyl glyceryl ether phosphorylcholine (platelet-activating factor) on ventricular preload, afterload and contractility in dogs. J Clin Invest 1984;74:1193-1203.
194. Handley DA, Van Valen RG, Melden MK, Saunders RN. Evaluation of dose and route effects of platelet activating factor-induced extravasation in the guinea-pig. Thromb Haemost 1984;52:34-46.
195. Sybertz EJ et al. Cardiac, coronary and peripheral vascular effects of acetyl glyceryl ether phosphorylcholine in anesthetized dogs. J Pharmacol Exp Therap 1985;232:156-162.
196. Boldt J et al. Platelet function in critically ill patients. Chest 1994;106:899-903.
197. Wahl SM. Transforming growth factor beta: The good, the bad, and the ugly. J Exp Med 1994;180:1587-1590.
198. McCartney-Francis NL, Wahl S. Transforming growth factor beta: A matter of life and death. J Leukocyte Biol 1994;55:401-409.
199. Herndon DN, Nguyen TT, Gilpin DA. Growth factors: Local and systemic. Arch Surg 1993;128:1227-1233.
200. Hamon G et al. Transforming growth factor-beta 1 lowers the CD 14 content of monocytes. J Surg Res 1994;57:574-578.
201. Galli SJ, Gordon JR, Wershil BK. Mast cell cytokines in allergy and inflammation. Actions Agents 1993;Suppl 43:209-220.
202. Pinsky MR. Multiple systems organ failure: Malignant intravascular inflammation. Crit Care Clin 1989;5:195-198.

CHAPTER 4

Coagulation and Disseminated Intravascular Coagulation

Tally N. Bell

Multiple organ dysfunction syndrome (MODS) is a significant threat to maintaining normal hemostatic function in the critically ill. Although hemostatic alterations commonly occur in severe disease or injury, they further insult the already compromised MODS patient. Disseminated intravascular coagulation (DIC) is a potentially life-threatening condition that results from the physiologic disequilibrium in MODS as it affects the hematologic system. Although end-organ failure of the hematologic system can manifest as DIC, more likely the development of DIC can be attributed to dysfunction of the complex physiologic interactions occurring among organ systems and the inflammatory/immune response. The purpose of this chapter is to review normal hemostatic mechanisms and the alterations that occur in these mechanisms during DIC, to explore the relationship of DIC and MODS, to examine diagnostic and clinical assessment parameters, and to identify current therapeutic interventions and management of the critically ill MODS patient with DIC.

DIC is an acquired coagulopathy that has been previously described in the literature by a variety of names, including defibrination syndrome, diffuse intravascular clotting, consumptive coagulopathy,[1] and intravascular clotting syndrome.[2-5] It never occurs as a primary disorder, but arises as an intermediary mechanism of disease in numerous underlying conditions.[5-9]

DIC is reported to occur in one out of every 900 to 2400 adults admitted to large urban hospitals.[10]

Because DIC is a complication of an underlying critical illness or produces other multisystem complications as a consequence, mortality rates can be high. Depending on the primary disorder of the patient, the mortality rate in DIC is estimated at 50% to 80%.[11] In patients with shock and infection as precipitating factors, the mortality rate can approach 90%.[11] Mortality and survival often depend more on the specific cause of DIC than the DIC itself.[9]

Feinstein defines DIC as "a dynamic pathologic process triggered by activation of the clotting cascade with the resultant activation of excess thrombin within the vascular system that leads to further activation of the coagulation system, shortened survival of certain hemostatic elements, deposition of fibrin in the microcirculation, and activation of the fibrinolytic system."[12] Paradoxically, this pathologic overstimulation of normal hemostasis produces a unique clinical situation where the patient develops microvascular thrombi and hemorrhage simultaneously.

Clinically, DIC can occur as an acute or chronic, generalized or localized process that is triggered by acute or chronic underlying disease states. Because coagulation is a systemic process, DIC can potentially affect all organ systems, producing multiple organ dysfunction, failure, or both. Although hemorrhagic and thrombotic manifestations occur more frequently in multiple organ systems, they can occur on an organ-specific basis.[13] Acute, generalized DIC occurs more frequently in the critical care setting and is the focus of this chapter.

73

NORMAL HEMOSTATIC MECHANISMS

Hemostasis is defined as the arrest of hemorrhage at the site of injury.[14] Normal hemostasis represents the outcome of integrated interactions among blood vessels, platelets, coagulation proteins, and the fibrinolytic system. Activation of endothelial cells,[15] neutrophils, monocytes, and macrophages is thought to be central to the process of coagulation.[16] When physical or chemical derangements occur in these interactions, the stage is set for untoward bleeding and/or inappropriate clotting.

Endothelium

The vascular endothelium plays a significant role in hemostasis. In its normal, intact state, the endothelial lining of the blood vessels provides a nonthrombogenic, nonadherent surface that prevents coagulation and maintains blood fluidity[17-20]; however, damaged or excited endothelial cells exhibit properties that are thrombogenic.[20-22] Damaged or excited endothelial cells respond by releasing tissue factor, allowing the endothelium to become a hemostatically active surface.[19,23,24] The endothelium also provides surface binding sites for thrombomodulin, a high-affinity thrombin receptor protein on the endothelial cell, and antithrombin III (AT III), a naturally occurring coagulation inhibitor. Additionally, the endothelium is a site for the synthesis and release of many other platelet, coagulation, and fibrinolytic activators and inhibitors, including protein C, protein S, and interleukin-1.[25] Because the endothelium is important in maintaining a sensitive balance between procoagulant and anticoagulant forces in both normal physiologic and pathophysiologic processes, its dynamic role is integrated throughout this section.

Vasoconstriction

When the integrity of a blood vessel is interrupted by rupture or incision, the blood vessel immediately goes into vasospasm, and adjacent blood vessels constrict as a result of sympathetic nervous system activation.[26] The initiation of this response is not well understood; however, it appears that multiple factors, including serotonin, the alpha-adrenergic system, thromboxane A_2 (TXA_2), and endothelin may contribute to the vasoconstrictive response.[14,22,23] Vasoconstriction promotes hemostasis by narrowing the blood vessel lumen and mechanically limiting blood flow at the site of injury.

The greater the extent of vessel trauma, the greater the extent of vasospasm. A crushing injury to a blood vessel produces more vascular spasm in that vessel than in one that has been cut.[27] Vasoconstriction contributes to hemostasis in the capillary bed, but alone it is insufficient to stop bleeding in larger vessels.[23,28] However, when larger blood vessels, particularly arteries, are traumatized, vasoconstriction is critical for preventing exsanguination.[29]

Platelet plug formation

Platelets do not adhere to intact endothelium. Endothelial cells secrete a prostaglandin called prostacyclin (PGI_2), a potent vasodilator that strongly inhibits platelet function by decreasing the reaction of the platelet to activating stimuli.[14,18,19,30] However, when the endothelial lining of the blood vessel is disrupted and subendothelial collagen of the basement membrane is exposed, the platelet reaction begins within seconds. This reaction initiates the formation of a platelet plug, an important step in hemostasis. When large vessels are damaged and vasoconstriction alone is ineffective in achieving hemostasis, platelet plug formation provides an essential element to slow blood loss.[28] As with vasoconstriction, platelet plug formation, in isolation, is insufficient to stop bleeding from major vessels.[30]

Shape change. Normal platelets at rest are disk-shaped and show little affinity toward one another or toward normal endothelial cells.[30] However, when platelet activation is triggered by endothelial disruption, drastic changes in platelet shape occur. Stimulated platelets rapidly become swollen and develop a spherical shape with numerous hairlike projections, known as pseudopods or filopodia, protruding from their surfaces. The shape change serves two important functions in the hemostatic process: it increases the surface area for adhesion, and it increases the likelihood of platelet aggregation.[31,32]

Platelet release reaction. During the shape change, the alpha-granules and dense-granules become centrally located within the platelet.[30,32] In the platelet release reaction that follows, the contents of the alpha granules and dense granules are discharged outside the platelet for use in coagulation and blood vessel repair. Adenosine diphosphate (ADP) is released from the dense granules and initiates platelet aggregation.[11,28] Among its many contents, the alpha granules release fibrinogen, factor

V, factor XI, factor VIII/von Willebrand factor, and thrombospondin.[32,33] During the release reaction, TXA$_2$ is extruded, as well as a platelet surface procoagulant that stimulates formation of a fibrin clot.[30] TXA$_2$ has potent vasoconstrictive properties and promotes platelet aggregation.[11,30,32]

Platelet aggregation. Platelet aggregation is essential for platelet plug formation. As platelet activation occurs, the platelets become sticky and, in the presence of von Willebrand factor, begin to adhere to one another and to the exposed collagen that underlies the damaged endothelium. Endothelial cells synthesize and secrete von Willebrand factor, thrombospondin, and fibronectin, all of which act as adhesion proteins for platelets.[17] Fibrinogen, from the platelet release reaction, also must be present for platelet aggregation to occur.[30]

The liberated ADP and TXA$_2$ from the release reaction activate more platelets, which undergo the same shape and chemical changes. These platelets recruit more platelets until the platelet aggregate grows large enough to effectively plug the damaged blood vessel.[30] Investigators postulate that the balance between the opposing actions of PGI$_2$ and TXA$_2$ regulates the growth of the platelet plug to prevent excessive platelet activation and aggregation.*

The resultant platelet plug is unstable and loosely formed but is usually successful in sealing small vascular disruptions to prevent blood loss. Over the next few hours, the aggregated platelets consolidate and lose their individual identities. Primary hemostasis concludes with the formation of the platelet plug. As the hemostatic process continues, a solid, nonsoluble fibrin clot enmeshes itself in the foundation of the platelet plug.

Role in fibrin formation. Although platelets are important in hemostatic plug formation they are also critical in subsequent steps of the coagulation cascade. Within their cytoplasm, platelets contain an important protein, known as fibrin-stabilizing factor, which is essential for forming a stable fibrin clot. Platelet factor 3 (PF3), secreted by activated platelets during the aggregation phase, participates in reactions of the intrinsic clotting cascade. Additionally, platelets that have undergone the release reaction are more potent than dormant platelets and demonstrate greater effectiveness in clotting cascade reactions.[30]

---

*References 14, 18, 19, 30, 32.

Clotting cascade

Secondary hemostasis begins with activation of the clotting cascade. The clotting cascade involves the sequential release and activation of clotting factors. As each reaction occurs, it produces a subsequent reaction in a cascade effect. Activation of the clotting cascade leads to the formation of thrombin and eventually to fibrin clot formation. Clotting factors are essential components of the clotting cascade and are consumed during the process of coagulation (Table 4-1).

The liver is the primary site for biosynthesis of the plasma clotting factors with the probable exception of factor VIII.[30,34] Factor VIII is synthesized from hepatic sinusoidal endothelial cells and megakaryocytes, as well as from mononuclear cells in the spleen, kidney, lungs, and lymph nodes.[30,32] The biosynthesis of factors II, VII, IX, and X requires vitamin K. Although production of these factors continues in the absence of vitamin K, the final step in biosynthesis cannot proceed in its absence, thus rendering these factors nonfunctional.[30,35] Vitamin K also is required for the production of two anticoagulant proteins: protein C and protein S.[30,35]

When the clotting cascade is activated, coagulation can proceed along two different pathways: the intrinsic pathway and the extrinsic pathway. Depending on the trigger that initiates the coagulation activity, one or both of the pathways can be involved. Although these pathways are stimulated differently and proceed differently, thrombin production and fibrin clot formation are the similar and ultimate outcomes. Both pathways are essential to ensure normal hemostasis.

Figure 4-1 presents a simplified schema of the intrinsic and extrinsic pathways of the clotting cascade. The concept of two separate and distinct pathways helps unravel the complex series of events that occurs in coagulation and facilitates discussion of the pathophysiologic alterations that occur in DIC. However, recent evidence suggests that many links between the intrinsic and extrinsic pathways occur.[11,14] More recently, two plasma proteins essential in the intrinsic pathway have been recognized but are currently not reflected in most traditional clotting factor schemas. These proteins are prekallikrein and high-molecular-weight kininogen (HMWK).

Intrinsic pathway. The intrinsic pathway is stimulated by direct damage to the red blood cells or

Table 4-1 Clotting Factors and Their Sites of Synthesis

Clotting factor	Name	Site of synthesis
I	Fibrinogen	Liver
II	Prothrombin	Liver
III	Tissue factor, thromboplastin	Tissue
IV	Calcium	—
V	Proaccelerin, labile factor, accelerator globulin (AcG)	Liver
VI	Not assigned	
VII	Proconvertin, serum prothrombin conversion accelerator (SPCA), autoprothrombin I	Liver
VIII	Antihemophiliac factor (AHF), antihemophiliac globulin (AHG)	Hepatic sinusoidal endothelial cells, megakaryocytes, mononuclear cells in spleen, kidney, lungs, and lymph nodes
IX	Plasma thromboplastin component, Christmas factor, autoprothrombin II	Liver
X	Stuart factor, Stuart-Prower factor, Prower factor	Liver
XI	Plasma thromboplastin antecedent	Liver
XII	Hageman factor, contact factor	Conflicting data
XIII	Fibrin stabilizing factor	Megakaryocytes, liver
—	Prekallikrein	Possibly liver
—	High molecular weight kininogen (HMWK)	Possibly liver

Data from Bell TN. Disseminated intravascular coagulation and shock: Multisystem crisis in the critically ill. Crit Care Nurs Clin North Am 1990;2:256; and Bithell TC. Blood coagulation. In: Lee GR, ed. Wintrobe's clinical hematology, ed 9. Malvern, PA: Lea & Febiger, 1993.

platelets or by blood coming into contact with negatively charged particles, such as exposed collagen, occurring in endothelial damage.[34] Any of these inciting events begins the contact phase of the intrinsic cascade.[14] Endothelial disruption and the subsequent exposure of the basement membrane promote several procoagulant activities. Although endothelial cells normally have little or no tissue factor production, their tissue factor production dramatically increases when the cells are exposed to thrombin. Endothelial cells synthesize factor V and possess binding sites for factors IX and X, all of which are involved in the coagulation cascade.

Additionally, the negatively charged surface attracts the circulating contact factors, factor XII and HMWK, which attach at the site of endothelial damage. HMWK is contained within endothelial cells and on their surfaces.[36] HMWK also exists in the plasma as a complex with prekallikrein and factor XI.

After factor XII binds to the negatively charged surface, it develops weak but highly specific activity that converts prekallikrein to kallikrein. Kallikrein then converts factor XII into activated factor XII (factor XIIa*) and activates the fibrinolytic system.

Factor XIIa activates both kallikrein and factor XI. The activation of kallikrein involves HMWK as a cofactor in the conversion of the precursor, prekallikrein, to the active kallikrein. A positive feedback loop exists as kallikrein cycles back to convert more factor XII to factor XIIa, and factor XIIa produces more kallikrein to accelerate the contact phase of coagulation[14,30,37] (Fig. 4-2).

The major consequence of activated factor XII is the subsequent activation of factor XI. Activated factor XI reciprocates by causing further production of factor XIIa. Factor XIa stimulates activation of factor IX in the presence of calcium. Factor IXa alone has no ability to continue the cascade. However, when factor IXa is complexed with factor VIII that has been converted to factor VIIIa in the presence of calcium and platelet phospholipids (PF3), it becomes a potent activator of factor X.

---

*The letter "a" denotes "activated."

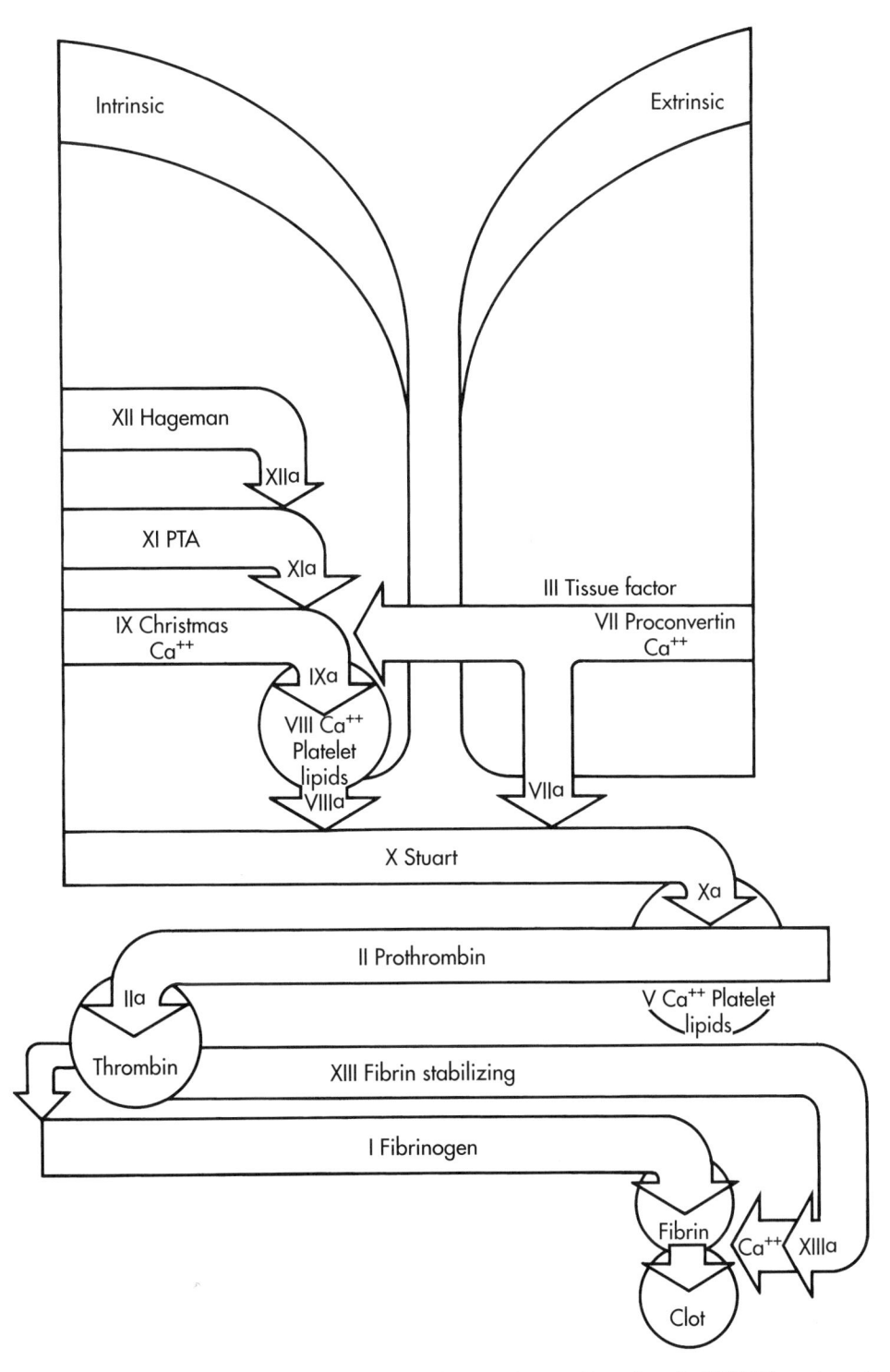

Fig. 4-1 The clotting cascade: intrinsic and extrinsic pathways. (Data from Bell TN. Disseminated intravascular coagulation and shock: Multisystem crisis in the critically ill. Crit Care Nurs Clin North Am 1990;2:257 and Quick D, Trowbridge AA. Use of anticoagulants: Therapy and prophylaxis for thromboembolic phenomena. Postgrad Med 1984;76:152.)

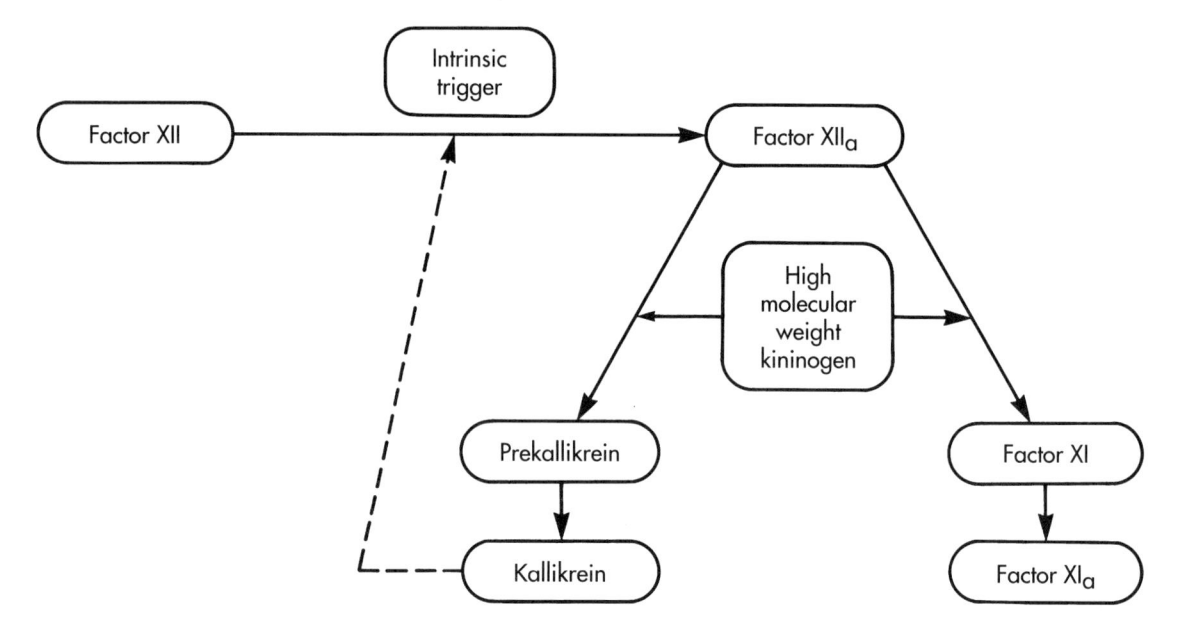

Fig. 4-2 Intrinsic system: factor XII reactions. (Data from Bell TN. Disseminated intravascular coagulation and shock: multisystem crisis in the critically ill. Crit Care Nurs Clin North Am 1990;2:2578 and Ravel R. Clinical laboratory medicine: clinical application of laboratory data. St. Louis: Mosby, 1989, 91.)

At this point, the intrinsic pathway enters the final common pathway of both the intrinsic and extrinsic pathways. Factor X is converted to factor Xa. Factor Xa alone slowly activates prothrombin (factor II), but in the presence of factor V, calcium, and platelet phospholipids, it rapidly stimulates conversion of prothrombin to thrombin (factor IIa). Research demonstrates that this factor Xa complex is inhibited by AT III.[14] Thrombin subsequently cleaves fibrinogen (factor I) to fibrin.

Cleavage of the fibrinogen molecule produces fibrin monomers. The fibrin monomers rapidly polymerize to produce a gelatinous mass of polymerized fibrin that adheres to the fused platelets. Initially the clot is held together by weak noncovalent bonds. Factor XIII, fibrin stabilizing factor, is released and converted to factor XIIIa by thrombin. Through the action of factor XIIIa and in the presence of calcium, the fibrin strands are crosslinked to produce a strong, stable, insoluble clot that is hemostatically effective. The fibrin fibers create a matrix that entraps blood cells, plasma, and platelets. The resultant fibrin clot adheres to the damaged vascular endothelium and prevents further bleeding. Clots are generally limited to the site of vascular injury and are proportional in magnitude to the extent of vascular damage.[38]

Two to six minutes are usually required for a clot to be produced through the intrinsic pathway. Within 1 hour of its formation, the clot retracts, releasing serum and further closing the traumatized blood vessel.

Extrinsic pathway. The release of tissue factor (tissue thromboplastin) from traumatized tissues activates the extrinsic pathway of the clotting cascade. Tissue factor is a membrane glycoprotein contained on most cells and certain tissues have particularly high concentrations of tissue factor, including the lungs, brain, bone marrow, liver, kidneys, placenta, and mesenteral fat.[29,39,40] Tissue factor is not normally present on the endothelial cell membrane; however, it is expressed when endothelial damage occurs.[15] Most tissue factor also contains large amounts of platelet phospholipid.[35] When the extrinsic pathway is activated after severe tissue trauma, blood clots begin to form within 15 to 20 seconds and are limited only by the amount of tissue factor present.[27]

Tissue factor complexes with factor VII and slowly activates factors IX and X. Factor VII, when complexed with calcium is converted to factor VIIa by factors IXa and Xa. Factor VIIa cascades to stimulate further activation of factor X, thereby joining the final common pathway.

Interactions of the clotting cascade. As mentioned above, interactions exist between the intrinsic and extrinsic pathways. The most important linkage is the ability of factor VIIa to activate factor IX.[11,32,41] Therefore, factor VII release can activate factor X through the extrinsic pathway or can activate factor IX with subsequent activation of factor X through the intrinsic pathway. Additionally, factors VIII, IX, and XI should be considered as amplification factors of the extrinsic pathway.[42]

Reactions also occur in the clotting cascade that cause it to further activate itself.[32] Trace amounts of factor Xa, in the presence of calcium and platelet phospholipid, cause rapid conversion of factor VII to factor VIIa. This cyclical reaction produces a dramatic increase in the activity of factor VII. Thrombin, in trace amounts, can activate factors V and VIII, as well as platelets. Thrombin also enhances factor VII activity.[35]

Thrombin. Thrombin serves several functions in the hemostatic process.* It cleaves fibrinogen into fibrin, forming the matrix mesh for a nonsoluble clot. Thrombin generation is localized to cell surfaces, but it diffuses from those surfaces where it acts on fibrinogen. Thrombin also stimulates platelet aggregation during platelet plug formation. Additionally, thrombin incites further platelet aggregation and fibrin formation around the platelet plug. Finally, thrombin serves a vital role by activating the fibrinolytic system to begin clot breakdown.

Normal coagulation cannot occur without thrombin; however, once thrombin is present, it has the ability to promote a vicious cycle of continued clot formation. In addition to its effect on fibrinogen, thrombin can convert prothrombin directly to more thrombin. Thrombin also accelerates the actions of factors VIII, IX, X, XI, and XIII and platelets[27] and converts factors V and VIII into forms that have a higher procoagulant activity.[14,30] In later stages of reaction, thrombin limits its own production by inactivating factor V.[14]

It quickly becomes evident that the positive feedback mechanism of thrombin can dramatically affect the coagulation process. Critical levels of thrombin produce a repetitive cycle of increased clotting, increased thrombin formation, and increased platelet aggregation. This cycle is an important component in the pathophysiology of DIC.

Fibrinolytic system

When a stimulus activates the coagulation system and subsequent fibrin clot formation, the fibrinolytic system is simultaneously activated to control and break down the blood clot to reestablish blood flow. Fibrinolysis represents an important anticoagulant process to balance coagulation and restrict the fibrin clot to the site of vessel wall injury. The process of fibrinolysis involves integrated interactions among four components: (1) plasminogen, (2) tissue plasminogen activator, (3) plasmin, and (4) fibrin (Fig. 4-3).

Fibrinolysis results in the enzymatic degradation of the fibrin clot by plasmin. As discussed previously, the fibrinolytic system is activated when factor XIIa activates kallikrein and when thrombin is produced. Factor XIIa initiates the release of two endogenous plasminogen activators: tissue plasminogen activator (t-PA) and urokinase plasminogen activator (u-PA).[20,43,44] The latter is responsible for keeping hollow organs clot free.[30] The former is the major physiologic activator of plasminogen[4] and is present in a variety of body cells, particularly the endothelium in the microcirculation.[35]

Plasminogen exists in all fibrin clots, having been incorporated into the clot during its formation. The t-PA converts plasminogen, an inactive proenzyme, to the active dissolving enzyme plasmin. The t-PA has a high affinity for fibrin, and its adsorption to a fibrin clot greatly enhances the conversion of plasminogen to plasmin.[4,11,32] Because the plasmin activation mechanism depends on the presence of fibrin, lysis can occur only at the site of clot formation, thereby preventing systemic fibrinolysis.

The fibrinolytic process continues when plasmin is released into the region of the clot, where it proteolytically degrades the fibrin strands. In the blood, plasmin also degrades other coagulation system components, including factors V, VIII, and XIII, and fibrinogen, the same elements that thrombin acti-

---

*References 4, 14, 29, 30, 32.

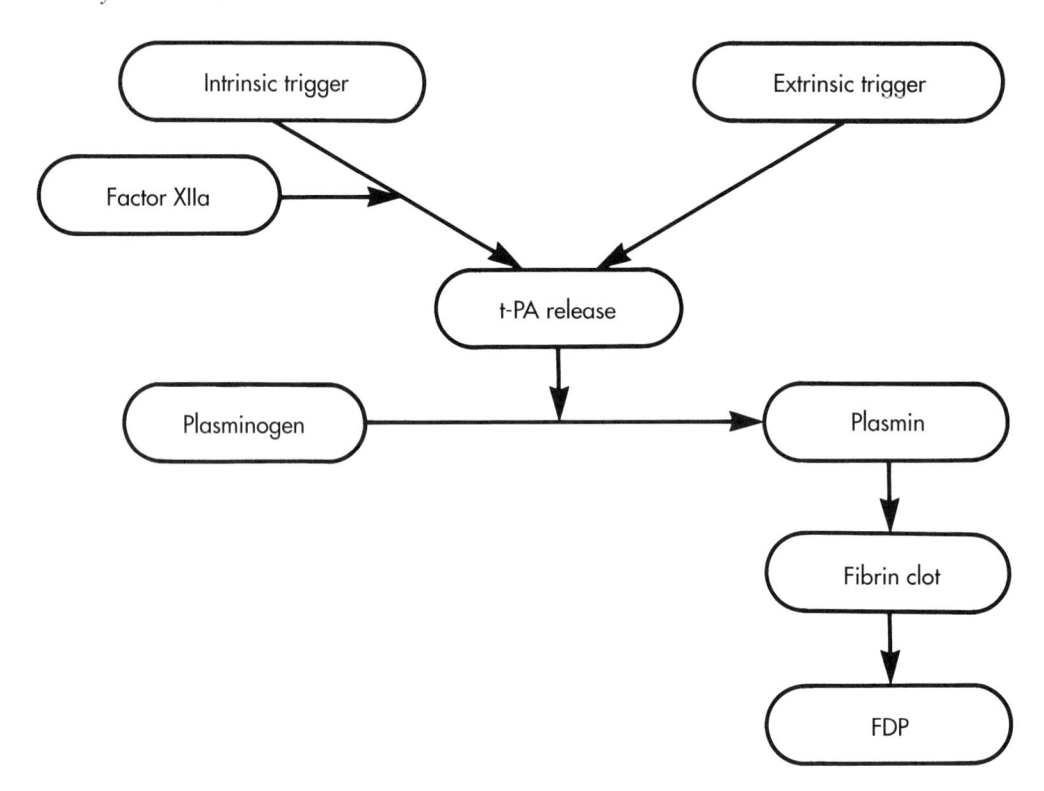

Fig. 4-3   The fibrinolytic system.

vates.[30,45,46] Plasmin that enters the free circulation is rapidly destroyed by two primary plasmin inhibitors: alpha$_2$-antiplasmin and alpha$_2$-macroglobulin. Plasmin inhibitors also ensure that the activity of plasmin is limited to the area of fibrin deposition. Plasmin that is adsorbed onto fibrin appears to be protected from the effects of plasmin inhibitors.[4]

As plasmin dissolves the clot, it releases breakdown products known as fibrinogen/fibrin degradation products (FDPs). As the crosslinked fibrin strands are proteolytically cleaved, they break off in fragments. The initial FDP fragment produced is fragment X. Fragment X then yields fragment Y and fragment D. Fragment Y is further degraded by plasmin to produce another D fragment and fragment E (Fig. 4-4). The identification of fragment D serves as the basis for a newer laboratory test to detect fibrin-specific degradation products. Additionally, plasmin rapidly releases specific peptides, fibrinopeptides A and B-β15-42, which serve as useful diagnostic markers.[5]

FDPs exert an inhibitory effect on the coagulation system by interfering with fibrin polymerization and, in high concentrations, inhibiting platelet aggregation and the release reaction.[4] Normally, however, FDP concentration in the blood is too small to produce an anticoagulant effect because FDPs are efficiently removed from the circulation by reticuloendothelial cells of the liver and the spleen. Once fibrin fibers are removed, blood flow through the newly healed blood vessel resumes.

Hemostatic control mechanisms

CLEARANCE. The procoagulant activities of the body are counterbalanced by a number of hemostatic control mechanisms, many of which are poorly understood. These mechanisms are essential for maintaining hemostatic homeostasis. An adequate blood flow rate is essential for eliminating activated clotting factors and clearing coagulation by-products. As blood moves through the circulatory network, activated coagulation factors and by-products are flushed from the site of injury and rapidly

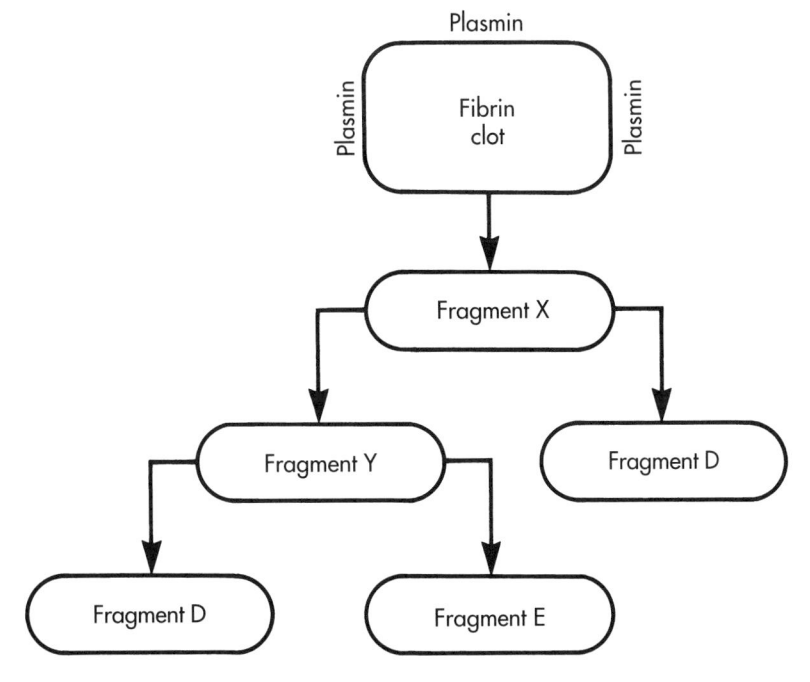

Fig. 4-4 Major fibrinogen/fibrin degradation products.

removed from the circulation by the hepatic system. The reticuloendothelial system, renal system, leukocytes, and the pulmonary circulation all assist in clearing activated coagulation factors, fibrin monomers, and small clots.

COAGULATION INHIBITORS. Several systemic coagulation inhibitors exist in the circulation. The action of these generally inactive inhibitors is limited to the coagulation factors that escape or dissociate from their procoagulant complexes.[38] These coagulation inhibitor plasma proteins include (1) AT III, (2) protein C and protein S, (3) alpha$_2$-antiplasmin, (4) alpha$_2$-macroglobulin, (5) alpha$_2$-antitrypsin, and (6) C-1 inactivator.[35] Tissue factor pathway inhibitor (TFPI) also has been described recently as a coagulation inhibitor.[47] Of these anticoagulants, the best described are AT III, the protein C and protein S systems, and alpha$_2$-antiplasmin.

AT III regulates the clotting cascade by chemically binding and slowly inactivating thrombin, as well as factors VIIa, IXa, Xa, XIa, and XIIa, plasmin, and kallikrein.[11,40,48-50] Heparin, which is endogenously secreted in small quantities by liver and lung mast cells, is another naturally occurring antithrombin agent. The binding of heparin to AT III heightens the affinity of AT III for thrombin and can increase its antithrombin effectiveness 1000-fold.[27] The speed at which AT III inactivates the clotting components depends on the amount of heparin present, but the degree of inactivation is solely dependent on the available amount of AT III.[50]

Protein C is a vitamin K-dependent coagulation inhibitor synthesized in the liver. Protein C exists in the circulation in an inactive form and is activated in the presence of thrombin. Thrombomodulin, the thrombin receptor of the endothelial cell, must complex with thrombin before protein C can exert any anticoagulant activity on the endothelium.[19,51,52] Activated protein C inactivates factors Va and VIIIa, thereby decreasing thrombin production.[28,30,32,43] Activated protein C may also enhance fibrinolytic activity by inactivating a t-PA inhibitor, thus increasing the rate of fibrin degradation.[32,53] Protein C is also thought to inhibit the shock response and to modulate the inflammatory response.[16] Since protein C requires thrombin for conversion to its active form, its effects are limited to areas of active clotting. Protein C and AT III have complementary effects because they each inactivate different coagulation factors.

Protein S, another vitamin K-dependent protein, functions as a cofactor for activated protein C and is required for activated protein C to bind to phospholipids on platelets and other cell surfaces. When protein S is present, the rate of factor Va inactivation is increased.[43] Protein S exists in the circulation in two forms.[42] Sixty percent of protein S in the circulation is bound to C4b binding protein, an acute-phase reactant complement protein.[16,32,53] The remaining 40% circulates in a free form. It is reported that a deficiency of protein S, in the presence of an inflammatory stimulus, can produce an abnormal coagulation response, such as DIC.[54] The protein C/protein S complex is important in controlling the inflammatory response.[16]

Increased information has become available about the fibrinolytic system.[19,55,56] Plasmin is regulated by the plasminogen activator inhibitors, plasminogen activator inhibitor type 1 (PAI-1) and plasminogen activator inhibitor type 2 (PAI-2). The dominant regulator of fibrinolytic activity, PAI-1, inactivates both t-PA and u-PA.[44] PAI-1 exists complexed with t-PA generated by the endothelium.

Alpha$_2$-antiplasmin is the major inhibitor of plasmin in the blood. Alpha$_2$-antiplasmin circulates in the plasma and is crosslinked with fibronectin into fibrin when fibrin is polymerized. Serving as a control for fibrinolysis, alpha$_2$-antiplasmin quickly binds and inactivates plasmin that detaches from the fibrin polymers.[57] Acute-phase reactions occurring in sepsis and trauma stimulate increased levels of alpha$_2$-antiplasmin.[58]

THROMBIN. The confinement of thrombin to the fibrin fiber assists in maintaining some degree of hemostatic control. Approximately 85% to 90% of thrombin formed during clotting is adsorbed to the fibrin fiber[27]; thus fibrin is restrained from moving downstream away from the injury site. Thrombin is also partially inactivated when adsorbed to fibrin.

ENDOTHELIUM. Although the primary role of endothelium in maintaining hemostatic homeostasis is anticoagulation, it has several other functions. Vascular endothelium provides surface binding sites for thrombomodulin and AT III. The endothelium also synthesizes and releases PGI$_2$, which decreases the responsiveness of platelets to activating stimuli. The synthesis and release of many activators, as well as inhibitors, of platelet aggregation, blood coagulation, and fibrinolysis occur from the vascular endothelium.

A delicate relationship must exist between procoagulant and anticoagulant activities to achieve hemostatic homeostasis. One can easily appreciate the potential for uncontrolled coagulation and hemorrhage without the body's integrated system of checks and balances.

ETIOLOGY OF DIC

A vast number of clinical conditions can precipitate DIC. Although DIC can occur with almost any illness or injury, several clinical events with known procoagulant effects predispose the patient to DIC. These events include (1) arterial hypotension, often associated with shock, (2) hypoxemia, (3) acidemia, and (4) stasis of capillary blood flow.[36,59] These clinical events promote pathophysiologic alterations that incite activation of the clotting mechanism. In critically ill patients, the factors promoting the development of DIC are often multiple and interrelated, because the pathophysiologic and etiologic origins of DIC have similarities to many other clinical conditions.[60]

In general, three groups of pathologic processes can promote the development of DIC. These include endothelial damage, release of tissue factor into the systemic circulation, and direct proteolytic activation of the clotting cascade at the level of factor X. However, in many clinical situations where DIC is present, the pathologic processes that incite development of DIC are often multiple and interrelated.[11] The box on p. 83 gives a representative list of clinical disorders that can be complicated by DIC.

Endothelial damage

Endothelial damage results in the exposure of the negatively charged basement membrane, which when denuded is a hemostatically active vascular surface.[23] Many clinical situations, including sepsis, hypoxia, and low-flow states such as cardiopulmonary arrest and shock, can damage the vascular endothelium and cause intrinsic pathway activation.[61,62] Venous stasis resulting from prolonged bed rest can also disrupt the vascular endothelium.[63] Any infectious process, including those caused by bacteria, viruses, rickettsiae, and fungi, can precipitate DIC. Gram-negative sepsis and septic shock are the most common causes of DIC* because endotoxin

---
*References 4, 11, 32, 36, 42, 60, 64, 65.

> **ETIOLOGY OF DIC**
>
> **Endothelial damage**
> Sepsis, particularly from gram-negative bacteria
> Hypoxia
> Cardiopulmonary arrest
> Shock: hemorrhagic, septic, cardiogenic, and traumatic
> Overwhelming inflammation
> Acidosis
> Alkalosis (less common)
> Adult respiratory distress syndrome
> Abdominal aortic aneurysm
> Rocky Mountain spotted fever
>
> **Tissue factor release**
> Trauma
> Burns
> Head injury
> Crush injuries
> Myocardial infarction
> Surgical procedures
> Dissecting aortic aneurysm
> Malignant disease, particularly acute promyelocytic and myelomonocytic leukemia
> Obstetric accidents
>
> **Direct activation of factor X**
> Acute pancreatitis
> Snake venom
> Hepatic disease
>
> **Miscellaneous**
> Massive blood transfusions
> Hemolytic transfusion reactions
> Anaphylaxis
> Freshwater near-drowning
> Hypothermia
> Renal disease
> Human immunodeficiency virus
> Diabetic ketoacidosis
> Acute fatty liver of pregnancy
> Malignant hyperthermia
> Pulmonary embolus
> Extracorporeal membrane oxygenation
> Aspirin toxicity
> Necrotizing enterocolitis

produces considerable activation of both the intrinsic and extrinsic pathways. Endotoxin activates factor XII, thereby inducing the platelet release reaction, endothelial sloughing through intrinsic pathway activity, or possible release of procoagulant granulocytic material.[5,13] Any one of these coagulation activators alone can trigger DIC. Overwhelming inflammation, common in both DIC and gram-negative sepsis, also activates the clotting cascade.

Many patients with meningococcal, pneumococcal, or staphylococcal septicemia experience acute DIC.[66] This is particularly true when the patient is asplenic or immunocompromised. Patients with meningococcemia may develop Waterhouse-Friderichsen syndrome, which is characterized by the rapid development of DIC with associated cutaneous and adrenal hemorrhage and shock.[6] The progressive organ system dysfunction that occurs in this syndrome corresponds to the severity of shock and associated intravascular coagulation.

Arterial aneurysm initiates DIC by activating the intrinsic pathway. Aortic aneurysm is most frequently associated with the development of DIC, although DIC with aneurysms in other locations has been reported.[6] The exact mechanism of stimulation is unknown, but it is thought that injury to the subendothelial layer of the aortic wall produces the trigger for the pathophysiologic events in DIC. Abdominal aortic aneurysm (AAA) repair is considered an effective treatment modality when DIC is present in patients with AAA; however, the surgical repair can result in massive hemorrhage.

Release of tissue factor

The second group of pathologic processes that can incite DIC is the group that causes the release of tissue factor into the circulation. Numerous conditions can activate the extrinsic pathway of the clotting cascade through the release of excessive amounts of tissue factor, including trauma, certain surgeries, malignancies, and obstetric accidents. Additionally, damaged endothelium, induced by the inflammatory mediator tumor necrosis factor, releases tissue factor.[67,68]

Damage to body tissues from traumatic injury can cause excessive tissue factor release into the circulation and subsequent activation of the extrinsic pathway at the level of factor VII. Fragments of damaged tissues and crushed cells enter the circulation and, in association with the circulatory stasis produced by hemorrhage, result in severe DIC.[6] Subsequent development of microthrombi contributes to the appearance of multisystem dysfunction. Traumatic tissue injury from burns, blunt trauma, crush injuries, traumatic brain injury, and myocardial infarction are examples of conditions that initiate DIC through tissue factor release.

Some surgical procedures place the patient at risk for developing DIC by precipitating the release of procoagulant material into the circulation. DIC has been identified as a complication of transurethral prostatic resections,[32] as well as of orthopedic procedures.[6] Surgical procedures that utilize cardiopulmonary bypass technology can precipitate DIC.[4] Use of an intraaortic balloon pump (IABP) to treat cardiogenic shock can contribute to low-grade DIC.[6] DIC can also occur in patients with dissecting aortic aneurysm and those experiencing transplantation and rejection crises.[60] DIC has been found to be a frequent complication in peritoneovenous shunt insertion for refractory ascites.[6]

Acute and chronic DIC often accompanies malignant disease. The appearance of DIC in acute promyelocytic leukemia (APL) is common.[23,32] Because the granules of the promyelocyte are rich in tissue factor, an increased frequency of DIC occurs in APL, particularly when the cells are lysed during chemotherapy. Mucin-secreting carcinomas of the pancreas, prostate, stomach, bowel, and lung release procoagulant tumor products with tissue factor activity into the circulation to promote DIC. DIC has been noted in numerous types of leukemia, Hodgkin's disease, adenocarcinomas, sarcomas, and metastatic solid tumors.[4,6,32,69] Additionally, administering certain chemotherapeutic agents to treat leukemia and other malignancies can precipitate the development of DIC secondary to increased cell debris.[70]

Obstetric accidents are a common etiologic factor in the development of DIC. DIC can occur as a complication of placenta previa, abruptio placentae, retained dead fetus, missed abortion, and hypertonic saline abortion, and it is a predictable feature of amniotic fluid embolism.* The release of tissue factor into the blood stream from these obstetric complications stimulates clotting cascade activity at the level of factor VII.

Direct proteolytic activation

The third group of pathologic processes precipitates DIC through direct proteolytic activation of the clotting cascade at the level of factor X. In acute

*References 4, 23, 30, 32, 60, 71.

pancreatitis, the introduction of pancreatic enzymes into the circulation can activate the clotting cascade at the level of factor X.[4,66] The venom of snakebites also infuses proteolytic enzymes into the blood stream, with the subsequent activation of factor X. Additionally, the numerous coagulation defects produced by hepatic disease can directly trigger the final common pathway at the level of factor X.

Miscellaneous conditions

Numerous other conditions exist that can be complicated by DIC. Complications arising from transfusion therapy can precipitate DIC in the critically ill patient. Massive blood transfusions dilute the clotting factors, as well as the circulating naturally occurring antithrombins, thus placing the patient at risk for developing DIC. In hemolytic transfusion reactions, antigen-antibody complexes promote the release of procoagulant material from disrupted platelets and red blood cells, contributing to diffuse bleeding and sudden hypotension in the patient.[30,60] Immune complexes are also responsible for initiating DIC following anaphylaxis.

PATHOPHYSIOLOGIC ALTERATIONS IN DIC

DIC is characterized by a pathologic overstimulation of the normal coagulation mechanism resulting in disseminated coagulation and excessive fibrinolysis. The abnormality of hemostasis in DIC is the extent to which the normal coagulation mechanism is overstimulated and normal inhibitory mechanisms are overwhelmed when triggered by an underlying pathologic condition. The coagulation mechanism itself remains normal. Overstimulation and dissemination of blood coagulation in DIC produce both thrombotic and hemorrhagic events, the two primary pathophysiologic alterations in DIC.

Excessive clotting cascade activation

Primary pathologic conditions can trigger the coagulation mechanism and the onset of DIC through either the intrinsic or the extrinsic pathway, although the predominant pathway in DIC appears to be the extrinsic pathway.[36,67] DIC resulting from overstimulation of the extrinsic pathway occurs when damaged tissues and cells release the potent procoagulant tissue factor into the circulation. In gram-negative bacterial infection, a common primary condition precipitating DIC, endotoxin is produced that stimulates generation of tissue factor on the surface of monocytes. Experimental data indicate that tissue factor expressed on the surface of endothelial cells or monocytes and macrophages is the most decisive procoagulant material.[36] Tissue factor release stimulates factor VII and activates the coagulation mechanism through the extrinsic pathway. Endotoxin also damages the vascular endothelium, resulting in release of factor XII and subsequent activation of the intrinsic mechanism, platelets, and the complement cascade.

In addition, to the pathophysiologic events that produce activation of the coagulation system, the interrelated cascades of kallikrein/kinin, complement, and fibrinolysis are activated. Subsequently, the complex series of local and systemic events that ensue activate one or more of the other cascades. These activated cascades further contribute to the thrombosis and hemorrhage produced by the primary events in DIC, as well as producing other complications.

Factor XII activation stimulates the kallikrein/kinin system. Bradykinin, a potent vasodilator, is liberated causing hypotension, increased vascular permeability, and shock.[14,72] Factor XII activation also stimulates the complement cascade, which contributes to the pathophysiologic events in DIC by producing anaphylatoxins. The cell lysis, increased vascular permeability, and platelet release reactions produced by complement activation all contribute more procoagulant material to perpetuate the clotting cycle and the inflammatory response.[9,72]

The pathophysiologic alterations and clinical manifestations in DIC are reflective of the balance between the amounts of thrombin and plasmin generated by the overstimulated coagulation mechanism. The excessive thrombin produced in DIC contributes significantly to the physiologic derangements that occur. The amount of thrombin that enters the systemic circulation during DIC far exceeds the ability of the naturally occurring antithrombins of the body, such as protein C and AT III, to control it. During the initial stages, 75% of DIC patients demonstrate a decrease in protein C, and almost all demonstrate a decreased level of protein C activity.[73]

Thrombosis

Thrombin is initially generated in DIC when the clotting cascade is activated, resulting in platelet aggregation and clotting factor consumption. The fibrin monomer then polymerizes into nonsoluble fibrin clots. Fibrin is formed as fibrinopeptides A and B are cleaved from fibrinogen, thus providing a basis for laboratory measurement. Because of the excessive thrombin present, a large number of fibrin clots are subsequently formed and deposited in the microcirculation. The circulatory obstruction that results from these intravascular microthrombi disrupts blood flow and creates widespread organ hypoperfusion, ischemia, infarction, and necrosis.

Thrombin, in addition to converting fibrinogen to fibrin, promotes platelet aggregation.[14,27] In DIC, when excessive amounts of circulating thrombin are present, numerous clumps of aggregated platelets develop and become trapped in the microvascular fibrin deposits.[5] Progressive accumulation of activated clotting factors and platelets in this low-flow state also contributes to the development of microvascular thrombi (Fig. 4-5).

In the critically ill patient, DIC can occur as a complication of shock, or shock can occur as a complication of DIC. Five aspects of shock that contribute to the development of DIC have been described. These include (1) sluggish blood flow caused by poor perfusion and capillary shunting, (2) metabolic acidosis, (3) release of ADP and phospholipids from traumatized cells, (4) hypoxemia of cells, and (5) endothelial damage.[26] These conditions create a physiologic imbalance, which results in an increased tendency to form clots.

Shock is produced in DIC when massive intravascular fibrin deposits create microthrombi that obstruct the intravascular circulation. The resultant stagnation of blood flow and tissue hypoxia produces lactic acidosis. Subsequent reactions increase clotting factor consumption and platelet aggregation. As the capillary blood flow progressively decreases, blood acidity rises, and cellular death occurs. Organ perfusion becomes increasingly compromised because of the increased blood acidity and cellular damage. As organ perfusion is impaired, manifestations of multisystem organ dysfunction or failure ultimately result.

The stasis of blood flow that occurs in shock potentiates the pathophysiologic processes in DIC, causing an accumulation of activated clotting factors in the circulation, which in part is the result of impaired clearance by the mononuclear phagocyte system.[30] In shock syndromes, the combination of tissue hypoxia, endothelial injury, and blood stasis

86 *Primary Events and Mediator Release*

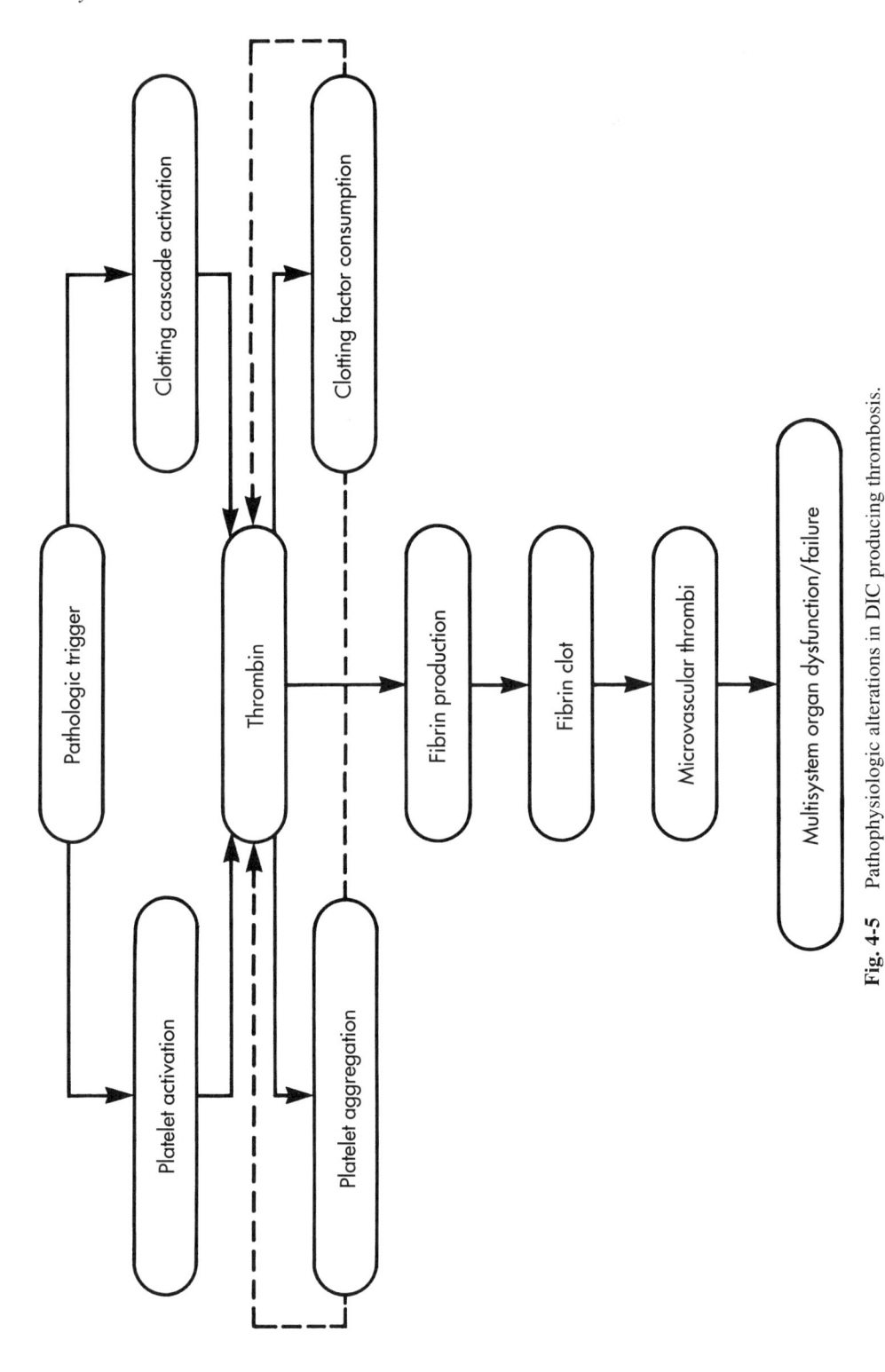

Fig. 4-5 Pathophysiologic alterations in DIC producing thrombosis.

accelerates the development of thrombosis in acute DIC.[61,65]

Red blood cells can be mechanically damaged or destroyed by the thrombotic events in DIC as the cells travel through the fibrin matrix in the intravascular circulation and are sheared. The erythrocytes become fragmented, and microangiopathic hemolytic anemia occurs. The resultant hemolytic anemia, although produced by thrombotic events, subsequently contributes to the hemorrhagic tendency in the patient. Red blood cell fragments known as schistocytes can also appear.

Hemorrhage

In addition to the microvascular thrombi, hemorrhagic complications also occur in DIC. Continual, repeated stimulation of the clotting cascade results in the consumption of clotting factors, particularly fibrinogen (factor I), prothrombin (factor II), and factors V, VIII, and XIII, at a rate greater than the body can replenish them. Hemorrhage and the potential for shock result when the demand for clotting factors outweighs the supply.

Again, excessive amounts of thrombin play a significant role in the pathologic alterations that produce hemorrhage in DIC. The increased quantities of thrombin produced during the accelerated cascading of clotting factors feed back into the clotting cascade to convert prothrombin into more thrombin, thus perpetuating this cycle. As clotting factors are consumed and not replaced, bleeding occurs. Thrombin-induced platelet aggregation produces thrombocytopenia and increases the risk of bleeding. Platelet activation exposes a binding site on the platelet surface that serves as a positive feedback mechanism to further accelerate the clotting cascade.[30] The platelets remaining in the circulation are dysfunctional and can contribute to clinically significant bleeding.[5,13] Additionally, thrombin activates the fibrinolytic system, producing increased fibrinolysis that results in increased bleeding.[66]

Excessive plasmin is also produced when the coagulation mechanism is overstimulated. Accelerated plasmin activity begins to degrade fibrin rapidly before a stable clot has formed. In the absence of a stable clot, the potential for bleeding and/or hemorrhage is greatly increased. The intensified breakdown of fibrinogen into fibrin causes microvascular clots to form randomly in the capillary bed, where they are not needed, and prevents stable clots from forming at the site of trauma, where they are needed (Fig. 4-6).

As fibrin is degraded by plasmin, FDPs are released. In DIC the normal hepatic, reticuloendothelial, and renal clearance mechanisms are saturated by increased FDPs, which contribute to the pathophysiologic events.[35] In particular, hepatic hypoperfusion resulting from hypostatic circulation impairs the clearance of hemostatic waste products.[23] DIC patients also have a decreased tissue macrophage clearing function that further aggravates the clearance problem.[46] As a result, increased levels of FDPs remain in the circulation. In high concentrations, FDPs are very potent anticoagulants; therefore, the bleeding diathesis in DIC is accelerated. Additionally, excessive plasmin contributes to hemorrhage by interfering with normal platelet function.[13]

It has been suggested that decreased tissue macrophage function may be caused by a decrease in the circulating levels of the opsonin fibronectin.[70] Fibronectin is a large glycoprotein with adhesive properties. Fibronectin mediates the reticuloendothelial or macrophage clearance of particulate matter such as fibrin clumps and collagen debris. Decreased fibronectin levels in patients with DIC have been associated with a poor prognosis.[74]

Summary

By examining the repetitive nature of the pathophysiologic events in DIC, one can appreciate the paradoxical clinical situation produced in a patient simultaneously experiencing thrombosis and hemorrhage. Although hemorrhage is the predominant presenting sign, there should be cognizance of coexistent microvascular occlusion from thrombi. The formation of microthrombi in DIC is the more irreversible of the two events and contributes significantly to the morbidity and mortality of the patient through multiorgan dysfunction, irreversible end-organ damage, and possible death.[5,13,72] The self-perpetuating cycle of thrombosis and hemorrhage persists until the underlying pathologic process that triggered the DIC is removed, or until appropriate therapeutic interventions halt the cycle (Fig. 4-7).

RELATIONSHIP OF DIC AND MODS

The interaction of the hematologic system with all other body systems contributes to the relationship of DIC and MODS. Similarly to shock, MODS

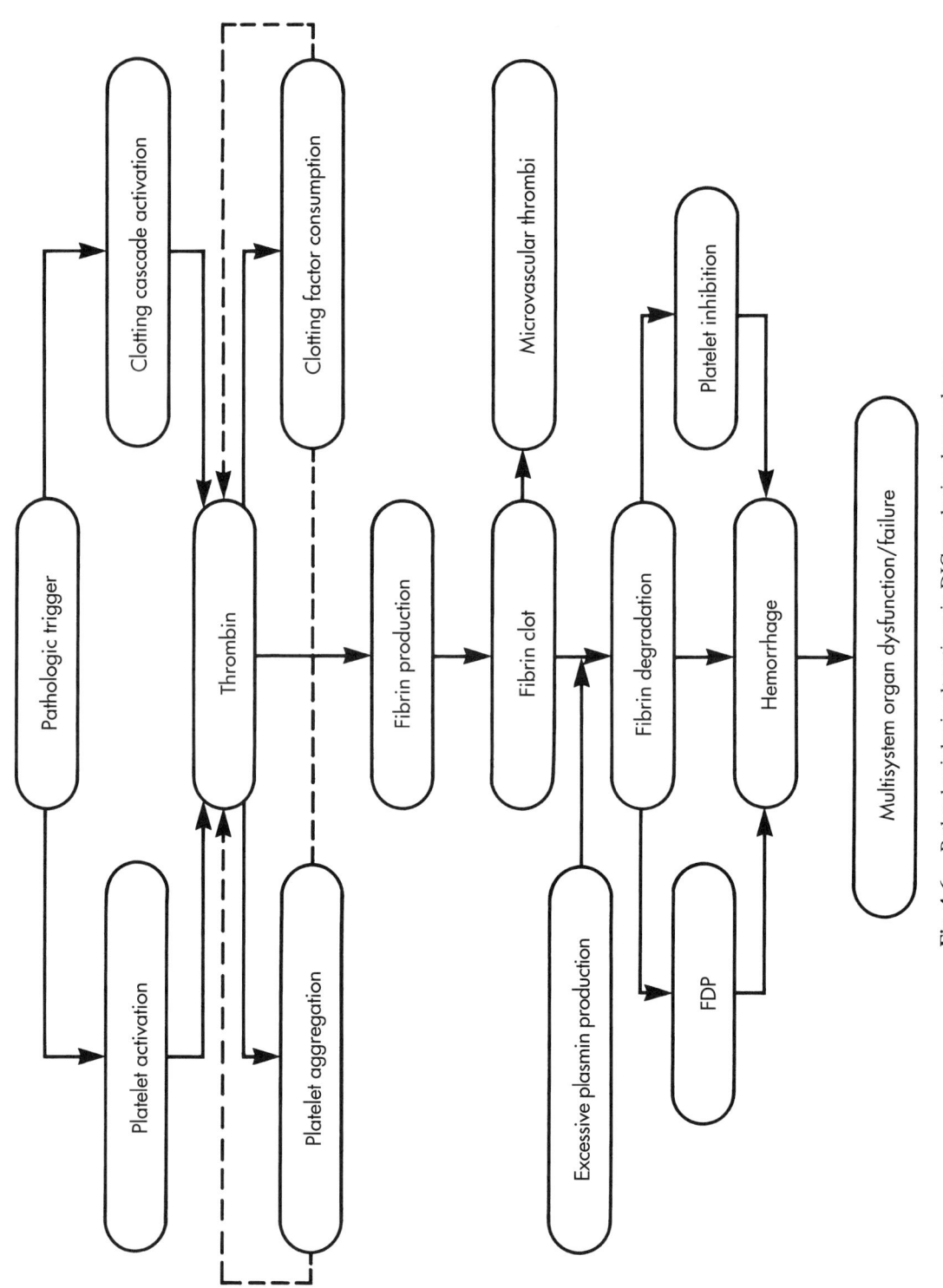

Fig. 4-6 Pathophysiologic alterations in DIC producing hemorrhage.

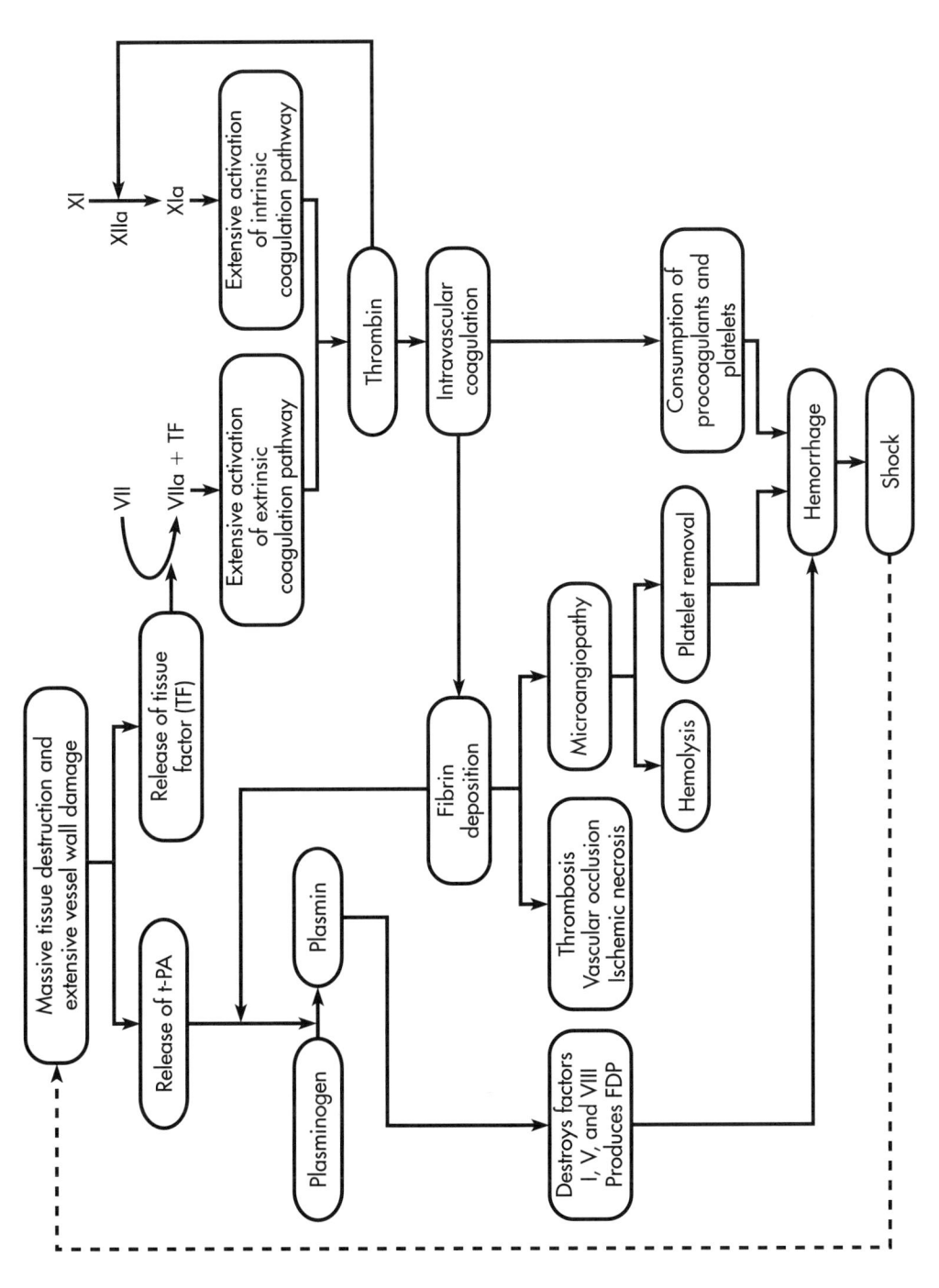

Coagulation and Disseminated Intravascular Coagulation   **89**

Fig. 4-7   Interacting pathophysiologic events in DIC.

can precipitate DIC, or DIC can precipitate or exacerbate MODS. DIC itself represents a functional failure of the hematologic system.[75] Although individual failure of the hematologic system (bone marrow exhaustion) can occur as MODS progresses sequentially, hematologic failure expressed by conditions such as DIC more commonly occurs as the result of the earlier occurring inflammatory response and pathophysiologic changes. Clinical observation suggests that DIC is an important pathogenic factor in the development of MODS.[42,53] Because DIC and MODS share common pathophysiologic and etiologic features, the two syndromes are commonly seen in the same patient.[76]

A rapidly emerging body of knowledge indicates that the vascular endothelium plays an integral, active role in the pathophysiologic derangements occurring in both DIC and MODS. Intact vascular endothelium serves an important homeostatic function by balancing procoagulant and anticoagulant activities.[17] When perturbations of the endothelium occur through influences such as inflammation or injury, the endothelium can actively contribute to subsequent hematologic alterations, including DIC.

Regardless of its etiology, inflammation is often associated with a state of hypercoagulation.[51] Sustained inflammatory/immune response (IIR) activity exhausts both the hematologic and immunologic systems and alters their activity by directly affecting the action of mediators on individual cellular components. In combination with the effects of sustained IIR on the bone marrow and spleen, a decreased ability to fight infection, form clots, and deliver oxygen to the cells results.[77] When the IIR is triggered, a number of humoral, cellular, and biochemical mediators common to both DIC and MODS are released.[78] The interrelated cascades of complement, kallikrein/kinin, coagulation, and fibrinolysis are intricately involved in both inflammation and coagulation.[44] Activation of one usually stimulates activation of the other.

Cellular responses to inflammation contribute to DIC and MODS. Activation of phagocytes, including macrophages and monocytes, leads to procoagulant activity and the deposition of fibrin at the site of the reaction.[60] Monocytes and macrophages produce interleukin-1 (IL-1), which plays a role in inflammation. Together with tumor necrosis factor (TNF), IL-1 acts on monocytes and endothelial cells to cause the release of tissue factor, a known procoagulant.[79] Recently, monocytes and endothelial cells have been shown to play an important role in the development of DIC.[80] Additionally, TNF is increasingly regarded as a possible mediator of DIC and MODS.[81] Platelet activation from endothelial damage and clotting cascade activation is another contributing factor to the common pathophysiologic events in DIC and MODS.

Fibrin deposition in the microvasculature from accelerated coagulation in DIC undoubtedly contributes to organ dysfunction or failure. Hypercoagulability causes widespread microemboli and is considered to be an important factor in the development of MODS.[36,72] Bredbacka and co-workers studied 101 medical and surgical ICU patients admitted for treatment of vital organ dysfunction to explore the relationship of hypercoagulation and organ failure.[82] The group of patients (n = 13) with higher levels of soluble fibrin (greater than 100 nmol/L) had a mean of 4.2 failing organ systems with an associated mortality rate of 85%. The group (n = 40) with low levels of soluble fibrin (less than 25 nmol/L) experienced 0.8% organ failures with a mortality rate of 18% and the group (n = 48) with intermediate levels of soluble fibrin (25 to 100 nmol/L) had 2.6% organ failures with a mortality rate of 27%. The pathophysiologic derangements in DIC produce thrombotic blood vessel occlusions and bleeding in the organs that contribute to the development of MODS.[20]

Asakura and co-workers studied changes in the plasma levels of soluble thrombomodulin in 66 cases of DIC to investigate the damage to vascular endothelial cells and its relationship to multiple organ failure.[52] The study found that plasma levels of soluble thrombomodulin were higher in DIC cases with multiple organ failure than in those without multiple organ failure, suggesting that endothelial cell damage is more prominent in DIC cases with multiple organ failure. The investigators believed that the liberation and resulting decrease in thrombomodulin on vascular endothelial cells may have some influence on further progression of multiple organ failure in DIC. Plasma levels of thrombomodulin decreased as the DIC improved, but remained high or increased in patients whose DIC did not improve. Other studies have examined the role of endothelin-1 and PAI in the development of MODS in DIC patients.[55,83,84]

Although MODS, sepsis, and DIC can be precipitated by a number of pathologic conditions, shock, hypotension, hypoxemia, and inadequate tissue perfusion are commonly implicated in the development of these conditions. Uncontrolled inflammation and sepsis are major underlying conditions in DIC.[85] Likewise, uncontrolled inflammation or infection is viewed by many as the primary etiologic factor in MODS.[75] Hematologic abnormalities are among the earliest manifestations in sepsis.[15] It is reported that DIC is an underestimated factor in the pathogenesis of organ failure in sepsis.[20] When hematologic homeostatic mechanisms fail, the potential for DIC and MODS heightens. In fact, MODS may be the direct consequence of DIC, becoming the fatal complication.[6]

CLINICAL PRESENTATION AND ASSESSMENT PARAMETERS

The critically ill DIC patient displays a wide spectrum of signs and symptoms because of the diversity of primary conditions that can precipitate DIC. Subtle clinical signs can rapidly progress to fulminant DIC accompanied by significant hemorrhage and/or thrombosis. The initial clinical manifestations of the patient are usually related to hemorrhagic involvement, although the initial pathologic events are thrombotic. Careful assessments of the various systems are needed to detect the life-threatening and limb-threatening thromboses that can occur.

In examining the clinical manifestations of DIC and determining appropriate assessment parameters, the critical care practitioner must consider the patient's medical history as well as current medical problems. Organ systems that have been compromised by chronic or acute pathologic conditions may demonstrate pathophysiologic aberrations resulting from DIC. It is important to emphasize that all organ systems have the potential to experience dysfunction or failure in acute DIC. Underlying factors, such as alterations in tissue or organ perfusion, alterations in macrophage clearance functions, preexisting or coexisting organ dysfunction (particularly the hepatic system), and competency of the coagulation and fibrinolytic systems, can all influence the clinical presentation in DIC.

The classic patient with acute, generalized DIC presents with the rapid evolution of bleeding at multiple sites. Ecchymoses, purpura, petechiae, hematomas, hemorrhagic bullae, and scleral and conjunctival hemorrhage can occur. Bleeding or oozing from past and present puncture or wound sites, tubes, drains, and body orifices can develop. Epistaxis and gingival bleeding are frequent occurrences. A decreased urinary output results from dehydration, hypotension, or renal microvascular obstruction. Hematuria secondary to renal infarction and genitourinary, intracranial, pleural, and pericardial bleeding often complicate the clinical situation. Pulmonary hemorrhage is usually accompanied by hemoptysis, tachypnea, dyspnea, and chest pain.[66] Additionally, bleeding into closed compartments and body cavities can result from increased capillary fragility.

Cutaneous manifestations can result from the hemorrhagic events in DIC. Changes in skin color, such as pallor, cyanosis, or jaundice can occur. Jaundice suggests that excessive red cell hemolysis associated with the underlying coagulopathy has occurred.[86] Hemorrhagic necrosis of the adrenal glands and skin is characteristic of the life-threatening Waterhouse-Friderichsen syndrome that can complicate DIC.

Changes in level of consciousness, unexplained behavior changes, focal neurologic deficits, headache, pupillary changes, paresis or paralysis of extremities, changes in mentation, confusion, and seizure activity can indicate cerebral hemorrhage or cerebral thrombosis, which are serious neurologic complications of DIC. Frequent neurologic assessments should be incorporated into the plan of care.

Tarry, bloody stools and hematemesis can indicate gastrointestinal bleeding. Hyperactive bowel sounds, abdominal tenderness or pain, and abdominal distention can also be present. Retroperitoneal bleeding can cause nerve compression at L2 to L3, resulting in impaired lower extremity movement.[87]

The bleeding in DIC usually arises from multiple, unrelated sites. Bleeding in a critically ill patient who has no history of bleeding or who experiences prolonged bleeding should alert the critical care nurse to investigate further, particularly if the patient has any of the four predisposing conditions: arterial hypotension, hypoxemia, acidemia, and stasis of capillary blood flow.[88] Less overt signs of bleeding, such as restlessness and vital signs tending toward hypotension and tachycardia, can be significant.

The sudden appearance of shock in the critical care patient or the presence of shock that is refractory to traditional therapy can indicate the onset of DIC. In severe DIC, the shock may be out of proportion to the blood loss.[11] Changes in level of consciousness, hypotension, tachycardia, tachypnea, and restlessness are among the clinical findings that can occur. The series of events in DIC and shock continues in a cyclic manner until appropriate therapeutic interventions are implemented.

Manifestations of multisystem organ dysfunction or failure resulting from microvascular occlusion can occur in the DIC patient. The skin, lungs, and kidneys have the highest incidence of microvascular thrombi[72]; however, all organ systems are at risk.[89] The underlying disease or injury of the patient plays a pivotal role in determining organ system dysfunction or failure from thrombosis. Although clot deposition occurs primarily in the microcirculation, the macrocirculation can also be involved.[9,72]

Cutaneous microvascular thrombi cause focal areas of infarction in the fingers and toes and subsequent gangrene. More extensive thrombi cause cold, mottled fingers, toes, and extremities that can progress to acrocyanosis or skin necrosis. Pallor, cyanosis, coolness, and diaphoresis may be noted during circulatory checks when peripheral tissue hypoperfusion from thrombosis is present in DIC. Peripheral pulses can be obliterated when excess fibrin deposition produces microvascular thrombi in the peripheral circulation. Pain results when tissue ischemia and necrosis are present in DIC.

The critical care practitioner must observe for trends in neurologic assessment and vital sign data that indicate neurologic decompensation and increasing intracranial pressure. Cerebrovascular infarctions may produce significant neurologic findings, including focal deficits and cerebrovascular accident (CVA)-like symptoms. Spinal artery thromboses producing quadriplegia and paraplegia can occur, but they are rare.[6]

Microvascular thrombi in the pulmonary system interfere with gas exchange at the alveolar level. Shortness of breath, hemoptysis, tachypnea, tachycardia, chest pain, cyanosis, hypoxemia, and acidosis may be present.[62]

Deposition of fibrin and thrombi in the renal microvasculature can produce oliguria, anuria, and hematuria. Ischemic renal cortical necrosis that develops can be complicated by concurrent acute tubular necrosis that develops secondary to hypotension, hypovolemia,[66] nephrotoxic inflammatory mediators, and use of therapeutic agents. Additionally, renal microvascular infarctions create fluid shifts that produce peripheral edema in the extremities.

DIAGNOSIS AND LABORATORY DATA

The diagnosis of DIC is based primarily on a high index of suspicion. The abrupt onset of bleeding in a patient with no previous history of an underlying coagulation defect, sudden organ dysfunction or failure(s), and refractory shock should alert the critical care practitioner to the possibility of DIC. Changes in laboratory values can occur before clinical evidence of bleeding appears, and laboratory values can improve before the patient stops bleeding.[87]

Laboratory data serve as useful indices in the diagnosis and the related therapeutic management of DIC (Table 4-2). Although laboratory data can be highly diagnostic of DIC, they can still be quite variable between patients, so it is important that the data are correlated carefully with the clinical situation.[5] The multiple abnormalities in the production and synthesis of coagulation factors when hepatic disease or failure is present make the subsequent diagnosis of DIC difficult. Diagnosis can also be difficult in the patient who has received multiple blood transfusions, because of the dilution of clotting factors and platelets that occurs.[70]

Acute, generalized DIC is associated with a characteristic pattern of laboratory abnormalities, although no one test is pathognomonic for DIC. Different patterns of laboratory results can develop depending on the underlying pathology, the triggering mechanism for the DIC, and the balance between the patient's inherent coagulation activators and inhibitors.[4] Laboratory values presented may vary from laboratory to laboratory.

Special techniques are often necessary when drawing and collecting blood specimens for hemostatic, platelet, and coagulation assays. Some of these laboratory tests require venous, not capillary, blood and some specimens must be placed on ice immediately after collection. The results of laboratory studies performed on blood specimens obtained from heparinized indwelling central venous catheters or arterial lines may be invalid because of contamination by the heparin. Organizational policy and procedure as to which blood samples can be obtained from heparinized lines, as well as special

Table 4-2 Common Laboratory Alterations in DIC*

Laboratory test	Alteration in DIC	Normal value
Platelet count	Decreased	150,000-400,000/μL
Activated partial thromboplastin time (aPTT)	Prolonged	25-38 seconds
Partial thromboplastin time (PTT)	Prolonged	60-90 seconds
Prothrombin time (PT)	Prolonged	11-16 seconds
Thrombin time	Prolonged	14-16 seconds
Fibrinogen levels	Decreased	170-400 mg/dL
Fibrinogen/fibrin degradation products (FDPs)	Increased	<10 μg
D-dimer assay	Elevated	<200 ng/mL
Antithrombin III level	Decreased	80-120% normal activity

*Laboratory values will vary from institution to institution.
From Bell TN. Disseminated intravascular coagulation: Clinical complexities of aberrant coagulation. Crit Care Nurs Clin North Am 1993;5:413.
Data modified from:
   Bick RL and Baker WF: Disseminated intravascular coagulation syndromes. Hematologic Pathology 6:1-24, 1992.
   Brandt JT: Hemostasis. In Howanitz JH and Howanitz PJ (eds): Laboratory Medicine: Test selection and interpretation. New York, Churchill Livingstone, 1991.
   Corbett JV: Laboratory tests and diagnostic procedures with nursing diagnoses, Norwalk, CT, Appleton and Lange, 1992.

collection techniques required to preserve the specimen need to be followed.

A decreased platelet count occurs in most cases of clinically apparent DIC.[10] A platelet count of less than 150,000/mm³ usually occurs in acute DIC. The thrombocytopenia that occurs in DIC is the result of rapid platelet consumption during the clotting cascade coupled with the inability of the body to replace them.

The activated partial thromboplastin time (aPTT) and partial thromboplastin time (PTT) can be prolonged in DIC. The aPTT and PTT both measure intrinsic pathway activity, but the aPTT is currently the more widely used test for monitoring heparin therapy. The aPTT is prolonged in only 50% to 60% of patients with DIC, so a normal result cannot rule out DIC.[9] Traumatic venipuncture can affect the aPTT results by contaminating the specimen with tissue factor, producing a falsely decreased value.[90]

The prothrombin time (PT) measures extrinsic pathway activity. The PT is prolonged when the triggering mechanism for DIC has activated the extrinsic pathway. The PT is prolonged in 50% to 75% of patients with DIC, and in up to 50% of DIC patients it may be normal or shortened; the PT thus may be an unreliable diagnostic test in this population.[9] PT values are usually prolonged when levels of factor II, V, VII, and X are less than 40% of normal.[90]

Thrombin time is prolonged in DIC. This test measures a late phase of coagulation when fibrinogen is converted to fibrin in the presence of thrombin. Because thrombin itself is so rapidly inactivated by AT III, it cannot be measured directly. The thrombin time test therefore allows the products of thrombin activity to be measured.

Because fibrinogen is consumed during activation of the clotting cascade, fibrinogen levels are less than 200 mg/dL. Fibrinogen levels, however, can be normal even in cases of severe DIC. Because fibrinogen is an acute phase reactant, it is elevated in numerous conditions, including inflammation, infection, tissue necrosis, pregnancy, and some malignancies. This increased rate of fibrinogen production can then be offset by the increased consumption of fibrinogen in DIC; hence, fibrinogen levels appear normal in the patient.[11,30,46]

FDPs are present at increased levels because of the excessive fibrinolysis that occurs in DIC. The usual test for FDPs does not distinguish between the breakdown products of fibrinogen and those of fibrin, therefore, the FDP measurement only indicates the presence and activity of plasmin, not true fibrin clot formation. Currently, FDPs are measured by a test that employs polyclonal antibodies; however, newer tests are being developed using monoclonal antibodies that do not cross-react with fibrinogen (see Chapter 16 for a description of monoclonal antibodies).

A more recent test, the D-dimer analysis, uses monoclonal antibodies to measure the fibrin-specific degradation fragment, fragment D.[11,91,92] D-dimer is formed as plasmin degrades fibrin that has been previously crosslinked through a thrombin-initiated process; the presence of D-dimer is therefore thought to represent both thrombin and plasmin generation. The D-dimer test does not detect fibrinogen or its degradation products and this test, therefore, has a major advantage over current laboratory tests for FDPs.[92]

In a series of 236 patients reported by Wilde and co-workers that included 43 DIC patients, all 43 were found to have elevated D-dimer levels.[93] In the other patient groups studied, D-dimer was rarely found to be elevated when FDPs were normal. Another study of 83 patients found that 93.7% of 48 patients with documented DIC had an elevated D-dimer level, whereas 83.7% of this same patient group had an elevated FDP titer.[94] It has been reported that the finding of elevated FDPs confirmed by an elevated D-dimer test has high predictive value in the detection of DIC.[94,95] One author suggests that the D-dimer assay appears to be the most reliable test for predicting abnormalities in patients with confirmed DIC,[5] although there continues to be variation in the literature, as well as ongoing research as to the most sensitive laboratory indicators to confirm a diagnosis of DIC.

Measurement of AT III levels is considered a key test in diagnosing and monitoring DIC treatment.[5,13] Antithrombin III levels are low in DIC because AT III complexes with thrombin and factor Xa to block the activity of thrombin.[4] Protein C and protein S are two other physiologic anticoagulants that can be decreased in DIC. The current utility of tests measuring protein C and protein S to diagnose DIC is not well documented.

The peripheral blood smear should be examined for the presence of schistocytes, helmet cells, burr cells, and fragmented red blood cells. Erythrocyte deformation occurs when the red blood cells are sheared as they travel through small blood vessels partially occluded by fibrin thrombi, resulting in microangiopathic hemolytic anemia.[30,46]

A clot tube should be drawn and examined in suspected cases of DIC. In DIC, the blood fails to clot in 1 hour or forms a small, poor clot that spontaneously lyses or breaks apart easily when the clot tube is shaken.

Investigators are examining the relative value of measuring thrombin–AT III (TAT) complex and plasmin–alpha$_2$-antiplasmin (PAP) complex to aid in diagnosis and management of the DIC patient.[96] TAT is a sensitive parameter of coagulation system activation, whereas PAP is an indicator of fibrinolytic system activation. The potential of these two tests for diagnostic and management purposes has not yet been fully evaluated. TAT and PAP have been found to be elevated in nearly all DIC patients.[97] Although the ratio itself varies with different underlying pathologic conditions, levels are significantly higher in nonsurvivors than in survivors.[97] However, it has also been reported that the TAT assay may be less effective than FDP values in detecting hypercoagulable states even though it is a more direct method of measurement.[96] The utility of measuring serum levels of fibrinogen/fibrin degradation fragment E (FgE) is being explored. One investigator reports the FgE assay to be 100% sensitive in detecting DIC.[96]

Carr recommends that measurement of platelets, PT, and fibrinogen be used as screening tests before the confirmatory tests of FDP and thrombin time are performed.[45] However, numerous other laboratory tests are used to detect DIC. The measurement of various clotting factors is possible, but is considered of little value in diagnosing DIC because of the variable behavior of the factors in DIC.[9,30] However, when hepatic disease is present, the measurement of factor VIII is necessary to diagnose DIC accurately. Interpretation of clotting factor assays is also difficult because several of the factors are acute-phase reactants.[19] The euglobulin lysis time, the protamine sulfate paracoagulation test, the ethanol gelation test, and the plasma euglobulin test are other laboratory tests that can be used to diagnose DIC, although they are not generally recommended.

Several molecular markers have been identified as being useful in diagnosing DIC.[5] The most reliable of these tests appear to be assays for D-dimer and fibrinopeptide A. Fibrinopeptide A demonstrates the action of thrombin on fibrinogen and the level of fibrinopeptide A is considered to be the gold standard measurement for thrombin generation.[98] Fibrinopeptide A is released from fibrinogen following augmented thrombin generation.[99,100] In addition to the molecular markers AT III and FDP, an elevated level of B-β 15-42 (from the B-β chain of fibrinogen) is another useful marker. Currently, measurement of B-β 15-42 is not a standard test because of its technical difficulty and long turnaround time.[9] In a study of 40 trauma patients with head injury, Gando and co-workers reported that the group that subsequently developed DIC (15 patients) had significantly higher levels of B-β 15-42, PAP complex, and D-dimer than did the non-DIC group.[100] Ongoing research continues as to the usefulness of these molecular markers in diagnosing and managing DIC.

THERAPEUTIC MANAGEMENT

The critically ill patient with DIC and MODS presents a true challenge in therapeutic management for the health care team. The galaxy of underlying pathologic conditions precipitating DIC and the potentially life-threatening multisystem problems it produces demand knowledgeable assessment, intervention, and evaluation to decrease the high morbidity and mortality rates associated with this clinical situation.[88,101] No treatment regimen is definitive for DIC. Therapeutic management of DIC encompasses three aspects: (1) removal of the underlying pathologic condition, (2) restoration of an appropriate balance between coagulation and fibrinolysis, and (3) maintaining organ viability.

In addition to clinical assessment data, laboratory results should be continually monitored to evaluate the effectiveness of the therapeutic regimen in resolving the DIC process. The coagulation profile, hemoglobin, and hematocrit provide important information in the DIC patient who is bleeding. Particular attention should be given to fibrinogen levels, which when decreased indicate increased clotting.

Removal of underlying pathology

The primary goal of therapeutic management is removal of the underlying pathology.* Removing the primary pathologic trigger halts the procoagulant stimulus and allows the DIC process to resolve. Once the underlying pathologic stimulus has been removed, the liver can replenish all plasma protein coagulation factors within 24 to 48 hours provided the patient has normal hepatic function.

As discussed in previous sections, numerous clinical situations cause the release of procoagulant material. Activation of factor XII by endotoxin perpetuates the clotting cascade and increases the propensity of the patient to bleed. Conscientious application of aseptic technique and adherence to universal protocols pertaining to blood and body secretion are necessary to prevent further infection that can seriously affect the prognosis of the DIC patient. Frequent aseptic dressing changes and wound débridement, as necessary, help prevent a nidus of infection. When DIC results from underlying infection with gram-negative bacteria, appropriate antimicrobial therapy, as well as management of concurrent septic shock, must be initiated.

Surgical intervention may be warranted to remove the procoagulant stimulus resulting from neoplasms, trauma, and obstetric accidents when DIC is present. Aggressive therapy must be instituted to correct shock, hypoxia, acidosis, and capillary blood flow stasis, which precipitate DIC by contributing to clotting cascade activation. Methylprednisolone has been shown to decrease the incidence of DIC that occurs after traumatic tissue injury or shock,[6] although its use is contraindicated in sepsis and MODS and remains controversial in many other conditions.

Restoration of balance

Heparin therapy. When the underlying procoagulant stimulus cannot be removed or when hemorrhagic or thrombotic events continue despite removal of the inciting cause, additional interventions are attempted to restore an appropriate balance between coagulation and fibrinolysis. The use of heparin therapy may be considered in some clinical situations; however, anticoagulant therapy in DIC remains controversial. Its efficacy is difficult to document, and although no randomized clinical trials exist to document the beneficial effects of heparin in decreasing the morbidity and mortality associated with DIC, numerous individual case studies exist in which heparin has dramatically improved the clinical picture.[30,45,60,66] However, another report has stated that in at least 95% of DIC patients, heparin did not prove beneficial and could, in fact, be harmful.[11]

There is a general consensus that heparin is indicated in the management of DIC when intravascular microthrombi produce signs and symptoms of ischemic organ dysfunction or when potential loss of life or limb exists.[4,10,102] The effectiveness of heparin is established in some conditions (acute

---

*References 4, 5, 11, 30, 63, 70, 72.

promyelocytic leukemia and retained dead fetus), but it is relatively contraindicated in other conditions (postoperative bleeding, peptic ulcer bleeding, central nervous system bleeding, and hepatic failure), and is the last recourse in others (refractory DIC).[10,37,72] In patients with DIC and septic shock, heparin is believed to be of no benefit.[72] Careful consideration is given to initiating heparin therapy in all DIC patients, particularly those with severe hepatic dysfunction, renal impairment, or vascular damage, because bleeding tendencies can be exacerbated.

Heparin produces two clinically important effects. In low doses, heparin markedly increases the activity of AT III, and together they neutralize free circulating thrombin with a resultant decrease in fibrin formation. The heparin-AT III complex also inhibits the activation of factors IXa, Xa, XIa, and XIIa. Since excessive thrombin generation stimulates the pathophysiologic alterations in DIC, heparin should theoretically interrupt the repetitive stimulation of the coagulation and fibrinolysis cycles. Additionally, the anticoagulant activity of heparin prevents the formation of microvascular thrombi and subsequent capillary bed obstruction, as well as excessive platelet aggregation. Again, the effectiveness of heparin is greatly enhanced when adequate amounts of AT III exist. Exogenous heparin administration does not affect preexisting clots; however, by slowing the coagulation process it allows restoration of the clotting factors.

The recommended dosage of heparin for DIC varies. The dosage must be adjusted when hepatic or renal dysfunction is present, and larger doses are necessary if the patient is febrile. Careful monitoring of serial laboratory data is essential to evaluate the effects of heparin therapy.

Current research has studied the effectiveness of low molecular weight heparin (LMWH) to treat DIC.[99,103] LMWH exhibits inhibitory effects on both factor Xa and thrombin. One study investigated the therapeutic response of 56 patients with DIC after continuous infusion with the LMWH, FR-850. The study concluded that administration of this agent was advantageous to the patient population. Another investigator suggested that LMWH may eventually replace unfractionated heparin in treating DIC.[19]

The practitioner should be alert for exacerbation of the bleeding diathesis, which can occur after heparin therapy is initiated. Any increase in bleeding must be reported immediately to the physician. A volume-control device must always be used with intravenous heparin drips. Protamine sulfate should be readily available in the intensive care unit as an antidote for heparin overdose.

Replacement therapy. Replacement therapy to reestablish therapeutic levels of deficient coagulation components is considered an important treatment modality once the procoagulant stimulus has been treated. Replacement of clotting factors, platelets, and other coagulation elements becomes increasingly more important when clinically significant bleeding occurs as a result of DIC.[104] Replacement therapy, in conjunction with heparin therapy, interferes with thrombin activity and prolongs the half-life of the circulating clotting factors. Even though the levels of clotting components may not be completely normalized through replacement therapy, normal hemostasis can still be achieved.

The use of replacement therapy in DIC has generated some debate. Central to the debate is concern that initiating replacement therapy "adds fuel to the fire" by increasing the availability of clotting factors and platelets to the repetitive cycles of coagulation and fibrinolysis in DIC, thus intensifying thrombus formation. Although theoretically plausible, no clinical studies support the "fuel to the fire" argument against replacement therapy, and some believe it is valuable in restoring hemostasis.* Bick, however, recommends that generally only concentrates and components devoid of fibrinogen be administered to patients with active DIC, particularly if the AT III level is depressed. These replacement products include washed packed red blood cells, platelet concentrates, AT III concentrates, and nonclotting proteins containing volume expanders, such as plasma fraction protein and albumin.[9]

Replacement of deficient clotting components can be achieved with a number of blood products.[105] Fresh whole blood provides stable coagulation factors, but not the labile factors V and VIII; however, it is generally unavailable.[104] Fresh whole blood can be used in cases of massive hemorrhage when volume replacement as well as clotting component replacement is necessary. In other clinical situations, replacement with fresh whole blood can place the patient at risk for circulatory overload. Fresh frozen plasma may be valuable in DIC, because it provides

---

*References 5, 9,11,13, 30, 46.

all of the plasma coagulation proteins, platelets, and AT III. Each unit of fresh frozen plasma should raise the level of clotting factors by approximately 5% to 10%. Fresh frozen plasma also aids in volume expansion.

Cryoprecipitated antihemophilic factor is an excellent replacement component for the hypofibrinogenemia associated with DIC, since it is rich in fibrinogen, factor VIII, AT III, protein C, fibronectin, and factor XIII.[4] Eight to 10 bags supply 2 g of fibrinogen.[106] Because the proteins contained in cryoprecipitate can initiate an allergic reaction, side effects such as fever, itching, and hives can develop. Premedication with 25 to 50 mg of diphenhydramine (Benadryl) helps prevent such reactions.[107]

Thrombocytopenia in DIC can be controlled through the administration of platelet concentrates. One platelet pack should raise the platelet count of a 70-kg adult by 5000-10000/mm^3.[106] Numerous factors diminish the responsiveness of the patient to platelet replacement therapy, including active bleeding, consumption, infection with fever, and the presence of antiplatelet antibodies.[32]

The patient must be closely monitored for signs of transfusion reaction. Appropriate measures must be taken to ensure that the patient's blood and the donor blood are properly matched. Although transfusion reactions can produce serious consequences in any patient, they are particularly problematic in the DIC patient because red cell hemolysis further intensifies bleeding episodes. Monitoring laboratory data provides valuable indices of the effectiveness of replacement therapy and the status of DIC resolution.

Fibrinolytic inhibitors. Fibrinolytic inhibitors, such as ε aminocaproic acid (EACA), generally have no value in the therapeutic management of DIC.[37,108] EACA slows the bleeding diathesis by preventing lysis of the intravascular microthrombi and the resultant release of FDPs. EACA acts to stabilize the microthrombi in DIC; however, it also impedes their clearance from the occluded microvasculature. EACA must *never* be administered to a DIC patient unless the patient concurrently receives heparin.[5] If administered in the absence of heparin therapy during DIC, EACA can precipitate a catastrophic exacerbation of the thrombotic condition. The use of EACA has been reported to produce several cases of MODS, perhaps related to EACA-induced microthrombi.[109]

Antithrombin III. The administration of AT III concentrate is a newer, controversial treatment in DIC, recently approved for clinical use in the United States. It is administered in an attempt to correct coagulation abnormalities and prevent thrombotic complications.[110] In a randomized series of 51 shock patients with DIC a distinct shortening of DIC was reported when only AT III was replaced.[111] In the same study, heparin therapy was found to be of no benefit, particularly when AT III levels were decreased. When heparin and AT III were administered simultaneously, thrombocytopenia and increased blood loss developed.

Another small study of 15 intensive care patients with shock and DIC found that heparin therapy should be started only when AT III activity was within normal limits and that primary replacement of AT III was indicated when AT III activity was less than 70% of normal.[50] This study found no benefits of simultaneous heparin and AT III administration and reported a higher incidence of blood loss during concurrent therapy. In cases of irreversible shock with DIC, the investigator reported that AT III administration could prove lifesaving. More randomized clinical trials with careful interpretation of the influence of other therapeutics need to be completed before the full value of AT III therapy in DIC will be known.

Investigational agents. A number of experimental drugs are being explored for use in DIC. Gabexate mesylate (FOY [Japan]) is an experimental synthetic antithrombin agent that is currently unavailable in the United States. Gabexate mesylate exerts an inhibitory effect on the clotting activity of thrombin and on other reactions in the clotting cascade. Gabexate mesylate may be of particular interest in DIC since its inhibitory effect on the clotting cascade occurs in the absence of AT III.[112]

Treatment with protein C and protein S is also being investigated. From a small study of 3 patients with DIC in Japan it was concluded that protein C or activated protein C administration significantly diminished the hypercoagulable state when therapeutic dosing with heparin was ineffective.[113] Nafamostat mesylate[114] and tranexamic acid[115] are other drugs currently under study for prevention of bleeding in DIC. Tranexamic acid is an antifibrinolytic agent considered to be more potent than other agents and is associated with fewer undesirable side effects.[5]

Hemostatic cofactor replacement. Hemostatic deficiencies need to be corrected in the DIC patient. Folic acid deficiency results in thrombocytopenia and is corrected by administering exogenous folic acid. Vitamin K deficiency results in the inability of the hepatic system to activate several important coagulation reactions involving the vitamin K–dependent clotting factors. The use of broad-spectrum antibiotics and lack of oral feedings in the critically ill patient potentiate a vitamin K deficiency.

Maintenance of organ viability

Impaired organ viability resulting from microvascular thrombotic occlusion and hemorrhage is a major threat to the DIC patient. Impaired organ viability in DIC results from deposition, after excessive fibrin production, of microvascular thrombi in the intravascular circulation. In the bleeding patient, decreased circulating blood volume, which produces hypovolemia and shock, also contributes to impaired organ function. Multisystem assessments are imperative to detect early signs of bleeding and thrombosis and to guide therapeutic management. It is imperative that the therapeutic regimen be individualized to support the presenting clinical problems and to minimize potential complications.

Thorough attention must be given to develop a plan of care that promotes organ viability and eliminates interventions that are deleterious to already compromised organ systems. The potential risks of therapeutic activities should be carefully weighed against the benefits of those activities for the patient.[88,101] In the critically ill DIC patient, the benefits may not outweigh the risks. Despite all precautions and gentle care, bleeding can occur.

When DIC occurs, particularly in MODS, aberrant bleeding can impair the viability of every organ system. The critical care practitioner must be cognizant that bleeding in DIC can be overt or covert, subtle or profuse. Although frank bleeding can occur, bleeding can also manifest as persistent oozing.

Adequate fluid replacement is imperative for restoring sufficient circulating blood volume to optimize maximal tissue perfusion. Hypovolemia from hemorrhage and microvascular obstruction prevents the delivery of adequate oxygen and nutrients to the organ systems, resulting in hypoperfusion, potential cellular hypoxia, and acidosis.

Massive fluid resuscitation may be required to restore blood pressure, cardiac output, and urine output to normal limits. Because of depressed capillary circulation in the patient, the practitioner must be alert to signs of fluid overload during fluid resuscitation.

Vital signs must be carefully monitored for signs of hypovolemia and impending shock. Persistent hypotension, tachycardia, tachypnea, and orthopnea are significant findings in the DIC patient. Insertion of an arterial line is recommended to monitor serial systolic and mean arterial blood pressure readings.[26] Although arterial-line insertion is an invasive procedure that can cause the DIC patient increased bleeding at the site of insertion, it also provides direct access for blood sampling, thus eliminating trauma from repeated arterial or venous punctures. If an arterial line is present, cuff measurements of blood pressure should be avoided because the pressure from cuff inflation can produce capillary rupture and superficial bleeding.

Hemodynamic monitoring to evaluate the patient's fluid status can be achieved through central venous pressure (CVP) or pulmonary artery (PA) readings. Pressure determinations, including pulmonary artery pressure (PAP), pulmonary artery wedge pressure (PCWP), or CVP, should be done every 2 hours, or more frequently as the patient's condition warrants. The data obtained from these measurements are vital for management of fluid replacement therapy. An abnormally high systemic vascular resistance (SVR) reading, decreased cardiac output (CO), decreased PCWP, or decreased cardiac index (CI) can indicate hypovolemia and potential hypoperfusion.[116] Hemodynamic support with dopamine and dobutamine may also be required.

The patient's medication profile must be evaluated to identify medications with anticoagulant and antiplatelet properties. Aspirin and aspirin-containing products interfere with platelet aggregation and inhibit coagulation. Many nonsteroidal antiinflammatory drugs also decrease platelet aggregation and intensify bleeding.[62] Other drugs known to interfere with platelet function include ethanol, tricyclic antidepressants, phenothiazines, furosemide, propranolol, and certain antibiotics.[60]

Other drugs intensify the bleeding tendency of the DIC patient by counteracting, to some degree, the anticoagulant effect of heparin. These drugs in-

THERAPEUTIC MANAGEMENT IN DIC: ADDITIONAL NURSING INTERVENTIONS

The collaborative management of DIC focuses on three major goals: (1) removal of underlying pathologic conditions, (2) restoration of coagulation/fibrinolysis balance, and (3) maintenance of organ viability as discussed in the text. Additional nursing interventions that enhance the patient response to therapy are outlined below.

Altered renal, cerebral, cardiopulmonary, gastrointestinal, or tissue perfusion related to hemorrhage from clotting factor consumption, thrombocytopenia, excessive circulating FDPs, and secondary fibrinolysis; impaired circulating volume from excessive fibrin deposition in the microvasculature; and fluid shifts from increased capillary permeability
Nursing interventions

Elevate lower extremities 15° to 20°
Measure calves every day
Avoid restrictive clothing
Evaluate for lower extremity bleeding if sequential compression hose ordered
Judiciously evaluate the need for and carefully perform turning and positioning
Use foam mattress pads, air mattresses, bed cradle, and therapeutic beds, as appropriate
Carefully inspect skin, particularly under extremity splinting devices
Use caution not to disrupt established clots
Minimize tape application to the skin. If necessary, use silk or paper tape. Use Montgomery straps (Johnson & Johnson) for frequent dressing changes
Measure abdominal girth as appropriate
Monitor for decreased urine output and increased specific gravity
Avoid limb restraints whenever possible
If invasive line not present, use small-gauge needles for venipuncture and venous cannulation unless replacement therapy requires a larger gauge
Apply local pressure for a minimum of 3 to 5 minutes for venipuncture and 10 minutes for arterial puncture
Apply cold compresses to bleeding sites as appropriate
Avoid IM injections
Perform care in a gentle manner
Ensure that all oxygen delivery is humidified
Use minimal amount of suction pressure for NT, ET, or oral suctioning
Prevent situations that produce a Valsalva maneuver, such as coughing, gagging, or straining
Use only electric razor
Gently use soft toothbrush, cotton or foam swabs and normal saline, diluted baking soda, or alcohol-free mouthwash for mouth care
Apply moisturizer frequently to lips
Adequately lubricate tubes before insertion
Apply antiembolism hose as ordered
Incorporate care of invasive lines and monitoring parameters into the plan of care
Evaluate continuous cardiac monitoring data for dysrhythmias or wave changes
Accurately document amounts of all oral, enteral, or parenteral intake and all output
Examine and test all outputs for occult blood as appropriate
Notify physician of abnormal systems assessments and of persistent hypotension, tachycardia, tachypnea, orthopnea, and significant blood loss

Pain related to tissue ischemia or bleeding into closed spaces
Nursing interventions

Assess for verbal and nonverbal indicators of pain
Assess and document character, intensity, location, and duration of any pain
Determine what activities contribute to or help relieve pain
Apply cold compresses to painful joints
Incorporate pharmacologic and nonpharmacologic interventions for pain control
Evaluate respiratory and circulatory status before administering narcotics
Document the effectiveness of pain control interventions
Notify the physician of significant or unrelieved pain

Anxiety related to critical illness, unfamiliar environment and events, and potential alteration in body image
Nursing interventions

Help the patient and family adjust to the critical care environment
Evaluate the impact of the therapeutic interventions on the patient and family's emotional status
Evaluate patient and family resources to determine if outside assistance needed
Identify patient and family coping strategies and encourage adaptive coping styles
Validate the patient and family's knowledge base
Provide honest, careful answers to questions to maintain realistic hope
Allow family sufficient time to visit, particularly when patient's prognosis is poor
Create opportunities for family to assist in planning and participating in the patient's care, should they desire

clude digitalis, nicotine, quinine, antihistamines, dextran, and tetracycline. Many drugs are known to have an effect on other aspects of the hematologic system.[117] The effects, side effects, and possible drug interactions of the patient's therapeutic regimen must be assessed on an ongoing basis.

Oxygen supply and transport must be maximized to promote organ viability in the DIC patient. The sudden onset of respiratory distress or adult respiratory distress syndrome is indicative of impaired lung perfusion. Supplemental oxygen or mechanical ventilation may be required to promote adequate tissue and organ oxygenation. Monitoring oxygen saturation with a pulse oximeter is a useful noninvasive measure.

Arterial blood gas data provide useful information about the existence or persistence of acidosis or hypoxia, two conditions that can trigger DIC. Pulmonary intravascular occlusion alters the dynamics of the pulmonary vasculature, predisposing the patient to pulmonary shunting and subsequent compromised gas exchange.[86] Pulmonary hypertension, evidenced by increased PA pressures, suggests intrapulmonary vascular clotting.[87] Pulmonary embolism can occur from microvascular obstruction and produce an increased alveolar-arterial (A-a) oxygen gradient greater than 30 mm Hg.[116]

Critical illness requires additional calories and protein to meet the increased metabolic demands of the body. Adequate nutrients are required, too, for production of new red blood cells to replace those lost through bleeding. Inadequate nutrition affects, and is affected by, the immune response, thus potentially increasing the occurrence and the severity of infection.[118] Additional nursing interventions to supplement the therapeutic management plan are found in the box on p. 99.

CONCLUSION

Dysfunction in the complex physiologic interactions occurring among organ systems and the IIR in MODS contributes to the pathophysiologic alterations in normal hemostatic function that produce the simultaneous thrombotic and hemorrhagic events in DIC. In the critically ill patient, DIC can also potentiate the development of MODS. Although numerous clinical conditions can precipitate DIC and MODS, uncontrolled inflammation and infection are commonly implicated in both conditions. Therapeutic management must focus on removing the underlying pathologic conditions, restoring an appropriate balance between coagulation and fibrinolysis, and maintaining organ viability. Intensive, knowledgeable assessment, planning, and intervention are vital to minimizing the high morbidity and mortality rates associated with DIC and MODS.

REFERENCES

1. Mammen EF. Perspectives for the future. Intensive Care Med 1993;19:S29-S34.
2. Bithell TC. Acquired coagulation disorders. Wintrobe's clinical hematology. 5th ed. Philadelphia: Lea & Febiger; 1993.
3. Johanson BC et al. Standards for critical care. 3rd ed. St. Louis: Mosby, 1988.
4. Lazarchick J, Krizer J. Interaction of fibrinolytic, coagulation, and kinin systems and related pathology. In: Pittiglio DH, Sacher RA, eds. Clinical hematology and fundamentals of hemostasis. Philadelphia: FA Davis, 1987.
5. Bick RL. Disseminated intravascular coagulation. Hematol Oncol Clin North Am 1992;6:1259-1285.
6. Baker WF. Clinical aspects of disseminated intravascular coagulation: A clinician's point of view. Semin Thromb Hemost 1989;15:1-57.
7. Gilbert JA, Ricciardetto PS. Disseminated intravascular coagulation. Hematologic/Oncologic Emergencies 1993;11:465-480.
8. Rubin RN, Colman RW. Disseminated intravascular coagulation: Approach to treatment. Drugs 1992;44:963-971.
9. Bick RL. Disseminated intravascular coagulation: Objective criteria for diagnosis and management. Med Clin North Am 7 1994;8:511-543.
10. Levitt LJ. Disseminated intravascular coagulation. In: Rippe JM, ed. Manual of intensive care medicine. Boston: Little Brown, 1989.
11. Logan LJ. Hemostasis and bleeding disorders. In: Mazza JJ, ed. Manual of clinical hematology. Boston: Little Brown, 1988.
12. Feinstein DI. Treatment of disseminated intravascular coagulation. Semin Thromb Hemost 1988;14:351-362.
13. Bick RL, Baker WF. Disseminated intravascular coagulation syndromes. Hematol Pathol 1992;6:1-24.
14. Saito H. Normal hemostatic mechanisms. In: Ratnoff OD, Forbes CD, eds. Disorders of hemostasis. Philadelphia: WB Saunders, 1991.
15. Bone RC. Modulators of coagulation: A critical appraisal of their role in sepsis. Arch Intern Med 1992;152:1381-1389.
16. Esmon CT, Taylor FB, Snow TR. Inflammation and coagulation: Linked processes potentially regulated through a common pathway mediated by protein C. Thromb Haemost 1991;66:160-165.
17. Bevilacqua MP, Gimbrone MA. Inducible endothelial functions in inflammation and coagulation. Semin Thromb Hemost 1987;13:425-433.
18. Stemerman MB, Colton C, Morell E. Perturbations of the endothelium. In: Spaet TH, ed. Progress in hemostasis and thrombosis. Orlando: Grune and Stratton, 1987.
19. Risberg B, Andreasson S, Ericksson E. Disseminated intravascular coagulation. Acta Anaesthesiol Scand 1991;35, supplementum 95:60-71.

20. ten Cate H, Brandjes DPM, Wolters HJ, et al. Disseminated intravascular coagulation: Pathophysiology, diagnosis, and treatment. New Horiz 1993:1:312-323.
21. Paraskevas F, Foerster J. Cell interactions in the immune response. Wintrobe's clinical hematology. 5th ed. Philadelphia: Lea & Febiger, 1993.
22. Shuman MA. Endothelial cell structure and function. In Hoffman R, Benz Jr EJ, Shattil SJ et al, eds. Hematology: Basic principles and practice. 2nd ed. New York: Churchill Livingstone, 1995.
23. Bithell TC. Disorders of blood coagulation. In: Thorup OA, ed. Leavell and Thorup's fundamentals of clinical hematology. ed 5. Philadelphia: WB Saunders, 1987.
24. Jaffe EA. Endothelial cell structure and function. In: Hoffman R, Benz Jr EJ, Shattil SJ et al, eds. Hematology: Basic principles and practice. New York: Churchill Livingstone, 1995.
25. Brozna JP. Shwartzman reaction. Semin Thromb Hemost 1990;16:326-332.
26. Perry AG, Potter PA. Shock: Comprehensive nursing management. St. Louis: Mosby, 1988.
27. Guyton AC. Textbook of medical physiology. 8th ed. Philadelphia: WB Saunders, 1991.
28. Van Dam-Meiras MCE, Muller AD. Blood coagulation as a part of the haemostatic system. In: Zwaal RFA, Hemker HC, eds. Blood coagulation. New York: Elsevier Science Publishers, 1986.
29. Thompson AR, Harker LA. Manual of hemostasis and thrombosis. 3rd ed. Philadelphia: FA Davis, 1983.
30. Babior BM, Stossel TP. Hematology: A pathophysiological approach. 2nd ed. New York: Churchill Livingstone, 1990.
31. Isenberg WM, Bainton DF. Megakaryocyte and platelet structure. In: Hoffman R, Benz Jr EJ, Shattil SJ et al, eds. Hematology: Basic principles and practice. New York: Churchill Livingstone, 1991.
32. Rapaport SI. Introduction to hematology. 2nd ed. Philadelphia: JB Lippincott, 1987.
33. Ware JA, Coller BS. Platelet morphology, biochemistry, and function. In: Beutler E, Lichtman M, Coller BS et al, eds. Williams hematology. 5th ed. New York: McGraw-Hill, 1995.
34. Bithell TC. Blood coagulation. Wintrobe's clinical hematology. 5th ed. Philadelphia: Lea & Febiger, 1993.
35. Bithell TC. Normal hemostasis and coagulation. In: Thorup OA, ed. Leavell and Thorup's fundamentals of clinical hematology. 5th ed. Philadelphia: WB Saunders, 1987.
36. Muller-Berghaus G. Pathophysiologic and biochemical events in disseminated intravascular coagulation: Dysregulation of procoagulant and anticoagulant pathways. Semin Thromb Hemost 1989;15:58-87.
37. Nanfro JJ. Anticoagulants in critical care medicine. In: Chernow B, ed. The pharmacologic approach to the critically ill patient. 2nd ed. Baltimore: Williams and Wilkins, 1988.
38. Sala N, Fontcuberta J, Rutllant MLL. New biological concepts on coagulation inhibitors. Intensive Care Med 1993;19: S3-S7.
39. Osterud B. Initiation mechanisms: Activation induced by thromboplastin. In: Zwaal RFA, Hemker HC, eds. Blood coagulation. New York: Elsevier Science Publishers, 1986.
40. Griffith MJ. Inhibitors: Antithrombin III and heparin. In: Zwaal RFA, Hemker HC, eds. Blood coagulation. New York: Elsevier Science Publishers, 1986.
41. Bach RR. Initiation of coagulation by tissue factor. CRC Crit Rev Biochem 1988;23:339-368.
42. Thijs LG et al. Coagulation disorders in septic shock. Intensive Care Med 1993;19:S8-S15.
43. Comp PC. Hereditary disorders predisposing to thrombosis. In: Coller BS, ed. Progress in hemostasis and thrombosis. Orlando: Grune and Stratton, 1986.
44. Idell S. Extravascular coagulation and fibrin deposition in acute lung injury. New Horiz 1994;2:566-574.
45. Carr ME. Disseminated intravascular coagulation: Pathogenesis, diagnosis, and therapy. J Emerg Med 1987;5:311-322.
46. Colman RW, Rubin RN. Disseminated intravascular coagulation due to malignancy. Semin Oncol 1990;17:172-186.
47. Rapaport SI. The extrinsic pathway inhibitor: A regulator of tissue factor-dependent blood coagulation. Thromb Haemost 1991;66:6-15.
48. Schwartz RS et al. Clinical experience with antithrombin III concentrate in the treatment of congenital and acquired deficiency of antithrombin. The antithrombin III study group. Am J Med 1989;87:53S-60S.
49. Hauptman TG et al. Efficacy of antithrombin III in endotoxin-induced disseminated intravascular coagulation. Circ Shock 1988;25:111-122.
50. Vinazzer H. Therapeutic use of antithrombin III in shock and disseminated intravascular coagulation. Semin Thromb Hemost 1989;15:347-352.
51. Esmon NL. Thrombomodulin. In: Coller BS, ed. Progress in hemostasis and thrombosis. Philadelphia: WB Saunders, 1989.
52. Asakura H et al. Plasma levels of soluble thrombomodulin increase in cases of disseminated intravascular coagulation with organ failure. Am J Hematol 1991;38:281-287.
53. Fourrier F et al. Septic shock, multiple organ failure, and disseminated intravascular coagulation: Compared patterns of antithrombin III, protein C, and protein S deficiencies. Chest 1992;101:816-823.
54. Taylor FB. Protein S, C4b binding protein, and the hypercoagulable state. J Lab Clin Med 1992;119:596-597.
55. Asakura H et al. Changes in plasma levels of tissue-plasminogen activator/inhibitor complex and active plasminogen activator inhibitor in patients with disseminated intravascular coagulation. Am J Hematol 1991;36:176-183.
56. Gettins P, Patston PA, Schapira M. Structure and mechanism of action of serpins. Hematol Oncol Clin North Am 1992; 6:1393-1408.
57. Moake J. Hypercoagulable states: New knowledge about old problems. Hosp Pract 1991;26:31-42.
58. Wolf P. The importance of alpha$_2$-antiplasmin in the defibrination syndrome. Arch Intern Med 1989;149:1724-1725.
59. Hudak CM, Gallo BM, Benz JJ, eds. Critical care nursing: A holistic approach. 6th ed. Philadelphia: JB Lippincott, 1994.
60. Baue AE. Multiple organ failure: Patient care and prevention. St. Louis: Mosby, 1990.
61. Ratnoff OD. Disseminated intravascular coagulation. In: Ratnoff OD, Forbes CD, eds. Disorders of hemostasis. Philadelphia: WB Saunders, 1991.

62. Thelan LA, Davie JK, Urden LD. Textbook of critical care nursing: Diagnosis and management. St. Louis: Mosby, 1990.
63. Suchak BA, Barbon CB. Disseminated intravascular coagulation: A nursing challenge. Orthop Nurs 1989;8:61-69.
64. Yurt RW, Lowry SF. Role of the macrophage and endogenous mediators in multiple organ failure. In: Deitch EA, ed. Multiple organ failure: Pathophysiology and basic concepts of therapy. New York: Thieme Medical Publishers, 1990.
65. Esparaz B, Green D. Disseminated intravascular coagulation. Crit Care Nurs Q 1990;13:7-13.
66. Brozovic M. Disseminated intravascular coagulation. In: Bloom AL, Thomas DP, eds. Haemostasis and thrombosis. 2nd ed. New York: Churchill Livingstone, 1987.
67. Aderka D. Role of tumor necrosis factor in the pathogenesis of intravascular coagulopathy of sepsis: Potential new therapeutic implications. Isr J Med Sci 1991;27:52-60.
68. Taylor FB. The inflammatory-coagulant axis in the host response to gram-negative sepsis: Regulatory roles of proteins and inhibitors of tissue factor. New Horiz 1994;2:555-565.
69. Young LM. DIC: The insidious killer. Crit Care Nurse 1990;10:26-33.
70. Griffin JP. Hematology and immunology: Concepts for nursing. Norwalk, CT: Appleton-Century-Crofts, 1986.
71. Poole J. HELLP syndrome and coagulopathies of pregnancy. Crit Care Nurs Clin North Am 1993;5:475-487.
72. Bick RL. Disseminated intravascular coagulation and related syndromes: A clinical review. Semin Thromb Hemost 1988;14:299-338.
73. Turgeon ML. Clinical hematology: Theory and procedures. Boston: Little Brown, 1993.
74. Hesselvik F et al. Fibronectin and other DIC-related variables in septic ICU patients receiving cryoprecipitate. Scand J Clin Lab Invest 1985;45:67-74.
75. Fry DE. Diagnosis and epidemiology of multiple organ failure. In: Deitch EA, ed. Multiple organ failure: Pathophysiology and basic concepts of therapy. New York: Thieme Medical Publishers, 1990.
76. Secor VH. Multisystem organ failure: Background and etiology. In: Secor VH, ed: Multisystem organ failure: Pathophysiology and clinical implications. 2nd ed. St. Louis: Mosby, 1996.
77. McFadden ME, Sartorius SE. Multiple organ failure in the patient with cancer: Part II-Nursing implications. Oncol Nurs Forum 1992;19:727-737.
78. Secor VH. Mediators of coagulation and inflammation: Relationship and clinical significance. Crit Care Nurs Clin North Am 1993;5:411-434.
79. Takahashi H et al. Tissue factor in plasma of patients with disseminated intravascular coagulation. Am J Hematol 1994;46:333-337.
80. Wada H et al. Plasma level of IL-1β in disseminated intravascular coagulation. Thromb Haemost 1991;65:364-368.
81. Wada H et al. Plasma level of tumor necrosis factor in disseminated intravascular coagulation. Am J Hematol 1991;37:147-151.
82. Bredbacka S, Blomback M, Wiman B. Soluble fibrin: A predictor for the development and outcome of multiple organ failure. Am J Hematol 1994;46:289-294.
83. Asakura H et al. Role of endothelin in disseminated intravascular coagulation. Am J Hematol 1992;41:71-75.
84. Ishibashi M et al. Endothelin-1 as an aggravating factor of disseminated intravascular coagulation associated with malignant neoplasms. Cancer 1994;73:191-195.
85. Tanaka T et al. Sepsis model with reproducible manifestations of multiple organ failure (MOF) and disseminated intravascular coagulation (DIC). Thromb Res 1989;54:53-61.
86. Dolan JT. Critical care nursing: Management through the nursing process. Philadelphia: FA Davis, 1991.
87. Moorhouse MF, Geissler AC, Doenges ME. Critical care plans: Guidelines for patient care. Philadelphia: FA Davis, 1987.
88. Bell TN. Disseminated intravascular coagulation and shock: Multisystem crisis in the critically ill. Crit Care Nurs Clin North Am 1990;2:255-268.
89. Hardaway RM. Organ damage in shock, disseminated intravascular coagulation, and stroke. Compr Ther 1992;18:17-21.
90. Tietz NW. Clinical guide to laboratory tests. 2nd ed. Philadelphia: WB Saunders, 1990.
91. Tomiya T et al. Plasmin alpha$_2$-plasmin inhibitor-plasmin complex and FDP D-dimer in fulminant hepatic failure. Thromb Res 1989;53:253-260.
92. Hafter R et al. Measurement of crosslinked fibrin derivatives in plasma and ascitic fluid with monoclonal antibodies against D-dimer using EIA and latex test. Scand J Clin Lab Invest 1985;45:137-144.
93. Wilde JT et al. Plasma D-dimer levels and their relationship to serum fibrinogen/fibrin degradation products in hypercoagulable states. Br J Haematol 1989;71:65-70.
94. Bick RL, Baker WF. Diagnostic efficacy of the D-dimer assay in disseminated intravascular coagulation (DIC). Thromb Res 1992;65:785-790.
95. Carr JM, McKinney M, McDonagh J. Diagnosis of disseminated intravascular coagulation: Role of D-dimer. Am J Clin Pathol 1989;91:280-287.
96. Boisclair M et al. A comparative evaluation of assays for markers of activated coagulation and/or fibrinolysis: Thrombin-antithrombin complex, D-dimer, and fibrinogen/fibrin fragment E antigen. Br J Haematol 1990;74:471-479.
97. Takahashi T et al. Thrombin vs. plasmin generation in disseminated intravascular coagulation associated with various underlying disorders. Am J Hematol 1990;33:90-95.
98. Prisco D. Markers of increased thrombin generation. Res Clin Lab 1990;20:217-225.
99. Deguchi K et al. Dynamic fluctuations in blood of thrombin/antithrombin III complex (TAT). Am J Hematol 1991;38:86-89.
100. Gando S, Tedo I, Kubota M. Posttrauma coagulation and fibrinolysis. Crit Care Med 1992;20:594-600.
101. Bell TN. Disseminated intravascular coagulation: Clinical complexities of aberrant coagulation. Crit Care Nurs Clin North Am 1993;5:389-410.
102. Cerra FB. Manual of critical care. St. Louis: Mosby, 1987.
103. Oguma Y et al. Treatment of disseminated intravascular coagulation with low molecular weight heparin. Semin Thromb Hemost 1990;16,supplement:34-40.
104. Pisciotto PT, Snyder EL. Use and administration of blood and components. In: Chernow B, ed. The pharmacologic approach to the critically ill patient. 2nd ed. Baltimore: Williams and Wilkins, 1988.

105. Coffland FI, Shelton DM. Blood component replacement therapy. Crit Care Nurs Clin North Am 1993;5:543-556.
106. US Department of Health and Human Services, National Institutes of Health. Transfusion therapy guidelines for nurses. NIH publication no. 90-2668, 1990.
107. Hamilton GC. Hemostasis out of order. Emerg Med 1985;17:82-88, 90, 92-93.
108. Stump DC et al. Pathologic fibrinolysis as a cause of clinical bleeding. Semin Thromb Hemost 1990;16:260-273.
109. Williams E. Plasma alpha$_2$-antiplasmin activity. Role in the evaluation and management of fibrinolytic states and other bleeding disorders. Arch Intern Med 1989;149:1769-1772.
110. Menache D. Antithrombin III concentrates. Hematol Oncol Clin North Am 1992;6:1115-1120.
111. Blauhut B, Kramar H, Vinazzer H. Substitution of antithrombin III in shock and DIC: A randomized study. Thromb Res 1985;39:81-89.
112. Umeki S et al. Gabexate mesylate as a therapy for disseminated intravascular coagulation. Arch Intern Med 1988;148:1409-1412.
113. Okajima K et al. Treatment of patients with disseminated intravascular coagulation by protein C. Am J Hematol 1990;33:277-278.
114. Takahashi H et al. Nafamostat mesilate (FUT-175) in the treatment of patients with disseminated intravascular coagulation. Thromb Haemost 1989;62:90-95.
115. Takada A et al. Prevention of severe bleeding by tranexamic acid in a patient with disseminated intravascular coagulation. Thromb Res 1990;58:101-108.
116. Swearingen PL, Sommers MS, Miller K. Manual of critical care: Applying nursing diagnosis to adult critical illness. 3rd ed. St. Louis: Mosby, 1994.
117. Fareed J et al. Drug-induced alterations of hemostasis and fibrinolysis. Hematol Oncol Clin North Am 1992;6:1229-1245.
118. McFarland GK, McFarlane EA, eds. Nursing diagnosis and intervention: Planning for patient care. St. Louis: Mosby, 1989.

Section 2

PATHOPHYSIOLOGIC CHANGES

Pathophysiologic changes occur at the systemic level following the primary events and overwhelming activation of mediators. The exaggerated mediator responses provoke maldistribution of circulating volume, imbalance of oxygen supply and demand, and alterations in metabolism. These three pathophysiologic changes incite ischemia, tissue damage, and organ dysfunction and failure.

5. Maldistribution of Circulating Volume
6. Imbalance of Oxygen Supply and Demand
7. Alterations in Metabolism

CHAPTER 5

Maldistribution of Circulating Volume

Elaine V. Robins

Multiple organ dysfunction syndrome (MODS) is the leading cause of mortality in the critically ill patient. Risk factors identified by Cerra in the development of MODS are sepsis; perfusion deficits, as with ruptured aneurysms; a persistent source of severe inflammation, for example, pancreatitis; and a persistent source of dead or injured tissue, as with multiple trauma or severe burns.[1] Maldistribution of circulating volume is a major component in the pathophysiology of MODS leading to organ failure. This chapter will focus on the cause of the maldistribution of blood flow and treatment modalities available in the treatment of MODS.

Primary MODS is directly associated with the initial insult and is usually caused by direct tissue trauma, impaired perfusion, or ischemia. The injury is characterized by a stress response that produces local inflammation. *Secondary* MODS is the perpetuation of the initial local inflammatory response that produces a systemic inflammatory response syndrome (SIRS) and an exaggerated neuroendocrine (stress) response causing distant organ dysfunction. These exaggerated responses produce blood flow maldistribution, cell injury, or cell death. The cause of the exaggerated inflammatory response is not well understood, but is probably due to an imbalance between mediators and their inhibitors, for example, oxygen-derived free radicals (which are oxidants) and antioxidant defenses targeted against them. The imbalance favors the mediator, such as the free radical, and the mediator activity becomes uncontrolled. This uncontrolled mediator activity is thought to cause the pathophysiologic derangements operating in MODS (Fig. 5-1).

PATHOPHYSIOLOGY

Impaired perfusion during the initial insult or the development of sepsis are the most common causes of MODS. In hypovolemia, a decrease in circulating blood or plasma volume is seen as a fall in cardiac output (CO) and a decrease in oxygen delivery. Septic shock is believed to directly cause a maldistribution of blood flow to the tissues because of the release of inflammatory mediators that trigger a variety of vasoactive responses. The defects in blood flow occur primarily in the microcirculation and may be perpetuated at this level by the local processes that occur in response to the initial defect in distribution.

In response to hypovolemia, direct sympathetic vasoconstrictor activity increases arteriolar tone. Other mediators, such as angiotensin and vasopressin, also increase arteriolar constriction. Other factors produce their effects only at the local level because of the short half-lives of these molecules. Factors known to constrict or dilate the arterioles are listed in Table 5-1.[2-5]

The venules have a thinner smooth muscle layer and constrict in response to mediators, but the degree of venoconstriction varies from organ to organ. This ability of the venule to constrict remains intact even during tissue ischemia and hypoxia. Venoconstriction increases capillary hydrostatic pressure; consequently, fluid shifts and edema formation occur.[2] Other factors that cause venoconstriction and venodilation are listed in Table 5-1.

The capillary bed, metarterioles, and precapillary sphincters have minimal innervation. The muscle fibers of the metarterioles and precapillary sphinc-

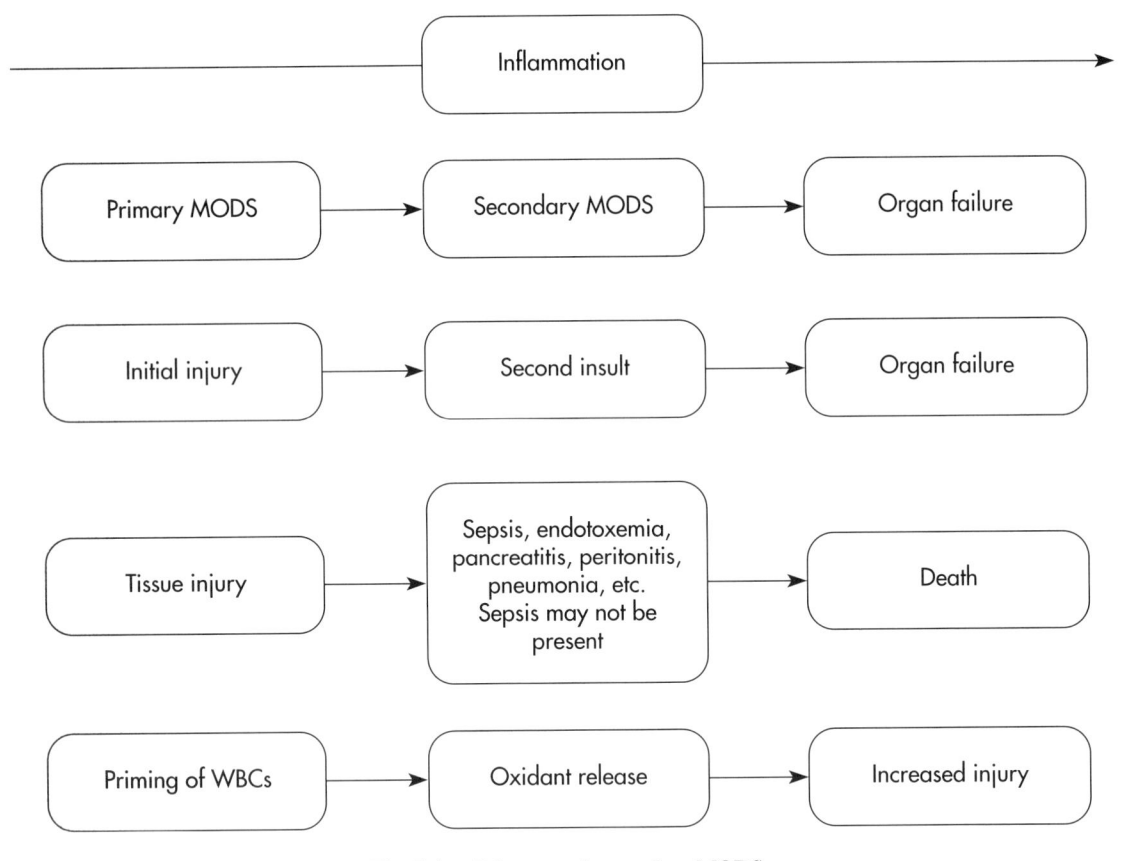

```
Inflammation ──────────────►

Primary MODS ──► Secondary MODS ──► Organ failure

Initial injury ──► Second insult ──► Organ failure

Tissue injury ──► Sepsis, endotoxemia, pancreatitis, peritonitis, pneumonia, etc. Sepsis may not be present ──► Death

Priming of WBCs ──► Oxidant release ──► Increased injury
```

Fig. 5-1 Primary and secondary MODS.

ters are controlled by local factors such as the concentrations of oxygen, carbon dioxide, hydrogen ions, and electrolytes rather than by sympathetic nervous system activity.[3] Dilatation of the capillary bed is affected by humoral mediators that are released locally upon tissue injury. As a passive exchange circuit, the capillary bed is vulnerable to extrinsic factors. Blood flow can be slowed or stopped by mechanical means such as thrombi, cell aggregates, and increased blood viscosity. Interstitial edema will also retard flow through the capillary bed because edema compresses the capillaries.

Release of vasoactive mediators with injury or inflammation

Vasoactive mediators are released immediately after tissue injury or inflammation. These mediators are derived from humoral, cellular, or biochemical pathways and initiate changes in the distribution of the circulating volume at the systemic, regional, and local levels.[6-14] The humoral response includes the plasma enzyme cascades of complement, kallikrein/kinin, coagulation, and fibrinolysis (Table 2-1).

The biochemical and cellular responses to sepsis, inflammation, and injury are intertwined with the humoral response. The humoral response and other factors activate numerous cells (neutrophils, macrophages, and lymphocytes), which in turn release many biochemical mediators that cause direct cell injury and maldistribution of circulating volume, such as oxygen-derived free radicals (ODFR), tumor necrosis factor (TNF), interleukin-1 (IL-1), platelet activating factor (PAF), proteases, and arachidonic acid metabolites (Fig. 5-2; Table 5-2).

Vasoactive mediators contribute to many of the vascular changes that occur with inflammation and

Table 5-1 Vasoactive Mediators

Mediator	Action	Site of action
Epinephrine	Dilatation at low doses Constriction at high doses (greater than 0.02 µg/kg/min)	Arterioles and veins of skeletal and cardiac muscle Systemic arterioles and veins
Norepinephrine	Constriction (strong)	All arterioles and veins
Angiotensin	Constriction	All arterioles and veins
Vasopressin	Constriction	Systemic arterioles
Serotonin	Constriction Dilatation	Systemic and pulmonary veins Precapillary sphincters
Bradykinin	Dilatation Constriction	Systemic arterioles Systemic veins
Histamine	Dilatation Constriction	Systemic arterioles, veins, and precapillary sphincters Pulmonary arterioles and veins
Endorphins	Dilatation	Systemic arterioles
Thromboxane A_2	Constriction	Peripheral, pulmonary, coronary, splanchnic, and renal arterioles
Prostaglandin $F_{2\alpha}$	Constriction	Pulmonary, renal, and splanchnic veins
Prostacyclin	Dilatation	Systemic arterioles and veins
Endothelium-derived relaxant factor	Local dilatation	Arterioles
Calcium, increased	Local constriction	Arterioles and veins
Potassium, increased	Local dilatation	Arterioles and veins
Magnesium, increased	Local dilatation (strong)	Arterioles and veins
Acidosis, severe	Local dilatation Constriction	Systemic arterioles and precapillary sphincters Pulmonary arterioles
Alkalosis, severe	Dilatation	Arterioles
Hypoxia	Dilatation Constriction	Systemic arterioles and precapillary sphincters Pulmonary arterioles
Hypercarbia	Dilatation	Systemic arterioles

Data for this table were derived from references 2-5.

injury.[6-14] Vasodilation is stimulated by histamine, bradykinin, TNF, and select prostaglandins. The powerful ability of bradykinin to increase blood flow and tissue edema in the area of its formation contributes to the disruption of the normal circulation. Vasoconstriction is mediated by leukotrienes, thromboxane, and many prostaglandins.

Prostacyclin (PGI_2) has generally been touted as a favorable prostaglandin because of its vasodilatory effects. It is a potent pulmonary and systemic vasodilator and has been reported to decrease pulmonary artery pressure and to relieve experimentally induced respiratory distress.[15] PGI_2 seems to work directly in opposition to thromboxane A_2 because it inhibits platelet aggregation and leukocyte adherence to damaged vascular endothelium,[16] while thromboxane A_2 promotes platelet aggregation and neutrophil adherence.

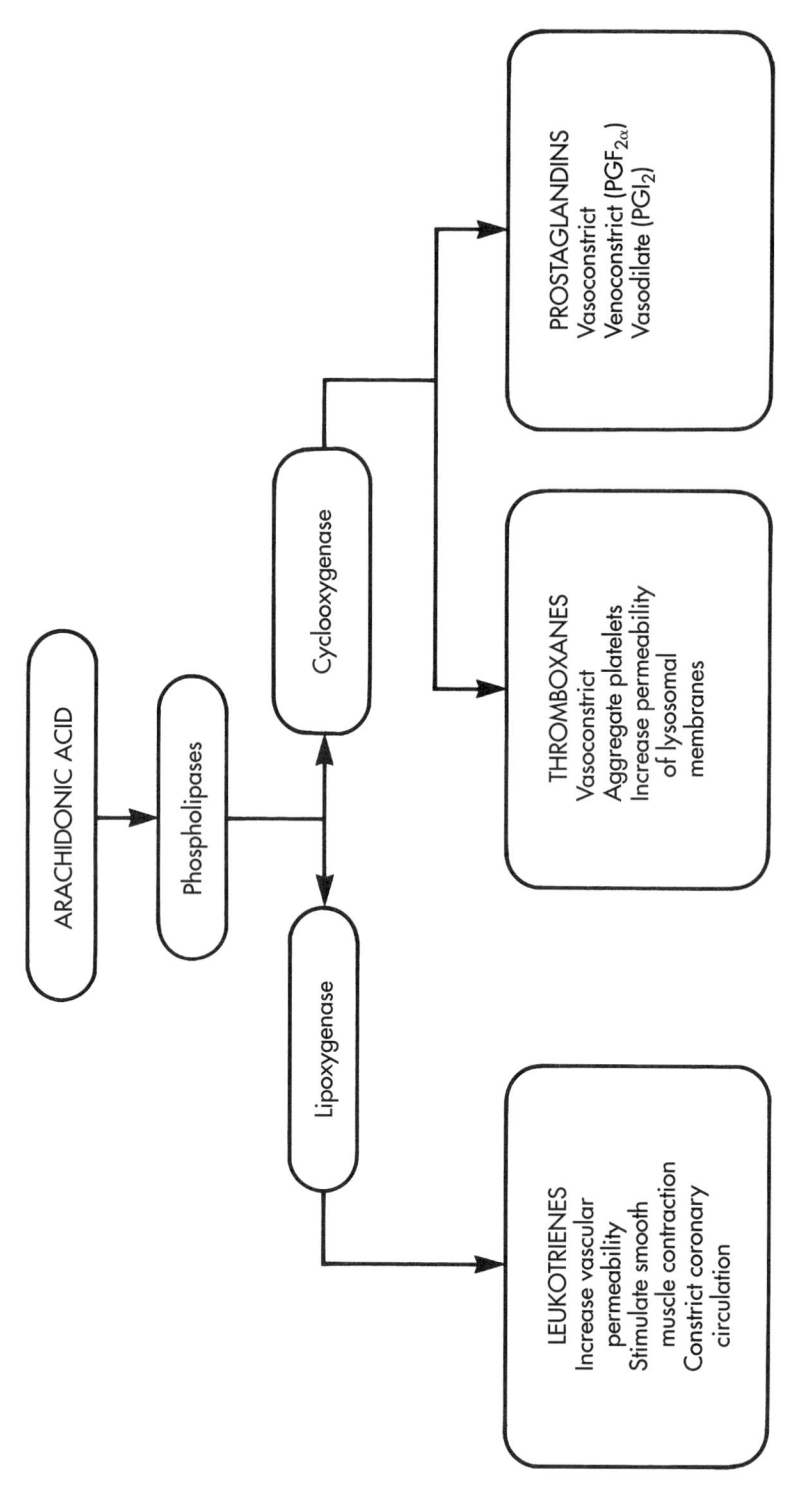

Fig. 5-2 Biologic activity of arachidonic acid metabolites.[4,14]

Table 5-2 Mediators Produced by Neutrophils and Macrophages

Cell type	Mediator	Action
Neutrophils	Platelet activating factor (PAF)	Increases capillary permeability Enhances neutrophil margination Induces platelet aggregation
Neutrophils and macrophages	Oxygen-driven free radicals (ODFRs)	Phagocytosis Damage endothelium when antioxidant defenses are depleted, thereby increasing permeability
	Proteases	Phagocytosis Destroy interstitial architectural proteins, thereby increasing permeability
	Arachidonic acid metabolites	See Figure 5-2
Macrophages	Interleukin-1 (IL-1)	Attracts neutrophils Stimulates lymphocytes Elicits fever as an endogenous pyrogen
	Tumor necrosis factor (TNF)	Induces IL-1 release from endothelial cells and macrophages Produces hypotension

Blood flow is blocked by microthrombi formation, which is stimulated by kallikrien, PAF, and thromboxane. Many of these mediators are produced by more than one cell type or biochemical reaction. In addition, some mediators are able to reactivate the process by which they were originally formed, leading to increased mediator activity. Chapter 3 presents an in-depth discussion of the systemic inflammatory response syndrome (SIRS) and inflammatory mediators.

Endothelial damage

Investigators postulate that the endothelial cell is the initial target cell in the acute septic injury and acute lung injury that occur in MODS.[17,18] The capillary endothelial cells are susceptible to damage by many different mechanisms. Direct mechanical trauma and mechanical stress, such as shear forces caused by changes in blood flow or pressure, will activate the endothelium causing the release of vasoactive mediators.[19] Other factors that affect endothelial integrity and function include coagulation, immune complexes, cellular activity, and mediator activity.

Coagulation. Surface coagulation occurs when the smooth lining of the endothelium is disrupted, thereby setting the intrinsic clotting system into motion. Exposure of the subendothelial collagen is a powerful initiator of the clotting process. Microorganisms, endotoxin, lipid moieties, and other bacterial products and toxins stimulate host cells to release endogenous proteins or cytokines that damage the endothelium. Human endothelial cells are reported to generate procoagulants in response to endotoxin.[17] In summary, coagulation taking place on the endothelial surface damages the endothelium, and endothelial damage promotes a procoagulant state.

Immune complexes and cellular interaction. Immune-complex formation enhanced by the complement cascade is believed to trigger production of vasoactive mediators by endothelial cells. Complement fragment C5a interacts with neutrophils and the endothelial membrane, resulting in activation and aggregation of these leukocytes.[17] Leukocyte aggregates, platelet aggregates, and microthrombi cause mechanical obstructions of the vasculature. Neutrophils also cause damage to the vascular endothelium through the generation of ODFRs.[17,20]

Macrophages generate IL-1 and TNF that damage the capillary endothelium. Each of these mediators can independently injure the vascular endothelium; however, studies have suggested that these cytokines may act synergistically to disrupt vascular endothelium.[17] IL-1 and TNF have many biologic activities, including the activation of macrophages, neutrophils, and endothelial cells; the induction of fever and the acute phase response; and the stimulation of wound healing.[17] TNF and IL-1 also trigger the production of adhesion molecules by the endothelium, which promote increased neutrophil adherence and obstruction in the microvasculature.[9,12]

Permeability changes. Capillary permeability is increased by mediator stimulation or by direct injury. Increased capillary permeability leads to third spacing and edema formation. Changes in capillary permeability occur either by mediator stimulation or by direct capillary endothelial damage. Mediators that stimulate increased capillary permeability include ODFRs, complement, histamine, bradykinin, and PAF. Direct cell damage is caused by the products of neutrophils and macrophages such as ODFRs, proteases, TNF, and IL-1. Many of the phagocytic neutrophils normally adhere to capillary walls, a phenomenon known as margination. Margination is enhanced by the kallikrein/kinin system, which increases the neutrophil attraction and adherence properties of the venular endothelial surface. Migration of additional neutrophils to the site of injury is dependent on local perfusion. Cell movement is impeded by diminished perfusion resulting from hemorrhage or burns, venous stasis resulting from shock states, and blocked vasculature as a result of microvascular thrombi. Neutrophil chemotaxis is compromised specifically in burn patients because complement component concentrations are reduced as a result of activation and consumption of complement in the burn wound.[21]

Vasomotor control. Endothelial cells are active participants in the regulation of blood flow.[18] Direct vasomotor control by endothelial cells is postulated to occur by stimulus-induced contraction and regulation or endothelial cell-to-cell signal transmission along the capillary lining.[19] In other words, endothelial cells must be intact for vasoactive mediators to be effective. Endothelium-derived relaxant factor (EDRF) is the name given to the humoral agent that mediates the action of vasoactive substances. Based on the ability of nitrovasodilators to mimic EDRF through their stimulation of nitric oxide release, it has been shown that EDRF and nitric oxide are the same substance.[22] ODFRs inactivate EDRF, resulting in disordered autoregulation of blood flow.

Neuroendocrine activation

The neuroendocrine response to trauma, sepsis, or shock includes the release of cortisol, catecholamines, glucagon, glucocorticoids, aldosterone, renin, and angiotensin. Endogenous catecholamines are released from the adrenal medulla and peripheral adrenergic nerve endings after trauma, sepsis, or ischemia. Epinephrine and norepinephrine generally induce vasoconstriction by stimulating alpha receptors and can produce redistribution of blood flow within a given vascular bed. Specific effects on regional blood flow will be discussed in the next section.

Catecholamines stimulate beta receptors that directly affect cardiopulmonary function, increase metabolic rate, and change the metabolism of protein, fat, and carbohydrate.[23] Glucagon secretion is increased in response to catecholamines. This hormone stimulates glycogenolysis, gluconeogenesis, lipolysis, and amino acid transport to the liver for conversion to glucose precursors. Glucocorticoids are released from the adrenal cortex and prepare the body for the stress caused by the insult of trauma or disease. This preparation includes anti-inflammatory effects such as stabilizing capillary, cellular, and lysosomal membranes, as well as the mobilization of nutritional components. Aldosterone is also released into the blood stream by the adrenal cortex in response to adrenocorticotropic hormone (ACTH) secretion by the anterior pituitary gland. This mineralocorticoid targets the distal renal tubules, sweat glands, salivary glands, and intestines to increase sodium reabsorption, thereby conserving extracellular fluid volume.[24]

The renin-angiotensin system is a complex humoral system with major cardiovascular effects including systemic vasoconstriction, positive inotropy, and increased capillary permeability.[24] Angiotensin II exhibits more potent cardiac activity than either angiotensin I or angiotensin III; however, this action is not as strong as that produced by the catecholamines. Vasoconstriction involves all vascular beds including the coronary circulation. Angiotensin can produce redistribution of blood flow, specifically in the kidney where flow is shifted from the cortical to the medullary regions.[24]

FAILURE OF COMPENSATORY MECHANISMS
Hyperemia

Skeletal muscle is relatively unaffected in sepsis. The vascular bed in striated muscle dilates with exercise, a process known as functional hyperemia. Functional hyperemia also occurs in other vascular beds such as the splanchnic and cerebral circulations when the tissue served becomes highly active.

Reactive hyperemia occurs when the blood supply to tissues is occluded for a period of time and is then restored.[3] Blood flow then increases to about five times normal for a few seconds to a few hours depending on the amount of time the flow was occluded. This phenomenon lasts long enough to repay, almost exactly, the oxygen debt accrued during the period of blockage.[3] Continued vasodilation in reactive hyperemia is proposed to occur according to the following mechanisms: (1) blood-flow dependent vasodilation, (2) endothelial cell-to-cell conduction of a vasodilatory stimulus along the vessel wall from the distal to the more proximal circulations, and (3) direct effects of a substance on vascular smooth muscle.[19] Reactive hyperemia is impaired in sepsis, and thus, ischemic tissues may not have their oxygen demands met even if volume and flow are restored.

Principle vasodilators considered to play a role in reactive hyperemia are intermediates of the kinin and prostaglandin systems: bradykinin and prostaglandin I_2.[25] These intermediates are activated during occlusion and cause dilatation of precapillary arterioles. Hartl and co-workers studied reactive hyperemia in 12 patients with septic conditions.[25] Nine of these patients developed MODS with the loss of reactive hyperemia. The two patients with MODS who survived were younger and demonstrated the return of reactive hyperemia upon recovery.[25] The investigators concluded that (1) the absence of reactive hyperemia in the septic state is not necessarily combined with impaired microvascular reactivity but may be related to generally poor clinical conditions, such as severe MODS; (2) the absence of reactive hyperemia precedes therapy-resistant hypotension, hypoxemia, and DIC, suggesting that these conditions are not responsible for the absence of reactive hyperemia; and (3) provocation of reactive hyperemia may be a useful method to detect microvascular derangements in high-risk patients.[25]

In other words, the loss of reactive hyperemia is an ominous sign in MODS; however, the absence of reactive hyperemia is not diagnostic, because other factors, such as age, will affect the outcome.

Peripheral vascular paralysis

Normal peripheral vascular autoregulatory mechanisms are overridden in a condition referred to as "peripheral vascular paralysis."[26] This condition is present in the early stage of sepsis that is characterized by increased cardiac output (CO), decreased systemic vascular resistance (SVR), altered metabolism with lactic acidosis, impaired oxygen utilization, and increased microvascular permeability. The CO is proposed to increase despite myocardial depression and decreased SVR because fluid resuscitation has expanded the intravascular volume or because blood flow has been redirected into shortened vascular circuits. Blood is travelling faster through the vascular tree because SVR is decreased and precapillary sphincters may be closed. Although this may contribute to an increased CO, it may also contribute to the defect in intraorgan blood flow distribution.[26] With capacitance reduced by venoconstriction, intravascular volume is redistributed centrally to the large vessels; increased venous return to the right heart results in increased CO. Although CO is often increased, hypotension is common.

Refractory hypotension frequently accompanies sepsis caused by gram-negative bacteria. Refractory hypotension is defined as hypotension that is unresponsive to fluid challenge and vasopressor therapy. Peripheral vascular unresponsiveness due to EDRF may have a role in causing refractory hypotension. Broner and co-workers have shown that inactivation of EDRF improves blood pressure in a model of septic shock.[27]

REGIONAL BLOOD FLOW

Regional circulation may be redistributed in sepsis, trauma, or shock in response to the many vascular mediators already discussed. In sepsis and inflammation, vasodilatation and increased vascular permeability are affected at the microcirculatory level by the complement cascade, the kallikrein/kinin system, histamine, and many other mediators. Vasodilatation in sepsis manifests as a decrease in SVR that then leads to a decrease in preload because of blood pooling in the periphery. The humoral systems stimulate the nonspecific immune response (inflammation), resulting in neutrophil chemotaxis, phagocytosis, and release of proteases and oxygen radicals. Neutrophil activity leads to a further increase in capillary permeability and production of monocyte/macrophage chemotactic substances. Proteases and arachidonic acid metabolites are common products of both neutrophils and macrophages. These products alter capillary permeability and generally cause vasoconstriction in various organ beds. However, SVR remains low in sepsis.

Systemic vasoconstriction, which is primarily mediated by catecholamines, is seen as an increase in SVR and will occur in cardiogenic or hypovolemic shock. Blood flow in either sepsis or hypovolemia is further disrupted by the formation of microthrombi and cell aggregates. Figure 5-3 depicts the many processes that contribute to maldistribution of circulating volume. This description of events is general because it is known that the regional blood flow within organs varies in sepsis. Table 5-3 outlines factors that change intraorgan blood flow.

Myocardium

Flow-dependent vasodilatation is a normal response to brief periods of ischemia in the myocardium.[19] In sepsis, myocardial blood flow is redistributed from the subendocardial to the subepicardial layer.[28] This redistribution may be caused by myocardial edema, increased end diastolic pressure, or a release of vasoactive substances. The left ventricular subendocardium, which receives most of its blood flow during diastole, is believed to be highly vulnerable to hypoperfusion resulting in ischemia because of redistribution of intramyocardial blood flow.[28] Adams and co-workers reported on several animal studies in which endotoxin was infused and the left ventricular subendocardial blood flow/left ventricular epicardial blood flow ratio remained normal or near normal despite a reduction in total coronary blood flow.[28] These findings were attributed to coronary autoregulation.

Human studies have been reported in which left ventricular coronary blood flow increased during septic shock.[29,30] These results were attributed to either excess coronary vasodilatation in relation to metabolic needs, suggesting abnormal autoregulation, or the presence of a defect in myocardial oxygen extraction in the septic heart.[29] In either case, an increase in coronary blood flow would result. Global myocardial ischemia, therefore, does not appear to be the causative factor of myocardial depression in individuals with sepsis as long as the mean arterial pressure remains equal to or greater than 60 mm Hg,[28,30] although patchy areas of ischemia and necrosis may occur.[29]

Right ventricular coronary blood flow also increased in animal studies; however, failing right ventricle autoregulation was suggested by a fall in the endocardial blood flow/epicardial blood flow ratio in the presence of mild pulmonary hypertension.[29] The right ventricle then becomes vulnerable to ischemia when adult respiratory distress syndrome (ARDS)-associated pulmonary hypertension occurs.

Coronary blood flow and myocardial ischemia provide only a partial explanation for myocardial dysfunction in shock. Another aspect to consider is that of contractility. Myocardial depression may be masked by the compensatory actions of epinephrine and norepinephrine on cardiac beta receptors. Beta-adrenergic receptor blockade with propranolol uncovers this underlying myocardial depression.[28] Contractility may also be affected by beta-adrenergic receptor dysfunction.[31] This type of dysfunction may be due to a decreased number of beta-adrenergic receptors, a decreased affinity of receptors for catecholamine agonists, or a dysfunction in the intracellular response to beta-adrenergic-receptor stimulation.

Myocardial depression is generally described in terms of left ventricular performance. The effect of endotoxin on left ventricular function has been well studied since endotoxin is one of the primary bacterial products present in patients with sepsis from gram-negative bacteria. Endotoxemia in humans produces a hyperdynamic state with a high cardiac index (CI) and a low SVR. In one study, left ventricular performance was depressed 5 hours after the administration of endotoxin and after volume loading as measured by decreased left ventricular ejection fraction and increased left end-diastolic and end-systolic volume indices.[32] Evaluation of left ventricular performance before and after volume loading in this same study demonstrated that left ventricular function is intrinsically abnormal in endotoxemia and that this is not simply related to preload or afterload.[32]

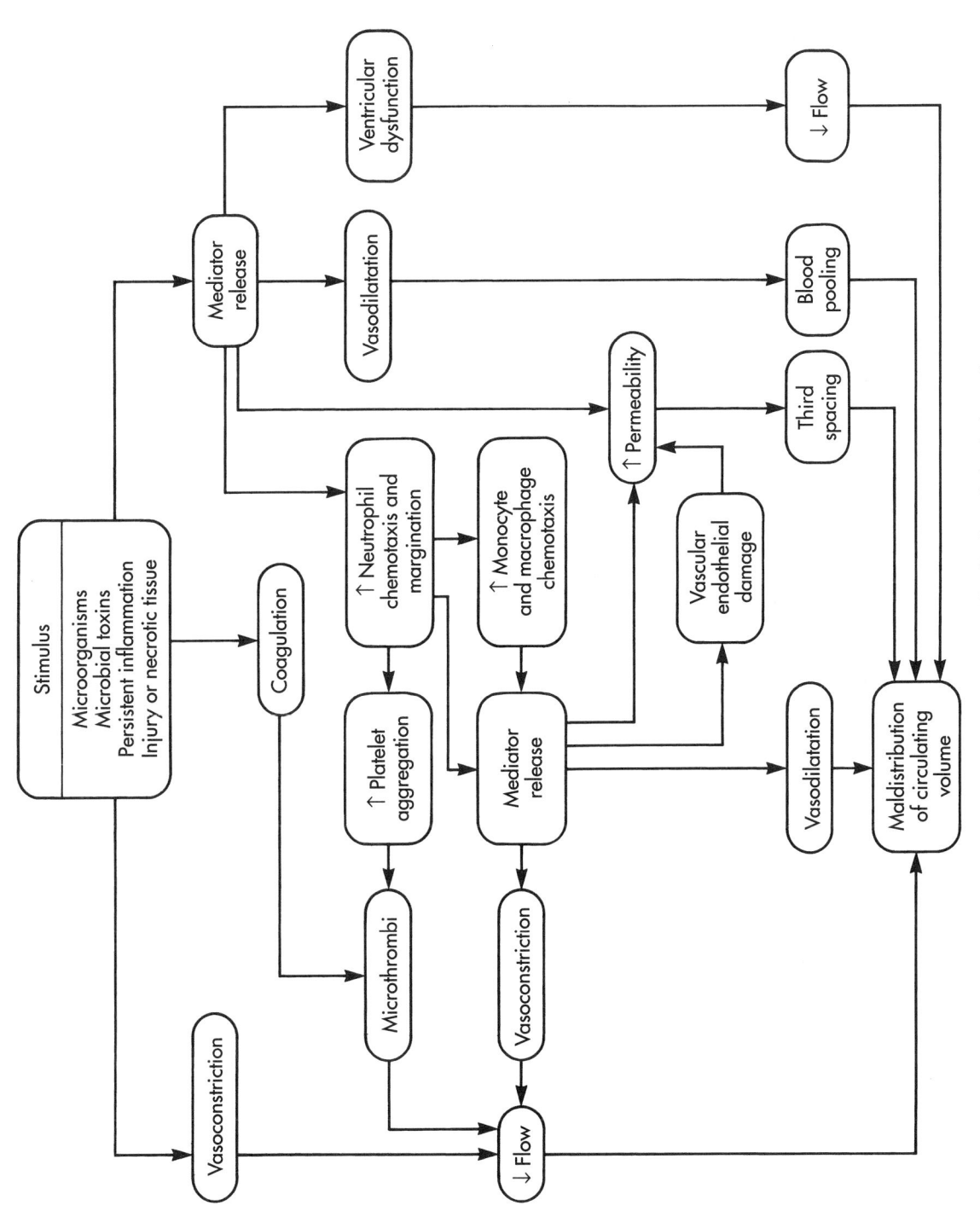

Fig. 5-3 Processes leading to maldistribution of circulating volume.

Table 5-3 Intraorgan Blood Flow

Organ	Abnormality	Consequence
Heart	Decreased subendocardial blood flow	Patchy ischemia
	Impaired β-adrenergic receptors	Decreased responsiveness to catecholamines
	Endotoxin-mediated damage	Depressed biventricular function
Lungs	Neutrophil and macrophage activity and mediator release	Destruction of pulmonary endothelium Increased capillary permeability
	Endotoxin-mediated damage	Vasoconstriction Bronchoconstriction Increased capillary permeability
	Hypoxia	Vasoconstriction
Gastrointestinal tract	Decreased splanchnic blood flow	Ileus Mucosal erosions Decreased liver function
	Endotoxin-mediated damage	Increased intestinal permeability
Kidneys	Decreased renal blood flow	Decreased glomerular filtration Tubular ischemia

Right ventricular performance has been studied less; however, myocardial depression is believed to be biventricular. Parker and co-workers studied a group of septic patients and found that changes in the right ventricular ejection fraction and end-diastolic volume index generally followed the same pattern as the comparable parameters of the left ventricle.[33] All patients were given intravenous fluids, and vasopressors were added if the mean arterial pressure remained below 60 mm Hg, thereby ruling out myocardial dysfunction caused by hypoperfusion. In their study, the authors included patients receiving vasopressors because they found no differences in the hemodynamic data between patients receiving or not receiving vasopressor therapy.[33]

Ventricular dilatation occurs in sepsis and returns to normal as patients recover.[34] In sepsis, ventricular dilatation is seen as an increase in the right and the left end-diastolic volume indices. The stroke volume index remains normal, yet ejection fraction is decreased, probably because of humoral factors and increased end-diastolic volume. The compensatory mechanisms of the Starling effect help to maintain ventricular performance.[34]

Vasoactive substances also affect cardiac performance. Platelet activating factor (PAF) is known to cause coronary constriction; however, its role in sepsis and MODS appears to be related to its negative inotropic effect. Animal studies indicate that myocardial ischemia may increase the local production of PAF and render the heart more susceptible to its action, thereby perpetuating ischemic cellular injury.[10] Myocardial depressant factor (MDF) is another substance hypothesized to cause decreased cardiac contractility. Patients with septic shock whose serum contains MDF activity have lower ejection fractions, larger end-diastolic volumes, higher pulmonary capillary wedge pressures (PCWP), and higher peak blood lactate concentrations than patients without MDF activity.[35] Leukotrienes have been shown to produce a dose-dependent coronary vasoconstriction in animal models that is prevented by the administration of a leukotriene receptor antagonist.[14] Leukotriene C_4 appears to be more potent than leukotriene D_4 in this regard; however, both leukotrienes produce a negative inotropic effect that is not blocked by leukotriene receptor antagonists.[14] More studies are required to define the effect of endogenously produced mediators on cardiac blood flow and performance.

Pulmonary vasculature

The pulmonary vascular response to endotoxin is a two-phase process consisting of the initial vasoconstrictive phase followed by the phase of increased microvascular permeability. Vasoconstriction of the pulmonary arterioles is measured by pulmonary artery pressure and pulmonary vascular resistance (PVR). This constriction is mediated by many substances that are released during shock and sepsis; pulmonary hypertension is common in experimental endotoxemia.[36] Endotoxin stimulates arachidonic acid metabolism that produces leukotrienes and thromboxane A_2 (Figure 5-2). Leukotrienes have been shown to affect contraction of the bronchial smooth muscle, enhance the action of histamine, and increase vascular permeability.[36] Thromboxane A_2 is a potent pulmonary vasoconstrictor thought to be responsible for some of the pulmonary hypertension seen early in acute lung injury.[36]

In animal studies, leukotrienes increase both PVR and vascular permeability; however, the change in PVR is transient and may be blocked by leukotriene receptor antagonists or indomethacin.[14] The pulmonary venoconstrictor effect of arachidonic acid metabolism is, therefore, likely to be mediated by cyclooxygenase products such as thromboxane, since venoconstriction is reported to be inhibited by cyclooxygenase and thromboxane synthetase inhibitors.[37,38] Ibuprofen has been shown to inhibit pulmonary hypertension and the hyperdynamic response to endotoxin in sheep.[39] In this study, ibuprofen did not attenuate the microvascular leak, leading the authors to conclude that the ibuprofen effect could be due to a response other than decreased prostanoid production.[39]

A study of normal volunteers administered endotoxin reported no changes in pulmonary artery pressure (PAP) or PCWP when compared with controls.[32] PAP and PCWP increased in both groups with volume loading; however, no significant differences were noted.[32] Another study of patients in septic shock reported a mean PAP of 22 mm Hg.[33] This value returned to normal in survivors but remained high in nonsurvivors.[33] The PVR index (PVRI) did not change significantly in either the survivors or the nonsurvivors.[33] The differences reported in these studies may reflect physiologic responses during different phases of sepsis; the normal volunteers received their first inflammatory stimulus with the endotoxin injection, whereas patients in septic shock were most likely already in an activated inflammatory state.

Alveolar hypoxia causes reflex pulmonary hypertension because precapillary arteries constrict and blood flow is directed to other areas of the lung. Although leukotrienes have been implicated as mediators of this response, this mediator role is unconfirmed. Studies with dogs demonstrated the expected increases in PVR and leukotriene concentrations in bronchoalveolar lavage fluid after induced alveolar hypoxia; however, administering a leukotriene inhibitor did not alleviate the pulmonary vasoconstriction even though leukotriene concentrations were controlled.[14] Reflex pulmonary hypertension resulting from alveolar hypoxia may be mediated by several substances, such as thromboxane, serotonin, and histamine, released by perivascular mast cell degranulation.[37]

Endotoxin-induced damage to pulmonary endothelium is caused through neutrophil release of leukotrienes, but this damage may also occur through alternative pathways.[36] Alveolar macrophages may be stimulated by endotoxin to produce ODFRs, proteolytic enzymes, or both.[36] Oxygen radical formation in the neutrophil occurs during a process known as the "respiratory burst" that is enhanced in the presence of alveolar macrophages. The result is an overwhelming imbalance in antioxidants and damage to the pulmonary vascular endothelium.[20] Oxidant injury is also perpetrated by the xanthine-hypoxanthine pathway that will be discussed in the section on postischemic reperfusion injury.

Neutrophils sequestered in response to the initial injury are hypothesized to cause oxidant-mediated lung injury by two mechanisms: first, neutrophil-produced peroxide diffuses directly into pulmonary endothelial cells; and, second, a more potent oxidizing agent, the hydroxyl radical, is produced when neutrophil peroxide is produced in the presence of free iron.[40] Catalase, an endogenous lung-tissue antioxidant, has been demonstrated to be greatly reduced after endotoxemia in sheep; therefore, lung tissue may be susceptible to subsequent peroxide injury before catalase activity is restored.[40] Endotoxin stimulates lymphocytes to produce cytokines, which have a chemotactant effect on neutrophils, thus increasing neutrophil activity and, consequently, endothelial damage in the septic lung.[11]

Thromboxane A_2 is also stimulated by endotoxin. Thromboxane causes pulmonary vasoconstriction, mediates bronchoconstriction, increases membrane permeability, and aggregates platelets and neutrophils.[4,11] Increased levels of thromboxane A_2 are reported to be associated with the pulmonary hypertension, hypoxia, and increased airway resistance that occur in endotoxemia.[4] A prospective study of 106 septic surgical patients revealed that the transpulmonary thromboxane B_2 gradient correlated with the degree of pulmonary hypertension.[4] Thromboxane B_2 is the stable, measurable end metabolite of the short-lived, physiologically active mediator thromboxane A_2.

PGI_2, another active metabolite from the cyclooxygenase pathway of arachidonic acid metabolism, inhibits thromboxane and is a potent pulmonary vasodilator.[11] This mediator has been used experimentally to treat the pulmonary hypertension associated with endotoxemia.[16] It is likely that, under normal circumstances, a balance among the endogenous constrictor and dilator prostaglandins may be necessary to maintain normal pulmonary and systemic vascular tone.

Increased pulmonary vascular permeability is the second phase occurring in traumatic and septic shock. As mentioned, this change is thought to be mediated by several substances including oxidants, leukotrienes, thromboxane, histamine, serotonin, and bradykinin. Conflicting studies have been reported regarding the role of leukotrienes in altering vascular permeability.[37] Further investigation is indicated to determine whether leukotrienes increase vascular permeability directly or increase transvascular fluid filtration by increasing the microvascular hydrostatic pressure.[37] Thromboxane A_2 inhibition has recently been shown to decrease lymph protein clearance in sheep that had received an infusion of endotoxin.[38] This study suggests that phase II increases in microvascular permeability may be attenuated by the specific inhibition of thromboxane A_2, whereas cyclooxygenase inhibition is unsuccessful.[38]

In summary, changes occurring in the pulmonary vasculature include vasoconstriction, increased hydrostatic pressure, increased capillary permeability, increased fluid movement, and microthrombi formation. These changes potentiate ventilation-to-perfusion mismatching, intrapulmonary shunting, and poor oxygenation status.

Splanchnic circulation

The splanchnic circulation serves the gastrointestinal (GI) tract, the spleen, the pancreas, and the liver. Blood flow to the splanchnic circulation is greatly reduced during trauma, shock, or sepsis. Sympathetic activity and catecholamine release trigger splanchnic vasoconstriction and shunting of blood away from the gut. Leukotrienes have also been shown to be potent mesenteric vasoconstrictors.[14,29] The bowel is reported to lose reactive hyperemia and, thus, the ability to augment blood flow after an ischemic event.[29] This finding supports the work of Hartl and co-workers who reported a loss of reactive hyperemia in septic patients before the development of MODS.[25]

Decreased blood flow to the GI tract results in an ileus; however, prolonged ischemia may result in mucosal erosions because of breakdown of the mucosal barrier, changes in intramural pH, and diminished epithelial regeneration.[41] These lesions are found primarily in the stomach, jejunum, and ileum and are presumed to occur because of high alpha receptor activity in the splanchnic vascular bed, which leads to a selective decrease in circulation to the mucosal layer.[42] Blunt and penetrating abdominal trauma can cause intestinal disruption and fecal contamination of the peritoneal cavity. Translocation of enteric bacteria and endotoxin from the bowel lumen to the portal circulation is reported to occur when bowel integrity is compromised by decreased blood flow.[17,26] The liver is then challenged to clear these bacteria and their toxins before they reach the central circulation.

Hepatic ischemia is believed to occur in sepsis despite the normotensive, high CO. In animal studies, a fall in hepatic blood flow was associated with a fall in energy charge and an elevation of the tissue lactate/pyruvate ratio.[29] Despite decreased blood flow, metabolic demands on the liver are increased in sepsis and shock as vasoactive mediators stimulate gluconeogenesis and protein synthesis, especially of acute-phase proteins. Decreased hepatic perfusion decreases the performance of vital functions of the liver, including phagocytosis by Kupffer cells, detoxification of drugs and hormones, and removal of activated clotting factors.[41]

Intraorgan hepatic blood flow is congested and associated with dilatation of sinusoids, particularly in the centrilobular region.[42] As blood moves from the periphery of the lobule to the central lobular region, the hepatocytes are continuously extracting oxygen; therefore, less oxygen may reach the centrilobular region and predisposes the region to ischemic damage.[42] Lipid accumulation in hepatocytes is another change seen in the ischemic liver.[42] This intracellular lipid accumulation, or fatty change, indicates an abnormality in the ability of the liver to process lipid. Fatty change may occur in other organs, but it is most commonly seen in the liver because it is the primary fat metabolizing organ.

Deficits in hepatic perfusion may stem from several mechanisms. Microcirculatory aggregates of platelets, leukocytes, and fibrin have been identified in the liver.[43] Thromboxane A_2 has been implicated in reducing hepatic blood flow in sepsis; however, the level at which this mediator produces its effect (prehepatic, hepatic vascular, mesenteric vascular, or intrahepatic) has not been determined.[44]

Following reperfusion of the splanchnic bed, many toxic mediators released by the liver and other GI organs during the ischemic period enter the circulation. After exposure to bacteria and endotoxin, hepatic macrophages release IL-1, which causes the liver to produce C-reactive protein.[41] This protein is considered to be proteolytic but its role in MODS is unclear. Two mediators released by the ischemic intestine, serotonin and thromboplastin, activate the clotting cascade and can promote the development of DIC. The ischemic pancreas is thought to release pancreatic enzymes and, possibly, myocardial depressant factor into the circulation during shock. Myocardial depressant factor is reported to further increase splanchnic vasoconstriction and depress myocardial contractility.[35]

Renal vasculature

Renal blood flow is normally greater than the metabolic needs of the kidneys in order to maintain glomerular filtration. In shock, the hypoperfused kidneys may lose the capacity for autoregulation if the mean arterial pressure falls below 70 mm Hg.[45] Blood flow is redistributed within the kidneys because of sympathetic stimulation, angiotensin production, and impaired prostaglandin synthesis.[46] The result of this redistribution is tubular ischemia. In sepsis, renal blood flow is reported to increase and, yet, does not meet the increased renal metabolic needs of the septic state.[29] Vasoconstricting prostaglandins are thought to be responsible for the increased renin/angiotensin activity; therefore, an increase in vasodilating prostaglandins, such as PGI_2, or a reduction in vasoconstricting prostaglandins, such as thromboxane, should increase glomerular filtration. Cumming and co-workers demonstrated an increase in glomerular filtration rate after infusion of a thromboxane synthetase inhibitor in septic sheep.[47]

Brenner and co-workers measured renal blood flow in septic and critically ill patients.[48] Their results showed (1) no direct correlation between renal blood flow and CI in septic patients, (2) increased renal blood flow during recovery from sepsis, and (3) unchanged renal vascular resistance throughout the study.[48] The authors concluded that the vasodilatation occurring in the systemic circulation during early sepsis was not matched in the renal circulation.[48] Consequently, the patients in the study had a lower fraction of their total blood volume delivered to the kidneys during early sepsis.

Cerebral circulation

The brain is one of the organs preferentially perfused in shock. Cerebral blood flow increases if arterial oxygen saturation (SaO_2) falls below 90% or if partial arterial pressure of oxygen (PaO_2) falls below 60 mm Hg. Autoregulatory mechanisms maintain a constant cerebral blood flow over a mean arterial pressure range of 50 to 130 mm Hg; however, global ischemia and partial ischemia will occur with cardiac arrest and shock, respectively. The brain relies on a continuous supply of oxygen; consequently, hypoperfusion permits a rapid depletion of the high energy substrates adenosine triphosphate (ATP) and phosphocreatine. The ATP-dependent sodium-potassium pump fails, allowing potassium to leak out of the cell. Calcium enters the cell at a critical level of extracellular potassium and activates phospholipase.[49]

Phospholipase activates arachidonic acid metabolism, which will produce thromboxane A_2, leukotrienes, and ODFRs in the case of partial ischemia because oxygen is available to support the reaction. Thromboxane and leukotrienes cause cerebral vasoconstriction, and ODFRs cause further damage to the cell membrane and vascular endothelium.

POSTISCHEMIC REPERFUSION INJURY
Xanthine oxidation

Postischemic reperfusion injury refers to alterations in cellular metabolism that occur during ischemic periods and the consequent inability to neutralize the toxic metabolites formed during reperfusion. The metabolites produced include ODFRs in which the oxygen has been reduced by one, two, or three electrons. Although neutrophils and macrophages form oxygen radicals through the reduced nicotinamide-adenine dinucleotide phosphate (NADPH) oxidase system during phagocytosis, another pathway involving ATP generates oxygen radicals during reperfusion injury. During ischemia, ATP is metabolized to hypoxanthine, and xanthine dehydrogenase is converted to xanthine oxidase (Fig. 5-4). Xanthine oxidase catalyzes the oxidation of hypoxanthine to xanthine and uric acid when reperfusion of the tissues supplies the oxygen to support the reaction.[50] Oxygen radicals are formed as byproducts of xanthine oxidation.[50]

Current research of oxidant-induced cell injury focuses on the early phase of trauma, because generalized inflammation and tissue changes are present very early after an injury has occurred.[51] Oxidant release in burn tissue is hypothesized to trigger systemic complement activation that results in inflammation in distant organs and further oxidant release.[51] Free iron is reported to react with the oxygen radicals generated by the xanthine oxidase pathway to produce a more potent oxidant, the hydroxyl ion.[52] This ion activates white blood cells to produce NADPH, which perpetuates ODFR production (Fig. 5-5).

Deferoxamine, an approved iron chelator, has recently been shown to provide protection from oxidant injury in a sheep model of burn injury.[52] This conclusion was reached because animals infused with deferoxamine complexed with hetastarch after a burn injury demonstrated improved cardiac function, decreased red cell hemolysis, and no evidence of lung or liver tissue lipid peroxidation as compared to animals receiving standard fluid management after a burn injury.[52] The resuscitation requirements of the animals decreased significantly, indicating less nonburn tissue fluid loss and increased oxygen consumption to meet the increased oxygen demands after the injury.[52]

Ibuprofen has also been examined for its antioxidant effects. Along with cyclooxygenase inhibition, ibuprofen protects lung tissue from septic injury by chelating iron.[53] Ibuprofen may then protect tissues from oxygen radicals in a dual fashion by preventing both the initial oxidant production early after an injury and the later generation of oxidants through the arachidonic acid pathway.

Individual organs differ in their ability to withstand ischemia reperfusion injury. Zhao-fan and co-workers studied the beneficial effects of three agents in reducing ischemia reperfusion injury.[54] Their results indicated that the protease inhibitor, leupeptin, protected the heart well and was somewhat effective in protecting the kidney; verapamil was also somewhat effective in protecting the kidney; superoxide dismutase, an ODFR scavenger, offered no protection to the three organs studied; and the liver showed no protective response with any of the therapies studied.[54]

Effects

Under normal conditions, intracellular antioxidant defenses protect tissues from the destructive effects of free radicals; however, these defenses are overwhelmed after ischemia followed by reperfusion, and excessive free radical activity and tissue damage result. The effects of the generation of oxygen radicals, listed in the box on p. 122, have been categorized into primary and secondary effects. Primary effects involve direct damage to the cell and its functions by breakdown of the cell membrane. Hydroxyl radicals induce changes in proteins and nucleic acids causing enzyme inactivation and DNA strand breaks. Secondary effects are those that activate proteases and phospholipases through a disturbance in cellular calcium homeostasis. Phospholipases destroy the cellular infrastructure and activate xanthine oxidase and NADPH oxidase, thereby perpetuating production of oxygen radicals.[50] Phospholipases also release free fatty acids which cause intracellular acidosis and increased arachidonic acid metabolism.

Myocardium

Postischemic reperfusion injury occurs primarily in the heart, the liver, the gut mucosa, and the kidneys. Evidence of reperfusion injury in the heart was reported by Bulkley and Hutchins at autopsies of patients who had died after coronary artery bypass graft surgery.[55] Two types of necrosis were described: a contraction band necrosis in areas that had been revascularized and a coagulation necrosis distal to obstructed vessels that were not bypassed.[55] Other processes in addition to ODFR production have been proposed to explain cardiac reperfusion injury. These processes include marked calcium entry into the cell at the moment of reperfusion, cell swelling resulting from influx of sodium and water, and white cell plugging of capillaries and arteri-

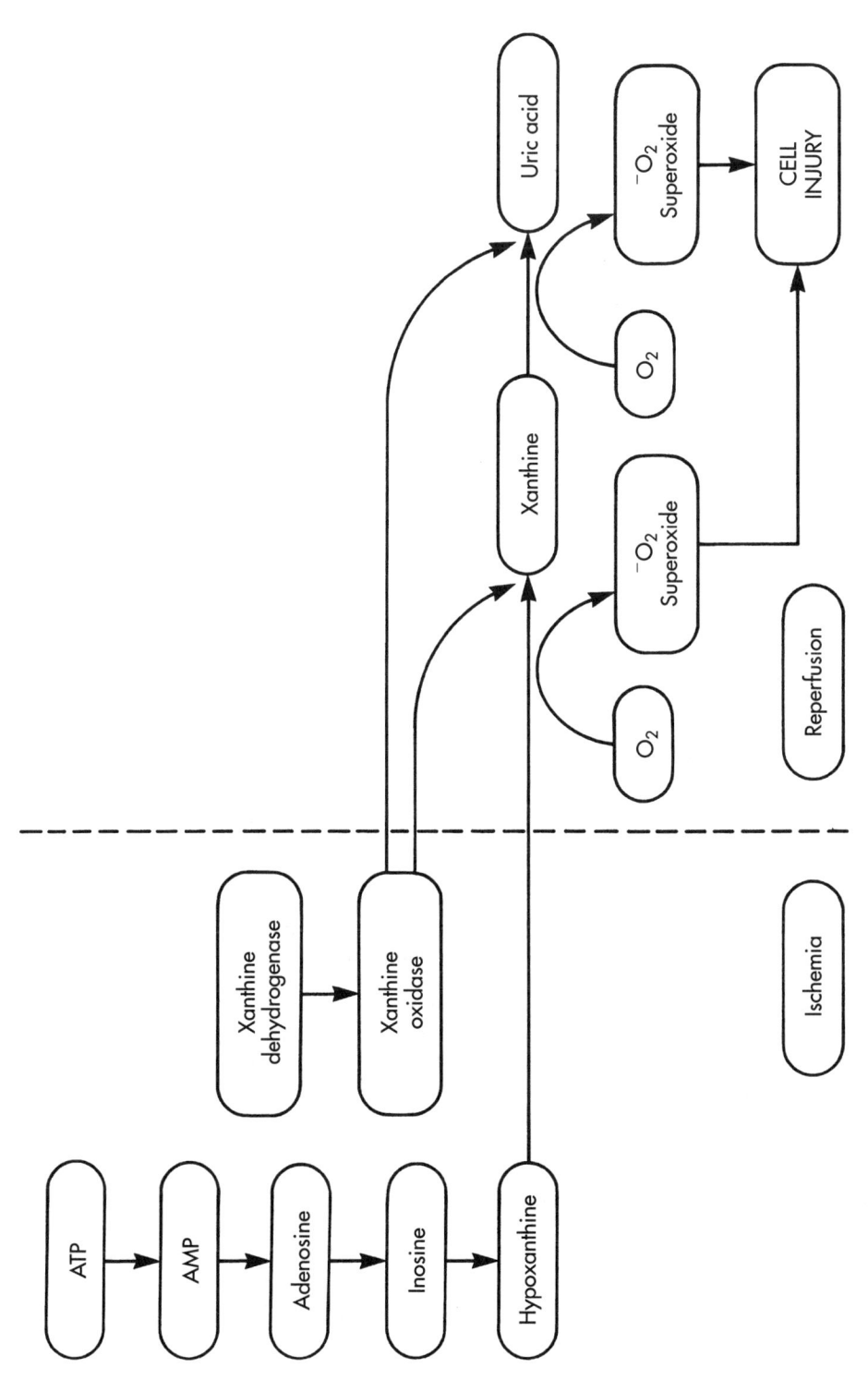

Fig. 5-4 Free radical production by xanthine oxidase pathway. *AMP*, Adenosine monophosphate; *ATP*, adenosine triphosphate. (From Black L, Coombs VJ, Townsend SN. Reperfusion and reperfusion injury in acute myocardial infarction. Heart Lung 1990; 19:279.)

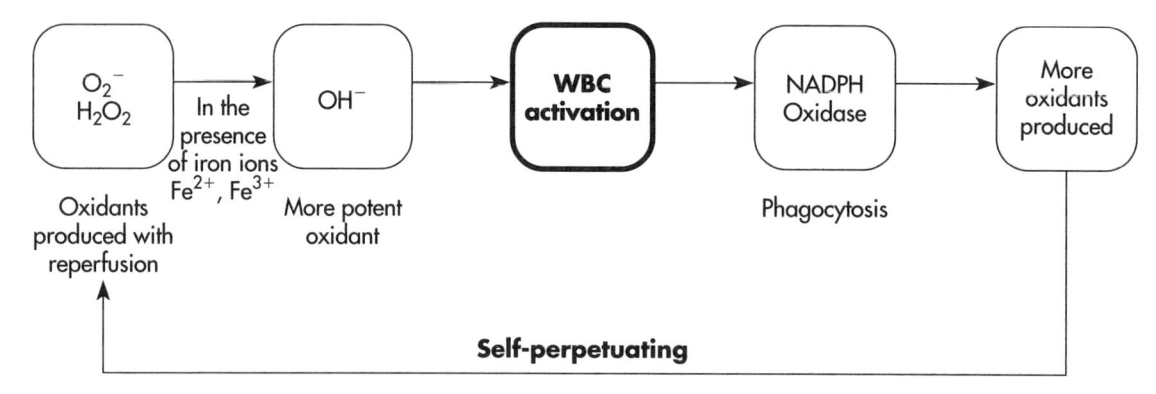

Fig. 5-5 White blood cell activation.

> **EFFECTS OF OXYGEN-DERIVED FREE RADICALS**
>
> Alteration in vascular permeability
> Peroxidation of cell lipid, altering cellular function
> Initiation and perpetuation of local and systemic inflammation
> Disruption of interstitial matrix
> Impairment of macrophage phagocytosis
> Alteration of cell DNA
> Initiation of arachidonic acid metabolism
> Triggering of red cell hemolysis
> Perpetuation of energy deficit

oles.[56] Oxygen radicals have also been implicated in depression of myocardial contractility after severe burns.[57]

Liver

Hepatic reperfusion after an ischemic period may produce not only liver injury but also widespread tissue injury, particularly in the lungs which are located "downstream" from the liver. The ischemic liver releases many cytoplasmic enzymes upon reperfusion. It has been shown that xanthine dehydrogenase and xanthine oxidase are included in this hepatocellular enzyme release, which stimulates the production of ODFRs.[58] The oxygen radicals produced from the activity of circulating xanthine oxidase could directly injure the vascular endothelium, activate oxidant-producing inflammatory cells that could travel to and injure tissues distal to the site of origin, and produce oxygen radicals in the plasma, which has limited antioxidant defense mechanisms.[58] Allopurinol, a xanthine oxidase inhibitor, may be beneficial in the case of systemic shock because of its extracellular antioxidant effects.[58]

Another mediator reportedly released from ischemic hepatic macrophages is TNF.[43] TNF has been shown in animals to be associated with both hepatic and pulmonary injury after hepatic lobular ischemia and reperfusion.[43] Pretreatment with anti-TNF monoclonal antibodies in the animals studied reduced serum glutamate pyruvate transaminase (SGPT) (currently known as alanine amino transferase [ALT]) levels and completely inhibited pulmonary edema.[43] This study suggests that TNF increases the susceptibility of the vascular endothelium to neutrophil-derived mediators such as ODFR; therefore, TNF may potentiate further pulmonary damage.[43]

Brain

The ischemia reperfusion sequence in the brain is followed by a prolonged postischemic hypoperfusion period associated with a profound increase in cerebral vascular resistance.[49] This cerebral vasoconstriction is attributed to cerebral edema, increased intracellular calcium, and increased levels of thromboxane A_2 in tissue as well as in the cerebral vasculature. Evidence exists to support the potential therapeutic effects of calcium channel blockers in cerebral ischemia. Postulated beneficial mechanisms include nonspecific cerebral vasodilatation, blockade of calcium activation of phospholipase, and antagonism of calcium-induced vasoconstriction.[49]

CLINICAL PRESENTATION AND ASSESSMENT

MODS has been defined by the American College of Chest Physicians (ACCP)/Society for Critical Care Medicine (SCCM) Consensus Conference Committee as the presence of altered organ function in an acutely ill patient such that homeostasis cannot be maintained without intervention.[59,60] As a syndrome, MODS describes a pattern of multiple and progressive signs and symptoms that are believed to be pathologically related and that develop over a period of time. Therapy in this syndrome is best begun before organ failure declares itself. The stages of syndrome progression as described by DeCamp and Demling are as follows: stage 1, clinical presentation of early sepsis; stage 2, multiple organ dysfunction; stage 3, late organ failure; and stage 4, the preterminal stage.[61] It is now recognized that, not only sepsis, but also uncontrolled systemic inflammatory response syndrome (SIRS) can initiate the progression of MODS to organ failure.

SIRS and sepsis

The first stage of MODS is defined by early sepsis or SIRS. Clinical symptoms for SIRS and sepsis are exactly the same according to the ACCP/SCCM Consensus Conference definitions[59,60] (see the box below). The primary difference is that SIRS is the response to a variety of severe clinical insults, and sepsis is the systemic inflammatory response to infection; thus sepsis presents as SIRS with infection. Sepsis develops along a continuum of clinical and pathophysiologic severity. Severe sepsis is associated with organ dysfunction, hypoperfusion, and hypotension. Septic shock occurs when hypotension and perfusion abnormalities are present despite adequate fluid resuscitation.[59,60] The clinical presentation of the sepsis continuum is outlined in Table 5-4.[62-64]

Septic shock has classically been divided into the two phases of hyperdynamic and hypodynamic shock. These terms are no longer useful given our improved knowledge and treatment of the pathophysiologic processes involved in septic shock. Research indicates that approximately 50% of patients with septic shock do not survive because of either unresponsive hypotension or MODS.[62] Less than 10% of the cases of unresponsive hypotension are attributable to a low CO and myocardial failure—a true hypodynamic state.[62] The falling CO commonly attributed to a hypodynamic phase of myocardial failure is more often related to volume status, and with adequate fluid resuscitation, most septic patients will maintain a high CO.[62] Myocardial failure, as indicated by a low CO in patients with adequate volume replacement, may be due to the presence of MDF or impaired beta-adrenergic receptor stimulation.[31,35] Hypotension unresponsive to aggressive therapy is usually caused by a very low SVR.[62] EDRF (nitric oxide) is postulated to contribute to this unresponsive hypotension.[27]

Organ dysfunction and failure

MODS describes a syndrome of multiple organ dysfunction that progresses to multiple organ failure if untreated. Currently, MODS is thought to occur by the "two hit" theory in which the first "hit" is a low flow state or direct injury producing local inflammation. The second "hit" may be one of several untoward events including sepsis, peritonitis, pancreatitis, pneumonia, or shock (Fig. 5-1). The second insult produces more inflammatory mediators and oxidants that activate WBCs to produce more mediators and oxidants (Fig. 5-5). The cycle becomes self-perpetuating.

Universal criteria for diagnosing failure of individual organs are not established. Organ dysfunction indicates a condition in which an individual organ is unable to maintain homeostasis but has not deteriorated to absolute failure. Many definitions for organ failure exist; however, it is possible to identify some consistency in the criteria used in the definitions. In cardiovascular failure, indicators generally include bradycardia, cardiac index less than 2.0 L/min/m^2, mean arterial pressure less than 50 or 60 mm Hg, and occurrence of a lethal ventricular dys-

---

CLINICAL SIGNS AND SYMPTOMS OF SIRS AND SEPSIS

Temperature greater than 38° C or less than 36° C
Heart rate greater than 90 beats/min
Respiratory rate less than 20 breaths/min or $PaCO_2$ less than 32 mm Hg
White blood cell count greater than 12,000/mm^3, less than 4,000/mm^3, or greater than 10% immature forms (bands)

Table 5-4 Clinical Presentation of the Sepsis Continuum

	Sepsis	Severe sepsis	Septic shock
Cardiovascular	Sinus tachycardia Bounding pulse CO/CI increased	Sinus tachycardia Warm, dry, flushed skin CO/CI normal or increased BP <90 mm Hg or 40 mm Hg below baseline PAP decreased PCWP decreased SI decreased SVR decreased PVR increased Mixed venous oxygen saturation increased	Tachycardia Dysrhythmias Cold, pale, clammy skin BP low or normal with vasopressors CO/CI normal or high PAP increased PCWP increased or decreased SI decreased SVR usually increased but may be decreased PVR increased Mixed venous oxygen saturation decreased
Pulmonary	Tachypnea Hyperventilation Respiratory alkalosis (if patient breathing spontaneously)	Tachypnea Respiratory depth decreased Hypoxemia while breathing room air Respiratory and metabolic acidosis Breath sounds diminished with crackles	Shortness of breath, if not ventilated Respiratory depth decreased Refractory hypoxemia Respiratory and metabolic acidosis Breath sounds diminished with crackles and wheezes
Renal	Urine output may be within normal limits	Urine output <0.5 ml/kg/hr Occasionally, inappropriate polyuria Osmolality increased	Oliguria Anuria BUN and creatinine increased
Metabolic	Temperature elevated or subnormal Hyperglycemia	Temperature elevated or subnormal Hyperglycemia Lactic acidosis (serum lactate >2.2-5 mmol/L)	Temperature subnormal Hyperglycemia or hypoglycemia Serum amylase, lipase, and LFTs elevated Lactic acidosis
Hematologic	Leukopenia, leukocytosis, or >10% bands	Leukopenia or leukocytosis Clotting factors decreased	Leukopenia or leukocytosis Clotting factors decreased Thrombocytopenia RBCs decreased
Central nervous system	Apprehension Mental cloudiness Delayed responses	Confusion Disorientation	Obtundation

BP, Blood pressure; *BUN*, blood urea nitrogen; *CO/CI*, cardiac output/cardiac index ratio; *LFT*, liver function tests; *PAP*, pulmonary artery pressure; *PCWP*, pulmonary capillary wedge pressure; *PVR*, pulmonary vascular resistance; *RBC*, red blood cell, *SI*, stroke index; *SVR*, systemic vascular resistance.

rhythmia, such as ventricular tachycardia, ventricular fibrillation, or asystole.[65,66] Other indicators associated with cardiovascular dysfunction are a decrease in right and left ventricular ejection fractions, an increase in left ventricular end-diastolic and end-systolic volumes, and a decrease in ventricular stroke work.[62,66]

Respiratory failure occurs from increased vascular permeability and direct endothelial damage. The lungs are the first organ to receive the toxic mediators released into the blood stream by the ischemic liver. Mediator-induced damage results in noncardiogenic pulmonary edema that is often followed by ARDS and nosocomial pneumonia. The clinical definition of respiratory failure used by Knaus and Wagner states that the patient would exhibit one or more of the following: respiratory rate ≤ 5 breaths/min or ≥ 49 breaths/min, $PaCO_2 \geq 50$ mm Hg, alveolar-arterial oxygen tension difference ≥ 350 mm Hg with fraction of inspired oxygen (FiO_2) = 1.0, or ventilator or continuous positive airway pressure (CPAP) dependence for more than 48 hours.[65] Other factors associated with respiratory dysfunction include chest radiograph changes, $PaO_2 < 50$ mm Hg with $FiO_2 > 40\%$, or changes in respiratory compliance.[67]

Failure of the liver is determined by an elevated bilirubin level, the presence of ascites, and evidence of encephalopathy. In the acute situation, dying hepatocytes release the enzymes aspartate aminotransferase (AST) (formerly known as serum glutamic-oxaloacetic transaminase [SGOT]), ALT (SGPT), and lactic dehydrogenase (LDH).[41] Prothrombin time will begin to increase and serum albumin levels will fall below 2.0 g/dL.[66] Hepatic dysfunction is indicated by an elevation in liver function tests to two times normal or a serum bilirubin level >2.0 mg/dL.[64]

The clinical signs of renal failure are generally agreed to be urine output ≤ 0.5 mL/kg/hr, serum BUN levels ≥ 100 mg/dL, and serum creatinine ≥ 3.5 mg/dL.[65] Renal dysfunction is identified with a urine output <0.5 mL/kg/hr, an increase in serum creatinine above normal levels with urinary sodium level <40 mmol/L, or a rise in the serum creatinine level by 2.0 mg/dL in the presence of preexisting renal insufficiency.[64]

Central nervous system dysfunction is manifested by changes in the level of consciousness. The patient may be confused, agitated, or respond slowly to verbal stimuli. Failure may be quantified by use of the Glasgow Coma Scale; a score less than or equal to 6 in the absence of sedation indicates neurologic failure.[65] The Glasgow Coma Scale may also be used to determine dysfunction if the score is <15 in instances where it had previously been normal or if the score is decreased by 1.[64]

Hematologic failure is more difficult to quantitate. A WBC count $\leq 1000/mm^3$, a platelet count $<50,000/mm^3$, and a fibrinogen level below 100 mg/dL have all been identified as measures of hematologic failure. Coagulation dysfunction is indicated by a confirmatory test for DIC, thrombocytopenia or a fall in platelet count by 25%, elevated prothrombin time and elevated partial thromboplastin time, or clinical evidence of bleeding.[64]

THERAPEUTIC MANAGEMENT

Therapeutic management of MODS begins as soon after the primary insult as possible. The goal is to prevent further cell injury. Correction of the maldistribution of circulating volume concentrates on restoring effective, circulating blood flow and oxygen transport to all tissues. In hypovolemic shock and the early stages of sepsis and inflammation, decreased preload must be treated along with its precipitating cause. Volume expansion and fluid challenges are used to correct decreased preload with the addition of inotropic support if fluid therapy alone does not improve the patient's status.

In sepsis, volume expansion is initiated along with empiric antibiotic therapy until the specific organism is identified. Inotropic and vasopressor support is often required in sepsis. Increased capillary permeability continues in the latter stages of sepsis, allowing intravenous fluids to cross into the interstitial space, which produces edema and compromises flow by compressing the microvasculature. Further manipulation of vascular tone by vasoactive agents is required. Many hemodynamic parameters are used to monitor cardiovascular status; however, optimal tissue perfusion is best monitored by oxygen delivery and consumption variables.[68] Chapters 6 and 17 provide a full discussion of oxygen supply and demand in sepsis, SIRS, and MODS.

Monitoring

In hypovolemic shock and early sepsis, monitoring is directed toward the assessment of preload, tissue perfusion, and tissue oxygenation. Defining optimal preload necessitates collecting data best obtained from a pulmonary artery catheter. Increases in filling pressures are required to generate a CO that is about one and one half times normal in order to provide adequate tissue oxygenation.[69] The Starling curve needs to be defined in sepsis so that the optimal filling pressure for the individual patient may be provided. PCWP also must be increased in order to optimize left ventricular function. The recommended value for PCWP is 12 to 18 mm Hg. Adequacy of perfusion may be signalled by a reversal of lactic acidosis, although some clinicians believe lactate levels and acidosis are affected by too many other factors and may not be true indicators of tissue oxygenation. Mean arterial blood pressure should exceed 80 mm Hg in order to maintain organ perfusion. Oxygenation is best monitored by evaluating oxygen delivery and oxygen consumption.

Prevention

The approach to prevention of postoperative organ failure has been stated by Waxman[70]; however, many of the points are applicable in the treatment of MODS from any cause. The recommendations include aggressive preoperative fluid resuscitation; monitoring of oxygen delivery and oxygen consumption; minimization of intraoperative oxygen deficits; assessment of cardiopulmonary reserve; support of physiologic compensatory mechanisms such as increases in CO, oxygen delivery, and oxygen consumption; prevention of sepsis; aggressive nutritional therapy; and support of individual organ systems.[70]

When this approach is generalized to treat trauma or sepsis, the major points include close monitoring of oxygen transport variables, especially in patients with decreased cardiopulmonary reserves as well as diminished reserves in other organ systems; aggressive support of oxygen delivery and oxygen consumption with timely and appropriate fluid resuscitation and support of individual organ systems; aggressive nutritional support; and prevention or resolution of sepsis. The prevention or resolution of sepsis requires that the source be controlled either by surgical intervention, if the source can be found, or by administration of antimicrobials if the septic source cannot be removed immediately, as in burns or peritonitis.

Fluid resuscitation

Crystalloids. Preload is increased by intravascular volume loading with intravenous fluids classified as crystalloids or colloids. Crystalloids are commonly the first resuscitation fluids administered after intravenous access is established in trauma patients.[71] Crystalloids, such as normal saline and lactated Ringer's solution, contain electrolytes but no plasma proteins and, consequently, will diffuse into the interstitial space causing edema. Diffusion of the crystalloid into the interstitial space necessitates that more fluid be administered than the amount lost. The American College of Surgeons Committee on Trauma advocates that crystalloid solutions be infused to replace three times the estimated blood loss because only one part will remain in the intravascular space while two parts will diffuse into the interstitial space.[71] Other authors recommend the prompt administration of 2 to 3 L of crystalloid during evaluation of the clinical situation.[69,71] Continued resuscitation and definitive diagnosis can then be guided by the patient's response to the fluid challenge. If more than 25% of the blood volume is lost, blood products must also be transfused in order to maintain intravascular volume; red blood cells are transfused to maintain oxygen carrying capacity.

Burn shock formulas in current use recommend crystalloid administration in the form of lactated Ringer's solution. Over the first 24 hours, the volume requirements are calculated as 2 to 4 mL/kg for each percent of total body surface area burned. One half of the calculated amount is given in the first 8 hours after burn injury, since this is the period when the greatest fluid, electrolyte, and protein shifts occur. Fluids are not bolused unless the patient develops grossly inadequate perfusion, because a bolus will increase capillary hydrostatic pressure transiently and increase the rate of loss into the burn wound.[72] If the patient does develop grossly inadequate perfusion due to delayed resuscitation, preexisting disease, or severity of injury, a bolus of colloid solution should be given.[73] Current studies demonstrate the advantages of addition of colloid to early postburn resuscitation regimens.[73,74] The advantage relates specifically to the nonburn tissue that regains normal permeability characteristics soon after injury. Hypoproteinemia accentuates edema formation in nonburn tissues, thereby increasing morbidity.[73]

Fluid resuscitation with crystalloids can potentially cause pulmonary, as well as peripheral edema. Colloid oncotic pressure reduction by dilution of plasma proteins with crystalloid solutions is the postulated mechanism for pulmonary edema formation.[75] When volume administration is monitored to prevent volume overload, there is no difference in lung function in fluid resuscitation of patients with shock using crystalloids or colloids.[75] According to Rainey and English the major pitfall to avoid in crystalloid resuscitation is inadequate fluid administration, since edema is expected with these fluids and is not considered a sign of intravascular volume overload.[75] Crystalloid resuscitation has the beneficial effect of reducing blood viscosity and thereby improving blood flow through the microvasculature. In addition, electrolyte solutions are beneficial because they are nonallergenic, inexpensive, and readily available.

Hypertonic saline. Hypertonic saline is another electrolyte solution used in fluid resuscitation. This solution produces a large osmotic force that pulls fluid from the intracellular space to the extracellular space in order to achieve an iso-osmolar state. Total fluid requirements are reduced with the use of hypertonic saline resuscitation. Complications of hypertonic saline resuscitation include excessive serum osmolality, hypernatremia, hypokalemia, and altered thermal regulatory set points.[76] Free water cannot be given during hypertonic saline resuscitation because it dilutes the solution to a more isotonic concentration necessitating an increase in the total amount of fluid infused.

Colloids. Colloids are generally considered to be plasma proteins; however, synthetic substitutes, such as dextran and hetastarch, are also included in this category. Plasma proteins are available in the form of albumin, plasma protein fraction, fresh frozen plasma, and whole blood. Fresh frozen plasma and whole blood carry the risk of disease transmission, whereas this risk is eliminated in heat-treated products such as albumin and plasma protein fraction. Heating also inactivates the clotting factors in albumin and plasma protein fraction. Plasma protein fraction, also known as plasmanate, differs from albumin because it contains some globulins in addition to albumin. Hypotension associated with plasmanate administration is attributed to kinins or prekallikrein activator present among the globulin proteins.[75]

Albumin. Albumin is a small protein that generates about 80% of the plasma oncotic pressure.[75] Endogenous albumin is present in both the intravascular and interstitial spaces. Interstitial albumin may be either tissue bound or nonbound. Free interstitial albumin returns to the intravascular compartment via lymphatic drainage, which increases during intravascular volume depletion.[75] Albumin is produced in the liver, but synthesis is depressed during injury or stress since hepatocytes increase the production of acute-phase reactants. In such situations, interstitial protein stores translocate into the intravascular space to correct up to a 50% depletion of intravascular albumin.[75]

Clinically, albumin is available as a 5% or a 25% solution. A comparison of the volumes of the two solutions containing 25 g of albumin shows that a 500-ml solution of 5% albumin is isooncotic and increases the intravascular space by 450 to 500 ml provided that microvascular permeability is normal. The 25% solution is 100 ml in volume and also increases the intravascular volume by about 450 ml; however, the additional 350 ml must translocate from the interstitial space.[75] In hypovolemic shock or early sepsis, this translocation of fluid does not occur rapidly enough, and the 5% solution, therefore, becomes the fluid of choice.

Dextran. Dextran and hetastarch are nonprotein colloids that generate oncotic force. Dextran is a high molecular weight polysaccharide produced from glucose and is commercially available as dextran 40 or dextran 70 with molecular weights of 40,000 and 70,000, respectively. The length of time that dextran molecules remain in the intravascular space is determined by their size. Although dextran solutions are labeled according to mean molecular weight, both solutions contain a range of molecular weights. Smaller particles are rapidly excreted by the kidney, causing an osmotic diuresis, but larger particles remain in the circulation longer than 24 hours.

Dextran improves microcirculatory blood flow by coating endothelial and cellular surfaces.[75] This reduces sludging and cell aggregation. The platelet functions of adherence and degranulation are inhibited by dextran, thus decreasing thrombus formation. By the same mechanism, aggressive dextran infusion can cause a clotting deficiency. Dextran has antigenic cross-reactivity with bacterial polysaccharide antigens and is reported to cause anaphylaxis.[75] A small portion of the population has circulating antidextran antibodies. Allergic reactions may be prevented with the previous infusion of a smaller dextran molecule, known as PROMIT, which will bind with circulating dextran antibodies.

Hetastarch. Hetastarch is another synthetic colloid with a volume-expanding capability comparable to that of 5% albumin.[2] This solution has an incidence of anaphylaxis similar to that of albumin and has the potential to cause bleeding complications if administered in amounts greater than 2 L/day.[76] As with dextran, hetastarch causes an osmotic diuresis and does not replace natural proteins. Hetastarch continues to expand the plasma volume for 24 to 36 hours after administration.[2]

Crystalloids versus colloids. The primary goal in fluid resuscitation is to increase the circulating volume without producing pulmonary edema. Given normal capillary permeability, colloids expand the plasma volume more effectively than do crystalloids. Whether crystalloid or colloid solutions are more effective in avoiding pulmonary edema has been debated, with beneficial and adverse effects demonstrated for each type of solution. Current knowledge indicates that expansion of plasma volume to a level above the preshock level improves survival significantly.[77] In sepsis, it is recommended that CO and oxygen delivery be increased to two times the normal levels in order to maintain oxygen consumption at about one and one half times the normal level, which is an initial estimate of the needs of the septic patient.[69] Overall, the outcome of resuscitation in shock is related to interacting factors, such as the type and severity of shock, selection and volume of infusion solution given, duration of infusion, and volume of infusion distribution over time.[77]

Neither crystalloid nor colloid solutions, excluding whole blood, replace the oxygen-carrying capacity of red blood cells. Fresh frozen plasma will replace clotting factors and is indicated in correcting specific coagulation deficiencies; however, plasma will not improve oxygen delivery. Packed red blood cells rather than whole blood are used to improve oxygen delivery because they provide specific therapy. The concept of optimal hematocrit relates to the ability of the circulation to provide optimal tissue oxygenation. Optimal tissue oxygenation must be balanced with promotion of flow through the microcirculation. The first goal is accomplished with an increased hematocrit and the latter by keeping the blood less viscous (i.e., with a lower hematocrit).

A range of hematocrit values, from 30% to 48%, have been reported as being optimal.[29,69,78] It is not yet established if one value is indeed optimal for all organs. The septic bowel is reported to have an increased hematocrit requirement of about 48%.[29] Dietrich and co-workers studied the benefit of red blood cell transfusion in critically ill, volume-resuscitated patients with circulatory shock resulting from sepsis and cardiogenic shock.[79] Transfusion significantly increased oxygen delivery, as expected, because hemoglobin is part of the arterial oxygen content equation as described in Chapter 6; however, oxygen consumption, CI, and PCWP did not change.[79] The authors concluded that isolated red blood cell transfusion after volume and inotrope resuscitation may not result in improved tissue oxygen utilization, although improvement did occur in some patients.[79]

Pharmacologic therapy

Pharmacologic therapy intended to correct the maldistribution of circulating volume in MODS involves manipulation of preload, afterload, and contractility. Initially, decreased preload is managed by fluid resuscitation techniques as previously described. If fluid therapy does not result in clear improvement, inotropic support is added to increase myocardial contractility and to reverse excessive vasodilatation. The majority of drugs that are used to support cardiovascular status in shock and MODS act on adrenergic receptors. A point to remember with all vasoactive medications is that patients respond differently to specific doses. The response of patients to vasoactive agents may also be influenced by the pathophysiologic changes that occur along the sepsis continuum. In other words, a drug that works well in the early phase of sepsis may be ineffective in the later phase as responsiveness to catecholamines decreases. Table 5-5 summarizes the different types of receptors and the vascular effects of their stimulation. Table 5-6 summarizes the activity of the vasoactive drugs discussed in this section.

Dopamine. Dopamine is generally infused to improve myocardial contractility and augment renal and mesenteric perfusion in the shock state. The effects of dopamine are dose dependent in that

Table 5-5 Vascular Effects of Adrenergic Receptor Stimulation

Receptor	Location	Effect
Alpha$_1$	Postsynaptic vascular smooth muscle receptors	Vasoconstriction in peripheral and pulmonary circulations
Alpha$_2$	Presynaptic receptor on sympathetic nerve ending	Inhibition of norepinephrine release
Beta$_1$	Postsynaptic myocardial receptors	Increased heart rate and contractility Increased coronary vasodilatation
	Renal juxtaglomerular cells	Release of renin
Beta$_2$	Postsynaptic vascular and bronchial smooth muscle receptors	Vasodilatation in peripheral circulation Bronchodilation
Dopaminergic	Postsynaptic renal and mesenteric vascular smooth muscle receptors	Vasodilatation of renal and mesenteric circulations

Table 5-6 Categories of Vasoactive Drugs

Drug	Chronotropic	Inotropic	Dopaminergic	Vasopressor	Vasodilator
Dopamine	Moderate dose	Moderate dose	Low dose	High dose	—
Dobutamine	High dose	Moderate dose	—	—	High dose
Epinephrine	All doses	Low dose	—	High dose	Low dose
Isoproterenol	All doses	All doses	—	—	All doses (cardiac, skeletal, and pulmonary circulations)
Norepinephrine	Low dose, may cause reflex bradycardia	Low dose	—	Moderate-to-high dose	—
Amrinone	—	All doses	—	—	All doses
Phenylephrine	May cause reflex bradycardia	—	—	All doses	—
Nitroprusside	May cause reflex tachycardia	—	—	—	All doses

dopaminergic receptors are stimulated at doses of 2 to 3 µg/kg/min. The improved blood flow to the renal and mesenteric vascular beds increases urine output and restores liver function.[41] The chronotropic and inotropic effects of increased heart rate and contractility predominate in the moderate dose range of 5 to 10 µg/kg/min. Vasopressor effects occur when the dose is in the high range of 10 to 15 µg/kg/min; alpha vasoconstriction predominates with minimal beta$_1$ activity and no dopaminergic effects.

Dopamine is not always successful in reversing the hypotension of sepsis.[27,80,81] Dopamine-resistant hypotension may occur as a result of the presence of vasodilatory mediators such as EDRF.[27] The ability of dopamine to stimulate peripheral alpha receptors may also be impaired in septic shock.[82] When dopamine is not used in vasoconstrictor doses, it is usually added at the low dopaminergic dose.

Dobutamine. Dobutamine has its major effect on contractility rather than on the heart rate or the blood vessels because it primarily stimulates beta$_1$ receptors. At higher infusion rates of 5 to 15 µg/kg/min, mild beta$_2$- and some alpha-receptor stimulatory activity cause slight vasodilatation and improved coronary blood flow.[83] Fluid requirements are reported to be increased when dobutamine is infused at a dose of 6 µg/kg/min; however, oxygen delivery and oxygen consumption improved significantly.[84] When dobutamine and dopamine were compared at the same dose, dobutamine reduced PCWP and improved oxygen delivery and oxygen consumption, whereas dopamine maintained wedge pressure without changing tissue oxygen variables.[85]

Not all studies have demonstrated a clinical benefit with the addition of dobutamine. Dobutamine may not be effective and, in fact, may be detrimental, in established sepsis.[78,86] Hayes and co-workers reported a 54% mortality (with a predicted risk of death of 34%) in patients receiving dobutamine therapy with the goal of achieving a CI >4.5 L/min/m^2, oxygen delivery >600 mL/min/m^2, and oxygen consumption >170 mL/min/m^2.[86] These results may be related to the timing of dobutamine therapy because the patients in this study were admitted to the ICU for therapy postoperatively and, often, after complications had already occurred.[86]

Combination therapy is frequently used to achieve an optimal cardiovascular effect. This approach avoids the administration of high dosages that are known to cause undesirable effects. Since dobutamine is shown to be beneficial in improving oxygen delivery and oxygen consumption, it is combined with a low dose of dopamine to perfuse the mesentery. Optimal tissue perfusion goals may then be attainable.[78,87]

Digoxin. Digoxin is indicated for improvement of myocardial contractility. The effect of digoxin is not immediate; however, it is an important addition because its action is not dependent on adrenergic receptors. Adrenergic receptor sensitivity is reported to be depressed during endotoxin shock.[31] Consequently, larger doses of vasoactive agents may be required in order to achieve the same effect. This depressed sensitivity does not affect the inotropic action of digoxin. Research has shown that digoxin improves left ventricular function in patients with severe sepsis as measured by significant increases in stroke output and work.[88]

Epinephrine. Epinephrine in low doses stimulates beta$_1$- and beta$_2$-adrenergic receptors, causing increased heart rate and force of contraction, which produces an increased CO. Other effects of epinephrine at this dose are dilatation of the bronchi and of the blood vessels of cardiac and skeletal muscle. In doses greater than 0.02 µg/kg/min, epinephrine stimulates alpha receptors, causing more constriction, thereby increasing afterload and blood pressure. Epinephrine is known to stimulate beta$_1$ receptors more than beta$_2$ receptors; therefore, it will increase cardiac work more than it increases coronary blood flow.[83] Myocardial ischemia may be a secondary result of this imbalance of oxygen supply and demand.

Epinephrine has been shown to improve CI and reverse hypotension in septic shock where dopamine had failed.[81] Infusion rates of epinephrine in septic shock must usually start at doses greater than 0.5 µg/kg/min in order to achieve the desired effect.[78,81] The side effects of ectopy and tachycardia are more common at this higher dose.

Isoproterenol. Isoproterenol is identified as a pure beta adrenergic drug because it stimulates only the beta receptors. Based on the actions produced by beta receptor stimulation, isoproterenol will improve contractility, increase heart rate, and produce vasodilatation in the cardiac, skeletal, and pulmonary circulations. This vasodilatation can be detrimental to the splanchnic bed and other organs that are not preferentially dilated. Because isoproterenol increases both fluid requirements by its vasodilatory effects and myocardial oxygen consumption, it is not generally recommended for use in shock.

Norepinephrine. Norepinephrine stimulates alpha$_1$ and beta$_1$ receptors. Again, low-dose and high-dose effects occur, so that beta receptor stimulation is seen at low doses and mixed effects of stimulation of both alpha and beta receptors occur at high doses. Norepinephrine increases cardiac work, and its potent vasoconstrictor effects can compromise blood flow to the kidney and other tissues and cause the movement of intravascular fluid into the interstitial space.[83] These considerations have limited the use of this drug in the shock state; however, current thinking suggests that patients in the past who had a poor outcome with norepinephrine had not been fully volume resuscitated.

The role of vasopressors in sepsis is being reconsidered. After fluid replacement guided by PCWP, norepinephrine, when compared to dopamine, has been shown to successfully maintain treatment outcomes of SVRI >1100 dynes/s/cm^5/m^2 or mean blood pressure >80 mm Hg, CI >4 L/min/m^2, oxygen delivery index >550 ml/min/m^2, and oxygen consumption index greater than 150 ml/min/m^2.[80] Urine output also improved with the use of norepinephrine. The authors speculate that the increase in urine output could be related to the improvement in CI or the decrease in antidiuretic hormone release that follows restoration of adequate central pressures.[80]

Amrinone. Amrinone is an inotrope that increases contractility by inhibiting phosphodiesterase. Its use in septic shock is limited because it decreases both preload and afterload through direct relaxation of both the venous and the arteriolar smooth muscle.[83] Reductions in preload and afterload are desirable in congestive heart failure but will exacerbate hypotension in sepsis unless adequate volume expansion is complete. Amrinone may be helpful in septic shock when SVR is elevated because it decreases afterload and increases contractility.[78] Because amrinone does not depend on adrenergic receptor activity, which is depressed in sepsis, it may be more effective than adrenergic drugs such as dopamine, dobutamine, and epinephrine.

Phenylephrine. Vasoconstrictor therapy may be indicated to increase vascular tone and SVR in distributive shock. Many of the inotropic agents previously discussed have vasoconstrictor properties when the dosage is increased. Phenylephrine is a pure alpha-adrenergic drug that constricts blood vessels in the skin, kidneys, lungs, and gastrointestinal tract. This drug increases coronary blood flow, but its use is limited to situations where the CO is adequate and vasoconstriction is necessary for blood pressure support.[83] Clinically, pure alpha-receptor agonists tend to reduce CO without improving peripheral blood distribution and oxygen availability.[78]

Nitroprusside. Vasodilators are used to decrease severe elevations of SVR that may occur in the preterminal hypodynamic phase of septic shock. The rationale for use of nitrates or nitroprusside is to increase CO by reduction of afterload. Nitroprusside is known as a balanced vasodilator because it reduces both the pulmonary venous and the systemic venous pressure.[89] Reduction of pulmonary venous pressure may override hypoxic pulmonary vasoconstriction, thereby increasing the shunt fraction. Nitroprusside causes direct relaxation of arterial and venous smooth muscle and is not dependent on adrenergic receptors to produce its effect.[89]

INVESTIGATIONAL THERAPIES

Unconventional pharmacologic therapy in shock includes the administration of glucagon, naloxone, and calcium antagonists. These agents are controversial because researchers have been unable to demonstrate consistently positive results with their use. A review of each agent is presented in order to provide a complete discussion of all agents used in shock.

Glucagon

Glucagon exerts an inotropic effect on the heart and is indicated in low-output states induced by blockade of beta receptors. The dose is 5 to 6 mg intravenously followed by an infusion of 2 to 10 mg/hr.[78] The mechanism of the inotropic effect of glucagon is thought to be activation of adenyl cyclase, thereby increasing the level of cyclic adenosine monophosphate (cAMP).[78] cAMP then induces cell contraction. Catecholamines are dependent upon the beta receptor in order to effect an increase in cAMP.

Naloxone

Naloxone is used only as adjunctive therapy in reversing the hypotension of septic shock. This narcotic antagonist is thought to be beneficial in shock because it antagonizes the cardiovascular actions of endogenous opiates. Factors reported to affect the success of naloxone therapy in septic shock include the length of time hypotension is present before naloxone administration and the amount of antagonist given.[90] The presence and concentration of other circulating mediators that contribute to cardiovascular instability may also contribute to the success of naloxone therapy. One study reported hemodynamic improvement with naloxone but found no overall effect on mortality.[91]

Calcium antagonists

Calcium homeostasis is disrupted in shock, resulting in increased intracellular calcium levels. Intracellular calcium accumulation activates several intracellular processes that can lead to cell destruction, organ dysfunction, and death.[92] Calcium antagonists have been used successfully in the treatment of myocardial ischemia. Researchers have demonstrated improved cardiovascular function and survival associated with the administration of calcium channel antagonists in endotoxin shock.[92]

Future therapy

Future therapy to correct maldistribution of circulating volume will focus on methods to maximize blood flow through the microcirculation. This may include infusing prostacyclin to dilate vascular beds or administering arachidonic acid metabolite inhibitors and antagonists. ODFR scavengers will reduce the damage done to the endothelium by toxic oxygen species. Anti-inflammatory therapy may include anti-TNF antibodies and neutralization of IL-1 and TNF. Many of these theoretical therapies may prove to be unworkable; however, new discoveries will occur to change our thinking about the etiology and prognosis of MODS.[93]

CONCLUSION

Maldistribution of circulating volume leading to MODS is a complex event involving treatment regimens, clinical conditions such as hemorrhage or inflammation, and the release of vasoactive mediators. These mediators, derived from humoral, cellular, and biochemical pathways, affect the microvascular, the organ, and the regional circulations through their effects on vasomotor tone, microvascular permeability, and coagulation. Neutrophil- and macrophage-generated mediators affect the heart, lungs, liver, kidneys, and brain. Reperfusion of these organs after shock may not result in a return to functioning normally but may instead initiate postischemic reperfusion injury. Current therapy of maldistribution of circulating volume concentrates on treatment of symptoms by restoring effective circulating blood flow and oxygen transport to all tissues. Attempts to accomplish these goals by fluid resuscitation and pharmacologic manipulation of the vasculature continue. Investigational therapy focuses on preventing mediator-induced cellular damage and maldistribution of circulating volume, which lead to organ dysfunction and failure.

REFERENCES

1. Cerra FB. Hypermetabolism-organ failure syndrome: A metabolic response to injury. Crit Care Clin 1989;5:289-302.
2. Whitman GR. Shock. In: Kinney MR, Packa DR, Dunbar SB, eds. AACN's clinical reference for critical care nursing. St. Louis: Mosby; 1993:133-172.
3. Guyton AC. Local control of blood flow by the tissues and humoral regulation. In: Guyton AC, ed. Textbook of medical physiology. 8th ed. Philadelphia: W.B. Saunders; 1991:185-193.
4. Petrak RA, Balk RA, Bone RC. Prostaglandins, cyclooxygenase inhibitors, and thromboxane synthetase inhibitors in the pathogenesis of multiple systems organ failure. Crit Care Clin 1989;5:303-314.
5. Ruffolo RR. Cardiovascular adrenoreceptors: Physiology and critical care implications. In: Chernow B, ed. Pharmacologic approach to the critically ill. 2nd ed. Baltimore: Williams and Wilkins; 1988:166-183.
6. Yurt RW, Lowry SF. Role of the macrophage and endogenous mediators in multiple organ failure. In: Deitch EA, ed. Multiple organ failure: Pathophysiology and basic concepts of therapy. New York: Thieme Medical Publishers; 1990:60-71.
7. Deitch EA, Mancini MC. Complement receptors in shock and transplantation. Arch Surg 1993;128:1222-1226.
8. Fletcher JR. Eicosanoids: Critical agents in the physiological process and cellular injury. Arch Surg 1993;128:1192-1195.
9. Secor VH. The inflammatory/immune response in critical illness: Role of the systemic inflammatory response syndrome. Crit Care Nurs Clin North Am 1994;6:251-264.
10. Lefer AM. Induction of tissue injury and altered cardiovascular performance by platelet-activating factor: Relevance to multiple systems organ failure. Crit Care Clin 1989;5:331-352.
11. Stroud M, Swindell B, Bernard GR. Cellular and humoral mediators of sepsis syndrome. Crit Care Nurs Clin North Am 1990;2:151-160.
12. Lowry SF. Cytokine mediators of immunity and inflammation. Arch Surg 1993;128:1235-1241.
13. Beutler B. Cachectin in tissue injury, shock, and related states. Crit Care Clin 1989;5:353-367.
14. Sprague RS et al. Proposed role for leukotrienes in the pathophysiology of multiple systems organ failure. Crit Care Clin 1989;5:315-329.
15. Bihari DJ, Tinker J. The therapeutic value of vasodilator prostaglandins in multiple organ failure associated with sepsis. Int Care Med 1988;15:2-7.
16. Bihari D et al. The effects of vasodilation with prostacyclin on oxygen delivery and uptake in critically ill patients. N Engl J Med 1987;317:397-403.
17. Deitch EA. Multiple organ failure: Pathophysiology and potential future therapy. Ann Surg 1992;216:117-134.
18. Schumacker PT, Samsel RW. Oxygen delivery and uptake by peripheral tissues: Physiology and pathophysiology. Crit Care Clin 1989;5:255-269.
19. Duling BR et al. Vasomotor control: Functional hyperemia and beyond. Fed Proc 1987;46:251-263.
20. Vaughan PP, Brooks Jr C. Adult respiratory distress syndrome: A complication of shock. Crit Care Nurs Clin North Am 1990;2:235-253.
21. Robins EV. Immunosuppression of the burned patient. Crit Care Nurs Clin North Am 1989;1:767-774.
22. Moncada S, Higgs A. The L-Arginine-nitric oxide pathway. N Engl J Med 1993;329:2002-2012.
23. Lawler DA. Hormonal response in sepsis. Crit Care Nurs Clin North Am 1994;6:265-274.
24. Gotch PM. The endocrine system. In: Alspach JG, ed. Core curriculum for critical care nursing. 4th ed. Philadelphia: WB Saunders; 1991:609-623.
25. Hartl WH et al. Reactive hyperemia in patients with septic conditions. Surgery 1988;103:440-444.
26. Pinsky MR, Matuschak GM. MSOF: Failure of host defense homeostasis. Crit Care Clin 1989;5:199-220.
27. Broner CW et al. Reversal of dopamine-refractory septic shock by diethyldithiocarbamate, an inhibitor of endothelium-derived relaxing factor. J Infect Dis 1993;167:141-147.
28. Adams HR, Parker JL, Laughlin MH. Intrinsic myocardial dysfunction during endotoxemia: Dependent or independent of myocardial ischemia? Circ Shock 1990;30:63-76.

29. Bersten A, Sibbald WJ. Circulatory disturbances in multiple systems organ failure. Crit Care Clin 1989;5:233-254.
30. Cunnion RE et al. The coronary circulation in human septic shock. Circ 1986;73:637-644.
31. Silverman HJ et al. Impaired beta adrenergic receptor stimulation of cyclic adenosine monophosphate in human septic shock: Association with myocardial hyporesponsiveness to catecholamines. Crit Care Med 1993;21:31-39.
32. Suffredini AF et al. The cardiovascular response of normal humans to the administration of endotoxin. N Engl J Med 1989;321:280-287.
33. Parker MM et al. Right ventricular dysfunction and dilatation, similar to left ventricular changes, characterize the cardiac depression of septic shock in humans. Chest 1990;97:126-131.
34. Parrillo JE. Pathogenetic mechanisms of septic shock. N Engl J Med 1993;328:1471-1477.
35. Reilly JM et al. A circulating myocardial depressant substance is associated with cardiac dysfunction and peripheral hypoperfusion (lactic acidemia) in patients with septic shock. Circ 1989;95:1072-1080.
36. Brigham KL, Meyrick BO. Endotoxin and lung injury. Am Rev Respir Dis 1986;133:913-927.
37. Garcia JGN et al. Leukotrienes and the pulmonary microcirculation. Am Rev Resp Dis 1987;136:161-169.
38. Henry CL et al. Attenuation of the pulmonary vascular response to endotoxin by a thromboxane synthesis inhibitor (UK-38485) in unanesthetized sheep. J Surg Res 1991;50:77-81.
39. Demling RH, LaLonde C, Pequet Goad ME. Effect of ibuprofen on the pulmonary and systemic response to repeated doses of endotoxin. Surg 1989;105:421-429.
40. Daryani R et al. Changes in catalase activity in lung and liver after endotoxemia in sheep. Circ Shock 1990;32:273-280.
41. Collins AS. Gastrointestinal complications in shock. Crit Care Nurs Clin North Am 1990;2:269-277.
42. Teplitz C. The pathology and ultrastructure of cellular injury and inflammation in the progression and outcome of trauma, sepsis, and shock. In: Clowes Jr GHA, ed. Trauma, sepsis, and shock: The physiological basis of therapy. New York: Marcel Dekker; 1988:71-120.
43. Colletti LM et al. Role of tumor necrosis factor-α in the pathophysiologic alterations after hepatic ischemia/reperfusion injury in the rat. J Clin Invest 1990;85:1936-1943.
44. Schirmer WJ et al. Imidazole and indomethacin improve hepatic perfusion in sepsis. Circ Shock 1987;21:253-259.
45. Lancaster LE. Renal response to shock. Crit Care Nurs Clin North Am 1990;2:221-233.
46. Price CA. Acute renal failure: A sequelae of sepsis. Crit Care Nurs Clin North Am 1994;6:359-372.
47. Cumming AD et al. The protective effect of thromboxane synthetase inhibition on renal function in systemic sepsis. Am J Kid Dis 1989;18:114-119.
48. Brenner M et al. Detection of renal blood flow abnormalities in septic and critically ill patients using a newly designed indwelling thermodilution renal vein catheter. Chest 1990;98:170-179.
49. Prough DS, DeWitt DS. Cerebral protection. In: Chernow B, ed. The pharmacologic approach to the critically ill. 2nd ed. Baltimore: Williams and Wilkins; 1988:198-218.
50. Ernster L. Biochemistry of reoxygenation injury. Crit Care Med 1988;16:947-953.
51. Demling RH, LaLonde C. Early postburn lipid peroxidation: Effect of ibuprofen and allopurinol. Surgery 1990;107:85-93.
52. Demling RH et al. Fluid resuscitation with deferoxamine prevents systemic burn induced oxidant injury. J Trauma 1991;31:538-543.
53. Kennedy TP et al. Ibuprofen prevents oxidant lung injury and in vitro lipid peroxidation by chelating iron. J Clin Invest 1990;86:1565-1573.
54. Zhao-fan X et al. Efficacy of leupeptin, superoxide dismutase, and verapamil in modulating delayed reperfusion damage after burn injury. J Burn Care Rehabil 1992;13:530-537.
55. Bulkley BH, Hutchins GM. Myocardial consequences of coronary artery bypass graft surgery: The paradox of necrosis in areas of revascularization. Circ 1977;56:906-913.
56. Black L, Coombs VJ, Townsend SN. Reperfusion and reperfusion injury in acute myocardial infarction. Heart Lung 1990;19:274-286.
57. Horton JW, White J, Baxter CR. The role of oxygen-derived free radicals in burn-induced myocardial contractile depression. J Burn Care Rehabil 1988;9:589-598.
58. Yokoyama Y et al. Circulating xanthine oxidase: Potential mediator of ischemic injury. Am J Physiol 1990;258:G564-570.
59. American College of Chest Physicians/Society of Critical Care Medicine Consensus Conference Committee. Definitions for sepsis and organ failure and guidelines for the use of innovative therapies in sepsis. Chest 1992;101:1644-1655.
60. American College of Chest Physicians/Society of Critical Care Medicine Consensus Conference Committee. Definitions for sepsis and organ failure and guidelines for the use of innovative therapies in sepsis. Crit Care Med 1992;20:864-874.
61. DeCamp MM, Demling RH. Posttraumatic multisystem organ failure. JAMA 1988;260:530-534.
62. Parillo JE et al. Septic shock in humans: Advances in the understanding of pathogenesis, cardiovascular dysfunction, and therapy. Ann Intern Med 1990;113:227-242.
63. Summers G. The clinical and hemodynamic presentation of the shock patient. Crit Care Nurs Clin North Am 1990;2:161-166.
64. Hazinski MF et al. Epidemiology, pathophysiology and clinical presentation of Gram-negative sepsis. Am J Crit Care 1993;2:224-237.
65. Knaus WA, Wagner DP. Multiple systems organ failure: Epidemiology and prognosis. Crit Care Clin 1989;5:221-232.
66. Dorinsky PM, Gadek JE. Multiple organ failure. Clin Chest Med 1990;11:581-591.
67. Vollman KM. Adult respiratory distress syndrome: Mediators on the run. Crit Care Nurs Clin North Am 1994;6:341-358.
68. Shoemaker WC. Pathophysiology, monitoring, and therapy of acute circulatory problems. Crit Care Nurs Clin North Am 1994;6:295-307.
69. Demling RH, Lalonde C, Ikegami K. Physiologic support of the septic patient. Surg Clin North Am 1994;74:637-658.
70. Waxman K. Postoperative multiple organ failure. Crit Care Clin 1987;3:429-440.
71. Maier RV. Evaluation and resuscitation. In: Moore EE, ed. Early care of the injured patient. 4th ed. Toronto: BC Decker; 1990:56-73.

72. Robins EV. Burn shock. Crit Care Nurs Clin North Am 1990;2:299-307.
73. Demling RH, LaLonde C. Restoration and maintenance of hemodynamic stability. In: Demling RH and LaLonde C. Burn trauma. New York: Theime Medical Publishers; 1989:24-41.
74. Carvajal HF, Parks DH. Optimal composition of burn resuscitation fluids. Crit Care Med 1988;16:695-700.
75. Rainey TG, English JF. Pharmacology of colloids and crystalloids. In: Chernow B, ed. The pharmacologic approach to the critically ill. 2nd ed. Baltimore: Williams and Wilkins; 1988:219-240.
76. Neff JA. Perfusion. In: Neff JA, Kidd PS. Trauma nursing: The art and science. St. Louis: Mosby; 1993:195-262.
77. Dawidson IJA et al. Lactated Ringer's solution versus 3% albumin for resuscitation of a lethal intestinal ischemic shock in rats. Crit Care Med 1990;18:60-66.
78. Conrad SA et al. Cardiovascular dysfunction in multiple organ failure. In: Dietch EA, ed. Multiple organ failure: Pathophysiology and basic concepts of therapy. New York: Thieme Medical Publishers; 1990:172-191.
79. Dietrich KA et al. Cardiovascular and metabolic response to blood cell transfusion in critically ill volume-resuscitated nonsurgical patients. Crit Care Med 1990;18:940-944.
80. Martin C et al. Norepinephrine or dopamine for the treatment of septic shock? Chest 1993;103:1826-1831.
81. Bollaert PE et al. Effects of epinephrine on hemodynamics and oxygen metabolism in dopamine-resistant septic shock. Chest 1990;98:949-953.
82. Scheuder WO et al. Effect of dopamine vs norepinephrine on hemodynamics in septic shock: Emphasis on right ventricular performance. Chest 1989;95:1282-1288.
83. Burns KM. Vasoactive drug therapy in shock. Crit Care Nurs Clin North Am 1990;2:167-178.
84. Vincent JL, DeBacker D. Initial management of circulatory shock as prevention of MSOF. Crit Care Clin 1989;5:369-378.
85. Shoemaker WC et al. Comparison of hemodynamic and oxygen transport effects of dopamine and dobutamine in critically ill surgical patients. Chest 1989;96:120-126.
86. Hayes MA et al. Elevation of systemic oxygen delivery in the treatment of critically ill patients. N Engl J Med 1994;330:1717-1722.
87. Yu M et al. Effect of maximizing oxygen delivery on morbidity and mortality rates in critically ill patients: A prospective, randomized, controlled study. Crit Care Med 1993;21:830-838.
88. Nasraway SA et al. Inotropic response to digoxin and dopamine in patients with severe sepsis, cardiac failure, and systemic hypoperfusion. Chest 1989;95:612-615.
89. Parrillo JE. Vasodilator therapy. In: Chernow B, ed. The pharmacologic approach to the critically ill. 2nd ed. Baltimore: Williams and Wilkins, 1988:346-364.
90. Schumann LL, Remington MA. The use of naloxone in treating endotoxic shock. Crit Care Nurs 1990;10:63-71.
91. Hackshaw KV, Parker GA, Roberts JW. Naloxone in septic shock. Crit Care Med 1990;18:47-51.
92. Malcolm DS et al. Calcium and calcium antagonists in shock and ischemia. In: Chernow B, ed. The pharmacologic approach to the critically ill. 2nd ed. Baltimore: Williams and Wilkins, 1988:889-900.
93. Natanson C et al. Selected treatment strategies for septic shock based on proposed mechanisms of pathogenesis. Ann Intern Med 1994;120:771-783.

CHAPTER 6

Imbalance of Oxygen Supply and Demand

Marguerite Littleton Kearney

To satisfy the energy requirements of tissues, oxygen must be supplied to the cells on a continous basis. Should cellular demands exceed the oxygen supply or should oxygen delivery reserves become exhausted then tissue hypoxia will ensue. Hypoperfusion, tissue injury, and ischemia remain prominent features of multiple organ dysfunction syndrome (MODS).[1-3] Pathophysiologic conditions that impair perfusion, initiate a systemic inflammatory response, or damage cells directly, lead to a pattern of sequential organ dysfunction.[2]

Systemic hypoperfusion presumably causes functional damage that primes specific target organs for the development of organ failure.[2,4] This has been termed the "first hit." Secondarily, an exaggerated stress response, superimposed on the initial organ injury affects normal homeostasis[5] and precipitates activation of the systemic inflammatory response syndrome (SIRS). These conditions may or may not be associated with bacterial infection, but they are strongly associated with the eventual dysfunction of one or more organs.[5] Disruption of normal physiologic control mechanisms could produce an acute oxygen debt,[4] believed to be a common denominator in MODS of various etiologies. Figure 6-1 depicts this proposed model. Regardless of the cause, oxygen deprivation impairs the bioenergetic work of the cell and ultimately leads to ischemia and cell death. This results in an inadequate supply of adenosine triphosphate (ATP) to run cellular processes.

CELLULAR BIOENERGETICS
ATP generation during cellular metabolism

To understand why interruption of oxygen supply or alterations in oxygen utilization affect organ function in MODS it is necessary to review the interrelationship between oxidative metabolism and ATP replenishment. Cells generate fuel for their metabolic processes via the formation of ATP. One of the most efficient mechanisms for ATP synthesis is through aerobic processing of glucose, proteins, and lipids via the Krebs cycle (also known as the citric acid cycle or the tricarboxylic acid cycle) as shown in Figure 6-2. Unresolved ischemia or an inability of the cell to use oxygen effectively results in inefficient substrate metabolism and poor energy production. The cell shifts its bioenergetic processes from aerobic to anaerobic metabolism at the expense of ATP production. Curtailment of cellular ATP synthesis leads to diminished active transport of ions across cell membranes, with the subsequent alteration of chemiosmotic gradients, resulting in cell swelling and eventual rupture.[6] The cell also requires ATP for synthesis of chemical compounds and mechanical work (e.g., muscle contraction); therefore, these processes will also be hindered by poor ATP production.

Normal substrate oxidation: aerobic metabolism

In the presence of oxygen, metabolism of energy substrates, such as glucose, results in a net gain of 36 moles of ATP per mole of glucose (38 moles of ATP are produced, but only 2 moles are used). Initially, glucose is converted to pyruvate in a process known as glycolysis that yields a net gain of 2 moles of ATP per mole of glucose. The pyruvate in the cell cytoplasm eventually reaches the mitochondria where it is converted to acetyl coenzyme A (CoA).[7] Acetyl CoA enters the Krebs cycle in the

136 *Pathophysiologic Changes*

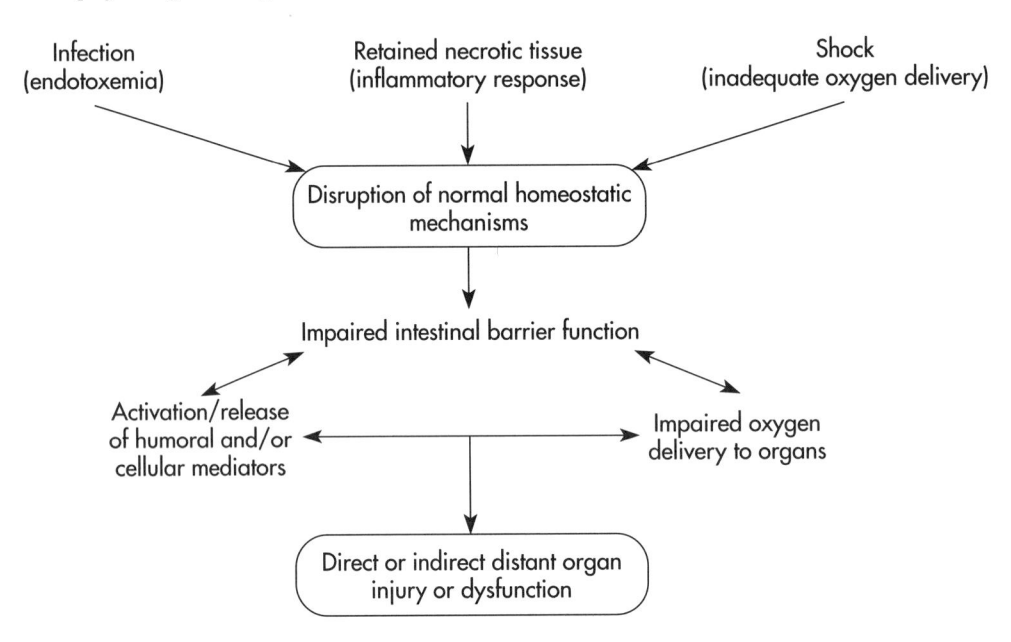

Fig. 6-1 Proposed relationships between triggers of MODS. (From Deitch EA. Multiple organ failure. Adv Surg 1993;26:339.)

mitochondrial matrix (Fig. 6-3) where aerobic metabolism and the bulk of ATP production take place. In the Krebs cycle four pairs of hydrogen atoms are removed from the intermediates formed during the cycle. Nicotinamide adenine dinucleotide (NAD) and flavin adenine dinucleotide (FAD) are coenzymes that function to accept these hydrogen ions and serve to transport electrons to the electron transport chain for oxidative phosphorylation (Fig. 6-4). Complete oxidation of glucose ultimately results in the formation of carbon dioxide and water. The carbon dioxide is eliminated by the lungs and the free oxygen is paired with hydrogen to form water during oxidative phosphorylation.

ATP replenishment

The reduced forms of the nicotinamide adenine dinucleotide (NADH) and flavin adenine dinucleotide (FADH) donate electrons that are shuttled along the electron transport chain for ultimate reduction of oxygen to water.[7] In the electron transport chain the electrons are carried first to ubiquinone (coenzyme Q), then along a series of heme-containing cytochromes embedded in the inner mitochondrial membrane.[7] Oxygen acts as the ultimate electron acceptor in the chain. As the electrons are ferried along the electron transport chain the free energy released is channeled into ATP synthesis via the attachment of inorganic phosphate to adenosine diphosphate (ADP). Thus, ATP synthesis is tightly coupled to electron transport.

The energy released as the electrons pass down the electron transport chain is used to establish a transmembrane gradient that depends on both an electric and an osmotic difference in the concentration of protons from the hydrogen ions. Hydrogen ions are believed to be pumped across the inner mitochondrial membrane creating this electrochemical gradient.[7] The higher concentration of hydrogen ions on the exterior of the inner mitochondrial membrane, as opposed to that of the matrix, establishes an electric potential (redox potential), as well as an osmotic difference. The energy contained in the electrochemical potential can be harnessed to generate ATP. Movement of the hydrogen ions back across the inner membrane to the matrix provides energy for the phosphorylation of ADP to form ATP during oxidative phosphorylation. ADP and NADH accumulate in the cytoplasm and, in the presence of an adequate oxygen supply, stimulate oxidative me-

Imbalance of Oxygen Supply and Demand **137**

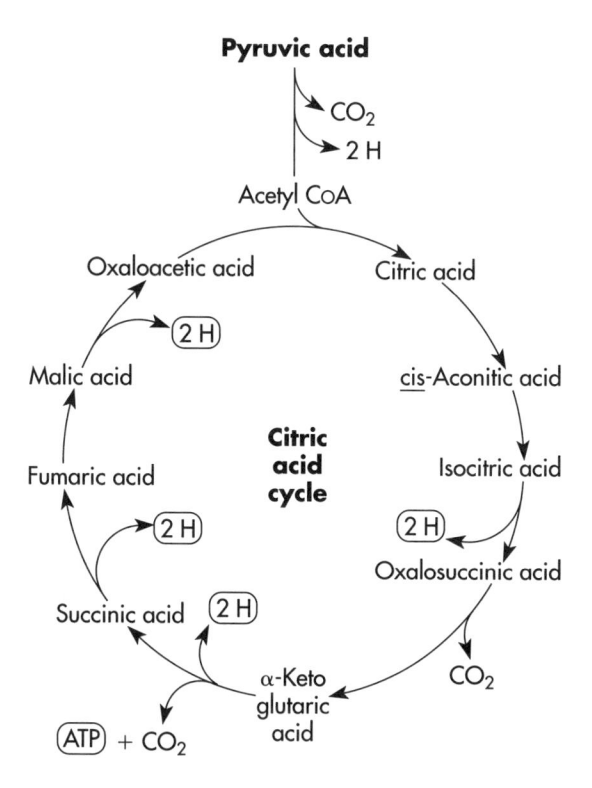

Fig. 6-2 Diagram of Krebs cycle. (From Porth CM, Curtis RL. Cell and tissue characteristics. In: Porth CM, ed. Pathophysiology concepts and altered states. 4th ed. Philadelphia: JB Lippincott, 1994:16.)

tabolism, increase oxygen consumption, and further ATP generation. ATP is then available to fuel the metabolic processes of the cell. As ATP is used it is broken back down to ADP and recycled for further ATP synthesis.

Anaerobic metabolism

As oxygen consumption falls, the cell shifts its bioenergetic processes from aerobic to anaerobic metabolism at the expense of ATP production.[6] In contrast to aerobic metabolism, anaerobic metabolism of glucose nets only 2 moles of ATP per mole of glucose burned. Glucose is preferentially metabolized during periods of low oxygen availability because in the absence of oxygen at least 2 moles of ATP can be generated via anaerobic metabolism. When oxygen is low, pyruvate, driven by the redox potential, is converted to lactate. Anaerobic metabolism can supply an extremely limited amount of ATP as compared to aerobic processing of pyruvate.[8]

Oxygen must be present to serve as the final electron acceptor as demonstrated in the following chemical reaction occurring during normal oxidative phosphorylation:

$$NADH + H^+ + 3\,ADP + 3\,P_i + \tfrac{1}{2}O_2 \rightarrow NAD^+ + 3\,ATP + H_2O$$

Diminished oxygen availability slows the process of oxidative phosphorylation and impairs synthesis of ATP, since mininal oxygen is available to accept electrons.[9] The by-product of anaerobic glycolysis, lactic acid, collects in the cell. High intracellular lactic acid levels are thought to inhibit enzymes, promote irreversible cell damage and enhance

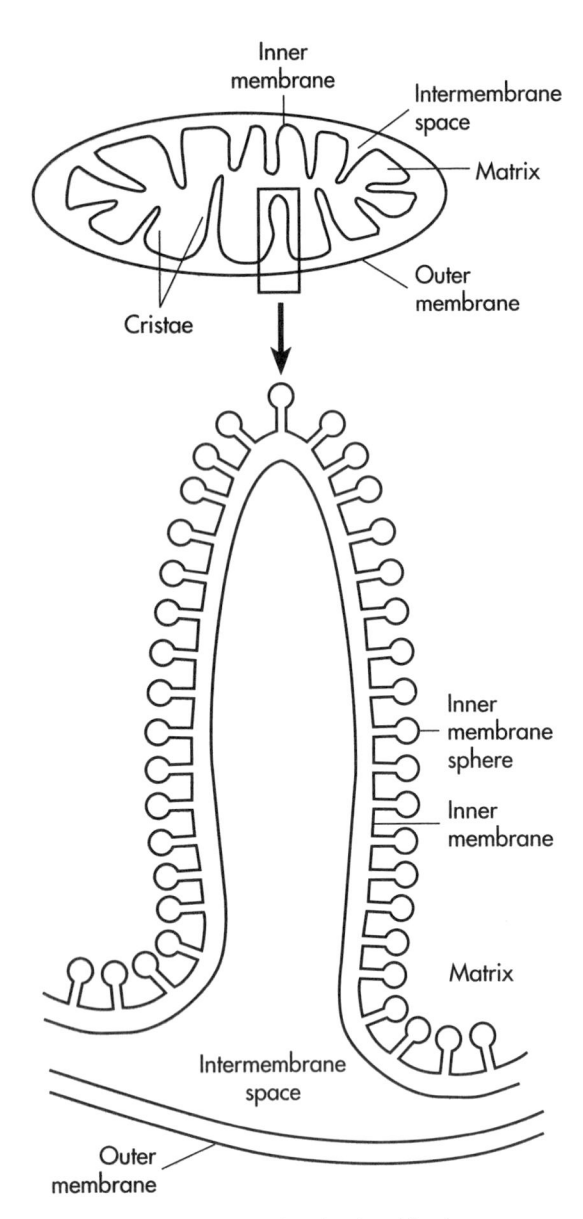

Fig. 6-3 Morphology of a mitochondrion in transverse section. (From Bhagavan NV. Medical Biochemistry. Boston: Jones and Bartlett Publishers, 1992:261.)

OXYGEN TRANSPORT AND UTILIZATION
Oxygen delivery and extraction

In healthy tissues oxygen delivery, defined as the amount of oxygen transported to tissues each minute, exceeds oxygen consumption by a ratio of approximately 5:1.[4] The perfusion in excess of demand serves as a physiologic cushion during short periods of increased cellular oxygen demand or hypoxia. However, normal oxygen delivery depends on several factors. First, there must be a vehicle to transport oxygen to the tissues since dissolved oxygen contributes minimally to the oxygen carrying capacity of the plasma. Therefore, hemoglobin loaded with oxygen functions as the principal vehicle for transportation of oxygen. Inherent to this fact is that hemoglobin levels remain constant and saturated with oxygen in the systemic arterial circuit. Reductions in arterial oxygen content affect the amount of oxygen the tissues can extract. Further, the degree of oxygen affinity for hemoglobin can be modified by various factors, including temperature, pH, and 2,3 diphosphoglycerate (DPG). Ideally, in times of greater oxygen need, the hemoglobin readily unloads the oxygen at the tissues. Oxygen content is discussed more extensively in Chapter 17.

Cardiac output constitutes the central driving force for tissue oxygen delivery. The arterial oxygen content, in combination with cardiac output, determines the quantity of oxygen carried to the peripheral tissues. Expanding tissue oxygen requirements can be met by elevation of cardiac output and maintenance of hemoglobin concentration and saturation within normal limits. In addition to central control of oxygen delivery, regional controls of distribution to and within the tissues also exist.

Ultimately, regional oxygen delivery is regulated at the level of the microcirculation. The pattern of blood vessel distribution,[11,12] as well as the diffusion distance between the microvasculature and the cells often limits how much oxygen eventually becomes accessible to the mitochondria in the tissues.[11]

Adequate local oxygen delivery depends on two mechanisms: (1) increasing the blood flow though the microvasculature and (2) increasing the number of vessels perfused. Microvascular regulation of vessel tone adjusts regional blood flow to fulfill oxygen uptake requirements.[13] Many tissues contain capillaries that are nonperfused or underperfused under normal conditions.[14] During periods of hypoxic stress these vessels open up to permit

breakdown of the phospholipid membrane of the cell.[10] Eventually, paralysis of membrane bound pumps (normally fueled by ATP) precipitates intracellular swelling, leading to loss of the cellular contents and liberation of proteolytic enzymes.[10,6]

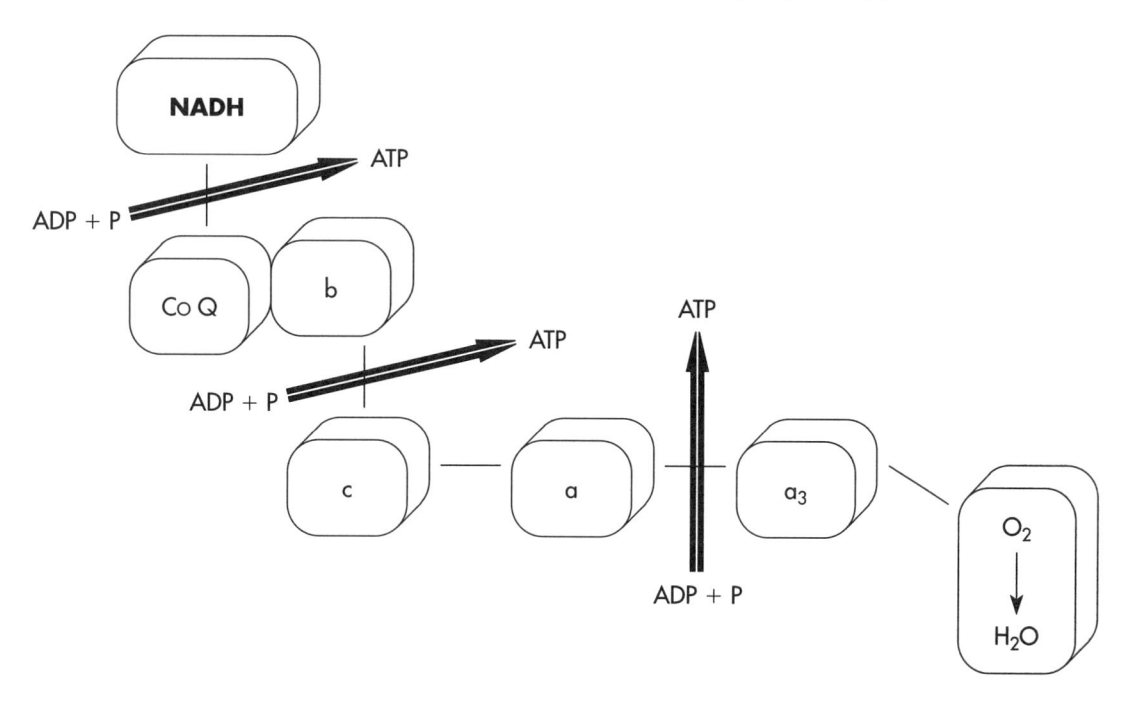

Fig. 6-4 Diagramatic representation of the electron transport system and ATP synthesis where oxidative phophorylation occurs. A, a_3, b, c, cytochromes; *CoQ*, ubiquinone (coenzyme Q).

greater oxygen delivery. This increase in capillary density subsequent to capillary recruitment reduces the diffusion distance for cellular oxygen uptake[15] and enhances delivery by increasing blood flow. Figure 6-5 depicts a typical capillary bed in the microcirculation.

Once oxygen reaches the tissues it must diffuse from the blood into the cell cytosol and enter the mitochondria. Under normal, resting conditions approximately 20% to 25% of the oxygen moving through the microcirculation of the tissues is extracted from the vessels. This percentage varies in some organs such as the heart, brain, and kidneys because of metabolic need. Ordinarily, the percentage of oxygen extracted is controlled by tissue oxygen demands. During periods of high demand, oxygen extraction increases to satisfy tissue metabolic requirements.[16,17] However, oxygen extraction can only be continually increased within certain limits. Once this physiologic end point is attained, cellular oxygen uptake can only increase if oxygen delivery increases.[18] Most organs, especially the heart, first increase the blood flow. If the higher blood flow remains insufficient to meet cellular oxygen demands, then oxygen extraction is increased.

Disturbances of microvascular blood flow distribution may be pivotal in determining the adequacy of oxygen delivery in MODS. Of particular importance are the effects of hypoxia on regional vascular regulatory mechanisms. At the local level hypoxia is associated with tissue acidosis. Hypoxia causes vascular relaxation and increases blood flow to the acidotic tissues. Additionally, some capillaries that normally receive little or no blood flow may be recruited to augment the number of nutrient vessels supplying specific organ beds. As a consequence, oxygen delivery is promoted through redistribution of capillary blood flow to tissues with the highest metabolic need. Local accumulation of metabolites during persistent hypoxia may induce further vasodilation. Consequently, regional blood flow is augmented[11] and oxygen delivery increased. Failure of these normal compensatory mechanisms to augment regional blood flow may produce an inequality between oxygen delivery and cellular oxygen consumption.

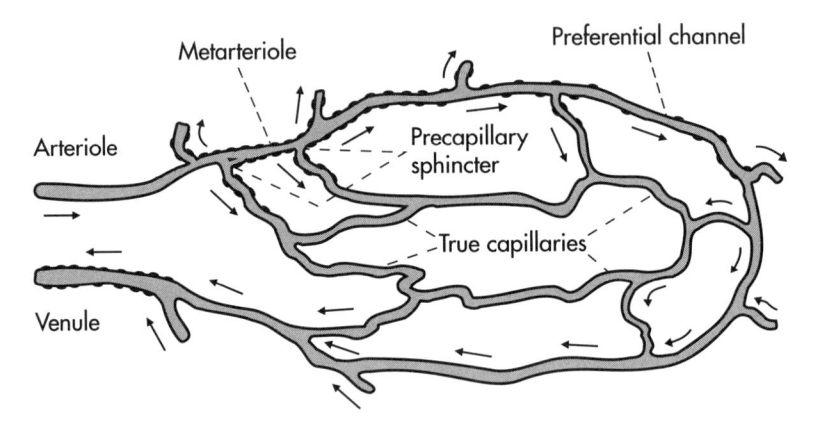

Fig. 6-5 Typical structure of a mesenteric capillary bed of the microcirculation. (From Guyton AC. Medical Physiology. Philadelphia: WB Saunders, 1991:171.)

Certain conditions may modify oxygen delivery and extraction because of disturbances in normal microvascular flow patterns. Opening of arteriovenous (A-V) shunts or inappropriate vasoconstriction will reduce oxygen transport to the surrounding tissues and effectively limit oxygen extraction.[19] Speculation regarding the presence of A-V shunts continues to exist. The opening of pathologic connections between the arterial and venous systems, thereby bypassing capillary beds is believed to decrease oxygen extraction. However, A-V shunting remains unsubstantiated because these physiologic shunts have not been detected in either animal models or in humans.[20]

The point at which oxygen delivery regulates oxygen consumption is termed critical oxygen delivery $DO_{2\,crit}$.[18] If a patient's DO_2 falls below the $DO_{2\,crit}$, metabolic processes begin the conversion from aerobic to anaerobic metabolism.[10] Further, the level of $DO_{2\,crit}$ for anaerobic metabolism differs depending on specific organs and can be modified in the presence of various physiologic stressors.[18] It is believed that the critical level where oxygen consumption becomes supply-dependent is connected to the cause of the physiologically stressed state. In fact, two separate studies demonstrated that the DO_{2crit} for anaerobic metabolism in septic patients[21] nearly doubles when compared to the $DO_{2\,crit}$ in patients following coronary artery bypass surgery.[22] However, a more recent investigation examining the difference in critical oxygen delivery between septic and nonseptic critically ill patients revealed a biphasic relationship between oxygen delivery and oxygen consumption.[23] In contrast to the earlier studies, Ronco and his colleagues[23] failed to show any difference between the septic and nonseptic groups. These studies emphasize the fact that a relationship between critical illness and critical oxygen delivery exists, but controversy remains regarding the exact effects of specific disease conditions.

Oxygen consumption

The metabolic needs of the various organs control the amount of oxygen actually consumed by cells and is reflected in the calculated oxygen consumption. Ordinarily, rising cellular requirements increase oxygen uptake from the blood. Initially the oxygen extraction ratio rises in response to the extra metabolic requirements of the cells. At this point consumption remains independent of delivery because delivery normally exceeds demands. However, as metabolic requirements increase or pathologic conditions causing persistent hypoperfusion or hypoxia evolve, a reciprocal relationship between oxygen delivery and consumption develops. That is, oxygen consumption (VO_2) cannot increase unless there is a rise in DO_2. Consumption is now "dependent" on delivery. This may be exhibited by sudden increases in systemic VO_2[24] after increases in oxygen delivery and is termed supply-dependent consumption (Fig. 6-6). Evidence indicates that tissue hypoxia or activation of a systemic inflammatory response produces this supply-dependent relationship

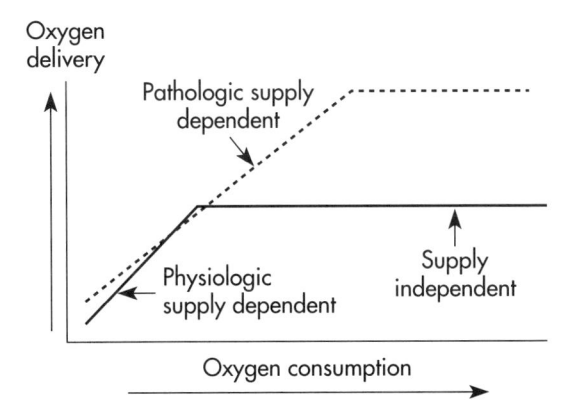

Fig. 6-6 Supply-dependent oxygen consumption. Theoretic relationship between oxygen delivery and oxygen consumption in MODS. (From Deitch EA. Multiple organ failure. Adv Surg 1993;26:341.)

between delivery and consumption.[25-27] However, in a recent study comparing indirect calorimetric and calculated measures of oxygen consumption from pulmonary artery data, calorimetry failed to substantiate a flow dependency in the majority of their critically ill patients. Oxygen delivery and consumption calculated from pulmonary catheter data may reflect errors arising from the mathematical coupling of delivery and consumption.[28] These findings have stimulated questions as to the exact nature of supply-dependent oxygen consumption during SIRS and MODS. An extensive discussion of this controversy is presented in Chapter 17.

OXYGEN SUPPLY-DEMAND RELATIONSHIPS
Tissue oxygen debt

Normally a balance exists between oxygen supply and oxygen demand. When oxygen supply and demand are equalized, as in normoxia, oxidative phosphorylation, oxygen consumption, and ATP turnover remain in a state of equilibrium.[29] If reduced oxygen availability occurs ATP synthesis is partially preserved because the anaerobic glycolytic pathway serves as a physiologic buffer for ATP supply. This condition involving very low ATP production is termed dysoxia with intact function.[2] If allowed to persist it eventually results in exhaustion of high-energy-phosphate reserves. The presence of creatine phosphate in tissues such as heart and skeletal muscle provides a reserve energy store.[2] Creatine phosphate provides the inorganic phosphate (P_i) that can be tapped to build ATP from ADP. However, these stores are relatively small and easily depleted in the face of a diminishing oxygen supply.

Typically, oxygen delivery exceeds cellular metabolic oxygen requirements.[19] Tissues extract the oxygen they need and the remainder is returned to the lungs unused. As tissue requirements grow, oxygen extraction escalates over time until the demand ultimately exceeds the supply, thus creating an oxygen debt.[30] Consequently, tissue oxygen consumption becomes dependent upon perfusion.[2,5] The severity of the incurred oxygen debt is related to specific organ oxygen needs. Some tissues, particularly the liver, are able to partially adapt necessary oxygen requirements by reducing energy demand in a process known as oxygen conformity.[31] As long as oxygen delivery continues above the critical levels, these tissues remain viable owing to reprioritized demand.[8] Nevertheless, once oxygen debt accumulates, repayment is not always successful.

Oxygen debt repayment

Restoration of normal tissue oxygen levels by increasing either perfusion or oxygen availability does not always ameliorate the existing oxygen debt. The debt repayment is evidenced by supranormal oxygen consumption by the tissues following restoration of perfusion after hypovolemia.[32] This excessive tissue oxygen consumption after ischemia or hypoxia, known as reactive hyperemia, is thought to be essential in the repayment of the incurred oxygen deficit.[30,33] Inadequate repayment of the oxygen debt appears to connect an oxygen supply-demand imbalance to development of MODS. Shoemaker and co-workers[15,34] have repeatedly demonstrated that tissue oxygen debt was greater and continued longer in patients eventually developing MODS. Further, Moore and his associates[4] observed that the oxygen debt incurred in one group of patients who developed MODS persisted more than 12 hours despite aggressive resuscitation and maximization of oxygen delivery. It remains unclear why patients with MODS possess an inability to achieve full repayment of the oxygen debt; possible reasons include hypoperfusion, flow maldistribution, and ineffective cellular oxygen metabolism.[4] Figure 6-7 depicts this pattern of oxygen debt with repayment.

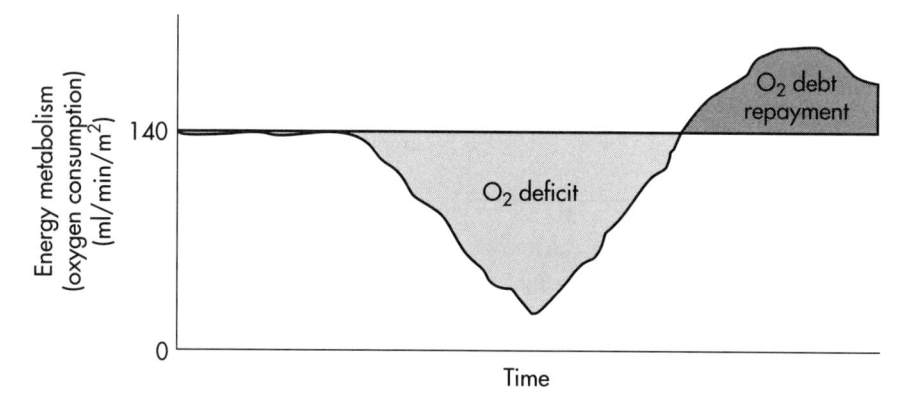

Fig. 6-7 Graphic representation of oxygen debt and oxygen debt repayment. (From Seigel JH, Linberg SE, Wiles CE. Therapy of low flow states. In: Seigel JH, ed. Trauma: Emergency surgery and critical care. New York: Churchill Livingstone, 1987:207.)

Conditions that increase oxygen demand

Clinical conditions such as hyperthermia, hypermetabolism, increased work of breathing, and pain all increase tissue oxygen demand and may potentiate the supply-demand imbalance of MODS. Fever frequently accompanies the systemic inflammatory response observed in patients with MODS and may intensify an existing oxygen debt. Because increased core body temperature can raise oxygen consumption 10% to 13% per degree of temperature above normal,[35] cellular oxygen demand increases proportionately. In fact acute infections can elevate oxygen consumption to as high as 60% above baseline.[36] Conversely, hypothermia lowers oxygen demand, but the rigors associated with rewarming markedly increase cellular oxygen requirements[16] and cause additional oxygen demands on an already physiologically stressed patient with MODS.

Patients who develop MODS and who are septic demonstrate marked hypermetabolism despite sedation or medical paralysis.[37] Consequently, these patients possess a higher resting energy expenditure that raises cellular oxygen demand still further. Moreover, the adult respiratory distress syndrome (ARDS) that accompanies MODS increases the work of breathing, which produces even greater oxygen demand. Pain or agitation may also raise tissue oxygen requirements because of sympathetic nervous system stress. Regardless of the cause, increased oxygen demand may also contribute to inadequate cellular oxygen delivery and processing in MODS.

PATHOPHYSIOLOGY OF OXYGEN SUPPLY-DEMAND IMBALANCE IN MODS

Myriad causes of multiple organ dysfunction exist, but the syndrome is characterized by ischemic tissue damage and activation of a systemic inflammatory response. The sequence of organ dysfunction maybe triggered by direct injury to specific organs (primary MODS)[2] or by infection or SIRS (secondary MODS).[2] Nevertheless, one of the common factors in the pathophysiologic progression of MODS appears to be an unrecognized mismatch between oxygen delivery, demand, and consumption.[2,4,5] The role of cellular oxygen deficit as a stimulus for MODS is well supported clinically by several studies documenting the association between high serum lactate levels and development of MODS.[4,38,39] The proposed causes of this acute cellular oxygen deficit focus on mechanisms of decreased supply or consumption including perfusion abnormalities such as widening of diffusion distances between the intravascular and intracellular spaces,[40,41] maldistribution of blood flow,[4] or increased intracellular oxygen utilization subsequent to altered cell metabolism.[2,41] An increased demand by hypermetabolic tissues also potentiates the oxygen deficit.

Perfusion abnormalities

Adequate oxygen uptake by the mitochondria depends on sufficient delivery and normal diffusion. Interstitial fluid accumulation frequently follows tissue trauma or local inflammation and can limit the oxygen uptake by widening the distance oxygen must passively diffuse before reaching the cell. Extending the distance between the capillary lumen and the cell as much as 40 µm still allows fairly rapid oxygen diffusion.[13,41] However, interstitial edema can widen these distances to the degree that higher partial pressures of oxygen become essential to preserve functional intracellular oxygen concentrations.[13] Edema affects oxygen diffusion because oxygen is not very soluble in water. Furthermore, reductions in capillary density increase the distance between capillaries with subsequent reductions in intraluminal oxygen tension. Finally, increased pressure of edema fluid can collapse the thin-walled capillaries with the result that some tissue beds receive little or no nutrient blood flow.

Furthermore, hyperdynamic increases in microcirculatory blood flow, as observed in SIRS, compound the problem because of the rapid transit of red blood cells through the microcirculation. Thus, insufficient time remains for complete unloading of oxygen from hemoglobin.[42] Consequently, conditions associated with interstitial edema, hypoperfusion, hyperdynamic blood flow, or hypoxia may disrupt oxygen delivery to the tissues and lead to the supply-dependent oxygen consumption implicated as a precipitating risk factor of MODS.

Microvascular blood flow distribution

Ordinarily, the regulation of the regional blood flow depends on the maintenance of the vasoconstrictor tone by the nervous system and is modulated by release of endogenous substances that possess local vasoactive properties. Geared to preserve blood flow during periods of hypoperfusion or hypoxia, these systems cause local vasodilatation to promote oxygen delivery to essential organs. However, some vascular beds may be inappropriately vasoconstricted or vasodilated because of impairment of normal nervous system control patterns or generation of toxic waste products and vasoactive mediators.

Conditions predisposing a patient to MODS such as multisystem trauma, ARDS, and sepsis could alter microcirculatory blood flow distribution, thus affecting the normal balance between oxygen delivery and oxygen consumption.[1,2,41] Loss of microvascular regulation subsequent to the accumulation of vasoactive mediators has been of particular interest to several investigators studying the pathogenesis of MODS. Current data suggest that sepsis-induced MODS correlates with elevations in complement split products, neutrophil adhesion, and reactive oxidant release.[43] Both neutrophils and the reactive oxygen species (O_2^-, OH^-, and H_2O_2) produced by neutrophils are known to alter microvascular blood flow either directly or indirectly.

Neutrophil adherence to the endothelium has been proposed to promote the formation of microvascular thrombi and subsequent maldistribution of flow.[1] During the respiratory burst, which occurs as neutrophils phagocytize foreign particles, oxygen-derived free radicals are generated. Because the neutrophils have adhered to the endothelium their released toxic products are concentrated locally. The local concentration of these toxic products of oxygen metabolism damage vascular endothelium and affect endothelial production of the vasodilatory prostaglandin, prostacyclin.[16] As a consequence, oxygen-derived free radical production could indirectly alter microvascular oxygen delivery by potentiation of thromboxane-induced regional vasoconstriction.[20,44,45] Because the effects of these mediatiors are local it is likely that patchy perfusion occurs in many tissues from local accumulation of thomboxane, a potent vasoconstrictor produced by activated platelets and white blood cells (WBCs).

The gut as an example of oxygen supply-demand imbalance

Recently, the gut has come under scrutiny as a potential motor driving the progression of MODS. Mythern and Webb[46] determined that gastric mucosal ischemia was present in 50% of their patients who developed MODS. Gut ischemia is thought to alter the barrier function of the mucosal lining so that bacterial translocation occurs.[5] Bacterial seeding of the portal system has been identified as a possible source of endotoxemic sepsis because plasma endotoxin levels have been observed to rise after restoration of perfusion.[47,48] Further, Nelson and his associates[49] demonstrated that gut vasoregulatory control was lost during endotoxemia. This impairment of vasoregulation may potentiate cellular ischemia.

Presumably, ischemic cell injury in the gut precipitates endothelial cell swelling, as well as neutrophil and macrophage infiltration. The phagocytic cells then generate inflammatory mediators (e.g., cytokines) that trigger the expression of adhesion molecules on their own cell surfaces and on those of the endothelial cells.[50] This increase in adhesion molecules promotes WBC accumulation in the vasculature and may further curtail cellular oxygen uptake through mechanical obstruction of blood flow. In the liver, macrophage-produced cytokines are thought to upregulate expression of E-selectin,[51] a cell adhesion factor, that may also contribute to microvascular obstruction by blood cells. Furthermore, endothelial cell edema obstructs capillary lumens and permits the accumulation of white cells and platelets that are then unable to change their shape enough to squeeze through the narrowed capillary channels.[50] The mechanical obstruction thus produced promotes hypoperfusion and intensifies cellular ischemia. Moreover, endothelial cell injury may stimulate the generation of numerous mediators that amplify the inflammatory response and further alter blood flow.

Roles of nitric oxide and endothelin

Recently, two endogenous vasoactive substances, nitric oxide and endothelin, have come under intense scrutiny because of their opposing actions and potential role as modulators of microvascular tone. The level of the vasoconstrictor peptide, endothelin, has been shown to rise in the plasma of septic patients[52,53] and is linked to the severity of the illness.[52] Endothelin production, probably stimulated by damaged endothelial cells, has been implicated as a contributor in the genesis of the microvascular perfusion defect associated with low flow and inflammatory states. Because the liver is one of the target organs in MODS, increased hepatic endothelin synthesis may precipitate sinusoidal constriction, leading to the formation of areas with patchy perfusion and focal ischemia.[54] In contrast, nitric oxide formed from its precursor amino acid, L-arginine, and initially identified as endothelial-derived relaxant factor (EDRF),[55] may increase hepatic perfusion by modulating presinusoidal vascular relaxation.[51] Therefore, at least in the liver, inflammatory states may upset the balance between nitric oxide and endothelin. In fact, some investigators theorize that proinflammatory amplification of nitric oxide synthesis by the vascular endothelium or activated white cells may be necessary to maintain sinusoidal blood flow.[51] It is likely that an increased production of the more stable endothelin promotes maldistribution of blood flow subsequent to regional vasoconstriction and hypoperfusion.[56]

Ischemia/reperfusion injury

An accumulating body of evidence suggests that restoration of cellular oxygen delivery after a period of hypoperfusion produces a reperfusion tissue injury.[57-59] Mechanistically, ischemic tissues produce large quantities of adenosine because of depletion of their high energy phosphate reserves as ATP is hydrolyzed.[7] Adenosine is eventually degraded to its purine base, hypoxanthine. Ischemia leads to conversion of the enzyme xanthine dehydrogenase to xanthine oxidase.[2] Once delivery of oxygen is restored the oxygen reacts with the xanthine and the xanthine oxidase to produce uric acid and oxygen-derived free radicals, such as the superoxide anion (O_2^-). The superoxide radical reacts with nitric oxide, if present. Peroxynitrites are then formed that degrade into the hydroxyl radical (OH^-).[60] Moreover, in the presence of free iron, the superoxide radical is reduced to the more potent reactive oxidants, the OH^- and hydrogen peroxide (H_2O_2). All of these reactive oxygen species are thought to induce cell membrane disruption.[61] Activated neutrophils produce additional oxidants as a result of the respiratory burst associated with phagocytic activity.[62]

Reactive oxidants presumably bring about tissue injury through lipid peroxidation of cell membranes.[50,63] Because cell membranes contain considerable amounts of phospholipids, they serve as prime targets for disruption by superoxide and hydroxyl radicals. The fatty acids located in cell membranes are structurally deranged by these oxidants.[64] Further, these toxic oxygen metabolites possess the ability to inactivate membrane-bound receptors and enzymes.[65] Consequently, the selective permeability of cell membranes may also become damaged so that ion leaks occur and intracellular processes are altered. In addition to membrane damage it appears that these toxic oxygen products activate the complement pathway through C5a.[66] These data demonstrate a potential link between reperfusion injury and activation of inflammatory processes that are frequently associated with MODS. Reperfusion injury has also been linked to altered cellular metabolism.

Altered cellular metabolism

While perfusion abnormalities have been documented in the development of sequential organ dysfunction, controversy over the existence of alterations in cellular metabolism remains because of conflicting results in several studies. Nevertheless, the oxygen supply-dependence observed in MODS has generated much interest in the pathophysiology of a potential metabolic defect. Because sepsis is commonoly associated with MODS, the results of many investigations examining these metabolic defects are largely based upon studies examining the effects of sepsis or endotoxemia.

Some investigators suggest that the tissue oxygen debt associated with MODS is related to an impairment of the functional ability of the mitochondria to maintain normal electron transport through the respiratory chain. The exact cause of mitochondrial injury is unclear, but it may be modulated via a common set of mediators, such as the reactive products of oxygen metabolism.[12,41] Ordinarily, ATP production increases with oxygen consumption (oxidative phosphorylation). This coupling of oxidation to phosphorylation depends on the normal activity of the cytochromes of the respiratory chain that may be altered during sepsis or MODS. Recently, Shaefer and associates[66] observed that the terminal set of respiratory chain cytochromes in intestinal cells were inhibited during experimental endotoxemia despite return of normal blood flow. These data indicate that the infection-induced inflammatory response promotes a defect in the ability of the terminal cytochromes to function.

Changes in mitochondrial respiratory chain activity occur during both ischemia and reperfusion in myocardial tissues.[67,68] Further, the duration of the period of ischemia determines the degree of mitochondrial damage.[68] In contrast to the injury associated with sepsis, reperfusion appears to harm the initial respiratory chain component, NADH-ubiquinone reductase[68] (Fig. 6-4), thereby impairing the electron transfer through the remaining respiratory chain cytochromes. Free radicals, which are normally produced in small amounts in all aerobically respiring cells,[61] are the putative mediators of myocardial injury.[41] These highly reactive oxidants are known to attack components of the cytochrome chain.[69]

Clinical measures of mitochondrial function have been attempted by measuring plasma acetoacetate and β-hydroxybutyrate levels that are thought to reflect mitochondrial redox potential.[70] Postburn MODS patients manifested higher plasma acetoacetate levels than did non-MODS patients, indicating functional mitochondrial defects. Furthermore, it is likely that widespread damage to mitochondria exists. Ultrastructural examination of various organs from several animal species with organ dysfunction reveals mitochondrial degeneration suggestive of free radical–mediated damage.[41] These mitochondrial disruptions include mitochondrial calcium deposits, as well as inner membrane edema[71,41] and are believed to partially explain the decline in high energy phosphate production. Impairment of normal mitochondrial electron transport effectively reduces ATP generation and has been proposed to cause the oxygen imbalance observed in MODS[66] as opposed to an oxygen transport malfunction. Insufficient production of high energy phosphates precipitates reduced substrate metabolism via aerobic processes. A limited quantity of pyruvate enters the Krebs cycle because of the intramitochondrial defect. Anaerobically derived lactate accumulates, resulting in elevated circulating lactate levels. Accordingly, the uncoupling of oxidation and phosphorylation, which can limit oxygen utilization, has been proposed as the basis for the high serum lactate levels reported in sepsis,[66,72] rather than, or in addition to, insufficient oxygen delivery.

CONCLUSION

Patients with MODS encounter a myriad of physiologic threats; a cellular oxygen supply-demand imbalance is one of the most severe alterations. Although oxygen supply-demand imbalance appears to be intrinsic to MODS regardless of the inciting event, incomplete understanding of the actual pathophysiology remains. Ordinarily, perfusion and oxygen delivery exceed the cellular oxygen requirements. However, during periods of hypoperfusion, hypoxemia, or tissue ischemia an oxygen debt is incurred. Once restoration of perfusion occurs, a reactive hyperemia ensues and oxygen consumption increases to repay the oxygen debt. Eventually, a normal balance between oxygen supply and demand returns with oxygen consumption once again becoming independent of oxygen delivery. With the development of MODS this relationship appears to be disturbed so that a condition of supply-dependent oxygen consumption ensues.

Investigators have identified several factors proposed to affect the oxygen supply-delivery relationship in MODS. Tissue injury and proinflammatory mediator generation that potentiate interstitial fluid accumulation are postulated to diminish regional capillary density and cause patchy perfusion. Regional blood flow maldistribution has also been presumed to contribute to the oxygen imbalance in MODS. Such factors as loss of microvascular regulatory control, opening of physiologic arteriovenous shunts, and mechanical obstruction have been implicated. Generation of proinflammatory mediators with vasodilator or vasoconstrictor properties, including thromboxane A_2, nitric oxide, the leukotrienes, and endothelin certainly affects microvascular vasomotor tone and potentially initiates a local oxygen debt. Sluggish microvascular blood flow presumably augments leukocyte and platelet margination and activation leading to mechanical blockade of the microvasculature. Moreover, activation of both cell types stimulates the release of vasoactive substances that may further amplify local blood flow abnormalities.

Finally, there is some evidence that intracellular oxygen utilization plays a role in the apparent oxygen supply-demand imbalance of MODS. Toxic damage to the cytochrome system or mitochondrial membranes could cause impaired oxygen utilization, which is reflected in poor oxygen consumption. Free oxygen radicals have been implicated in this mitochondrial dysfunction.

Substantial evidence points to the existence of an oxygen-supply demand imbalance; however, currently, there is no clear understanding of its etiology and effects in MODS. It is likely that numerous factors affect tissue oxygen extraction, utilization, and consumption during the genesis and progression of multiple organ dysfunction and failure.

REFERENCES

1. Beal AL, Cerra FB. Multiple organ failure syndrome in the 1990s. JAMA 1994;271:226-233.
2. Demling R et al. Multiple-organ dysfunction syndrome in the surgical patient: Pathophysiology, prevention and treatment. Curr Probl Surg 1993;30:357-414.
3. Shoemaker WC et al. Hemodynamic and oxygen transport monitoring to titrate therapy in septic shock. New Horiz 1993;1:154-159.
4. Moore FA et al. Incommensurate oxygen consumption in response to maximal oxygen availability predicts postinjury multiple organ failure. J Trauma 1992;33:58-67.
5. Deitch EA. Multiple organ failure. Adv Surg 1993;26:333-357.
6. Grum CM. Cellular energetics. In: Zelenock GB et al, eds. Clinical ischemic syndromes. St. Louis: Mosby; 1990:47-62.
7. Lehninger AL, Nelson DL, Cox MM. Principles of biochemistry. 2nd ed. New York: Worth Publishers; 1993:542-597.
8. Jones DP, Kennedy FG. Intracellular oxygen supply during hypoxia. Am J Physiol 988;243:C247-C253.
9. Gutierrez G, Lund N, Bryan-Brown CW. Cellular oxygen utilization during multiple organ failure. Crit Care Clin 1989;5:271-287.
10. Gutierrez G. Cellular energy metabolism during hypoxia. Crit Care Med 1991;19:619-625.
11. Pinsky MR, Schlichtig R. Regional oxygen delivery in oxygen supply-dependent states. Intensive Care Med 1990; 16:S169-S171.
12. Vincent JL. The relationship between oxygen demand, oxygen uptake, and oxygen supply. Intensive Care Med 1990;16:S145-S148.
13. Shumacker PT, Samsel RW. Oxygen delivery and uptake by peripheral tissues: Physiology and pathophysiology. Crit Care Clin 1989;5:255-269.
14. Duling BR. Local control of microvascular function: Role in tissue oxygen supply. Ann Rev Physiol 1980;42:373-383.
15. Shoemaker WC, Appel PL, Fram HB. Tissue oxygen debt as a determinant of post-operative organ failure. Prog Clin Biol Res 1989;308:133-136.
16. Buran MJ. Oxygen consumption. In: Snyder JV, Pinsky MR, eds. Oxygen transport in the critically ill. Chicago: Year Book; 1987;16-21.
17. Russell JA, Phang PT. The oxygen delivery/consumption controversy. Am J Respir Crit Care Med 1994;149:533-537.
18. Pinsky MR. Beyond global oxygen supply-demand relations: In search of measures of dysoxia. Intensive Care Med 1994;20:1-3.
19. Tuchschmidt J, Oblitas D, Fried JC. Oxygen consumption in sepsis and septic shock. Crit Care Med 1991;19:664-671.
20. Mangino MJ et al. Mucosal arachidonate metabolism and intestinal ischemia-reperfusion. Am J Physiol 1989; 257:G299-G307.
21. Tuchschmidt J et al. Early hemodynamic correlates of survival in patients with septic shock. Crit Care Med 1989;17:719-724.
22. Shuibutani K et al. Critical level of oxygen delivery in anesthetized man. Crit Care Med 1983;11:640-645.
23. Ronco JJ et al. Identification of the critical oxygen delivery for anaerobic metabolism in critically ill septic and nonseptic humans. JAMA 993;270:1724-1730.
24. Shoemaker WC. Monitoring and management of acute circulatory problems: The expanded role of the physiologically oriented critical care nurse. Am J Crit Care 1992;1:38-53.
25. Schlichtig R, Kramer D, Pinsky MR. Flow redistribution during progressive hemorrhage is a determinant of critical O_2 delivery. J Appl Physiol 1991;70:169-178.
26. Schlichtig R et al. Hepatic dysoxia commences during O_2 supply dependence. J Appl Physiol 1992;72:1499-1505.
27. Nelson DP et al. Pathologic supply dependency of O_2 uptake during bacteremia in dogs. J Appl Physiol 1987; 63:1487-1492.
28. Hanique G et al. Evaluation of oxygen uptake and delivery in critically ill patients: a statistical reappraisal. Intensive Care Med 1994;20:19-26.
29. Connett RJ et al. Defining hypoxia: A systems view of VO_2, glycolysis, energetics and intracellular PO_2. J Appl Physiol 1990;68:833-842.
30. Vary TC, Kearney MTL. Pathophysiology of traumatic shock and multiple organ failure. In: Cardona V et al, eds. Trauma nursing from resuscitation to rehabilitation. Philadelpha: WB Saunders; 1994:114-150.
31. Schlichtig R, Gayowski T. Liver dysoxia and its detection. In: Matuschak GM, ed. Multiple systems organ failure: Hep-

atic regulation of systemic host defense. New York: Marcel Dekker, Inc.; 1993:193-213.
32. Seigel JH, Linberg SE, Wiles CE. Therapy of low-flow states. In: Seigel JH, ed. New York: Churchill Livingstone; 1987:201-284.
33. Fahey JT, Lister G. Oxygen transport in low cardiac output states. J Crit Care 1987;2:288-305.
34. Shoemaker WC, Appel PL, Kram HB. Role of oxygen debt in the development of organ failure, sepsis, and death in high-risk surgical patients. Chest 1992;102:208-215.
35. Beisel W, Wannemacher RW, Neufield HA. Relation of fever to energy expenditure. In: Assessment of energy metabolism in health and disease. Columbus: Ross Laboratories; 1980:144.
36. Kinney JM et al. Tissue fuel and weight loss after injury. J Clin Pathol 1970;23(suppl 4):65-72.
37. Frankenfield DC et al. Relationships between resting and total energy expenditure in injured and septic patients. Crit Care Med 1994;22:1796-1804.
38. Hanique G et al. Significance of pathologic oxygen supply dependence in critically ill patients: Comparison between measured and calculated methods. Intensive Care Med 1994;20:12-18.
39. Roumen RM et al. Scoring systems and blood lactate concentrations in relation to the development of adult respiratory distress syndrome and multiple organ failure in severly traumatized patients. J Trauma 1993;35:349-355.
40. Parillo JE. Pathogenic mechanisms of septic shock. N Engl J Med 1993;328:1471-1477.
41. Crouser ED, Dorinsky PM. Gastrointestinal tract dysfunction in critical illness: Pathophysiology and interaction with acute lung injury in adult respiratory distress syndrome/multiple organ dysfunction syndrome. New Horiz 1994;2:476-487.
42. Dantzker D. Oxygen delivery and utilization in sepsis. Crit Care Clin 1989;5:81-98.
43. Goya T, Morisaki T, Torisu M. Immunologic assessment of host defense impairment in patients with septic multiplc organ failure: Relationship between complement activation and changes in neutrophil function. Surgery 1994;115:145-155.
44. Myers SI et al. Splanchnic prostanoid production: Effect of hemorrhagic shock. J Surg Res 1990;48:5879-593.
45. Myers SI, Taylor BJ, Stanislawska M. Reperfusion inhibits elevated splanchnic prostanoid production following hemorrhagic shock. Ann Surg 1991;212:688-693.
46. Mythern MG, Webb AR. Intra-operative gut mucosal hypoperfusion is associated with increased post-operative complications and cost. Int Care Med 1994;20:99-104.
47. Caty ML et al. Evidence for tumor necrosis factor-induced pulmonary microvascular injury after intestinal ischemia-reperfusion injury. Ann Surg 1990;212:694-700.
48. Turnage RH, Guice KS, Oldham KT. Endotoxemia and remote organ injury following intestinal reperfusion. J Surg Res 1994;56:571-578.
49. Nelson DP et al. Pathologic supply dependence of systemic and intestinal oxygen uptake during endotoxemia. J Appl Physiol 1988;64:2410-2419.
50. Fantone JC. Pathogenesis of ischemia-reperfusion injury: An overview. In: Zelenock GB et al, eds. Clinical ischemic syndromes. St. Louis: Mosby; 1990:137-145.
51. Clemens MG et al. Hepatic intercellular communication in shock and inflammation. Shock 1994;2:1-9.
52. Pittet JF et al. Elevated plasma endothelin-1 concentrations are associated with the severity of illness in patients with sepsis. Arch Surg 1991;213:260-264.
53. Voerman H et al. Plasma endothelin levels are increased during septic shock. Crit Care Med 1992;20:1097-1101.
54. Clemens MG, Bauer M, Pannen BHJ. Heterogeneity of hepatic perfusion in shock. In: Vincent JL, ed. Yearbook of intensive care and emergency medicine. Berlin: Springer-Verlag; 1995:767-776.
55. Dinerman JL, Lowenstein CJ, Synder SH. Molecular mechanisms for nitric oxide regulation: Potential relevance to cardiovascular disease. Circ Res 1993;73:217-222.
56. Traber DL. Tumor necrosis factor and endothelins: Team players in shock? J Lab Clin Med 1994;124:746-747.
57. McCord JM. Oxygen-derived radicals: A link between perfusion injury and inflammation. Fed Proc 1987;46:2402-2406.
58. Granger D. Role of xanthine oxidase and granulocytes in intestinal ischemia-reperfusion. Am J Physiol 1988;255:2169-1275.
59. Hernandez LA et al. Role of neutrophils in ischemia/reperfusion-induced microvascular injury. Am J Physiol 1987; 253:H699-H703.
60. Beckman JS et al. Apparent hydroxyl radical production by peroxynitrite. Implications for endothelial injury from nitric oxide and superoxide. Proc Natl Acad Sci U S A 1990;87: 1620-1624.
61. Haglund U, Gerdin B. Oxygen free radicals (OFR) and circulatory shock. Circ Shock 1991;34:405-410.
62. Turnage RH, Guice KS, Oldham KT. Pulmonary microvascular injury following intestinal reperfusion. New Horiz 1994;2:463-475.
63. Powell RJ et al. Effect of oxygen free radical scavengers on survival in sepsis. Am Surg 1991;57:86-90.
64. Bonventure JV, Malis CD, Cheung JY. Calcium. In: Zelenock GB et al, eds. Clinical ischemic syndromes. St. Louis: Mosby; 1990:232-325.
65. Goode HF, Webster NR. Free radicals and antioxidants in sepsis. Crit Care Med 1993;21:1770-1776.
66. Shaefer CF, Lerner MR, Biber B. Dose-related reduction of intestinal cytochrome a,a_3 induced by endotoxin in rats. Circ Shock 1991;33:17-25.
67. Rouslin W. Persistence of mitochondrial competence during myocardial autolysis. Am J Physiol 1987;252:H985-H989.
68. Veitch K et al. Global ischemia induces a biphasic response of the mitochondrial respiratory chain. Biochem J 1992; 281:709-715.
69. Narabayshi H, Takeshige K, Minakami S. Alteration of inner-membrane components and damage to electron-transfer activities of bovine heart submitochondrial particles induced by NADPH-dependent lipid peroxidation. Biochem J 1982;202:97-105.
70. Dong YL et al. Metabolic abnormalities of mitochondrial redox potential in postburn multiple system organ failure. Burns 1992;18:283-286.
71. Natanson C et al. Selected treatment strategies for septic shock based on proposed mechanisms of sepsis. Ann Intern Med 1994;120:771-783.
72. Groeneveld ABJ et al. Relation of arterial blood lactate to oxygen delivery and hemodynamic variables in human shock states. Circ Shock 1987;22:35-53.

CHAPTER 7

Alterations in Metabolism

Joy Davis Kimbrell

The insults and complications that precede multiple organ dysfunction syndrome (MODS) are complex, multifactorial, and challenging syndromes that provoke alterations in the normal metabolic response. Specific clinical conditions associated with the evolution of the hypermetabolic response include injured or necrotic tissue, inflammation, sepsis, and perfusion deficits.[1,2] Initially, alterations in metabolism are compensatory mechanisms, aimed at meeting the increased needs of the body. Over time, however, metabolic changes may result in significant detrimental effects on the patient's prognosis and duration of illness.[3]

Neuroendocrine responses are at least partially responsible for the alterations of protein, carbohydrate, and lipid metabolism that occur after a major insult. Other possible contributing factors to the metabolic response are less clearly understood and remain under investigation. Activation of inflammatory mediators, such as interleukin-1, may play a pivotal role[4,5,6] (see Chapter 3).

Because there are major alterations in metabolism with marked increases in resting energy expenditure (REE) and catabolism of lean body mass and visceral organs, nutritional and metabolic support serves as a primary therapeutic tool in managing the patient with MODS. For this reason, knowledge of current methods of metabolic assessment and support with parenteral and enteral nutrition is essential.

PATHOPHYSIOLOGY OF THE METABOLIC RESPONSE

The altered metabolic regulation typical of major insults such as trauma and sepsis includes a neuroendocrine response mediated primarily by the sympathetic nervous system and the hypothalamus[7-9] (Fig. 7-1). This response serves as a compensatory mechanism to provide substrates for increased energy demands, and it is characterized by hypermetabolism, hyperglycemia, and hypercatabolism. Initially, the "ebb phase," normally lasting 48 to 72 hours, occurs with little change or with a slight depression in the metabolic response.[10] At the end of this period of relative metabolic rate stability, the "flow phase" begins,[10] characterized by hypermetabolism. The classic features seen in the hypermetabolic response include an increase in the resting energy expenditure (to 170% to 200 % of the baseline value), increase in cardiac output, increase in oxygen consumption, and increase in carbon dioxide production.[11,12]

The sympathetic nervous system is stimulated by the initiating stress and, in turn, it stimulates the adrenal medulla to release the catecholamines epinephrine and norepinephrine. Epinephrine release increases cardiac output, blood pressure, pulse, and rate and depth of respirations. Epinephrine also stimulates hepatic glycogenolysis (breakdown of glycogen to re-form glucose) and gluconeogenesis (formation of glucose from amino acids and fat). In addition, epinephrine inhibits insulin secretion and the uptake of glucose in the peripheral tissues and stimulates the hydrolysis (breakdown) of fat. The other catecholamine released, norepinephrine, also increases metabolic activity and fat hydrolysis and stimulates peripheral vasoconstriction.[8,13]

After stress or insult, the hypothalamus becomes excited and releases corticotropin releasing hormone (CRH), which stimulates the anterior pituitary

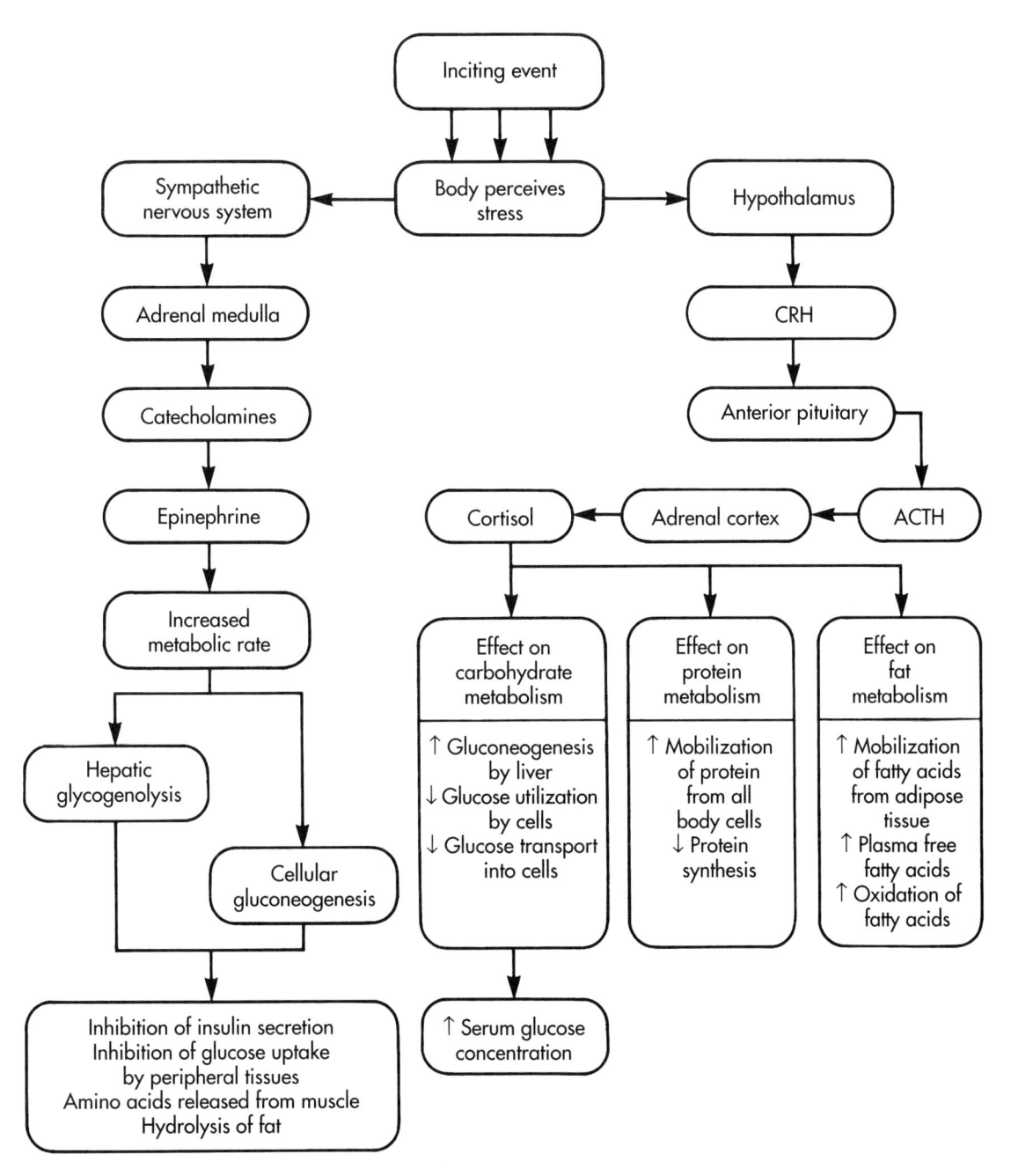

Fig. 7-1 Neuroendocrine effects on metabolism. As the body perceives stress or insult, neuroendocrine compensatory mechanisms are triggered to provide more energy to meet the body's needs. *ACTH,* Adrenocorticotropic hormone; *CRH,* corticotropin releasing hormone.

to secrete adrenocorticotropic hormone (ACTH). ACTH stimulates the adrenal cortex to release cortisol,[8,13] a glucocorticoid with a powerful ability to alter metabolism, primarily increasing the production of glucose. Cortisol stimulates the mobilization and transport of amino acids from muscle stores, to be used by the liver to produce glucose (gluconeogenesis). In addition, cortisol stimulates an increase in the enzymes required to convert amino acids to glucose.[14]

In many stress states other than MODS, the hypermetabolic "flow" phase normally peaks in 48 to 72 hours and abates completely in 7 to 10 days. With MODS, conditions such as uncontrolled inflammation or a continued focus of sepsis trigger a "reactivation" phase.[15] Hypermetabolism then continues until the source of inflammation or sepsis is controlled or the organ failure stage begins.[16] In MODS, the liver, kidneys, and other organs fail progressively, and the body may not be able to continue to manufacture substrates for energy. Metabolism then plummets as decompensation occurs, leading progressively to cellular damage and irreversible injury.[17] If the inflammation or the uncontrolled focus of sepsis persist, the ultimate outcome is death (Fig. 7-2). Whether metabolic failure is the *cause* of MODS or the *outcome* of sepsis, inflammation, and multiple organ damage remains to be determined.

Carbohydrate metabolism

The metabolic response preceding actual organ failure includes a significant alteration in carbohydrate metabolism. In conditions of simple starvation, the initial primary source of energy is glucose from its stored form of glycogen. Glycogen stores are limited (there is enough glycogen to generate about 1200 kcal),[18] and after these are depleted, the substrate for body energy changes to fatty acids and ketones derived from fat. With superimposed stress states and organ failure, there is mixed substrate oxidation (the breakdown of a substance, often for the purpose of energy production). The fraction of energy obtained from glucose is significantly reduced,

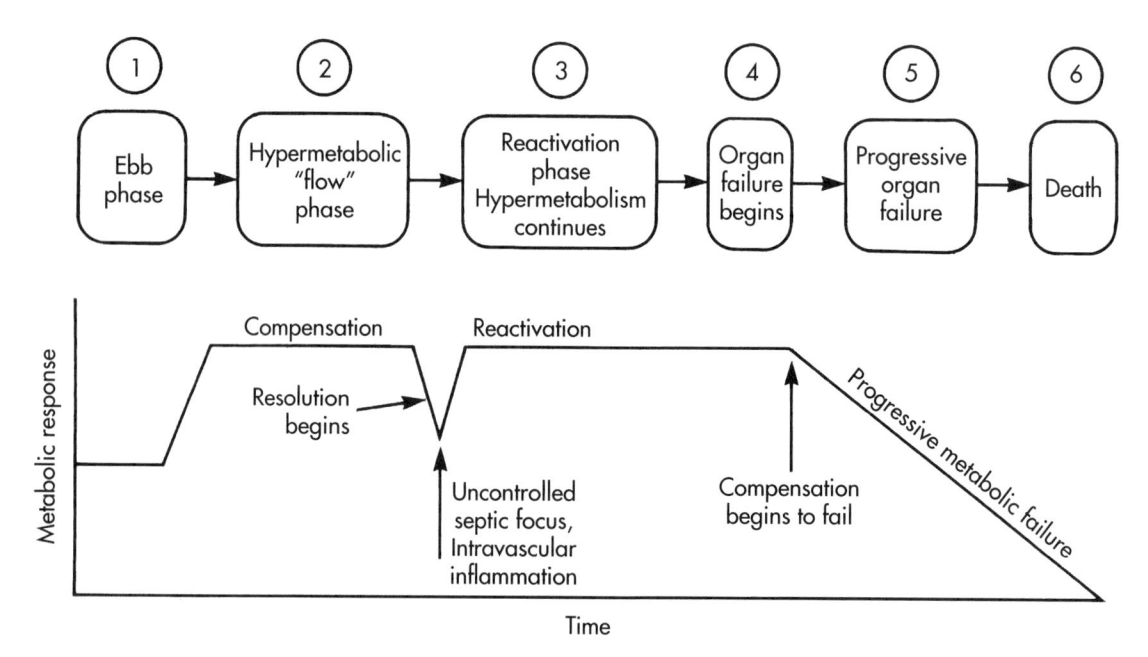

Fig. 7-2 Metabolic response in MODS. The metabolic response seen in MODS can be broken down into six steps. The multileveled horizontal line in the center of the graph represents the increases and decreases in metabolism that occur as the patient progresses through the steps. The patient may recover at any point with the metabolism returning to near normal.

while the fraction obtained from oxidation of amino acids and fat increases.

The altered metabolism in stress states is reflected by changes in the respiratory quotient (R/Q), which is the ratio of carbon dioxide production to oxygen consumption. The normal R/Q varies depending on the substrate metabolized.[19-21] In simple starvation states, the R/Q is 0.70, reflecting metabolism of fat stores for energy. In hypermetabolic states, the R/Q may be 0.8 to 0.85, reflecting oxidation of mixed substrates of fat, carbohydrate, and amino acids for energy.[11] This reflects the increased reliance on amino acids for energy production during stress states.

In stress states, after the initial stores of glycogen are depleted (within 6 to 12 hours), the liver converts amino acids to glucose (gluconeogenesis). The body catabolizes skeletal muscles to obtain these amino acids (proteolysis). Catabolism results in a mild to moderate hyperglycemia, which is mediated by increased secretion of epinephrine and cortisol. In addition, epinephrine inhibits insulin secretion and promotes the development of insulin resistance.[22] Other poorly defined mechanisms may also contribute to insulin resistance. The compensatory attempt to keep the blood glucose elevated is thought to occur in part because of the preference of the body for glucose as the substrate for wound repair[23] and also because glucose is necessary to supply the needs of the brain, the red and white blood cells, the bone marrow, and the cardiac muscle.

As the hypermetabolic response progresses, lactic acid is produced from muscle glycogen oxidation and carried to the liver, where it is converted back to glucose. As organs fail and the liver becomes dysfunctional, the plasma lactate level rises. Some tissues, such as the myocardium, can use lactate as an energy substrate by allowing direct entry of the lactate into mitochondria.[11] However, most tissues, such as those in the central nervous system, are glucose dependent and are unable to utilize lactate as an energy source. Lactic acidosis usually results as lactate production increases and adenosine triphosphate (ATP) breaks down and is not recycled. With further progression of hypermetabolism and a continued need for increased energy, either substrate stores are exhausted or the body is unable to use them, and the mitochondria fail to produce ATP for energy. Without energy available to carry out their functions, organs progressively fail.[17] The compensatory mechanisms for producing substrates for fuel become useless. In the later stages of MODS the liver is unable to produce glucose through gluconeogenesis and hypoglycemia occurs.[11] This hypoglycemia is considered by many clinicians to be an ominous sign and often heralds the onset of liver failure and death.

Lipid metabolism

Injury and sepsis, as well as other conditions that incite organ failure, produce significant alterations in lipid metabolism.[24-26] With increased catecholamine secretion and decreased insulin levels, triglycerides are catabolized to free fatty acids and ketone bodies for energy sources. There is increased turnover and oxidation of medium- and long-chain fatty acids, which can meet the energy needs of cardiac and skeletal muscles. In this manner, up to 80% of the energy needs of the body can be provided for the tissues that are not solely glucose-dependent. Glucose is spared for use by those tissues, such as the central nervous system, that can only use glucose for energy. Specific processes such as cell-mediated immune activity and wound healing are also exclusively dependent on glucose for energy. This alteration in lipid metabolism may actually help to conserve protein by signalling muscle tissue to minimize the release of amino acids during prolonged stress and sepsis.[8]

As the organ dysfunction progresses, there is an increase in hepatic lipogenesis reflected by a progressive rise in the R/Q, which eventually exceeds 1.0.[27] Triglyceride clearance decreases, and a spontaneous lipemia or hypertriglyceridemia may occur secondary to increased hepatic lipogenesis and decreased fat uptake by the peripheral adipose tissue. Both tumor necrosis factor and interleukin-1 have been implicated in these alterations of fat metabolism.[28,29] The alteration in fat metabolism contributes to weight loss, depletion of subcutaneous fat stores, and may contribute to acidosis.[8]

Protein metabolism

Protein, in the form of amino acids, becomes an important energy source during stress.[8] Amino acids are used as the fuel for hepatic conversion to glucose during gluconeogenesis. Unfortunately, the primary site for obtaining amino acids is skeletal muscle, connective tissue, and the unstimulated gut.[27] This mechanism causes autocannibalism, with rapid loss of skeletal muscle mass as the body breaks down muscle protein to provide an energy substrate. As skeletal muscle mass is depleted catabolism of visceral organs occurs to provide amino acids to the liver. Autocannibalism causes decreased muscle strength, seriously compromises the respiratory system, and limits the amino acids available for protein synthesis, immune system functions, and wound healing. Eventually, as the visceral organs are catabolized, organ function may be impaired leading to progressive organ failure.[30]

As muscles are broken down, a relative deficiency of essential amino acids, particularly branched-chain amino acids (BCAA), develops. This occurs because there is an elevation in the oxidation of BCAA during stress states; BCAA are used as an energy source by skeletal muscles and as a substrate for gluconeogenesis by the liver.[8]

A measure to quantify the degree of stress and protein breakdown is urea nitrogen excretion. Nitrogen, a byproduct of protein breakdown and gluconeogenesis, is converted to urea in the liver (ureagenesis). The amount of nitrogen lost from protein breakdown may be measured in the urine as urea nitrogen and is proportional to the degree of stress. Thus the clinician may measure the degree of protein catabolism for a specific patient. The measurement and quantification of stress will be discussed further in the section on assessment of metabolic requirements.

As MODS progresses, total body and hepatic protein synthesis fail and amino acid clearance decreases, particularly clearance of aromatic amino acids. The body is unresponsive to the exogenous administration of amino acids. With poor hepatic clearance, plasma levels of all amino acids, including BCAAs, increase. There is continued catabolism, and levels of urine urea nitrogen rise.[31] The failing kidneys are unable to excrete the excess amino acids, resulting in prerenal azotemia and further damage.[11,28]

Consequences of alterations in metabolism

The metabolic response described above is a compensatory mechanism for maintaining organ viability by producing energy for metabolic reactions. However, it is intended to be a short-term response. Prolonging the hypermetabolic response by the reactivation that occurs in MODS can produce the rapid detrimental effect of excessive catabolism with resulting protein-calorie malnutrition. The lean body mass can become significantly depleted in as short a time as 7 days,[30] so early measures must be initiated to meet metabolic requirements. In MODS, excessive catabolism of protein and fat stores and a decrease in overall body protein synthesis cause a negative nitrogen balance with multiple adverse effects.

Weight loss, fatigue, and overall muscle weakness occur. The ability to turn, cough, and breathe deeply is dramatically affected, and ventilatory reserves are decreased. Protein-calorie malnutrition decreases the ability to mount an immune response, and the alterations in metabolism may adversely affect wound healing, although the latter effect is currently, an area of controversy.

Overall, malnutrition resulting from the metabolic response and subsequent failure is associated with delayed recovery,[32-34] increased susceptibility to infection,[35,36] and increased morbidity and mortality.[37]

METABOLIC SUPPORT
Benefits of metabolic support

Metabolic support refers to the nutritional support and monitoring of the critically ill patient. Although the hypermetabolic response cannot be prevented, providing adequate metabolic support can preserve lean body mass, prevent visceral malnutrition, and control nutrient deficiencies.[22,27] Even though nutritional repletion is difficult or impossible during periods of extreme stress, it is possible to maintain body stores,[3] thereby emphasizing the importance of beginning metabolic support at the earliest possible opportunity.

Cerra[38] has outlined the principles or goals for metabolic support during the management of conditions associated with the development of MODS. His principles are the following:
 1. Do no harm.
 2. Prevent substrate-limited metabolism.
 3. Support organ structure and function.
 4. Attempt to alter the disease course.
 5. Attempt to reduce morbidity and mortality.

Assessment of metabolic requirements

From the discussion of metabolic alterations and their negative consequences, it is clear that the judicious use of metabolic support is an important adjunctive tool in supporting the patient at risk for

MODS. It is prudent to point out that a clinician cannot determine the exact degree of catabolism and risk for malnutrition just by looking at the patient. Delivering too many calories may produce many respiratory and hepatic complications, as well as detrimental effects on metabolism, organ structure, and function. Therefore, it is extremely important to determine the calorie and protein needs of the patient accurately and to estimate the degree of hypermetabolism for each patient. This is best accomplished by a complete metabolic assessment.[39]

The most logical approach to a comprehensive metabolic assessment is a multidisciplinary one.[7,40,41] If the metabolic or nutrition support team are available, they should be consulted early in the clinical course. The registered dietitian on the team is equipped with the education and experience to conduct a comprehensive nutritional assessment and collaborate with the physician as to disease-specific enteral and parenteral formulas. The registered nurse can offer input concerning gut function and fluid and electrolyte status and monitor the tolerance of the patient for nutritional support. Important components of a comprehensive nutritional assessment are described in the accompanying box on p. 154 and Table 7-1.[42,43]

Methods of metabolic support

Enteral vs. parenteral. Deciding on the proper route of metabolic support is a complex process and requires careful collaboration between the nurse, physician, dietitian, and pharmacist. The decision tree in Figure 7-3 may be used as a tool to assist with this process. For the critically ill hypermetabolic patient, metabolic support should be initiated at the earliest possible opportunity.

Enteral route

Advantages. The use of the enteral route for metabolic support has received renewed interest because it is simpler, safer, and cheaper.[44,45] Also, nutrients delivered by the enteral route are used more efficiently by the body and serve to maintain structural and functional integrity of the bowel.[46,47] Several investigators[38,48-57] have concluded that enteral nutrition appears to have a role in preserving the gut mucosal barrier and preventing translocation of bacteria, thus ultimately decreasing sepsis and enhancing the immune response. This phenomenon is discussed in Chapter 10.

In addition, other investigators[58,59] have found that enteral feedings eliminate the problems of biliary sludge and cholestasis in many patients. The enteral route also provides improved nitrogen retention when compared to identical solutions given intravenously,[60,61] and enteral feedings can successfully prevent stress ulcerations without the addition of other stress prophylaxis therapies.[62-64] One group of investigators[65] even demonstrated improved survival rates in an animal burn model, in the group that received early enteral feedings versus another group that received total parenteral nutrition, although extrapolation of these conclusions to human populations is controversial.[66]

Complications. Even though there are many potential benefits, the use of the enteral route in the critically ill population has been hindered by the problems of ileus, diarrhea, obstruction of feeding tubes, and aspiration pneumonia.

ILEUS. The gut is often overlooked as a route for providing early metabolic support because of the inherent problem of ileus associated with critical illnesses. However, several studies[67-70] indicate that most of the atony occurs in the stomach and colon and that the small bowel is resistant to the development of ileus. Small intestinal motility usually returns within the first 24 hours after an insult.[68,69] Cerra and co-workers[67] also found that even when an ileus is present, nutrient absorption occurs in the small bowel without an increase in the rate of diarrhea. Therefore, feeding tubes placed distal to the pylorus into the duodenum or jejunum can be successfully used for early enteral metabolic support. These tubes may be placed either surgically, fluoroscopically, endoscopically, or passed at the bedside, with the position confirmed by radiography.

DIARRHEA. Several authors have described diarrhea as being the most frequent complication of enteral feedings.[71-74] Although there is no standard definition of diarrhea, many researchers have investigated the problem. Flynn, Norton, and Fisher[71] found that 60% of patients who were studied experienced diarrhea for an average of 2.6 days. This finding will not surprise any nurse who has cared for patients receiving enteral feedings. Diarrhea causes great concern for critical care practitioners because it may initiate multiple complications, many of which may be life-threatening for critically ill patients.[72] Complications of diarrhea include dehydration, electrolyte imbalances, skin breakdown,

COMPONENTS OF A COMPREHENSIVE NUTRITIONAL ASSESSMENT

1. Review of medical, social, and dietary history
2. Clinical assessment
3. Anthropometric measurements to provide information about muscle and fat stores
4. Visceral protein measurements (Table 7-1)
   a. Serum albumin
   b. Serum transferrin
   c. Prealbumin
   d. Retinol-binding protein
5. Tests of immune competence
   a. Total lymphocyte count = (% lymphocytes × WBC) ÷ 100
      Normal = >2000/mm^3
      Mild depletion = 1200 to 2000/mm^3
      Moderate depletion = 800 to 1199/mm^3
      Severe depletion = <800/mm^3
   b. Cell-mediated immunity—tested by administering common skin test antigens and measuring reactions:
      Normal = Ability to react to one or more antigens
6. Nitrogen balance study—24-hour urine collection to monitor nitrogen losses
   a. Nitrogen balance = Nitrogen intake minus total urinary nitrogen minus insensible losses minus gastrointestinal losses
   b. Positive balance is indicative of an anabolic state
   c. Negative balance is indicative of a catabolic state
      Mild = −5 to −10 g/day
      Moderate = −10 to −15 g/day
      Severe = >−15 g/day
7. Determination of caloric needs
   a. Estimation of total caloric needs:
      1) Estimation of basal energy expenditure (BEE) is most frequently calculated by using the Harris-Benedict equation

      Female: BEE = 655 + (9.56 × W) + (1.85 × H) − (4.7 × A)

      Male: BEE = 66 + (13.75 × W) + (5.00 × H) − (6.75 × A)

      (W = Weight in kg; H = Height in cm: A = Age in years)

      2) Estimation of activity factor and injury factor:[30]
         Activity factor: Confined to bed = 1.2
         Ambulatory = 1.3
         Injury factor:

Surgery	**Trauma**
Minor = 1.1	Skeletal = 1.35
Major = 1.2	Head = 1.6
	Blunt = 1.35
Infection	**Burns**
Mild = 1.2	40% = 1.5
Moderate = 1.4	100% = 1.95
Severe = 1.8	

      3) Estimation of total caloric needs:
         BEE × Activity factor × Injury factor = Caloric needs for 24 hours
   b. Measured energy expenditure
      1) Indirect calorimetry (metabolic cart studies)—Calculated energy expenditure by measurement of oxygen consumed and carbon dioxide produced. Based on the assumption that oxygen consumed (Vo_2) and carbon dioxide produced (Vco_2) represent intracellular metabolism.
      2) This method requires expensive, bulky equipment and trained operators and is currently not widely available. However, preliminary evidence points to the fact that there may actually be a significant cost savings with this method because of the associated lower caloric needs reported, compared to the Harris-Benedict equation, which is an estimate. Many clinicians believe indirect calorimetry will improve patient care and become more widely used in the next decade.
8. Determination of protein needs
   a. Calculated on the basis of ideal body weight
   b. Estimated protein needs:
      Healthy adult = 0.8 g/kg/day
      Moderate stress = 1.5 g/kg/day
      Severe stress = 1.5 to 2.5 g/kg/day
      Peritoneal/hemodialysis = 1.2 to 2.5 g/kg/day
      Burns = 1.5 to 3.0 g/kg/day
   c. Factors to consider
      1) Visceral protein status—reflects internal organ mass (see Table 7-1)
      2) Protein losses—drains, wounds, diarrhea, or fistulas
      3) Disease status—hepatic and renal function
      4) Urinary nitrogen losses

Table 7-1 Visceral Proteins

Name	Normal range / Half-life	Function	Notes	Significance of abnormalities
Serum albumin	>3.5 g/dL 20 days	Maintains plasma oncotic pressure Carrier protein	Long half-life does not reflect acute protein status changes Values affected by hydration status	Mild depletion 3.0 to 3.5 g/dL Moderate depletion 2.4 to 2.9 g/dL Severe depletion <2.4 g/dL
Serum transferrin	>200 mg/dL 8 to 10 days	Carrier protein for iron	Shorter half-life more sensitive indicator of protein status	Mild depletion 150 to 200 mg/dL Moderate depletion 100 to 150 mg/dL Severe depletion <100 mg/dL
Prealbumin	20 mg/dL 2 to 3 days	Carrier protein for retinol-binding protein	Very sensitive to acute changes in protein status	Mild depletion 10 to 15 mg/dL Moderate depletion 5 to 10 mg/dL Severe depletion <5 mg/dL
Retinol-binding protein	3 to 5 mEq/dL 10 to 18 hours	Carrier protein for retinol	Extremely sensitive to acute changes in protein synthesis	

and, ultimately, sepsis. Severe diarrhea may cause fluid losses of 5 to 10 L/day,[75] and losses of this magnitude exacerbate the problems of poor perfusion of vital organs and maintenance of blood pressure.[76]

Recognizing that diarrhea may be a major problem with enteral feedings, nurse researchers have studied many of the possible contributing factors. Two researchers have studied the effects of formula temperature on the incidence of diarrhea. When Williams and Walike[77] compared the delivery of cold, room-temperature, or warm enteral formulas in rhesus monkey models, they found that temperature variations in the formula caused only brief and inconclusive effects on gastric motility and concluded that the temperature of the formula did not contribute to diarrhea.

Kagawa-Busby and co-workers[78] used human subjects to investigate differences in development of diarrhea with cold, room temperature, or warm enteral formulas. Their results again showed no significant association between the temperature of enteral feedings and gastric motility and diarrhea.

The implications for practice from these findings are that the temperature of the enteral formula is not a significant factor in the incidence of diarrhea. Some investigators[72] have suggested that feedings may be refrigerated after opening and administered without rewarming. This practice has the advantage of being potentially time-saving for the nurse and thus cost-effective for the hospital.

Heitkemper and associates[79,80] studied the effects of the rate of formula delivery and formula volume on gastrointestinal symptoms in their human subjects. They studied bolus feeding and found that the rate of formula delivery had little effect on mean gastric motility or return time of motility. Therefore, when delivering bolus tube feedings, moderate rates such as 60 mL/min are recommended to decrease the subjective feelings of discomfort.[72] Others have suggested that when delivering continuous tube feedings, the rate should be increased slowly, fol-

156 *Pathophysiologic Changes*

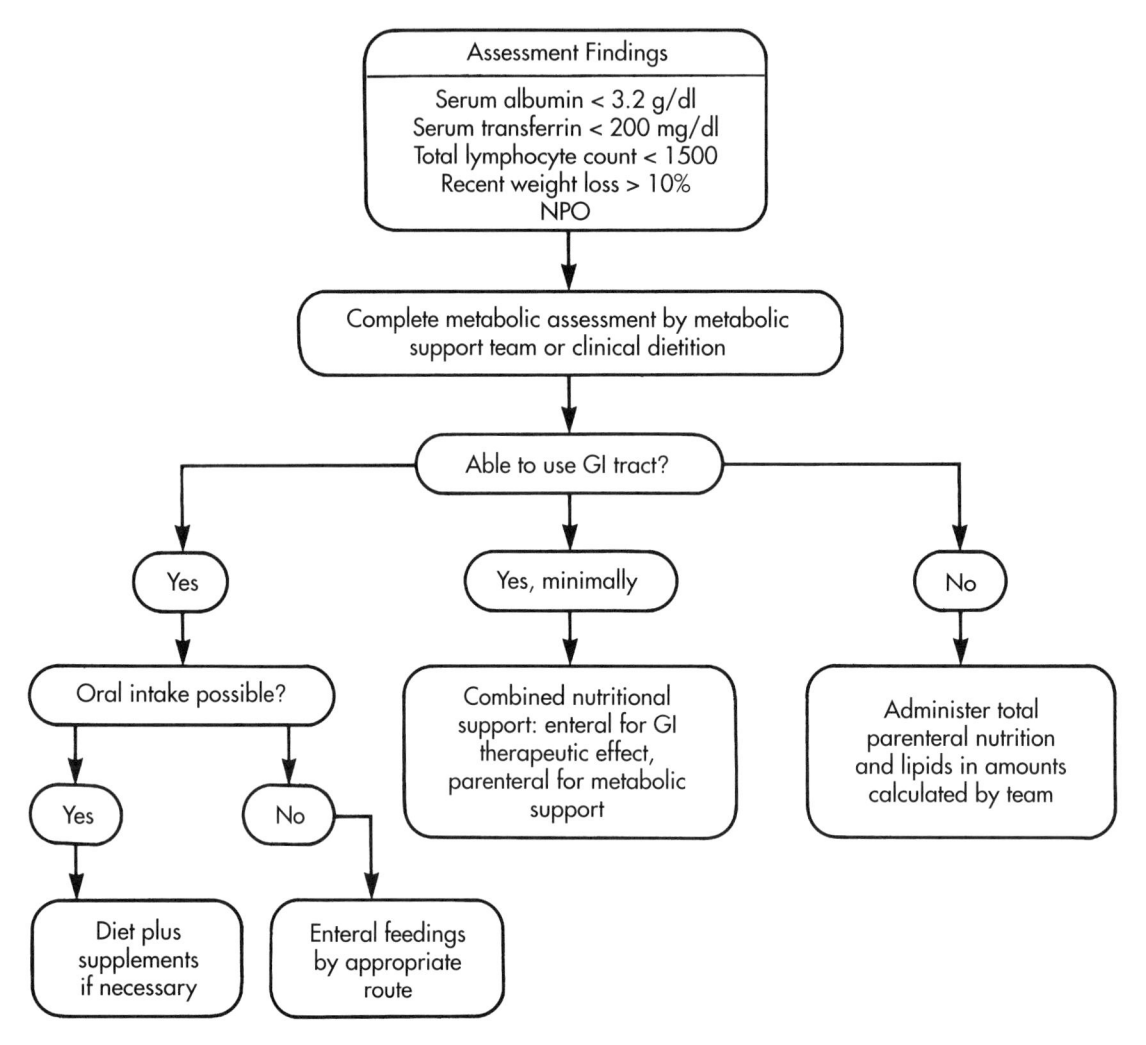

Fig. 7-3 Decision tree for enteral and parenteral nutrition to assist in determining the appropriate route of metabolic support for a particular patient. *GI*, Gastrointestinal.

lowed by an increased concentration of formula over a period of 4 to 7 days.[81,82]

Researchers have studied the incidence of diarrhea with intermittent versus continuous administration of enteral formulas and report conflicting results. Heibert and co-workers[83] compared continuous and intermittent feedings in adult burn patients. They found significantly fewer stools and subjective complaints of abdominal discomfort with continuous tube feedings. They also found that the time required to reach the calculated nutritional goals was significantly reduced in the continuously fed group. This study supports the current practice of delivering enteral formulas by continuous drip.

Keohane and co-workers[84] investigated the relationship between the osmolality of the enteral feeding and the gastrointestinal side effects. In the investigation, 118 subjects were given either hypertonic, isotonic, or hypotonic formulas by continuous nasogastric infusion. The results showed that diarrhea was not related to the administration of full-strength hypertonic enteral feedings. The investigators further concluded that using diluted formula as a starter or using isotonic formulas decreased nutrient intake and nitrogen balance and did not reduce diarrhea. This conclusion remains controversial and the area continues to be researched.

Bacterial contamination of enteral products or delivery sets as a cause of diarrhea has been studied.[85-87] The implications for practice from these studies are that containers and tubing should be changed on a daily basis to avoid bacterial contamination.[88]

TUBE OBSTRUCTION. A major advance in enteral metabolic support was the advent of the small-bore, pliable, weighted feeding tube. These small tubes are much more comfortable for the patient and their weighted ends facilitate passage into the small bowel. One of the disadvantages of these tubes is that they often become occluded. Replacement leads to increased costs related to additional nursing and physician time, exposure to radiation for confirmation of tube position, and trauma for the patient. Marcuard and Perkins[89] studied major formulas that were frequently used to determine if the type of formula used contributed to obstruction of the feeding tubes. Obstruction was observed in all tubes in which intact protein formulas were being delivered. The formula that caused the most obstruction was Pulmocare, followed by Ensure Plus and Osmolite. Diluting these formulas to half-strength helped decrease the obstruction. The researchers concluded that the acidity of the stomach contents led to precipitation of certain proteins and was an important factor in the obstruction of tubes. They offered the following suggestions to prevent obstruction of feeding tubes:

1. Flush the feeding tube before and after aspirating for residual gastric contents to eliminate acid precipitation of formula in the feeding tube.
2. Advance the feeding tube into the duodenum (the pH in the duodenum is higher and is less likely to cause precipitation).
3. Avoid mixing enteral products with liquid medications having a pH value of 5.0 or lower.[89]

Nurses have tried many innovative, creative methods to unclog feeding tubes. Meat tenderizer, warm coffee, cola products, and cranberry juice are a few of the products frequently mentioned. The use of these products has come under scrutiny, particularly the use of meat tenderizer, because it may be associated with significant complications, such as electrolyte imbalances. Metheny, Eisenberg, and McSweeney[90] studied the effectiveness of three irrigant fluids (cranberry juice, cola, and water) in preventing tube obstruction. Their results demonstrated that water and cola were consistently superior to cranberry juice as irrigating fluids, with no difference between water and cola noted. They also investigated the tube material and found that polyurethane was consistently superior to silicone in preventing tube obstructions. Finally, they found that tube diameter had no effect on the incidence of obstruction.

Treating feeding tube obstructions with activated pancreatic enzyme has been identified as a successful method when water has failed to clear the obstructions. Marcuard and Stegall[91] found that injecting activated pancreatic enzyme into the obstructed feeding tube was successful in clearing the obstruction in 96% of the cases in which formula clotting was identified as the cause of the obstruction.

ASPIRATION. Aspiration pneumonia is a potentially fatal complication of enteral feeding, and much of patient care is geared toward its prevention. One group of researchers found that the incidence of aspiration in patients fed via nasogastric tubes was five times greater than in those fed via nasointestinal tubes.[92] Tubes can also be placed accidentally in the lung or can become dislodged from the stomach by coughing, vomiting, and movement. Traditionally, the correct position of the nasoenteral tube is initially confirmed by radiography (an extremely accurate method). However, follow-up confirmation on an intermittent basis is usually accomplished by aspirating stomach or intestinal contents or by auscultating for noise while insufflating bursts of air through the tube. Both of these methods may be very deceiving and lead to false assurances of tube position.[93,94] Recognizing this, Metheny and co-workers[95] studied the effectiveness of pH readings in differentiating between gastric and intestinal placement. They also found that it was possible to aspirate enough fluid for pH testing in more than 90% of nasogastric or nasointestinal tubes. They found that in cases in which they were unable to obtain enough fluid to test for pH, insufflation of small bursts of air through the tubes facilitated aspiration of fluid through the syringe, reportedly by forcing the ports away from the mucosa. Tubes in the stomach had aspirate pH values ranging from 1 to 4, and those in the small bowel had values of 6 or higher.

Tubes that had inadvertently been placed in the lung had aspirates with an alkaline pH.[95] This method of tube position confirmation seems to hold promise and deserves further study; it may prove to be an acceptable nursing practice.

Metheny and co-workers[95] studied the incidence of aspiration pneumonia in tube-fed patients and found that 5.7% of the group studied demonstrated pulmonary aspiration directly related to the tube feedings. Most of those who aspirated had their feeding tubes in the stomach rather than in the small bowel. It was also interesting that in 83% of the group that aspirated, the head of the bed had been lowered recently before aspiration occured. Two researchers[71,92] have also investigated the practice of elevating the head of the bed to protect the patient from aspiration pneumonia. Both concluded that although this practice is recommended, it is not consistently practiced in the clinical setting. This inconsistency may contribute to the incidence of aspiration pneumonia.

Flynn, Norton, and Fisher[71] also investigated practices associated with enteral tube feedings in the acutely ill population and found that only 15% of the study group had a nutritional assessment completed before or during the period they were being fed. When they calculated the patients' caloric needs, the investigators found that most of the patients were being fed in hypocaloric concentrations. They also found that a standard protocol was not used in most of these patients. This again demonstrates the need for consultation with a nutrition support team to calculate the caloric needs of specific patients and to provide guidance for developing standard protocols.

Formulas. A wide variety of enteral formulas are available on the market, including many organ- or disease-specific formulas. Research on the efficacy of these formulas is ongoing and is promising. These formulas are constantly being developed and refined; therefore, selecting the proper formula is a very complicated process that involves many variables. A report by Eisenberg[96] offers an excellent review of indications, formulas, and delivery techniques as well as a sample protocol. It is strongly recommended that collaboration with a clinical dietitian or metabolic support team occurs when selecting the appropriate formula for a specific patient with organ failure.

Parenteral route. Many times the enteral route is not appropriate or available for use for problems with bowel obstruction or when there is a need for bowel rest. When this occurs the parenteral route is indicated for metabolic support.

Advantages. The use of this route for delivery of total parenteral nutrition (TPN) has increased tremendously over the past 15 years. The ability to precisely deliver a prescribed daily intake of calories, carbohydrates, fat, protein, vitamins, and minerals is very desirable in the critically ill patient. In addition, with TPN, the clinician has the ability to infuse high osmolar solutions and, therefore, minimize the volume, while optimizing rapid caloric delivery.

Complications. The complications associated with the use of TPN include technical problems with the vascular access: pneumothorax, arterial laceration, venous thrombosis, air embolism, and cardiac dysrrhythmias. Other complications, such as fluid overload, electrolyte imbalances, hyperglycemia, and septic complications, and the nursing measures aimed at their identification and prevention have been discussed extensively in the literature and will not be reviewed here.

In the beginning, metabolic support through TPN was accomplished primarily with glucose-based solutions. This type of support produced many detrimental effects, including increased resting energy expenditure, increased carbon dioxide production, elevated R/Q with resulting increased ventilatory demand, fatty liver syndrome, hyperglycemia, hyperosmolar states, increased body fat mass, stimulation of catecholamine release, elevated lactate formation, bowel distention, and increased gas production.* These problems have been attributed to the delivery of excess calories or excess glucose calories.

Investigators have reported that when more than 5 mg/kg/min of glucose is infused, only 50% to 70% of the glucose is directly oxidized for energy.[99] Others report that glucose in excess of 7 mg/kg/min is metabolized to fat and leads to fatty infiltrates of the liver and derangement of hepatic enzymes.[100] Duncan, Bistrain, and Blackburn[3] also reported that the body can oxidize infused glucose up to 4 to 5 mg/kg/min (400 to 500 g of glucose/day for a 70-kg adult). Excess infused glucose is converted to fat. The lipogenesis from glucose produces large quantities of water and carbon dioxide. This may exac-

---

*References 11, 31, 38, 97, 98.

erbate pulmonary dysfunction, so limitation of glucose administration is recommended.[3]

To prevent the described problems of overfeeding, it is extremely important to deliver only as many calories as are needed by the individual patient. This goal may be accomplished by calculating the patient's needs based on the techniques discussed under "Assessment of Metabolic Requirements."

One solution to delivering too many calories from glucose is to meet caloric needs by supplementing with intravenous fat emulsions. These fat emulsions are produced from soybean or safflower oil. The solutions not only serve to prevent essential fatty acid deficiency but may also be used as a calorie source. Studies of sepsis using animal models show better preservation of lung architecture, surfactant composition, and pulmonary function with the use of fat emulsions.[11] In addition, Nordestrom and co-workers[101,102] and Askanazi and co-workers[103] compared the effects of TPN delivered as a "glucose system" (all nonprotein calories supplied via carbohydrates) versus TPN delivered as a "lipid system" (nonprotein calories supplied via equal amounts of glucose and fat). All patients were given equal quantities of protein. The investigators compared nitrogen balance in the two groups and found there was no difference between the groups, but they did demonstrate that the "lipid system" group had a lower metabolic response and lower levels of norepinephrine excretion.[101-103]

Cerra[11] concluded that standard TPN with caloric loads greater than 50 kcal/kg caused increased organ failure resulting from increased carbon dioxide production, increased minute ventilation, ventilatory failure, hepatic steatosis, suboptimal nitrogen retention, hyperglycemia with hyperosmolar problems, and elevations in resting energy expenditure.

From these findings it is recommended that TPN be delivered as a mixed substrate solution of carbohydrate, fats, and protein in the form of amino acids. However, it is also recommended that no more than 30% to 40% of non-protein calories be delivered as fat calories.[104,105] It is very important to monitor lipid clearance by measuring serum triglyceride levels when providing calories in this manner. Excess fat may block reticuloendothelial activity and thus impair overall immune function, but this theory is controversial.[3] In organ failure, determining the exact mix of the three major substrates depends on the needs of the individual patient and the specific organs involved. Research on improved TPN usage in organ failure is ongoing and consultation with a metabolic support team or clinical dietitian is critical when making decisions regarding an individual patient with organ failure. An excellent review of composition and administration of formulas, vascular access, and care of the patient with TPN has been reported by Worthington and Wagner.[106]

Disease- or organ-specific formulas. Some areas of ongoing research in delivering TPN to patients with organ failure include the following:

HEPATIC FAILURE. Some authors suggest that with fulminant hepatic failure, TPN solutions should contain only the branched chain amino acids and decreased levels of aromatic amino acids. They propose that this will help reduce endogenous protein breakdown without increasing encephalopathy because the aromatic amino acids have been identified as contributing to encephalopathy.[107-109] Fischer[110] and Freund and co-workers[111] found that solutions of BCAAs given to patients with hepatic encephalopathy were well tolerated and caused no worsening of the hepatic encephalopathy. However, these formulas are very expensive and their efficacy is questioned by many practitioners; more research is indicated.

RENAL FAILURE. Studies indicate the mortality rate in acute renal failure may be decreased if nutritional status is maintained,[112] but careful manipulation of fluid, electrolyte, and protein levels is required. Specialized formulas used for patients with renal failure include Aminosyn-RF, Nephramine, and RenAmin. Aminosyn-RF contains only the essential amino acids and arginine. Nephramine contains only the essential amino acids. RenAmin contains more nonessential amino acids. For renal failure patients not on dialysis, 250 mL of these solutions may be mixed with 500 mL of 70% dextrose and administered at a rate of 1 L/day. Patients on dialysis may tolerate rates of 2 to 2.5 L/day.[113,114] There are also reports of using continuous arteriovenous hemofiltration in conjunction with metabolic support. In this case, aggressive metabolic support can be provided without worry of protein and fluid loads adversely affecting blood urea nitrogen (BUN) and creatinine levels.[115]

CARDIOPULMONARY FAILURE. Adequate metabolic support is essential to maintain adequate cardiopulmonary function, maintain host defenses against pulmonary infections, and provide energy to recover from ventilatory failure. As described earlier, calories from carbohydrates must be limited and caloric needs must be met through an appropriate mix of carbohydrates and fats.[113,115]

Monitoring of metabolic support

Table 7-2 lists the recommendations for monitoring of parenteral and enteral nutrition. Specific time frames and components monitored vary from institution to institution.

INVESTIGATIONAL THERAPIES

Other areas of research in metabolic support of MODS include the following.

Growth hormone therapy

While studying the effects of growth hormone on metabolic support, Manson, Smith, and Wilmore[116] found that growth hormone favored nitrogen retention and protein synthesis when a hypocaloric parenteral glucose solution was given. Another study demonstrated improved nitrogen retention when growth hormone was given with TPN.[117] Promising research is ongoing in the area of combining growth hormone with metabolic support.[118]

Glutamine therapy

The major amino acid in the plasma and cells is glutamine. The kidneys and small intestine are the major organs that utilize glutamine. Patients receiving TPN with glutamine demonstrated a significantly lower loss of nitrogen than did control patients.[119,120] Souba[121] demonstrated that animals fed a glutamine-supplemented diet had a significantly lower incidence of bacterial translocation of the gut and speculated that glutamine may support intestinal metabolism, structure, and function.

Other areas of research

Research is ongoing to determine more precisely the caloric needs and ideal substrate mix for the MODS patient. Indirect calorimetry provides vital information in this area. Research is also promising in the area of combined enteral and parenteral nutrition for the patient whose gut cannot support the entire nutritional requirement but for whom the therapeutic effects of gut stimulation are advantageous.

CONCLUSION

The metabolic alterations and ultimate metabolic failure seen in patients with MODS are not yet clearly understood. The hypermetabolic state is a compensatory mechanism initially triggered to help meet short-term increased energy needs. In MODS, continued hypermetabolism places tremendous demands on the skeletal muscle mass, the liver, and other organs. Whether this overwhelming demand

Table 7-2 Monitoring for Parenteral and Enteral Nutrition

Parameter	Parenteral nutrition	Enteral nutrition
Weight	Daily	Daily
Intake and output	Every shift	Every shift
Electrolyte levels	Daily	Daily until stable, then as indicated
Complete blood count	First day, then Mondays and Thursdays	First day, then Mondays and Thursdays
Nitrogen balance	Weekly	Weekly
Nutritional assessment	Weekly	Weekly
Blood glucose levels	q4-6h (or more if unstable)	q4-6h until stable, then daily
Urine glucose and acetone levels	q6h	q6h
Tube position	n/a	q4h
Transferrin levels	Weekly	Weekly
SMA12 panel	First day, then Mondays and Thursdays	First day, then Mondays and Thursdays
Magnesium levels	Weekly	Weekly
Vitamin levels	As indicated by metabolic support team	As indicated by metabolic support team

is the cause of progressive organ failure or whether the ongoing hypermetabolic response is the result of other mechanisms triggered by failing organs remains to be elucidated. Clearly, no matter what the cause-and-effect relationship is between nutrition and metabolism, aggressive metabolic support is a vital adjunctive weapon in the arsenal of treatment modalities currently available in management of patients suffering from or at risk for MODS.

REFERENCES

1. Lekander BJ, Cerra FB. The syndrome of multiple organ failure. Crit Care Nurs Clin North Am 1990;2:331-342.
2. Barton RG. Nutrition support in critical illness. NCP 1994;9:127-139.
3. Duncan JL, Bistrian BR, Blackburn GL. Septic stress. Nutritional management of the patient. Consultant 1982;22:235-247.
4. Pomposelli JJ, Flores EA, Bistrian BR. Role of biochemical mediators in clinical nutrition and surgical metabolism. JPEN 1988;12:212-218.
5. Dinarello CA. Interleukin-1 and the pathogenesis of the acute phase response. N Engl J Med 1984;311:1413-1418.
6. Graham P, Brass NJ. Multiple organ dysfunction: Pathophysiology and therapeutic modalities. Crit Care Nurs Q 1994;16:8-15.
7. Buckner MM. Perioperative nutrition problems: Nursing management. Crit Care Nurs Clin North Am 1990;2:559-566.
8. Leupold C. Critical care—Stress, trauma, burns, and sepsis. In: Kennedy-Caldwell C, Guenter P, eds. Nutrition support nursing, core curriculum. 2nd ed. Silver Springs: ASPEN; 1988:413-453.
9. Baue AE. Nutrition and metabolism in sepsis and multisystem organ failure. Surg Clin North Am 1991;71:549-565.
10. Cuthbertson DP. Post-shock metabolic response. Lancet 1942;1:433-437.
11. Cerra FB. Hypermetabolism, organ failure, and metabolic support. Surgery 1987;101:1-14.
12. Beal AL, Cerra FB. Multiple organ failure syndrome in the 1990s. JAMA 1994;271:226-233.
13. Guyton AC. Textbook of medical physiology. 9th ed. Philadelphia: WB Saunders Co.; 1995.
14. Johnson D. Metabolic and endocrine alterations in the multiply injured patient. Crit Care Nurs Q 1988;11:35-41.
15. Barton R, Cerra FB. The hypermetabolism multiple organ failure syndrome. Chest 1989;96:1153-1160.
16. Cerra FB. Hypermetabolism-organ failure syndrome: A metabolic response to injury. Crit Care Clin 1989;5:289-302.
17. Gutierrez G, Lund N, Bryan-Brown CW. Cellular oxygen utilization during multiple organ failure. Crit Care Clin 1989;5:271-287.
18. Barrocas A, Webb G, St. Romain C. Nutritional considerations in the critically ill. South Med Jour 1982;75:848-851.
19. Kovacerich D. Nutritional alterations in illness: Pulmonary. In Kennedy-Caldwell C, Guenter P, eds. Nutrition support nursing core curriculum. 2nd ed. Silver Springs: ASPEN, 1988.
20. Guenst JM, Nelson, LD. Predictors of total parenteral nutrition-induced lipogenesis. Chest 1994;105:553-559.
21. Liposky JM, Nelson LD. Ventilatory response to high caloric loads in critically ill patients. Crit Care Med 1994;22:796-802.
22. Kinney JM. Nutrition in the intensive care patient. Crit Care Clin 1987;3:1-10.
23. Wilmore DW et al. The gut: A central organ after surgical stress. Surgery 1988;104:917-923.
24. Heath DF, Stoner HB. Studies on the metabolism of shock. Non-esterified fatty acid metabolism in normal and injured rats. Br J Exp Pathol 1968:49:168-169.
25. Babgy GJ et al. Lipoprotein lipase-suppressing mediator in serum of endotoxin-treated rats. Am J Physiol 1986:251:E470-E476.
26. Fitzsimmons L, Hadley SA. Nutritional management of the metabolically stressed patient. Crit Care Nurs Q 1994;17:1-13.
27. Cerra FB. Hypermetabolism-organ failure syndrome: A metabolic response to injury. Crit Care Clin 1989;5:289-302.
28. Cerra FB et al. Autocannibalism, a failure of exogenous nutritional support. Ann Surg 1980;192:570-574.
29. Lindholm M, Rossner S. Rate of elimination of the intralipid fat emulsion from the circulation in ICU patients. Crit Care Med 1983;10:740.
30. Lekander BJ, Cerra FB. The syndrome of multiple organ failure. Crit Care Nurs Clin North Am 1990;2:331-342.
31. Cerra FB. The syndrome of multiple organ failure. In: Cerra FB, Binati D, eds. New Horizon Series. Cell injury and organ failure. Fullerton: Society of Critical Care Medicine; 1988.
32. Hill GL et al. Malnutrition in surgical patients: An unrecognized problem. Lancet 1977;1:689-692.
33. Woolfson AMJ. Artificial nutrition in the hospital. Br Med J 1983;287:1004-1006.
34. Dempsey DT, Mullen JL, Buzby GP. The link between nutritional status and clinical outcome: Can nutritional intervention modify it? Am J Clin Nutr 1988;47:352-356.
35. Law DK, Dudrick SJ, Abdou NI. The effects of protein-calorie malnutrition on immune competence of the surgical patient. Surg Gynecol Obstet 1974;139:257-266.
36. Stoddart JC. Multiorgan failure and its management in the intensive therapy unit. Br Med Bull 1988;44:475-498.
37. Kuhn MM. Nutritional support for the shock patient. Crit Care Nurs Clin of North Am 1990;2:201-220.
38. Cerra FB. The hypermetabolism organ failure complex. World J Surg 1987;11:173-181.
39. Littleton MT. Pathophysiology and assessment of sepsis and septic shock. Crit Care Nurs Q 1988;11:30-47.
40. Champangne MT, Ashley ML. Nutritional support in the critically ill elderly patient. Crit Care Nurs Q 1989;12:15-25.
41. Lehmann S. Nutritional support in the hypermetabolic patient. Crit Care Nurs Clin North Am 1993;5:97-103.
42. Curtis S. Nutritional assessment. In: Kennedy-Caldwell C, Guenter P, eds. Nutrition support nursing core curriculum. 2nd ed. Silver Springs: ASPEN; 1988:29-42.
43. Gianino S, St. John RE. Nutritional assessment of the patient in the intensive care unit. Crit Care Nurs Clin North Am 1993;5:1-16.
44. Silk DBA. Enteral nutrition. Post Grad Med J 1984;60:779-790.

45. Cataldi-Betcher E et al. Complications occurring during enteral nutrition support: A prospective study. JPEN 1983;7:546-552.
46. Levine GM et al. Role of oral intake in maintenance of gut mass and disaccharide activity. Gastroenterology 1974;67:975.
47. Deitch EA. Multiple organ failure. Advan Surg 1993;26:333-356.
48. Andrassy RJ. Practical rewards of enteral feeding for the surgical patient. Contemp Surg 1989;35(5-A):20-23.
49. Kever AJH et al. Prevention and colonization of infection in critically ill patients: A prospective, randomized study. Crit Care Med 1988;16:1087-1094.
50. Kripke SA et al. Stimulation of mucosal growth with intracolonic butyrate infusion. Surg Forum 1987;38:47-49.
51. Alverdy JC. The GI tract as an immunologic organ. Contemp Surg 1989;35(5-A):14-19.
52. Phillips MC, Olson LR. The immunologic role of the gastrointestinal tract. Crit Care Nurs Clin North Am 1993;5:107-120.
53. Van Leeuwen PA et al. Clinical significance of translocation. Gut 1994;Supplement 1:S28-S34.
54. Heyland DK, Cook DJ, Guyatt GH. Does the formulation of enteral feeding products influence infections morbidity and mortality rates in the critically ill patient? A critical review of the evidence. Crit Care Med 1994;22:1192-1202.
55. Keithley JK, Eisenberg P. The significance of enteral nutrition in the intensive care unit patient. Crit Care Nurs Clin North Am 1993;5:23-29.
56. Heyland DK, Cook DJ, Guyatt GH. Enteral nutrition in the critically ill patient: A critical review of evidence. Inten Care Med 1993;19:435-442.
57. Lord LM, Sax HC. The role of the gut in critical illness. AACL Clin Issues Crit Care Nurs 1994;5:450-458.
58. Barracos V, Rodemann HP, Dienarello C. Stimulation of muscle protein degradation on PGE2 release by leukocyte pyrogen. N Engl J Med 1983;308:553-558.
59. McClave SA, Lowen CC, Snider HL. Immunonutrition and enteral hyperalimentation of critically ill patients. Dig Dis Sci 1992;37:1153-1161.
60. Allardyce DB, Groves AC. A comparison of nutritional gains resulting from intravenous and enteral feedings. Surg Gynecol Obstet 1974;139:180-184.
61. Hindmarch JT, Clark RG. The effects in intravenous and intraduodenal feeding on nitrogen balance after surgery. Br J Surg 1973;60:589.
62. Pingleton SK, Harmon GS. Nutritional management in acute respiratory failure. JAMA 1987;257:3094-3099.
63. Saito H, Trock O, Alexander J. Comparison of immediate postburn enteral versus parenteral nutrition. [Abstract]. ASPEN Clinical Congress,1985.
64. Baue AE. The role of the gut in the development of multiple organ dysfunction in cardiothoracic patients. Ann Thorac Surg 1993;55:822-829.
65. Cerra FB et al. Branched chain metabolic support. Ann Surg 1984;199:286-291.
66. Cerra FB et al. Enteral nutrition does not prevent multiple organ failure syndrome (MOFS) after sepsis. Surgery 1988;104:727-733.
67. Cerra FB et al. Enteral feeding in sepsis: A prospective, randomized, double-blind trial. Surgery 1985;98:632.
68. Rothnie NG, Harper RAK, Catchpole BN. Early postoperative gastrointestinal activity. Lancet 1963;2:64.
69. Wells C et al. Postoperative gastrointestinal motility. Lancet 1964;1:4.
70. Anderson JD, Moore FA, Moore EE. Enteral feeding in the critically injured patient. NCP 1992;7:117-122.
71. Flynn KT, Norton LC, Fisher RL. Enteral tube feeding: Indications, practices and outcomes. Image 1987;19:16-19.
72. Zimmaro DM. Diarrhea associated with enteral nutrition. Focus Crit Care 1986;13:58-63.
73. Posa PJ. Nutritional support of the critically ill patient: Bedside strategies for successful patient outcomes. Crit Care Nurs Q 1994;16:61-70.
74. Posa PJ. Nutritional support strategies: A case study approach. AACN Clin Issues Crit Care Nurs 1994;5:436-449.
75. Groer M, Shekleton M. Basic pathology, a conceptual approach. St Louis: Mosby; 1979.
76. Walike BC et al. Patient problems related to tube feeding. Communicating Nurs Res 1975;7:89-112.
77. Williams KR, Walike BC. Effect of the temperature of tube feeding on gastric motility in monkeys. Nurs Res 1975;24:4-9.
78. Kagawa-Busby K et al. Effects of diet temperature on tolerance of enteral feedings. Nurs Res 1980;29:276-280.
79. Heitkemper M, Hanson R, Hansen B. Effects of rate and volume of tube feeding in normal human subjects. Communicating Nurs Res 1977;10:71-89.
80. Heitkemper M et al. Rate and volume of intermittent enteral feeding. JPEN 1981;5:125-129.
81. Hersh R, Rudman D. Nasogastric hyperalimentation through a polyetheylene catheter. Am J Clin Nutrition 1979;32:1112-1120.
82. Hoover HC et al. Nutritional benefits of immediate post-operative jejunal feeding of an elemental diet. Am J Surg 1980;139:153-159.
83. Heibert J. et al. Comparison of continuous versus intermittent tube feedings in adult burn patients. JPEN 1981;5:73-75.
84. Keohane PP et al. Relation between osmolality of diet and gastrointestinal side effects in enteral nutrition. Br Med J 1984;288:678-680.
85. Hosteller C et al. Bacterial safety of reconstituted continuous drip tube feeding. JPEN 1982;6:232-235.
86. Scheimer RL et al. Environmental contamination of continuous drip feedings. Pediatrics 1979;63:232-237.
87. Schroeder P et al. Microbial contamination of enteral feeding solutions in a community. JPEN 1983;7:364-367.
88. Koruda MJ, Guenter P. Enteral nutrition in the critically ill. Crit Care Clin 1987;3:133-153.
89. Marcuard SP, Perkins AM. Clogging of feeding tubes. JPEN 1988;12:403-405.
90. Metheny N, Eisenberg P, McSweeney M. Effect of feeding tube properties and three irrigants on clogging rates. Nurs Res 1988;37:165-169.
91. Marcuard S, Stegall K. Unclogging feeding tubes with pancreatic enzyme. JPEN 1990;14:198-200.
92. Metheny N, Eisenberg P, Spies M. Aspiration pneumonia in patients fed through nasoenteral tubes. Heart Lung 1986;15:256-261.
93. Kohn CL, Keithley JK. Enteral nutrition. Potential complications and patient monitoring. Nurs Clin North Am 1989;24:339-353.

94. Boyes RJ, Kruse JA. Nasogastric and nasoenteric intubation. Crit Care Clin 1992;8:865-878.
95. Metheny N et al. Effectiveness of pH measurements in predicting feeding tube placement. Nurs Res 1989;38:280-285.
96. Eisenberg P. Enteral nutrition. Indications, formulas, and delivery techniques. Nurs Clin North Am 1989;24:315-338.
97. Shaw JHF, Wolfe RR. Glucose and urea kinetics in patients with early and advanced gastrointestinal cancer: The response to glucose infusion, parenteral feeding, and surgical resection. Surgery 1987;181:191.
98. White RH et al. Hormonal and metabolic responses to glucose infusion in sepsis studies by the hyperglycemic clamp technique. JPEN 1987;11:345-353.
99. Wolfe BR, Allsop JR, Burke JF. Glucose metabolism in man: Response to intravenous glucose infusion. Metabolism 1979;28:210.
100. Sheldon GF, Peterson SC, Sanders R. Hepatic dysfunction during hyperalimentation. Arch Surg 1978;113:504.
101. Nordenstrom J, Jeevanandam J, Elwyn DH. Increasing glucose intake during total parenteral nutrition increases norepinephrine excretion in trauma and sepsis. Clin Physiol 1981;1:525.
102. Nordenstrom J et al. Nitrogen Balance during total parenteral nutrition: Glucose versus fat. Ann Surg 1983; 197:27.
103. Askanazi J et al. Influence of total parenteral nutrition on fuel utilization in injury and sepsis. Ann Surg 1980;191:40-46.
104. Macho, J, Luce, J. Rational approach to management of multisystems organ failure. Crit Care Clinics 1989;5:379-392.
105. Evans NJ. The role of total parenteral nutrition in critical illness: Guidelines and recommendations. AACN Clin Issues Crit Care Nurs 1994;5:476-484.
106. Worthington PH, Wagner BA. Total parenteral nutrition. Nurs Clin North Am 1987;24:355-371.
107. Wahren J, Davis J, Desurmont P. Is intravenous administration of branched chain amino acids effective in the treatment of hepatic encephalopathy? A multicentre study. Hepatology 1983;3:294-304.
108. Millikan WJ, Henderson JM, Warren WD. Total parenteral nutrition with F080 in cirrhosis with subclinical encephalopathy. Ann Surg 1983;3:294-304.
109. Zaloga G, Ackerman MH. A review of disease-specific formulas. AACN Clin Issues Crit Care Nurs 1994;5:421-435.
110. Fischer JE. Portasystemic encephalopathy. In: Wright R et al, eds. Liver and biliary disease: Pathophysiology, diagnosis, management. Philadelphia: WB Saunders Co; 1979:973-1001.
111. Freund H et al. Infusion of branched-chain enriched amino acid solution in patients with hepatic encephalopathy. Ann Surg 1982;196:209-220.
112. Baek SM et al. The influence of parenteral nutrition on the course of acute renal failure. Surg Gynecol Obstet 1975; 141:405-408.
113. Baue AE. Multiple organ failure. Patient care and prevention. St Louis: Mosby; 1990:390.
114. Varella L, Utermohlen V. Nutritional support for the patient with renal failure. Crit Care Nurs Clin North Am 1993;5: 79-96.
115. Bessey PQ. Nutritional support in critical illness. In: Deitch E, ed. Multiple organ failure. Pathophysiology and basic concepts of therapy. New York: Thieme Medical Publishers, 1990:126-149.
116. Manson JM, Smith RJ, Wilmore DW. Growth hormone stimulates protein synthesis during hypocaloric parenteral nutrition: role of hormonal-substrate environment. Ann Surg 1988;208:143-149.
117. Ziegler TR et al. Metabolic effects of recombinant human growth hormone in patients receiving parenteral nutrition. Ann Surg 1988;208:6-16.
118. Ziegler TR, Gatzen C, Wilmore DW. Strategies for attenuating protein-catabolic responses in the critically ill. Annu Rev Med 1994;45:459-480.
119. Hammarqvist F et al. Addition of glutamine to total parenteral nutrition after elective abdominal surgery spares free glutamine in muscle, counteracts the fall in muscle protein synthesis, and improves nitrogen balance. Ann Surg 1989;84:224-230.
120. Grant, JP. Nutritional support in critically ill patients. Ann Surg 1994;220:610-616.
121. Souba WW. The gut—a key metabolic organ following surgical stress. Contemp Surg 1989;35(5-A):5-13.

Section 3

ORGAN INVOLVEMENT AND CLINICAL PRESENTATION

As the pathophysiologic changes continue, organ dysfunction occurs, often remote from the initial site of injury or inflammation. The organs do not suffer damage in isolation but within the entire presentation of the systemic inflammatory response syndrome and multiple organ dysfunction syndrome. Organ-organ interaction is thought to be a principal contributor to the progression of both syndromes, with organ ischemia and damage further stimulating the uncontrolled inflammatory/immune response. As each additional organ fails, morbidity and mortality escalate.

8. Adult Respiratory Distress Syndrome
9. Hepatic Dysfunction, Hypermetabolism, and Multiple Organ Dysfunction Syndrome
10. Gastrointestinal System: Target Organ and Source of Multiple Organ Dysfunction Syndrome
11. Acute Pancreatitis and Multiple Organ Dysfunction Syndrome
12. Myocardial Dysfunction in Sepsis and Multiple Organ Dysfunction Syndrome
13. The Kidney in Multiple Organ Dysfunction Syndrome
14. Central Nervous System Dysfunction in Multiple Organ Dysfunction Syndrome

CHAPTER 8

Adult Respiratory Distress Syndrome

Margaret T. Morris

Adult respiratory distress syndrome (ARDS) is responsible for respiratory failure in as many as 150,000 patients a year and has an overall mortality rate of 10% to 90%. These figures are controversial and exact numbers have always been difficult to obtain because of a lack of a specific definition for ARDS, lack of definition of the underlying disease processes, the abundance of different management strategies, and the failure to define the subset of patients that is diagnosed with ARDS.[1-4] The exact cause of death in patients with ARDS is difficult to determine because various underlying pathologic conditions are often present: systemic inflammatory response syndrome (SIRS), disseminated intravascular coagulation (DIC), and multiple organ dysfunction syndrome (MODS). Furthermore, death may not be from failure of gas exchange alone, but rather from the multisystem organ failure (MSOF) often associated with ARDS. Some reseachers believe that death in a specific subset of ARDS patients is more often caused by inadequate tissue perfusion and maldistribution of blood flow that is not identified early or that is treated inadequately.[5]

ARDS can occur in isolation, but it occurs more frequently in the setting of MODS and MSOF. ARDS can incite the development of MODS, or it may develop secondary to the pathophysiologic derangements accompanying the MODS. Whether the culprit or the victim, ARDS contributes to the self-perpetuating nature of MODS by exacerbating tissue hypoxia and activating mediators of the inflammatory cascade. ARDS is a complex syndrome manifested by increased capillary permeability, atelectasis, and intraalveolar and interstitial noncardiogenic pulmonary edema, all of which cause a derangement in gas exchange and refractory hypoxemia.

Acute lung injury, noncardiogenic pulmonary edema, and shock lung are terms used to describe the scenario of respiratory failure in the setting of SIRS, MODS, and critical illness. The American-European Consensus Conference (AECC) on ARDS held in 1992 created a definition for acute lung injury (ALI) and ARDS that is discussed in the section on Definition and Diagnosis. The syndrome of ARDS is the primary focus of this chapter because it is the condition most commonly associated with the etiology of MODS.

Since the ARDS syndrome was first described by Ashbaugh and co-workers more than 20 years ago, the understanding of the mechanisms of lung injury and its clinical manifestations has evolved considerably.[6] It is now clear that a cascade of inflammatory/immune reactions, including activation of the coagulation system, greatly contributes to lung injury. The exact role of each mechanism has not been fully defined.

A variety of clinical conditions are responsible for initiating the cascade of events that cause lung injury, ARDS, and MODS. Causes can be differentiated as direct (pulmonary) or indirect (systemic) (see the box on p. 168).[7] Overt signs and symptoms can be evident immediately or as late as 48 to 72 hours after the initial insult. Clinical features of ARDS include refractory hypoxemia, decreased pulmonary compliance, radiographic evidence of noncardiogenic pulmonary edema, and normal pulmonary capillary wedge pressures (PCWP).[8] However, the PCWP may be elevated because of cardiac dysfunction related to hypoxemia or other causes of

ETIOLOGY OF ARDS

Direct causes
Inhalation of toxins
Aspiration of gastric contents
Pulmonary contusion
Thoracic trauma
Bacterial or viral pneumonia
Oxygen toxicity
Fat emboli
Near drowning

Indirect causes
Septic shock
Other shock states
Multiple trauma
Disseminated intravascular coagulation
Pancreatitis
Thermal injuries
Anaphylaxis
Multiple blood transfusions

From Vaughan P, Brooks C. Adult respiratory distress syndrome: A complication of shock. Crit Care Nurs Clin North Am 1990;2:236.

cardiac pathology, such as myocardial ischemia or infarction, chronic congestive heart failure, or congenital cardiomyopathies. In the critically ill patient, it is sometimes difficult to determine when the initial injury precipitating the development of ARDS occurred. Distinguishing ARDS from other causes of respiratory failure in these patients is also difficult, especially in the presence of underlying chronic disease and other host-related factors such as age, immunosuppression, and previous infection.

The purposes of this chapter are (1) to review the definition and diagnosis of ARDS; (2) to discuss principles of ventilation, perfusion, and gas transport; (3) to describe the pathophysiology of ARDS; (4) to discuss the clinical presentation; and (5) to outline therapeutic strategies used in the management of ARDS.

DEFINITION AND DIAGNOSIS

Definitions of both acute lung injury and ARDS describe the syndrome of severe respiratory failure that can occur in both children and adults. The syndrome of respiratory failure can be viewed as a dynamic continuum, with patients ranging from those with acute lung injury without ARDS to others who progress to the advanced stage of severe ARDS. In an effort to simplify and create a common language for clinicians and researchers, the AECC developed a definition for ALI and ARDS.[1,9,10] Table 8-1 summarizes the criteria for defining ALI and ARDS.

Definition

The definitions of acute lung injury and ARDS include three components: (1) oxygenation, (2) chest radiograph, and (3) PCWP[1,9] (Table 8-1). The oxygenation status is measured by the partial arterial pressure of oxygen (PaO_2)/fraction of inspired oxygen (FiO_2) ratio regardless of the presence of positive end-expiratory pressure (PEEP). The effects of PEEP over a period of time are difficult to predict; therefore, it has been eliminated from this definition as a variable in assessing oxygenation. A frontal chest radiograph should demonstrate bilateral infiltrates. The PCWP should be greater than 18 mm Hg in the absence of clinical evidence of left ventricular dysfunction.

The PCWP has been a useful tool in differentiating between cardiogenic and noncardiogenic pulmonary edema. However, the practitioner should remember that ventricular dysfunction may be an underlying disease process already present in some patients or, more frequently, that may develop as a result of profound hypoxemia and MODS. Therefore, these specific patients may have a PCWP ≥18. This high PCWP does not negate a diagnosis of ARDS, but instead, it reflects the fact that these patients will then have an additional pathologic process contributing to their pulmonary edema.

Diagnosis

Diagnosing ARDS should include identifying the clinical disorder associated with the development of the syndrome. In the causes outlined previously, the most common is SIRS.[1,7,11,12] In addition to defining ALI and ARDS and identifying the etiology, recognizing any nonpulmonary organ failure also is important in determining management strategies. This system for examining the ARDS patient shifts the focus of management from the treatment of an isolated, severe lung injury to treating the severe lung injury, underlying systemic process, and multisystem organ involvement.[10] The combination of ARDS with another organ failure carries a much greater mortality than either occurring in isolation.[13] Most patients who develop ARDS in conjunction

Table 8-1 Definition Criteria for Acute Lung Injury and Adult Respiratory Distress Syndrome

	ALI	ARDS
Oxygenation (PaO_2/FiO_2)	≤300	≤200
Chest radiograph	Bilateral infiltrates	Bilateral infiltrates
PCWP (No evidence of left atrial hypertension)	≤18 mm Hg	≤18 mm Hg

PaO_2/FiO_2, Partial arterial pressure of oxygen/fraction of inspired oxygen ratio; *PCWP*, pulmonary capillary wedge pressure.

with other organ failures are considered by some investigators to have had inadequate or maldistributed blood flow that was not adequately corrected.[5]

PULMONARY PHYSIOLOGY

The respiratory system provides oxygen for transport to the tissues through the process of gas exchange. Oxygen moves from the atmosphere into the blood, and carbon dioxide moves from the blood out to the atmosphere. The respiratory process can be divided into three different phases: (1) ventilation, (2) diffusion/perfusion, and (3) gas transport. Disorders of the respiratory system can include abnormalities of one or all of these phases. An understanding of normal pulmonary physiology is an integral step in the appreciation of the pathophysiology of ARDS.

VENTILATION

Ventilation involves movement of air from the atmosphere through all branches of the airway to the terminal alveoli. The involuntary process of ventilation involves active motion of the thorax during inspiration and passive elastic recoil of the lungs and the thoracic cage during expiration.

Muscles of ventilation. The diaphragm and the external intercostal muscles perform most of the work of normal, quiet ventilation. The diaphragm, a dome-shaped muscle located between the thorax and the abdomen, is innervated by the phrenic nerve of the autonomic nervous system.[14,15] When the diaphragm contracts, the lower portions of the lungs are pulled downward, increasing the vertical dimension of the chest. Contraction of the external intercostal muscles during inspiration increases the anteroposterior diameter of the thorax. Both of these muscular activities decrease the intrathoracic and intraalveolar pressure and increase lung volume. Slightly negative intraalveolar pressure with respect to atmospheric pressure causes air to flow inward from the mouth through the lungs.

Exhalation occurs passively through elastic recoil of the lungs and the thorax. The lungs return to the resting volume, intraalveolar pressure increases above atmospheric pressure, and air rushes out of the lungs.

Ventilatory control. Ventilation is regulated by neuronal and chemical control. Other factors that contribute to the control of ventilation are changes in body temperature, pressoreceptors responding to changes in the blood pressure, stretch receptors located in the lungs, and pharmacologic agents.

Neuronal control. Spontaneous involuntary ventilation occurs through innervation of the respiratory muscles. The respiratory center is located in the medulla oblongata and the pons, and impulses travel down the phrenic nerve to stimulate contraction of the diaphragm.

Chemical control. Central chemoreceptors located in the medulla and peripheral chemoreceptors located in the carotid bodies and aortic bodies are the two main components of chemical control for respiration. In chemical regulation, changes in respiratory neuronal activity occur in response to the concentration of carbon dioxide (CO_2), hydrogen ions (H^+), and oxygen (O_2) in the body fluids.[14,15]

Distribution of ventilation. In the healthy lungs of a person standing or sitting, the alveoli in the apex remain more distended than those in the base. The alveoli at the base are slightly compressed by the weight of the tissue in the upper portions of the lung. Because the apical alveoli are more distended, they expand less during inspiration compared to the alveoli located in the base.[15,16] In the supine position, the alveoli in the apex and the base are ventilated equally, with the dependent portions of the lungs most affected by gravity and the weight of the tissue. Ventilation and perfusion are more equally matched in the supine position[15] (Fig. 8-1).

170 *Organ Involvement and Clinical Presentation*

anatomic dead space and alveolar dead space is termed physiologic dead space.[14,15] Increased dead space, such as that occuring in shock states and with pulmonary emboli, contributes to ventilation-perfusion (V/Q) mismatching and impaired gas exchange. The addition of ventilator tubing and artificial airways increases the calculated dead space.

Lung mechanics

Compliance. Lung compliance refers to the distensibility of the lungs. The pressure required to achieve a change in the lung volume is the lung compliance, and it is opposed by the elastic recoil of the lung.[14-16] The greater the elastic recoil or stiffness of the lung secondary to pathologic changes, the lower the compliance.

The compliance of the entire respiratory system is influenced by the lung compliance and chest-wall compliance. Chest-wall compliance decreases with age (the chest wall becomes stiff), obesity, and chest deformities such as kyphoscoliosis.[16]

Surface tension. Forces between molecules of a liquid are very strong (stronger than at gas-liquid interface), so the liquid surface area becomes as small as possible. Because the alveoli have a liquid film lining, relatively large forces of surface tension have the potential to cause alveolar collapse. Pulmonary surfactant, a surface layer phospholipid produced by type II alveolar epithelial cells, decreases the surface tension of the alveolar sac.[16] By decreasing surface tension, surfactant stabilizes patent alveoli and increases lung compliance.

Airway resistance. Four major factors determine airway resistance: the cross-sectional area of the airways, the velocity of gas flow, the density of gas, and the total lung volume.[16] Airway resistance increases secondarily to pathologic obstruction to airflow resulting from secretions, inflammation, edema, airway collapse or constriction, or mass lesions in the airways. Normally, most of the energy expended for ventilation is used to overcome the elasticity and airway resistance of the respiratory system.[17] However, if an underlying pathologic condition is present, energy is expended to overcome this frictional resistance to airflow as well. The pathologic conditions causing respiratory failure can affect both airway resistance and lung compliance. Artificial airways, such as endotracheal tubes, and mechanical ventilation also increase airway resistance and the work of breathing.

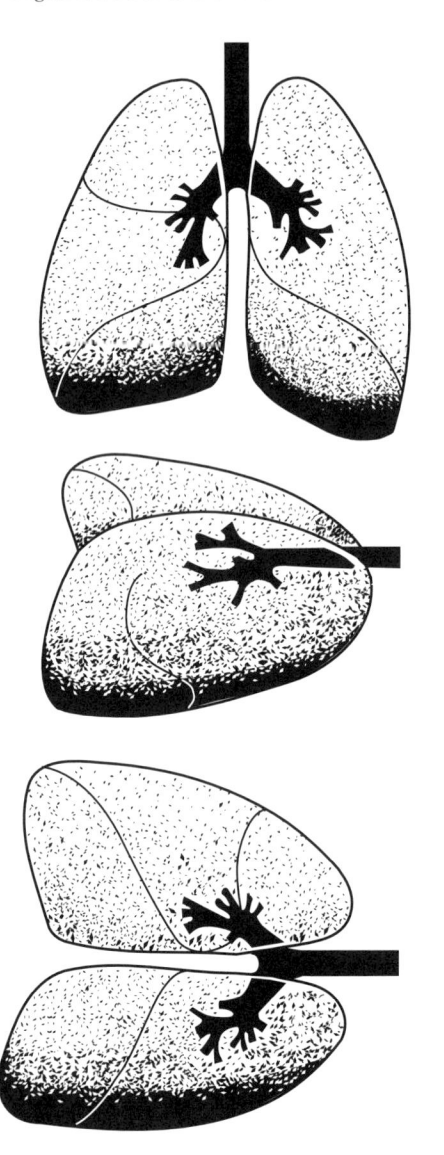

Fig. 8-1 The effects of position on pulmonary blood flow and gas exchange. (From Shapiro BA, Harrison RA, Walton JR. The physiology of external respiration. In: Shapiro BA, Harrison RA, Walton JR, eds. Clinical application of blood gases. 3rd ed. St Louis: Mosby, 1982;56.)

Dead-space ventilation. Anatomic dead space refers to that portion of ventilation in the tracheobronchial tree that is not involved in gas exchange. Alveolar dead space refers to alveoli that are ventilated but not perfused.[14,15] The combination of

The work of breathing for a normal individual at rest consumes approximately 5% of the total oxygen uptake of the body. Voluntary exercise may increase this value to 25% to 30%.[18] When there is significant pulmonary disease, the oxygen consumption of the work of breathing may exceed 30% of the total body consumption.[18]

Lung perfusion

Gas exchange occurs at the level of the pulmonary capillary bed. The capillary bed is a low pressure system that contains approximately 50 to 60 mL of flowing blood. The pulmonary capillary endothelium is one cell layer thick and has very little support from surrounding structures; therefore, the capillaries may collapse or expand depending on internal or external pressures. Only 25% to 35% of the pulmonary capillaries are open under normal resting conditions.[15] This percentage can increase dramatically through the process of recruitment (opening of capillaries not previously opened) and dilatation (expansion of currently opened capillaries) to accommodate changes in the cardiac output.[15] These mechanisms are responsible for decreased pulmonary vascular resistance as blood flow through the lungs increases. Conversely, vasoconstriction or collapse of capillaries resulting from increased surrounding pressures will cause increased pulmonary vascular resistance.

Patient positioning affects blood flow to lung regions in the same way that it affects ventilation (Figure 8-1). The blood flow is greater in the dependent portions of the lung, which may not match the areas that have the greatest number of ventilated alveoli (see the section on ventilation/perfusion matching). Blood flow may also be affected by positive-pressure ventilation, PEEP, exercise, or a change in cardiac output.[15]

Diffusion

Diffusion is a passive process involving gas transfer across the alveolar-capillary membrane in the presence of a concentration gradient. The factors that affect diffusion include (1) the pressure difference between the alveolar gas and the gas in the capillary blood, (2) the surface area of the alveolar-capillary membrane, (3) the membrane thickness and integrity, (4) the diffusion coefficient of the gas, and (5) the amount of hemoglobin in the blood.[14]

The alveolar-capillary membrane includes (1) the surfactant lining, (2) the alveolar epithelium and its basement membrane, (3) the tissue in the intercalated interstitial space, and (4) the capillary endothelium and its basement membrane.[19] The alveolar epithelium is composed of two important cell types. Alveolar type I cells are large, thin cells with very little cytoplasm, and they provide the major structural support of the alveolus. They are vulnerable to injury from direct or indirect causes. Alveolar type II cells produce surfactant and are also damaged easily.

Another important cell abundant in the lung is the alveolar macrophage, which constitutes the most important mechanism for fighting pulmonary infection. Macrophages release several mediators as part of the inflammatory process. A deficiency in function or the inability to down regulate inflammatory activity can facilitate injury and infection in the lung. This injury and infection can alter both diffusion and V-Q matching.

Ventilation-perfusion matching

Ventilated alveoli must come into contact with perfused capillaries for gas exchange to occur. Total lung perfusion slightly exceeds ventilation because normally there is some perfusion of nonventilated alveoli; therefore the normal ventilation/perfusion ratio (V/Q) is approximately 0.8 rather than 1.0 (a ratio of 1.0 would indicate an exact match between ventilation and perfusion).[14,20]

The V/Q differs in various zones of the lungs. Intravascular hydrostatic pressures change in different areas of the pulmonary capillary bed in relation to the vertical distance from a particular capillary to the heart. The intraalveolar pressure also differs at any particular point in relation to gravity. As described by West,[21] in zone I, intravascular pressure is lower than the intraalveolar pressure, and the capillary is totally collapsed because of pressure from surrounding alveoli.

In zone II, the intravascular inflow (arterial) pressure exceeds intraalveolar pressure, but alveolar pressures are higher than intravascular outflow (venous) pressures. The result is narrowed capillaries and intermittent flow regulated, in part, by the cardiac cycle.

In zone III, greater intravascular inflow and outflow pressures are unaffected by alveolar pressures, and the capillaries remain fully dilated throughout the respiratory and cardiac cycle[21] (Fig. 8-2). High levels of PEEP decrease the number of perfused

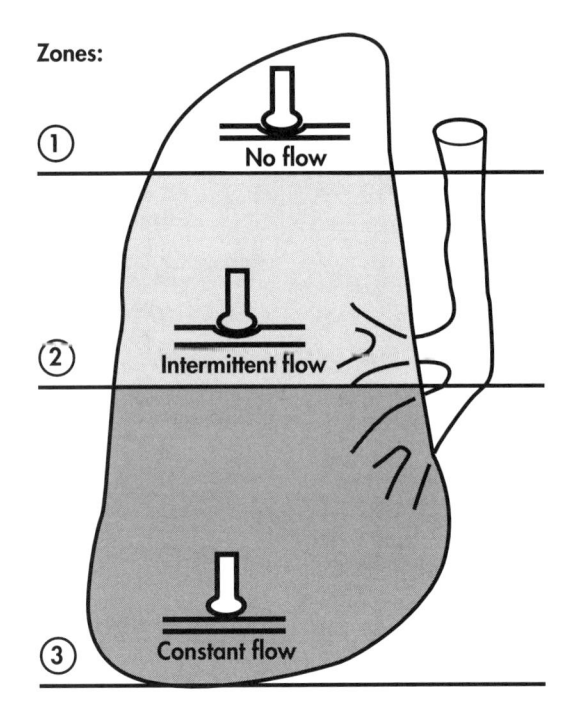

172 *Organ Involvement and Clinical Presentation*

Fig. 8-2 A three-zoned model illustrating the effects of gravity on the alveolar/pulmonary capillary blood flow relationship. (From LouAnn Johnson.)

capillary beds and increase the area of zones I and II as the increased intraalveolar and intrathoracic pressures compress the poorly supported capillaries.

Alterations in ventilation, perfusion, or their matching impair gas exchange (Fig. 8-3). For example, if ventilation is decreased because of conditions such as pulmonary edema, mucous plugging, atelectasis, or pneumonia, V/Q is less than 0.8 and may produce hypoxemia.[22] If perfusion becomes impaired, in instances such as pulmonary emboli, vasoconstriction secondary to hypoxia, low cardiac output, or loss of capillary flow, V/Q will be greater than 0.8, also potentiating hypoxemia.

Intrapulmonary shunt. A pulmonary shunt is the component of pulmonary blood flow that is perfusing unventilated alveoli and, therefore, not participating in gas exchange.[14] Pulmonary shunting is a severe form of V-Q mismatch. Normally, a shunt of 3% to 5% exists secondary to the venous drainage of the bronchial, pleural, and thebesian veins mixing with oxygenated blood in the pulmonary veins and left atrium. Also, perfusion slightly exceeds ventilation.[14]

In ARDS, intrapulmonary shunts may exceed 15% to 20% of pulmonary blood flow, because perfusion of collapsed and poorly functioning alveolar units does not contribute to gas exchange.[16] The shunt percentage can be estimated by dividing the FiO_2 into the PaO_2. The normal PaO_2/FiO_2 ratio is greater than 300 to 400.[20] A lower value usually indicates the presence of a shunt. Large shunt fractions indicate that a large percentage of the cardiac output is returning to the left side of the heart unoxygenated. Poor oxygen content and tissue oxygen delivery are the ultimate results.

Gas transport

Approximately 98% of oxygen transported in the blood is bound to hemoglobin, with the remaining 2% dissolved in the plasma.[14] The amount dissolved in the plasma (measured by the PaO_2) determines the saturation of hemoglobin. Oxygen combined with hemoglobin is referred to as oxyhemoglobin, and the percent saturation (SaO_2) refers to the amount of oxygen actually carried by the hemoglobin in relation to the total oxygen-carrying capacity of hemoglobin.

Adult Respiratory Distress Syndrome 173

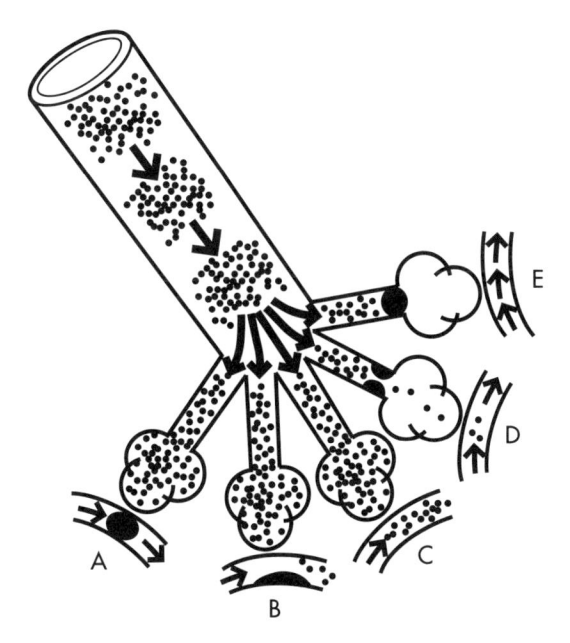

Fig. 8-3 Examples of ventilation-perfusion relationships. **A**, Alveolar deadspace. **B**, Alveolar deadspace effect. **C**, Normal. **D**, Venous admixture. **E**, Absolute shunts. (From LouAnn Johnson.)

Oxygen saturation and the partial pressure of oxygen have a curvilinear relationship. On the steep portion of the curve (PaO_2 less than 50 to 60 mm Hg), saturation of hemoglobin dramatically decreases with small changes in PaO_2. Factors that affect the oxyhemoglobin dissociation curve and thus the SaO_2 are pH, temperature, 2,3-diphosphoglycerate (2,3-DPG) levels, and partial arterial pressure of carbon dioxide ($PaCO_2$).[14]

Carbon dioxide is the end-product of cellular metabolism. It is transported in the blood in three forms: (1) a dissolved state measured as the $PaCO_2$ (5% to 10%), (2) as carbamino compounds (10% to 20%), and (3) as bicarbonate (70% to 90%). In the pulmonary circulation, the bicarbonate combines with hydrogen ions to form carbonic acid, which dissociates into carbon dioxide and water.[15] The carbon dioxide diffuses out of the plasma and red blood cells into the alveoli under the influence of a pressure gradient. Carbon dioxide diffuses 20 times more readily than oxygen does and is the most accurate indicator of minute ventilation (respiratory rate $\times$ tidal volume)[20]; therefore alterations in ventilation result in abnormal carbon dioxide levels.

There is an intricate relationship between PaO_2 and $PaCO_2$ loading and unloading, both in the peripheral tissues and in the lung. At the tissue level, increased carbon dioxide levels shift the oxyhemoglobin dissociation curve to the right, which facilitates oxygen unloading by the hemoglobin (Fig. 8-4).[14] In the lungs, the level of carbon dioxide and hydrogen ions decrease rapidly as carbon dioxide diffuses into alveoli; the pH increases, and the curve shifts to the left. The affinity for oxygen and hemoglobin increases, thus facilitating the uptake of oxygen in the lung.

Adequate tissue oxygenation involves ventilation, diffusion, and oxygen transport. ARDS primarily affects ventilation and diffusion. Refractory hypoxemia causing inadequate tissue oxygenation at the cellular level is the severe consequence of ARDS.

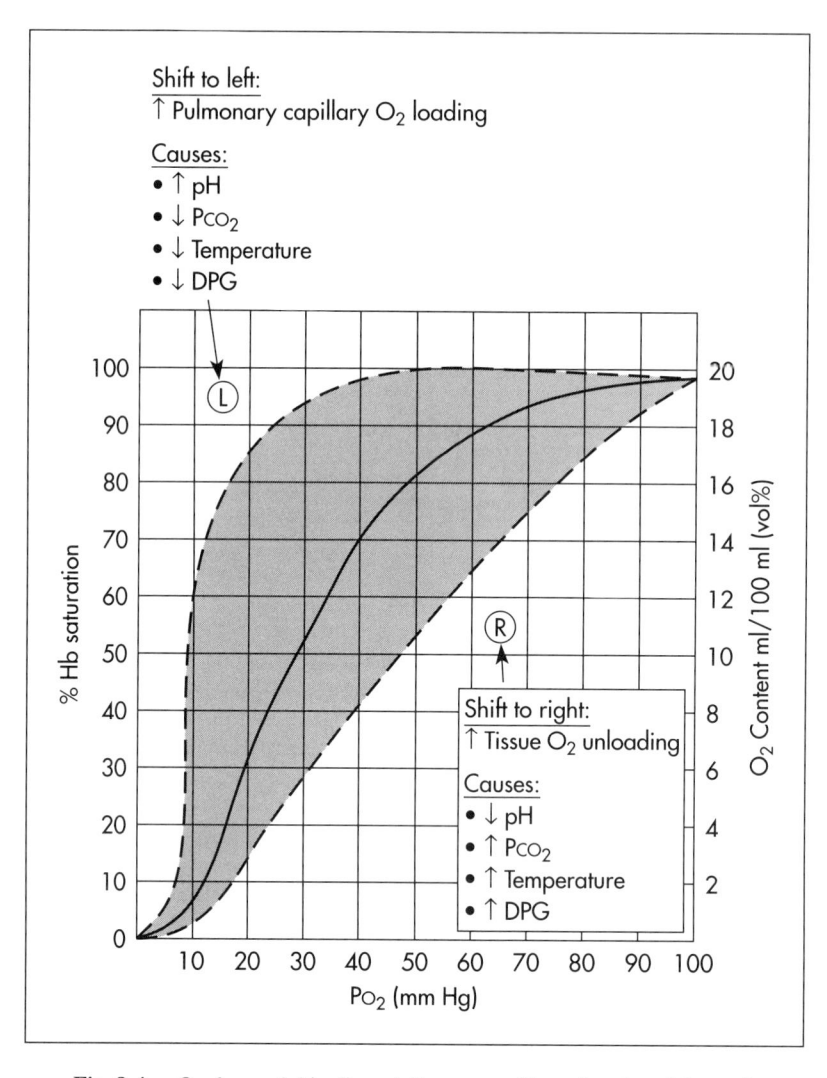

Fig. 8-4 Oxyhemoglobin dissociation curve. (From LouAnn Johnson.)

PATHOPHYSIOLOGY

The cascade of events responsible for the acute lung injury seen in ARDS and other organ dysfunction represents the host response to injury. Both cellular and humoral activities contribute to microvascular permeability, pulmonary hypertension, cellular necrosis, epithelial hyperplasia, inflammation, and fibrosis. The exact sequence of mediator activation and release is unknown. Investigators postulate that the initial event precipitating ARDS may determine the progression of mediator responses.[8] It is important to remember that various inflammatory/immune processes contributing to lung injury are initially activated to maintain host defense homeostasis; however, persistent activation (or absence of downregulation) and multiple inflammatory responses combine to cause damage to healthy tissue (such as the endothelium), as well as the targeted injured tissue or foreign substances.[7]

Endothelial damage results in increased capillary permeability, which allows protein-rich fluid to move into the interstitial and the alveolar spaces. Pulmonary hypertension and microvascular obstruction contribute to the fluid shifts, overwhelming the lymphatic vessels. Pulmonary edema and alveolar flooding occur, further disrupting gas exchange.[23-25] The damaged endothelium releases mediators, such as eicosanoids, complement split products, and tissue factor. Endothelial cell–white blood cell interaction is often accompanied by further mediator release. The following paragraphs summarize the cells and mediators responsible for these changes and their mechanism of action. For an indepth discussion of the inflammatory mediators, refer to Chapter 3.

Neutrophils

The neutrophils are thought to play a key role in the pathogenesis of ARDS. Within hours after major systemic insults, large numbers of neutrophils are sequestered in the pulmonary vasculature, where they marginate along the endothelial lining. Expression of adhesion molecules by the neutrophil and endothelium plays a major role in the sequestration and adherence of neutrophils in the pulmonary microcirculation. Neurophils are also sequestered in the interstitium and the alveolar spaces.

Activated neutrophils phagocytize injured tissue and foreign debris. This process requires an increased consumption of oxygen and is referred to as the "respiratory burst." Oxygen-derived free radicals (ODFRs) and other toxic oxygen species are produced as metabolites. In large amounts, ODFRs damage the pulmonary endothelium, contributing to the increased capillary permeability and coagulation abnormalities. Neutrophil aggregation also can cause direct damage to the pulmonary vasculature through vascular obstruction or endothelial damage; tissue ischemia and inflammation result.[7,26] Although ARDS can occur in the neutropenic patient,[27] the majority of research demonstrates a strong correlation between increased neutrophil activity and pulmonary damage.

Alveolar macrophages

Macrophages located in the alveoli, the interstitium, and the pulmonary vasculature are stimulated by bacteria, foreign substances in the alveoli, activated neutrophils, or endotoxin. Once stimulated, macrophages produce two potent cytokines: tumor necrosis factor (TNF) and interleukin-1 (IL-1).[28] Macrophages also produce lysozymes, ODFRs, and arachidonic acid metabolites.[28,29] In the past, the alveolar macrophage was thought to play a role only in the latter phases of ARDS, particularly in uncontrolled fibrosis. However, increasing evidence supports the activity of an uncontrolled inflammatory response triggered by cytokines in the pathogenesis of ARDS and MODS. Because the macrophage is such a major producer of inflammatory mediators, it may well have an earlier role in the pathogenesis of ARDS.

Tumor necrosis factor

Tumor necrosis factor is a cytokine produced primarily by macrophages. It is believed to be the major mediator in the development of ARDS, sepsis, and MODS. Direct adverse effects of TNF include enhanced release of ODFRs by neutrophils, indirect endothelial damage, decreased vascular responsiveness to catecholamines, and increased capillary permeability.[30-32] The importance and pathologic potential of TNF stem not only from its direct toxic effects but also from its ability to promote the elaboration of many secondary mediators of inflammation.

Interleukin-1

Interleukin-1 is produced primarily by macrophages, but it can also be synthesized by fibroblasts, natural killer cells, and damaged endothelium.[33] Its major contribution to ARDS is related to its synergistic activity with TNF. Both TNF and IL-1 are believed to contribute to increased vascular permeability and the development of microthrombosis.[7] TNF and IL-1 may also indirectly contribute to vascular or tissue damage by causing increased neutrophil aggregation and adhesion to the endothelium.[33]

Arachidonic acid metabolites (eicosanoids)

Arachidonic acid (eicosatetraenoic acid) is present in most cell membranes. When stimulated by tissue injury, endotoxin, or other substances, arachidonic acid is released and metabolized through one of two pathways. Prostaglandins (PGs) and thromboxanes (TXs) are produced through the cyclooxygenase pathway, and leukotrienes (LTs) are produced through the lipoxygenase pathway.[34,35] Many different eicosanoids are produced within these three major classes. In the lung, prostacyclin (PGI_2) causes vasodilatation and decreased platelet aggregation. It acts in opposition to thromboxane A_2 (TXA_2), which causes pulmonary vasoconstriction, platelet aggregation, and bronchoconstriction.[36] Leukotrienes cause vasoconstriction and bronchoconstriction and facilitate increased pulmonary capillary permeability. In ARDS, the ratio of PGI_2 to TXA_2 may shift to an increase in TXA_2 production.[34,37]

Proteolytic enzymes

Activated neutrophils and macrophages are responsible for the elaboration of proteolytic enzymes at the site of injury. Elastase is abundant in acute lung injury. Normally, antiproteases inactivate the elastase. In ARDS, there is an imbalance in the protease/antiprotease ratio, resulting in high levels of protease activity.[38] The proteases cause direct injury to the vasculature as well as to lung parenchyma. ODFRs have been implicated in damaging or inhibiting antiprotease activity, thus perpetuating the damage caused by the proteases.[39]

Platelet activating factor

Platelet activating factor (PAF) is present in cell membranes and is released by neutrophils, alveolar macrophages, mast cells, platelets, and damaged endothelium.[8] PAF stimulates platelet activation and aggregation, and it also enhances neutrophil adhesion and respiratory burst activity.[40,41] Excessive PAF activity incites increased endothelial damage, increased clot formation, bronchoconstriction, increased pulmonary artery pressure, and further exacerbation of coagulopathics.[36]

Platelets

Activated platelets release eicosanoids, serotonin, PAF, and platelet-derived growth factor.[41] These substances attract and activate neutrophils and cause vasoconstriction and bronchoconstriction. Platelet activation is thought to contribute to pulmonary vascular damage and pulmonary hypertension.

Complement

The complement cascade operates through enzymatic reactions involving more than 20 different plasma proteins. The complement system initiates, facilitates, and enhances the inflammatory/immune response[42] and becomes activated in response to tissue injury, antigen-antibody complexes, endotoxin, and bacteria. Complement contributes to the development of ARDS by increasing neutrophil activity, increasing microvascular permeability, and directly lysing target cells.[43,44] The C5a component of complement has been isolated from the plasma and bronchoalveolar lavage fluid of patients with ARDS.[44]

Other vasoactive substances

The kallikrein/kinin system produces metabolites such as bradykinin, which is a potent vasodilator and promoter of capillary permeability. The kinins also stimulate neutrophil chemotaxis, phagocytosis, and respiratory burst activity.[45]

Histamine

Histamine, a vasoactive amine, is released by mast cells during the inflammatory/immune response. A potent bronchoconstrictor, histamine, also increases vasodilatation and capillary permeability.

Summary

Regardless of the precipitating event, the combined effects of numerous inflammatory mediators are ultimately responsible for the vascular and lung tissue changes that result in the development of ARDS. Pulmonary hypertension occurs early in ARDS, secondary to pulmonary vascular occlusion and uncontrolled vasoconstriction. Bronchoconstriction also occurs in response to various eicosanoids and humoral substances.

Increased capillary permeability, the hallmark of ARDS, allows protein-rich fluid to leave the intravascular space and fill the surrounding interstitial area. The lymphatic system of the lungs is overwhelmed and may be unable to reabsorb fluid adequately. This interstitial fluid increases interstitial pressure, facilitating the movement of fluid through the enlarged epithelial junctions of the alveoli. The protein-rich fluid creates an osmotic gradient in lung tissue, which further enhances fluid movement out of the vasculature. Atelectasis occurs as a result of interstitial edema compressing alveoli and decreased surfactant production. Without surfactant, surface tension increases and the alveoli collapse. Reexpanding the collapsed alveoli becomes even more difficult.

Lung parenchymal damage results from direct injury by macrophages and various mediators, in addition to cellular necrosis from hypoxia. Eventually, fibrotic tissue replaces the altered lung tissue, and the compliance decreases further.[46] Hyaline membranes may form as macrophages attempt to digest this extracellular protein and cellular debris.[46] Figure 8-5 diagrams the pathophysiologic cascade of ARDS.

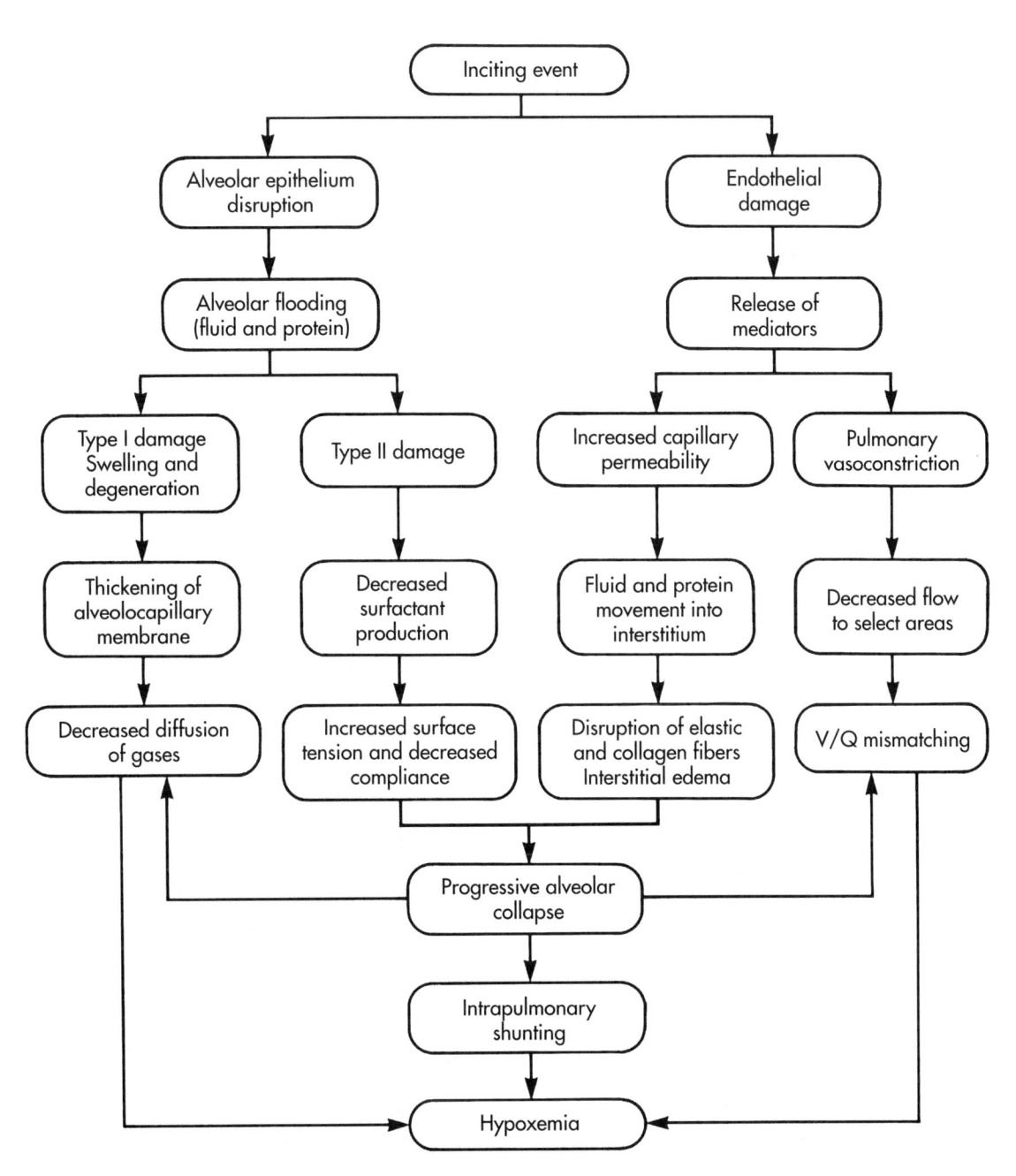

Fig. 8-5 Pathophysiologic cascade mechanism of ARDS. (From Huddleston VB. Pulmonary problems. Crit Care Nurs Clin North Am 1990;2:531.)

The pathology described above is the result of an exaggerated inflammatory/immune response to some initial event. As endothelial damage continues, more mediators are released, and this contributes to further endothelial damage. Current management focuses on supportive care and the prevention of secondary injury related to treatment methods. The future direction of management involves therapies that block or modulate the uncontrolled production and activity of local or systemic mediator described above.

CLINICAL PRESENTATION AND ASSESSMENT

Patients present in various stages of ARDS. Their signs and symptoms indicate respiratory compromise or failure, but a definitive diagnosis of ARDS and injury severity score may not be possible until the lung injury progresses and oxygenation worsens.

Signs and symptoms

In general, the patient in early phases of acute respiratory failure will experience dyspnea, tachypnea, tachycardia, and restlessness.[47] An increased use of accessory muscles and a discoordinated respiratory pattern (abdominal muscle movement in opposition to chest wall expansion) may be seen. Lung sounds will vary from clear, isolated or generalized crackles to wheezes. Overall, physical signs and symptoms are specific to hypoxia and decreased pulmonary compliance (Table 8-2). The following paragraphs discuss specific diagnostic findings.

Radiographic findings

Patients with impending or acute respiratory failure typically are too ill to undergo upright posterior/anterior (PA) or lateral chest roentgenograms (CXRs). Usually, only CXRs obtained using portable machines are available for review. Early in the course of ARDS, CXR findings are nonspecific. Lung fields that are almost clear, scant infiltrates, unilateral lobar consolidations, and diffuse lung involvement have all been noted.[48,49] Large pleural effusions are typically absent, but diffuse alveolar consolidation appears later in the course of ARDS.[48,49] Low lung volumes may also be present.[47-49]

Computed tomography. Computed tomography (CT) may provide additional information about areas of infiltrate mixed with normal lung tissue present in lungs that, on CXRs, appear to have total involvement. A CT scan can reveal barotrauma or localized infection that may not be seen on plain films.[49-51] The risks of transporting an unstable patient to undergo CT must be weighed against the benefit of obtaining additional information.

Laboratory findings

Laboratory values in ARDS are often nonspecific, especially in the early stages. White blood cell counts may be high or low. Early arterial blood gas analysis reveals a normal or slightly alkaline pH and low-to-normal carbon dioxide tension with hypoxemia. As the lung injury progresses and respiratory failure worsens, the carbon dioxide tension increases, hypoxemia becomes refractory, and respiratory and metabolic acidosis are both present.[18] Circulating inflammatory mediators such as complement split products and TNF are also present.[44]

Bronchoalveolar lavage (BAL) can be performed to assist in diagnosing nosocomial or opportunistic infections. One abnormal finding found frequently in the BAL fluid of ARDS patients is an increased number of polymorphonuclear leukocytes that may constitute as much as 80% of the total cell population.[52] The presence of eosinophilia may have important implications for steroid management.[53]

Alterations in lung mechanics

Patients with ARDS have increased extravascular lung water (EVLW). This pathologic process decreases the lung compliance; thus, more pressure is required to ventilate the lungs. Normal dynamic lung compliance is approximately 100 mL/cm H_2O, and static effective compliance (SEC) is greater than 50 mL/cm H_2O.[20] Patients with ARDS have a reduced SEC of 20 to 30 mL/cm H_2O or an even lower value.[20] Decreased lung compliance contributes to the difficulty in ventilating the lungs. Each tidal volume delivered by the ventilator requires a higher pressure as compared to the same tidal volume delivered to healthy lungs. Atelectasis, secretions, and fibrosis further contribute to the poor lung compliance and decrease the amount of alveolar surface area available for gas exchange.[20] Decreased lung compliance contributes to increased work of breathing.

Respiratory failure occurs when a patient's work of breathing becomes excessive and the patient be-

Table 8-2 Assessment of Tissue Hypoxia

Central nervous system	Cardiovascular	Pulmonary	Renal	Gastrointestinal/hepatic	Musculoskeletal
Restlessness	Tachycardia	↑ Respiratory rate	↓ Urine output	↓ Bowel sounds	Muscle tremors
Agitation	↑ BP	↑ Tidal volume	Edema	Abdominal distention	Muscle fatigue
Confusion	Widened pulse pressure	Dyspnea	↑ BP	Vomiting	Muscle aches
Irritability	Dysrhythmias	Use of accessory muscles	↑ BUN	Jaundice	Generalized fatigue
Headache	ST- and T-wave changes	Cyanosis (late)	↑ Creatinine	Lactic acidosis	
↓ LOC	↑ CO	↑ PAP	Hyperkalemia	Anorexia	
Impaired judgment and memory	Bounding pulse	Respiratory alkalosis (early)	Metabolic acidosis	Nausea	
Altered sleep patterns	Diaphoresis	Respiratory acidosis (late)		Constipation	
Lethargy	Angina	↓ PaO_2		Abdominal pain	
Drowsiness		↓ SaO_2		Liver tenderness	
Coma					
Seizures					

Modified from Rice V. Clinical hypoxia. Crit Care Nurs 1980;1(1):21-29.
BP, Blood pressure; *BUN*, blood urea nitrogen; *CO*, cardiac output; *Hct*, hematocrit; *Hgb*, hemoglobin; *LOC*, level of consciousness; *PaO₂*, arterial pressure of oxygen; *PAP*, pulmonary artery pressures; *SaO₂*, arterial oxygen saturation.

comes too fatigued to sustain the necessary effort to maintain oxygenation and ventilation. The percentage of oxygen consumed by the respiratory muscles in a resting normal adult is approximately 5% of the total body consumption. In patients with ARDS, the percentage of oxygen consumed in the respiratory muscles alone may exceed 30% of the total body consumption.[18]

Ventilation-perfusion mismatching

Ventilation-perfusion matching is a heterogenous process throughout the lung fields in both normal and abnormal conditions. V-Q mismatching occurs secondary to venous admixture, shunting, and increased alveolar dead space and is the source of hypoxemia in the ARDS patient (Fig. 8-3).[54]

Venous admixture. Venous admixture occurs when partially ventilated alveoli receive blood flow.[54] Alveolar compression and secretions impair oxygen diffusion; therefore, the blood leaving the dysfunctional alveoli has a lower oxygen tension. It mixes with oxygenated blood draining from other areas of the lung, and the overall SaO_2 decreases. In venous admixture, increasing the FiO_2 will improve the defect.[20]

Intrapulmonary shunt. In the region of a true shunt, unventilated alveoli are still receiving a blood flow.[54] Distinguishing a true shunt from venous admixture is helpful for two reasons: determining the severity of lung injury and deciding on treatment. The presence of a large shunt indicates severe lung injury. In the partially ventilated alveoli, some gas exchange still occurs. In areas that have a true shunt, no gas exchange occurs. Therefore, if a large shunt is present, high oxygen concentrations will not increase the PaO_2. This is referred to as refractory hypoxemia, and other methods of ventilator management, such as PEEP, are more beneficial in this situation (see the section on therapeutic management).

Alveolar dead space. When alveoli continue to inflate in regions of poor or absent perfusion, increased alveolar dead space occurs. Mediators such as serotonin and thromboxane A_2 contribute to increased pulmonary vasoconstriction and platelet aggregation. Other inflammatory mediators incite neutrophil adhesion and aggregation, endothelial damage, and microvascular permeability. The combination of mechanical obstruction, edematous tissue compression of vessels, and vascular constriction, along with low flow states of shock and decreased cardiac output contributes to poor perfusion through the lung fields and leads to alveolar dead space. The result is hypoxemia. Increasing the FiO_2 may do very little to improve this condition.

Hemodynamic parameters

Pulmonary hypertension is usually present early in the development of ARDS. Mediators such as TXA_2 and serotonin, as well as decreased levels of PGI_2 contribute to pulmonary vasoconstriction. Pulmonary systolic and diastolic pressures are elevated, but the PCWP will usually be normal unless there is abnormal cardiac function present or underlying chronic pulmonary disease.[55] A third heart sound indicates the possibility of heart failure as a cause for the respiratory failure.

THERAPEUTIC MANAGEMENT

The goals of management for ARDS with or without MODS are to maintain adequate gas exchange, prevent nonpulmonary organ failure, and prevent further lung injury while the lungs heal. Achieving these goals involves a management strategy that includes a balance of ventilatory techniques, pharmacologic intervention, hemodynamic support, and nutritional support.

Mechanical ventilation in ARDS

Goals. Different philosophies abound concerning the use of mechanical ventilation in the patient with ARDS. The controversy focuses on the balance between using components of mechanical ventilation that cause the least additional injury to the lungs and attempting to maintain adequate gas exchange. Some practitioners view ventilatory management for the ARDS patient as falling into two categories: full support and partial support. Full support is recommended during the acute phase and partial support during the recovery and weaning phases of ARDS.[46-56]

A consensus conference held in 1993 and sponsored by the American College of Chest Physicians and other organizations developed guidelines on mechanical ventilation for the ARDS patient.[57] The AECC supported the same guidelines during its conferences held in 1992.[1] The mechanical ventilation guidelines are as follows:

1. Choose a ventilator mode that has been shown to be capable of supporting oxygenation and

ventilation in patients with ARDS and one with which the clinician has experience.
2. Maintain an acceptable SaO₂ (usually ≥90%).
3. Maintain plateau pressure ≤35 mm Hg when possible. Tidal volumes of 5 to 10 mL/kg may be used to achieve this goal.
4. Allow for increased PaCO₂ (permissive hypercapnea) unless the risk of increased intracranial pressure or other complications exists, which requires a more normal pH. Rapid rises in PaCO₂ should be avoided. Slow reduction of tidal volume may allow for renal system–induced compensatory metabolic alkalosis.
5. Utilize PEEP. The level should be minimized because it is associated with complications such as barotrauma, further lung injury, and myocardial depression. Increase PEEP in small increments.
6. Minimize the FiO₂ (≤0.6). When high plateau pressures and high FiO₂s are present, the complications of pulmonary barotrauma and oxygen toxicity are likely. Accepting an SaO₂ somewhat less than 90% may be considered.
7. Consider sedation, paralysis, and position changes to achieve adequate oxygenation. Other factors (cardiac output and hemoglobin) involved with oxygen delivery should be examined.

The two goals of mechanical ventilation are maintaining gas exchange and avoiding secondary injury associated with mechanical ventilation, specifically barotrauma, oxygen toxicity, and structural damage to the airways.[56] Table 8-3 compares the various modes of ventilation.[56,58]

Complications

Barotrauma. Barotrauma refers to damage caused by excessive airway or alveolar pressures. Alveolar rupture, producing a tension pneumothorax, pneumomediastinum, subcutaneous air, and air emboli is a common results of barotrauma. Pulmonary edema may also occur secondary to excessive intrathoracic pressures.[18,57,59-63] In ARDS, some lung regions are stiff and noncompliant, but other areas may be relatively unaffected. The high pressures required to ventilate the injured lung tissue and recruit alveoli are transmitted to unaffected compliant areas as well, causing further damage. The literature suggests that both high peak inspiratory pressures, high mean airway pressures, and elevated plateau pressures (static pressure during a no-flow state) are responsible for causing barotrauma to the lungs.[1,57,59-64]

Oxygen toxicity. High FiO₂ levels are believed to increase oxygen radical formation, decrease surfactant production, contribute to reabsorptive atelectasis, contribute to the formation of hyaline membranes, and facilitate pulmonary fibrotic changes.[1,57,65,66] Although increased FiO₂ is often necessary, the use of PEEP can enhance arterial oxygenation and allow reduction of FiO₂.

Structural damage. Structural damage to the airway can occur secondary to the insertion and presence of artificial airways. Long-term use of endotracheal tubes and mechanical ventilation has been shown to cause permanent changes in the upper airway.[67,68]

Depressed myocardial function. Myocardial function in the ARDS patient can be adversely affected either as a direct result of the underlying pathologic conditions of the lung or as a result of mechanical ventilation. Positive pressure mechanical ventilation with or without high airway pressures, pressure support, PEEP, or inverse ratio ventilation increases intrathoracic pressure. Impaired venous return, decreased filling pressures on the right side of the heart, and decreased cardiac output can result.[55,69] Because decreased cardiac output can contribute to decreased delivery of oxygen to the tissues, this adverse effect of positive pressure ventilation is an important concept to consider when deciding on a strategy for ventilation.

Considerations for the patient treated with mechanical ventilation. Airway management of mechanical ventilation. Specific patient care issues for the ARDS patient being treated with mechanical ventilation are similar to those for all patients undergoing respiratory failure. A pulmonary toilet regimen consisting of airway suctioning as needed, in-line bronchodilatation treatments, and frequent repositioning is important.[20] Frequently, patients with ARDS are "PEEP-dependent," and they do not tolerate suctioning while off of PEEP. Several suctioning systems and ventilator circuits are available that maintain PEEP during suctioning.

The ARDS patient is at greater risk for "ventilator-associated pneumonia".[70] The rigid suction catheter and high suction pressures used can traumatize the airways[18] and increase the likelihood of bacterial contamination; therefore suctioning is performed only when indicated.

Table 8-3 Ventilator Strategies

	Assist control (AC)	Synchronized intermittent mandatory ventilation (SIMV)	Positive end-expiratory pressure (PEEP)	Pressure support ventilation (PSV)	Pressure control ventilation (PCV)	Inverse ratio ventilation (IRV)	High-frequency ventilation (HFV)
Respiratory rate	Machine set plus patient-triggered breaths	Machine set in synchrony with patient-triggered breaths	May be used with any mode and all settings	Patient determined	Patient determined	Patient determined or machine set	Machine set 30-600 BPM
Apnea protection				Depends on model	Depends on model	Depends on mode and model	Continuous ventilation
Tidal volume	Machine set for both preset and patient's breaths	Machine set for machine breaths only		Patient determined	Patient determined	Patient determined or machine set	Machine set (very small)
Peak flow	Machine set	Machine set		Patient determined	Patient determined	Patient determined	Machine set

Inspiratory time	Machine set	Machine set		Patient determined	Machine set (used with IRV)	Machine set
Peak airway pressure	High	High	High	Lower	Lower	Lower	Very low
Advantages	Full and partial support	Full and partial support	Full and partial support, keeps alveoli open, redistributes intraalveolar fluid	Allows spontaneous breathing, full and partial support, low pressures	Allows spontaneous breathing, full and partial support, low pressures	Full and partial support, gas trapping keeps alveoli open	Full support
Spontaneous breathing	Present, patient initiated-machine set TV delivered	Present with patient's own rate and TV	May or may not be present			Present	Not present
Complications	Can facilitate respiratory alkalosis and ↑WOB	↑WOB	↑Barotrauma, ↓CO, ↑ICP, overdistention of alveoli compressing capillaries	Used with severe ARDS as partial support causes ↑WOB. PSV + PEEP = ↓CO	Same as for PSV and IRV	I:E ratios of 2:1 and 3:1 allow gas trapping causing "autoPEEP" and ↓CO	No major complications. Controversial as to benefit.

BPM, Breaths per minute; *CO*, cardiac output; *E*, expiration; *I*, inspiration; *ICP*, intracranial pressure; *TV*, tidal volume; *WOB*, work of breathing.

Repositioning. Repositioning the patient frequently facilitates blood flow to all lung regions, which may contribute to intermittent periods of decreased shunting (more blood flows to ventilated areas of the lungs). Recent evidence demonstrates the positive effects of the prone position on oxygenation in patients.[71] The primary mechanism for the success of this position is believed to be related to decreased shunting. Despite the practical difficulties of caring for patients in a prone position, this may be an important component of ventilation strategies used to improve oxygenation in the future. Since ARDS affects the lungs heterogeneously, it is impossible to know which areas of the lung contribute the most to gas exchange. Unlike the patient with a unilateral lung injury where placing the "good lung" down facilitates gas exchange, the ARDS patient may benefit most from frequent repositioning. Monitoring the oxygen saturations of a patient during repositioning gives the practitioner information about the best position to facilitate gas exchange.

Work of breathing. Management theories related to the problem of "increased work of breathing" have changed through the years. The goal is to prevent the work of breathing from increasing oxygen consumption by respiratory muscle. The balance between that concept and the theory that maintaining active use of respiratory muscles prevents atrophy is difficult to maintain.[17,59,72] Stoller and Kacmarek[56] promote the use of full ventilatory support to decrease the work of breathing in early ARDS.

Falling oxygen saturations may reflect excessive work of breathing. If the patient increases respiratory effort or becomes restless for other reasons and the oxygen saturation decreases, a change in the ventilatory strategy or sedation should be considered.

Another tool recently employed in critical care areas is the continuous end-tidal carbon dioxide monitor (etCO$_2$). As with any form of respiratory failure, monitoring indicators of effective ventilation (Paco$_2$ values and minute ventilation) can provide information about increased work of breathing and worsening respiratory failure.[20] The etCO$_2$ monitor provides an in-line estimate of the patient's Paco$_2$ (carbon dioxide tension in the alveolus). In the absence of chest trauma, fistulas, and other anomalies, the etCO$_2$ values are considered to be an accurate reflection of the patient's Paco$_2$.[73,74] Changes in the ventilation process of the patient, as a result of either ventilator changes or the condition of the patient, can be identified immediately.

Pharmacologic support

Currently, the use of most of the pharmacologic agents in patients with ARDS is considered supportive therapy. Several drugs that block or inhibit various mediators are under investigation in vitro, in vivo, and in clinical studies.

Specific supportive drug therapy includes the use of antibiotics, bronchodilators, and paralytic agents. Antibiotics are used to treat specific infections. Bronchodilators can be administered to reverse airway obstruction secondary to inflammation and mediator-induced bronchoconstriction. Neuromuscular blocking agents and sedatives relieve discomfort, decrease anxiety, and decrease oxygen consumption. The use of neuromuscular blocking agents is usually restricted to patients with severe ARDS and subsequent problems with oxygen delivery and oxygen consumption. Disadvantages of paralytic therapy include development of respiratory muscle atrophy and lethal consequences of ventilator equipment malfunction.

Cardiovascular support

One of the more difficult aspects of ARDS management is maintenance of cardiovascular function. Maximizing cardiac output and oxygen delivery with the appropriate combination of fluids, adequate hemoglobin levels, and inotropic support is critical. However, several clinical studies demonstrate better outcomes in patients who are treated with diuretics or maintained on fluid restriction during the first few days after the onset of ARDS.[53,75,76]

Maintaining an adequate cardiac output to sustain end-organ perfusion is critical and can only be monitored accurately by looking at the oxygen consumption (V̇o$_2$) and oxygen delivery (Do$_2$). Although the normal values for both are generally agreed upon, it is not clear what the minimally acceptable value is for preventing organ failure. Inducing hypovolemia is not recommended.[1] Maintaining adequate filling pressures can be achieved through the use of fluids and inotropic agents.

A great deal of controversy remains concerning the use of crystalloids or colloids in fluid therapy (see Chapter 5). Crystalloids third-space more easily but may be used more frequently because of the theory that leaky pulmonary capillaries will also leak plasma albumin and other colloids. The increased oncotic pressure secondary to colloid movement into the interstitium would then facilitate further fluid accumulation in the interstitial and intraalveolar space. Some reseachers believe that there is no evidence to support this theory, and in fact believe that there is evidence to suggest that saline would not stay in the intravascular space for more than a few seconds and could enhance the expansion of the interstitial space significantly.[5] It should also be noted that the cost of colloids far exceeds the cost of crystalloids; however, patient needs and responses to therapy should dictate the type of fluid used.

A combination of vasoactive and inotropic agents is also used to treat the derangements of cardiac output, systemic vascular resistance, and pulmonary vascular resistance. In ARDS patients, the use of these agents can have a significant impact on matching ventilation and perfusion. Vasodilators may increase pulmonary flow to areas of injured lung with poor ventilation. However, vasoconstrictors may decrease blood flow to areas of injured lung that have lost the protective "hypoxic vasoconstrictive mechanism" and better match ventilation to perfusion. Kollef and Schuster recommend that the use of these drugs be limited to systemic hemodynamic indications.[53,77]

Hemodynamic monitoring plays a critical role in the ability of the practitioner to assess and treat variations in cardiac function accurately. Mixed venous oxygen saturation monitoring will also assist the practitioner in diagnosing problems with oxygen transport and use, unless the patient demonstrates a pathologic oxygen supply dependency (see Chapter 6). This tool is helpful in assessing the effect of various nursing care procedures on patient status.[47]

Nutritional support

Early, aggressive nutritional support should be implemented. Patients with ARDS generally need 35 to 45 kcal/kg/day, and that level will increase if an additional systemic injury or illness is present.[78] The distribution of calories will vary depending on the presence of nonpulmonary organ failure; however, high levels of the appropriate type of protein should be included. These patients remain in a catabolic state that contributes to further metabolic and infectious complications.[47,79] Large feedings of high-carbohydrate solutions may contribute to fluid overload and increased carbon dioxide production. A multidisciplinary approach is needed to accurately assess patient need and response to therapy[80] (see Chapter 7).

Infection control and management

The injury caused by the inflammatory process may facilitate a magnified response to bacteria. However, infections are not always present in patients with ARDS. A common cause of infection in the ARDS patient is "ventilator-associated pneumonia," which plays a major role in morbidity and mortality. The most significant and possibly the most preventable causes of the pneumonia include poor infection control measures and the use of multiple invasive devices that lead to oropharyngeal and tracheal colonization with organisms such as gram-negative bacilli.[70] Prevention strategies include using proper hand washing technique, optimizing nutritional status, minimizing the use of nasogastric and endotracheal tubes, avoiding excessive sedation, and decontaminating respiratory equipment properly. Although some studies have demonstrated that selective decontamination of the digestive tract reduces upper airway colonization and pneumonia, the overall mortality rates in the studies were not reduced. The cost of this therapy can be prohibitive, and the risk of developing resistant strains with the use of prophylactic antibiotics also limits the promise of this therapy. Instead, emphasis is placed on obtaining accurate specimens through bronchoscopy and using specific narrow-spectrum antibiotics.[70,81] The empiric use of antibiotics should be avoided unless overwhelming sepsis is suspected.

INVESTIGATIONAL THERAPIES

Experimental studies of newer therapies used to provide prophylactic immunotherapy, block inflammatory effects, provide antibody protection against endotoxin, and inhibit effects of various activated mediators are ongoing. Laboratory animal studies and clinical trials using these investigational agents are currently under way, but it may be several years before findings demonstrate significant decreases in mortality related to the administration of these therapies in the ARDS patient.[82]

Prostaglandin E$_1$

Prostaglandin E$_1$ inhibits platelet aggregation, neutrophil chemotaxis, and macrophage activity.[83]

It also causes vasodilatation and may actually increase V-Q mismatching. Studies report conflicting results in ARDS patients receiving PGE_1. Improvement in overall oxygen delivery has been noted, but it may be at the expense of a further V-Q mismatch.[82,84,85] Investigation continues to further define the role of vasodilatory prostaglandins in the pathogenesis and management of ARDS.

Antilipid mediators

Lipid mediators associated with inflammation include metabolites of arachidonic acid (PGs, TXs, LTs) and platelet-activating factor. All of these compounds contribute to pulmonary hypertension, V-Q mismatching, and further mediator activation. Agents such as ibuprofen have been shown to blunt the production of these mediators in both in vitro and in vivo models.[86] Clinical trials are ongoing.

Antioxidant therapy

Both neutrophil and macrophage activation contribute to the respiratory burst and resultant release of oxygen-derived radicals. These compounds contribute to significant endothelial injury. Glutathione protects the lung tissue against oxidative stress but is thought to be rapidly depleted in vital cells in the ARDS patient. Administration of N-acetylcysteine may replenish the stores of glutathione and has been shown to reduce tissue injury in both cell and animal models.[86] Human clinical trials are ongoing.

Exogenous surfactant

Surfactant is a naturally occurring phospholipid that reduces surface tension in the alveoli. The use of exogenous surfactant (Exosurf) in neonates with premature hyaline membrane disease has been studied for several years. Some studies report positive effects, and others report no change in mortality rates. However, the use of surfactant is increasing in neonatal intensive care units. The benefits of surfactant in adult ARDS patients have not been demonstrated, but research continues.[83,87]

Monoclonal antibodies to white blood cell adhesion molecules

Autopsied lungs from ARDS patients show large numbers of white blood cells (WBCs) in both the parenchyma and the pulmonary vasculature. Various efforts have been made to prevent adherence of WBCs to the pulmonary endothelium through their adhesion molecules. Investigators have developed monoclonal antibodies against the adhesion molecules on the WBC,[88] and these monoclonal antibodies have decreased the incidence of tissue injury and inflammation in several animal studies.[89-91]

Ketoconazole

Ketoconazole is a potent inhibitor of thromboxane synthesis, which leads to pulmonary vasoconstriction and contributes to platelet and WBC aggregation. Limited studies have demonstrated a reduction in ARDS in a certain subset of patients receiving ketoconazole, but further studies are needed before definitive recommendations can be made.[92,93]

Nitric oxide

Inhaled nitric oxide reduces pulmonary hypertension and improves arterial oxygenation in some ARDS patients. This occurs through the mechanisms of pulmonary vasodilatation and reduced intrapulmonary right-to-left shunting. Clinical studies have documented no significant changes in central venous pressure, PCWP, or systemic blood pressure.[94] Further controlled studies are recommended before the use of inhaled nitric oxide can be promoted.

Extracorporeal membrane oxygenation

Extracorporeal membrane oxygenation (ECMO) is a form of extracorporeal bypass used to oxygenate the blood of critically ill patients. It, previously, had been investigated in adult patients with ARDS, with disappointing results,[95,96] although it had positive results in neonates. The adult studies demonstrated no significant decline in mortality rates but instead, showed a greater number of associated complications with the ECMO. A more recent study supported by the National Institutes of Health demonstrated the same results.[97] Recent technology has allowed the development of more sophisticated techniques in ECMO administration, and ECMO is once again being investigated in adults in Europe.[97]

RECOMMENDATIONS FOR MANAGEMENT WITH INVESTIGATIONAL THERAPIES

ARDS is a complex syndrome that can occur in isolation or in conjunction with multiple organ dysfunction. Management strategies can be diverse based on the multitude of ongoing research studies.

Complications of management include barotrauma, nosocomial pneumonia, stress-related gastrointestinal bleeding, hemodynamic instability, and overwhelming financial costs. Goals of management should be focused on providing adequate gas exchange, preventing nonpulmonary organ failure, and preventing further lung injury or any complications that may be associated with therapies.

One guideline for management, described by Kollef and co-workers,[53] includes a grading system for therapies based on the quality of the evidence demonstrated in studies. Tables 8-4, 8-5, and 8-6, summarize these recommendations for the treatment of ARDS.

RESEARCH AND MANAGEMENT IN THE FUTURE HEALTH CARE ENVIRONMENT

Extensive research on ARDS has been pursued over the last decade, contributing to an increase in the overall cost of healthcare but not to a reduction in mortality or morbidity. The United States House of Representatives Committee on Appropriations reported in the budget for fiscal year 1993 that critical care costs accounted for approximately 28% of total

Table 8-4 The Quality of the Evidence and the Grading of Recommendations in ARDS

Quality of the evidence

Level 1: Randomized, prospective, controlled investigation of ARDS
Level 2: Nonrandomized concurrent-cohort investigations, historical-cohort investigations and case series of ARDS
Level 3: Randomized, prospective, controlled investigations of sepsis or other relevant conditions with potential application in ARDS
Level 4: Case reports of ARDS

Grading of recommendations

A: Supported by at least two level 1 investigations
B: Supported by only one level 1 investigation
C: Supported by level 2 investigations only
D: Supported by at least one level 3 investigation
Ungraded: No available clinical investigations

Table 8-5 Recommendations for the Nonpharmacologic Treatment of ARDS*

Treatment	Recommended	Grade
Mechnical ventilation		
Initial settings: AC mode; Fio$_2$ 1.0; PEEP <5 cm; inspiratory flow 60 L/min	Yes	Ungraded
Initial tidal volume, 6-10 mL/kg	Yes	C
Prophylactic PEEP	No	B
Least PEEP with Sao$_2$ >0.9 and Fio$_2$ <0.6	Yes	Ungraded
Permissive hypercapnia (pressure-targeted ventilation) for peak airway pressure >40-45 cm H$_2$O	Yes	C
Inverse ratio ventilation for persistent hypoxemia or peak airway pressures >40-45 cm H$_2$O	Yes	C
Airway-pressure-release ventilation	No	—
High-frequency ventilation	No	B
Extracorporeal membrane oxygenation	No	B
Extracorporeal carbon dioxide removal	No	B
Patient repositioning (except prone)	Yes	C
Early fluid restriction or diuresis	Yes	B
Optimization of oxygen	—	—

*Grades based on criteria in Table 8-4.

Table 8-6 Recommendations for the Pharmacologic Treatment of ARDS*

Treatment	Recommended	Grade
Exogenous surfactant	No	B
Early corticosteroids	No	A
Late corticosteroids	Yes	C
Acetylcysteine	No	B
Ketoconazole	—	—
Nitric oxide	—	—
Ibuprofen	No	D
Alprostadil	No	B
Pentoxifylline	No	—
Antiendotoxin and anticytokine therapy	No	D
Prophylactic antibiotics (including selective digestive decontamination)	No	D

*Grades based on criteria in Table 8-4.

acute care hospital costs.[98] Most admissions to the intensive care unit are because of acute events such as ARDS, SIRS, MODS, trauma, burns, and asthma.

The appropriations committee urged the National Heart, Lung and Blood Institute (NHLBI) "to consider the potential benefits to society of enhanced research on effective practices and treatments in this technology-dependent field."[98] The NHLBI convened a task force on Research in Cardiopulmonary Dysfunction in Critical Care Medicine. The committee is charged with the job of developing a plan, including setting scientific priorities for research. Research will be examined in basic, clinical, and epidemiologic areas. One tool that may assist with research, cost containment, and overall management strategy is protocol management or development of critical pathways.

Protocol management

Protocol management can provide a standardized plan or set of guidelines that also allows for individualized goal-directed care. This approach can define patient selection (ARDS versus ALI), treatment modalities, and the process for delivering the selected treatment.[99] Several institutions have taken this idea one step further and developed "critical pathways" as a multidisciplinary tool used to deliver individualized care. One example developed by Vanderbilt University Medical Center, Nashville, Tennessee, is shown in Table 8-7, with general information and the instructions on its use shown in Table 8-8.[100] This critical pathway design is based on phases and the approximate days that the patient may be in the ICU during each particular phase. The document is intended to offer guidelines and should be adapted for individual needs.

CONCLUSION

Adult respiratory distress syndrome represents a major insult to the host, either as an isolated event or as a part of the overall MODS picture. Refractory hypoxemia and further stimulation of the inflammatory cascade exacerbate maldistribution of circulating volume, imbalance of oxygen supply and demand, and alterations in metabolism, contributing further to organ failure. Some data suggest that lung injury occurs before other organ failure, but does this indicate that the lung is the major site for the stimulation and release of inflammatory mediators, or is the inflammatory process caused by the initial insult affecting all organs at the same time?[101] Another factor contributing to organ failure may be the sensitivity of individual organs to the inflammatory response. Whether ARDS is the source of damage to remote organs or the victim of the existing MODS process, acute lung injury greatly contributes to the increased morbidity and mortality seen in this patient population. Prevention, early identification of respiratory deterioration, and prompt, aggressive intervention are key factors in minimizing the morbidity and mortality of ARDS in the critically ill patient.

Table 8-7 Vanderbilt University Medical Center
Acute Respiratory Distress Syndrome

Inclusion criteria: P/F Ratio ≤ 300 mm Hg and 2 quadrants with infiltrate on CXR

MICU Admission Date: _____
Pathway Initiation Date: _____
Pathway Completion Date: _____
DRG Number: _____
ELOS: __18 days__

THIS DOCUMENT IS INTENDED AS A GUIDELINE AND SHOULD BE ADAPTED FOR INDIVIDUAL PATIENT NEEDS.

	PHASE I: Stabilization (ICU 2 days)	PHASE II: Chronic Respiratory Support (ICU 10 days)	PHASE III: Pre Extubation (ICU 2 days)	PHASE IV: Post Extubation (ICU 1 day → Floor)	PHASE V: Discharge (Floor 3 days → Home)
Entrance Date/Time	Date: ___ /Time: ___	Date: ___ /Time: ___	Date: ___ /Time: ___	Date: ___ /Time: ___	Date: ___ /Time: ___

Goals	Hemodynamically stable:
	• HR >60<140
	• PCWP <18
	• BPS >90<180
	• Evidence of adequate perfusion per clinical exam and/or high normal cardiac index
	Respiratory status stable:
	• pH >7.25-7.50
	• O₂ Sat ≥88%
	• RR 15-35
	Ventilatory targets achieved:
	  - FiO₂ ≤.80
	  - Plateau pressure ≤35
	  - Accept early hypercapnia to maintain plateau pressure ≤35 (except in head injury)
	Ensure patient comfort and rest
	Family oriented to unit/hospital and communication mechanism established
		Hemodynamically stable without high dose vasoactive drips:
		• HR >60<120
		• BPS >90<150
		• U/O >30 cc/hr
		• Stable Cr
		• PCWP <18/CO >3.5
		Respiratory status stable:
		• pH >7.30
		• CO₂ <60
		• O₂Sat ≥88%
		Progress to pre extubation phase when meets criteria:
		• MV <12 • RR <30
		• PEEP ≤10 • FiO₂ ≤.5
		• NIF ≤ -20
		
		Consider: Trach at 14 days if weaning does not seem possible Family information and support needs are met
			Extubate patient when meets criteria × 2 hours:
			• SaO₂ ≥88%
			• PaO₂ ≥55 • RR ≤30
			• PCO₂ ≤50 • f/Tv <100
			• Compensated pH
			• Maintain airway protection
			On ventilatory settings of:
			• PEEP ≤5
			• Pressure support ≤5
			• FiO₂ ≤.5
				Patient tolerates extubation:
				• RR >12<30
				• O₂Sat >88%
				• FiO₂ <40%
				• Effective cough and gag
				D/C from ICU when meets criteria:
				• Overnight observation
				• Hemodynamically stable
				• No upper airway obstruction
				• Effectively clearing secretions
				• Stable, spontaneous respiratory rate
					No readmit to ICU
					D/C from hospital when meets criteria:
					• Effectively clearing secretions
					• O₂Sat ≥88% on nasal cannula ≤3L/min
					• Home care assistance coordinated as indicated
					• Able to transfer from bed to chair
					• Patient/family teaching is completed/documented
					• F/U appointment scheduled

Individualized Goals					

Continued.

190 Organ Involvement and Clinical Presentation

Table 8-7 Vanderbilt University Medical Center—cont'd
Acute Respiratory Distress Syndrome

	PHASE I: Stabilization (ICU 2 days) Date: ___ /Time: ___	PHASE II: Chronic Respiratory Support (ICU 10 days) Date: ___ /Time: ___	PHASE III: Pre Extubation (ICU 2 days) Date: ___ /Time: ___	PHASE IV: Post Extubation (ICU 1 day → Floor) Date: ___ /Time: ___	PHASE V: Discharge (Floor 3 days → Home) Date: ___ /Time: ___
Assessments & Evaluations	History and physical exam Nursing assessment Continuously monitor and record q1°: • VS • SaO$_2$ • I&O • FiO$_2$ Monitor and record q3°: • PIP • MV • TV • Plateau pressure	Continuously monitor and record q 2-4°: • VS • I&O • SaO$_2$ • FiO$_2$ • PIP • MV • TV • Plateau pressure	Assess q 30" to 4 hours during peri extubation process to guide ventilary support reduction: • Patient comfort • LOC • O$_2$ Sat • RR • Secretions • HR, BP • Secretions • Respiratory muscle effort	Monitor for airway obstruction and laryngeal edema VS continuously monitored × 30 minutes post extubation, then q1 hour × 2, then per routine	↑
Tests & Labs	On admit and daily: • SMA 7 • ABG • SMA 12 • CXR • CBC with diff, plts • EKG • PT, PTT For fever of unknown origin: • Blood culture q 3 days • Urine dipstick • Sputum for gram stain/culture • If w/u negative and fever persists → change lines	Q3 days: • SMA 7 • SMA 12 • CBC with plts, diff pm • CXR ABG for O$_2$ sat <90%, respiratory distress (RR >30) or change in LOC3	Day of extubation • CXR • CBC • SMA 7 • ABG pre extubation	ABG for O$_2$ sat <88% or respiratory distress (RR >30) Or decreased LOC	↑
Treatments	Orotracheal intubation and total ventilatory support Arterial line if indicated: • Frequent blood draws • Hemodynamic instability GI access Foley catheter Suction prn for ↑ PIP/secretions/↓ V$_T$/adventitious breath sounds Pulmonary artery catheter if: • Diagnosis uncertain • Hemodynamic instability Pulse oximeter Daily weight Routine ICU care Therapeutic bed if meet criteria (order)	Decrease IMV pressure support	Begin extubation maneuvers—adjust parameters by 0-50% q 30" to 4° as tolerated → extubation as appropriate Establish day/night orientation Reassess need for therapeutic bed	O$_2$ via nasal cannula (mask PRN O$_2$ sat <88%) Remove ventilator 2 hours post extubation if stable Cough and deep breathe—no tracheal suctioning (may suction oropharynx) D/C Pulse oximeter 6 hours post extubation if stable	↑

Adult Respiratory Distress Syndrome   191

Table 8-7 Vanderbilt University Medical Center—cont'd
Acute Respiratory Distress Syndrome

	PHASE I: Stabilization (ICU 2 days) Date: ___ /Time: ___	PHASE II: Chronic Respiratory Support (ICU 10 days) Date: ___ /Time: ___	PHASE III: Pre Extubation (ICU 2 days) Date: ___ /Time: ___	PHASE IV: Post Extubation (ICU 1 day → Floor) Date: ___ /Time: ___	PHASE V: Discharge (Floor 3 days → Home) Date: ___ /Time: ___
Entrance Date/Time / **Individualized Treatments**					
Diet	NPO	Enteral feedings: • 30 Kcal/kg • Basic Formula: Ultracal—Standard with fiber Perative—High Protein Needs Osmolyte HN—Standard with Lower Protein Needs	Hold feeding 2 hours prior to extubation	Assess swallowing (nursing) Begin PO feeding with soft (pureed) diet then advance as tolerated	Regular
Meds/IV	IV access • NS for fluid resuscitation • Albumin only if serum albumin <2.0 • Blood transfusion for Hgb <10 Antibiotics as indicated for fever: • Broad spectrum AP coverage Heparin 5000 units SQ q12° for DVT/pulmonary embolus prophylaxis (if cannot anticoagulate, then SCD) Analgesia: MSO₄ (IV) use as indicated to lower impact on GI motility Sedatives: Diazepam or Lorazepam (IV) Haldol 2 mg IV/PO as adjunct to sedation as needed Gastric bleeding prophylaxis: • with gastric feeding → optional • with gastric tube/no feeding → sucralfate • with duodenum tube →H₂ blocker Paralytic agents (Pavulon-intermittent) only if: • refractory ventilator dyssynchrony • short term use with selective procedures Individualized Meds—see MAR	Reassess need for and response to antibiotics in 72 hours: • D/C if no indication • Initiate appropriate antibiotics for known infections for 7-10 day intervals	Adjust analgesia and sedatives to enhance LOC and resp drive during weaning/extubation	Heparin or saline lock IV Analgesia as indicated	

Continued.

192 *Organ Involvement and Clinical Presentation*

Table 8-7 Vanderbilt University Medical Center—cont'd
Acute Respiratory Distress Syndrome

	PHASE I: Stabilization (ICU 2 days)	PHASE II: Chronic Respiratory Support (ICU 10 days)	PHASE III: Pre Extubation (ICU 2 days)	PHASE IV: Post Extubation (ICU 1 day → Floor)	PHASE V: Discharge (Floor 3 days → Home)
Entrance Date/Time	Date: ____ /Time: ____	Date: ____ /Time: ____	Date: ____ /Time: ____	Date: ____ /Time: ____	Date: ____ /Time: ____
Activity	BR Increase HOB if hemodynamically stable	ROM (active and passive) per RN ↑	OOB as tolerated (minimum BID) Elevate HOB with weaning	OOB TID and as tolerated Ambulate q day	
Consults	Pulmonary/Critical Care Respiratory Care Case Manager	Physical Therapy (assessment and plan) Dietary as indicated DT (splints)		Social Services for D/C planning	
Teaching/ D/C Plan	Code Status written w/in 24° of admit Pt/Family assessment Pt/Family oriented to ICU & hospital Pt/Family support Provide information to family regarding procedures/plan of care	↑ Explain goals for total respiratory support phase to patient/family	Explain weaning procedure/goals to patient/family	Prepare family for move to next level of care Coordinate transfer with floor staff Explain post extubation care/goals	Home care as indicated F/U appointment scheduled in 3 weeks ↑↑
Individualized Teaching D/C Plan					
Equipment	Routine ICU set up Pulse Oximeter Ventilator (pressure preset) Arterial line (per criteria) PA/central line (per criteria) GI access Foley catheter Bag/PEEP valve IV pump (per criteria) Therapeutic bed (per criteria)	↑↑	—(Reassess need)— —(Reassess need)— T-Piece Blow-By set up O₂ administration set up (Nasal cannula)	D/C 6 hours post extubation ↑ D/C 2 hours post extubation ↑↑↑ Heparin/saline lock ↑ Yankauer ↑	↑ ↑ ↑

Table 8-8 Guidelines for Using the Collaborative Pathway and Nursing Documentation Tool

I. Purpose:
1. To provide a mechanism for the provision and documentation of a plan for consistent, coordinated, high quality, cost effective, individualized patient care.
2. To facilitate communication among health care providers to direct care toward achievement of desired patient goals.
3. To guide the health care team in the evaluation of patient progress toward desired patient goals.

II. General information:
1. The pathway is intended as a guideline and should be customized for *individual patient needs*.
2. The pathway will be initiated when the patient has met the inclusion criteria and an order is written in the medical record.
3. The pathway is a permanent chart document and should *never* be discarded.
4. All entries must be written in blue or black ink.
5. The pathway will be used and reviewed during ICU collaborative rounds and change of shift report to facilitate discussion of goals and plan of care.
6. Standard individual goals may be utilized when specific problems are present.
7. Individualized goals, treatments, D/C plan that are ongoing will be arrowed over to the next phase.
8. Individualized treatments which are no longer applicable should be stricken with a single line using blue or black ink. The health professional making the change should initial and date the change.
9. If a patient should regress on the pathway a new one will be initiated. The old pathway will be clearly marked "Patient Returned to Phase _____."
10. Each goal for that particular phase will be documented on every 24 hours when criteria for that goal are not met, or support is required in order to meet those criteria. Documentation will be written in the nursing progress notes.
11. The phase will be documented on the nursing assessment at the beginning of each shift (under other, i.e., ARDS Phase I).
12. Patients can progress to the next phase when all goals are achieved. The progression will be documented in the nursing progress notes. The date and time of phase entrance will be documented on the pathway.

III. Instructions:
1. Stamp the pathway with patient's addressograph plate.
2. Complete all sections on top of page 1.
3. Complete sections on individualized goals, treatments, teaching, D/C plan if applicable.
4. Enter date and time of phase entrance.

REFERENCES

1. Bernard GR, Artigas A, Brigham KL. The American-European consensus on Adult Respiratory Distress Syndrome: Definitions, mechanisms, relevant outcomes and clinical trial coordination. Am J Respir Crit Care Med 1994;149:818-24.
2. Villar J, Slutsky AS. The incidence of adult respiratory distress syndrome. Am Rev Respir Dis 1989;14:814-16.
3. Thomsen GE et al. Incidence of the respiratory distress syndrome in Utah (abstract). Am Rev Respir Dis 1993;147 (4part2):347.
4. Murray JF, Matthay MA, Luce J. An expanded definition of the adult respiratory distress syndrome. Am Rev Respir Dis 1988;138:720-723.
5. Shoemaker WC, Appel PL, Bishop MH. Temporal patterns of blood volume, hemodynamics and oxygen transport in pathogenesis and therapy of postperative adult respiratory distress syndrome. New Horiz 1993;1:522-37.
6. Ashbaugh DG et al. Acute respiratory distress in adults. Lancet 1967;2:319-323.
7. Bersten A, Sibbald WJ. Acute lung injury in septic shock. Crit Care Clin 1989;5:49-79.
8. Vaughan P, Brooks C. Adult respiratory distress syndrome: A complication of shock. Crit Care Nurs Clin North Am 1990;2:235-253.
9. Hyers TM. Prediction of survival and mortality in patients with adult respiratory distress syndrome. New Horiz 1993;1: 466-70.
10. Hyers TM. Adult respiratory distress syndrome. In: Zapol W, LeMaire F, eds. New York: Marcel Dekker;1991:23-26.
11. Petty TL. Adult respiratory distress syndrome: Refinement of concept and redefinition. Am Rev Respir Dis 1988;138: 724-742.

12. Matthay MA. The adult respiratory distress syndrome: New insights into diagnosis, pathophysiology and treatment. West J Med 1989;150:187-194.
13. Dorinsky PM, Gadek JE. Multiple organ failure. Clin Chest Med 1990;11:581-591.
14. Guyton AC. Pulmonary ventilation: Textbook of medical physiology. Philadelphia: WB Saunders, 1986:466-525.
15. Brooks-Brunn J. Respiration. Critical care nursing: A physiologic approach. St Louis: Mosby; 1986:168-251.
16. Murray JF. Ventilation: The normal lung. St Louis: Mosby; 1986:83-107.
17. Marini JJ. Strategies to minimize breathing effort during mechanical ventilation. Crit Care Clin 1990;6:635-661.
18. Marini JJ. Lung mechanics. Respiratory medicine and intensive care. Baltimore: Williams & Wilkins; 1985:1-10.
19. Crapo JD et al. Cell number and cell characteristics of the normal lung. Am Rev Respir Dis 1982;125:740-745.
20. Marini JJ, Wheeler AP. Respiratory failure. Critical Care Medicine: The essentials. Baltimore: Williams & Wilkins; 1989:175-184.
21. West JB, Dollery CT, Naimark A. Distribution of blood in isolated lung: Relation to vascular and alveolar pressures. J Appl Physiol 1964;19:713-724.
22. Murray JF. Circulation: The normal lung. Philadelphia: WB Saunders; 1986:139-150.
23. Freudenberg N. Reaction of the vascular intima to endotoxin in shock. Prog Clin Biol Res: Second Vienna Shock Forum 1989;308:77-89.
24. Del Vecchio PJ, Malik AB. Thrombin-induced neutrophil adhesion. Prog Clin Biol Res: Second Vienna Shock Forum 1989;308:101-112.
25. Muller-Berghaus G. Septicemia and the vessel wall. In: Verstraete M, Vermylen J, Lijnen R, Arnout J, eds. Thrombosis and haemostasis. Belgium: Leuven University Press; 1987:619-671.
26. Brigham KL, Meyrick B. Interactions of granulocytes with lungs. Circ Res 1984;54:623-635.
27. Ognibene FP et al. Adult respiratory distress syndrome in patients with severe neutropenia. N Engl J Med 1986;315:547-551.
28. Ford HR et al. Characterization of wound cytokines in the sponge matrix model. Arch Surg 1989;124:1422-1428.
29. Lazarou SA et al. The wound as a possible source of posttraumatic immunosuppression. Arch Surg 1989;124:1429-1431.
30. Beutler B. Cachectin in tissue injury, shock, and related states. Crit Care Clin 1989;5:353-368.
31. Tracey KJ et al. Shock and tissue injury induced by recombinant human cachectin. Science 1986;234:470-474.
32. Debets JM et al. Plasma tumor necrosis factor and mortality in critically ill patients. Can J Surg 1988;31:172-176.
33. Dinarello CA. Biology of interleukin-1. FASEB J 1988;2:108-115.
34. Sprague RS et al. Proposed role for leukotrienes in the pathophysiology of multiple systems organ failure. Crit Care Clin 1989;5:315-330.
35. Petrak RA, Balk RA, Bone RC. Prostaglandins, cyclooxygenase inhibitors, and thromboxane synthetase inhibitors in the pathogenesis of multiple systems organ failure. Crit Care Clin 1989;5:302-314.
36. Yellin SA et al. Prostacyclin and thromboxane A2 in septic shock: Species differences. Circ Shock 1986;20:291-297.
37. Brigham KL, Sheller JR. Leukotrienes and adult respiratory distress syndrome. Intensive Care Med 1989;15:422-423.
38. Rinaldo JE, Christman JW. Mechanisms and mediators of the adult respiratory distress syndrome. Clin Chest Med 1990;11:621-632.
39. Weiss SJ. Tissue destruction by neutrophils. N Engl J Med 1989;320:365-376.
40. Lefer AM. Induction of tissue injury and altered cardiovascular performance by platelet-activating factor: Relevance to multiple systems organ failure. Crit Care Clin 1989;5:331-352.
41. Braquet P, Hosford D. The potential role of platelet-activating factor (PAF) in shock, sepsis and adult respiratory distress syndrome. Prog Clin Biol Res: Second Vienna Shock Forum 1989:425-439.
42. Walport M. Complement. In: Roitt I, Brostoff J, Male D, eds. Immunology. 2nd ed. London: Gower Medical Publishing; 1989:13.1-13.16.
43. Bengtson A, Heideman M. Anaphylatoxin formation in sepsis. Arch Surg 1988;123:645-649.
44. Langlois RF et al. Accentuated complement activation in patient plasma during the adult respiratory distress syndrome: A potential mechanism for pulmonary inflammation. Heart Lung 1989;18:71-84.
45. Ichinose M, Barnes PJ. Bradykinin-induced airway microvascular leakage and bronchoconstriction are mediated via a bradykinin B2 receptor. Am Rev Respir Dis 1990;1104-1107.
46. Pratt PC. Pathology of the adult respiratory distress syndrome. In: Thurlbeck WM, Abell MR, eds. The lung: Structure, function and disease. Baltimore: Williams & Wilkins; 1978:44-57.
47. Mims BC. Adult respiratory distress syndrome. Lewisville, Tx: Barbara Clark Mims Associates, 1990.
48. Aberle DR, Brown K. Radiologic considerations in the adult respiratory distress syndrome. Clin Chest Med 1990;11:737-754.
49. Wheeler AP, Carroll FE, Bernard GR. Radiographic issues in adult respiratory distress syndrome. New Horiz 1993;1:441-477.
50. Gattinoni L, Pesenti A. Computed tomography scanning in acute respiratory failure. In: Zapol WM, Lemaire F, eds. Adult respiratory distress syndrome. New York: Marcel Dekker; 1991:199-221.
51. Maunder RJ et al. Preservation of normal lung regions in the adult respiratory distress syndrome: Analysis by computed tomography. JAMA 1986:255:2463-2465.
52. Idell S, Cohen AB. Bronchoalveolar lavage in patients with the adult respiratory distress syndrome. Clin Chest Med 1985;6 459-71.
53. Kollef MH, Schuster DP. The acute respiratory distress syndrome. N Engl J Med 1995;332:27-37.
54. Shapiro BA, Harrison RA, Walton JR. Clinical application of blood gases. 3rd ed. St Louis: Mosby; 1982.
55. Biondi JW et al. Mechanical heart-lung interaction in the adult respiratory distress syndrome. Clin Chest Med 1990;11:691-714.
56. Stoller JK, Kacmarek RM. Ventilatory strategies in the management of the adult respiratory distress syndrome. Clin Chest Med 1990;11:755-772.

57. Slutsky AS. (chairman) Consensus Conference on Mechanical Ventilation. Intensive Care Med 1994;20:64-79.
58. Sassoon LS, Mahutte CK, Light RW. Ventilatory modes: Old and new. Crit Care Clin 1990;6:605-634.
59. Marini JJ. New options for the ventilatory management of acute lung injury. New Horiz 1993;1:489-503.
60. Marini JJ, Culver BH. Systemic gas embolism complication mechanical ventilation in the acute respiratory distress syndrome. Ann Intern Med 1989;110:699-703.
61. Tsuno K, Prato P, Kolobow T. Acute lung injury from mechanical ventilation at moderately high airway pressures. J Appl Physiol 1990;69:956-961.
62. Hickling KG, Henderson SJ, Jackson R. Low mortality associated with low volume pressure limited ventilation with permissive hypercapnia in severe ARDS. Intensive Care Med 1990;16:372-377.
63. Tuxen DV. Permissive hypercapnic ventilation. Am J Respir Crit Care Med 1994;150:870-874.
64. Pierson DJ. Complications associated with mechanical ventilation. Crit Care Clin 1990;6:711-724.
65. Lodato RF. Oxygen toxicity. Crit Care Clin 1990;6:749-765.
66. Jenkenson SG. Oxygen toxicity. New Horiz 1993;1:504-511.
67. El-Naggar M et al. Factors influencing choice between tracheostomy and prolonged translaryngeal intubation in acute respiratory failure: A prospective study. Anesth Analg 1976;55:195-210.
68. Elliott CG, Rasmussen BY, Crapo RO. Upper airway obstruction following acute respiratory distress syndrome: An analysis of 30 survivors. Chest 1988;94:526-530.
69. Pinsky MR. Multiple systems organ failure: Malignant intravascular inflammation. Crit Care Clin 1989;5:195-198.
70. Leeper KV. Diagnosis and treatment of pulmonary infections in ARDS. New Horiz 1993;1:550-562.
71. Langer M et al. The prone position in adult respiratory distress syndrome patients: A clinical study. Chest 1988;94:103-107.
72. Dreyfuss D, Saumon G. Should the lung be rested or recruited? Am J Respir Crit Care Med 1994;149:1066-1068.
73. Von Rueden KT. Noninvasive assessment of gas exchange in the critically ill patient. Clin Issues Crit Care Nurs 1990;6:679-709.
74. Tobin MJ. Respiratory monitoring during mechanics of ventilation. Crit Care Clin 1990;6:679-709.
75. Bone RC. Treatment of ARDS with diuretics, dialysis and positive end-expiratory pressure. Crit Care Med 1978;68:136-139.
76. Humphrey H et al. Improved survival in ARDS patients associated with a reduction in pulmonary capillary wedge pressure. Chest 1990;97:1176-80.
77. Schuster DP. ARDS: clinical lessons from the oleic acid model of acute lung injury. Am J Respir Crit Care Med 1994;149:245.
78. Pingleton SK. Nutritional support in the mechanically ventilated patient. Clin Chest Med 1988;9:101-112.
79. Cerra FB. Hypermetabolism, organ failure and metabolic support. Surgery 1987;101:1-14.
80. Holtzman GM et al. Nutritional support of pulmonary patients: A multidisciplinary approach. Clin Issues Crit Care Nurs 1990;1:300-312.
81. Meduri GU et al. Management of bacterial pneumonia in ventilated patients. Chest 1992;101:500-506.
82. Goldstein G, Luce JJ. Pharmacologic treatment of the adult respiratory distress syndrome. Clin Chest Med 1990;11:773-787.
83. Bone RC et al. Randomized double-blind multicenter study of prostaglandin E_1 in patients with the adult respiratory distress syndrome. Chest 1989;96:114-119.
84. Silverman HJ et al. Effects of prostaglandin E_1 on oxygen delivery and consumption in patients with the adult respiratory distress syndrome. Chest 1990;98:405-410.
85. Melot C et al. Prostaglandin E_1 in the adult respiratory distress syndrome: Benefit for pulmonary hypertension and cost of pulmonary gas exchange. Am Rev Respir Dis 1989;139:106-110.
86. Christman BW, Bernard GR. Antilipid mediator and antioxidant therapy in adult respiratory distress syndrome. New Horiz 1993;1:623-630.
87. Seejer W et al. Alveolar surfactant and adult respiratory distress syndrome. Clin Investig 1993;71:177-190.
88. Wegner CD et al. Intercellular adhesion molecule-1 (ICAM-1) in the pathogenesis of asthma. Science 1990;247:456-459.
89. Tuomanen EI et al. Reduction of inflammation, tissue damage, and mortality in bacterial meningitis in rabbits treated with monoclonal antibodies against adhesion-promoting receptors of leukocytes. J Exp Med 1989;170:959-968.
90. Mileski WJ et al. Inhibition of CD18-dependent neutrophil adherence reduces organ injury after hemorrhagic shock in primates. Surgery 1990;108:206-212.
91. Wortel CH, Doerschuk CM. Neutrophils and neutrophil-endothelial cell adhesion in adult respiratory distress syndrome. New Horiz 1993;1:631-37.
92. Slotman GJ et al. Ketaconazole prevents acute respiratory failure in critically ill surgical patients. J Trauma 1988;28:648-54.
93. MiHae YU, Tomasa G. A double-blind, prospective, randomized trial of Detoconazole, a thromboxane synthesis inhibitor in the prophylaxis of the acute respiratory distress syndrome. Crit Care Med 1993;21:1635-1643.
94. Zapol WM, Hurford WE. Inhaled nitric oxide in the acute respiratory distress syndrome and other lung diseases. New Horiz 1993;1:638-650.
95. Zapol WM et al. Extracorporeal membrane oxygenation in severe acute respiratory failure. JAMA 1979;242:2193-2196.
96. Villar G, Winston B, Slutsky AS. Nonconventional techniques of ventilatory support. Crit Care Clin 1990;6:579-603.
97. Morris AH et al. Randomized clinical trial of pressure controlled inverse ratio ventilation and extracorporeal CO_2 removal for acute respiratory distress syndrome. Am J Respir Crit Care Med 1994;149:295-305.
98. Lenfant C. Task Force on Research in Cardiopulmonary Dysfunction in Critical Care Medicine. Am J Respir Crit Care Med 1995;151:243-48.
99. Morris AH. Protocol management of ARDS. New Horiz 1993;1:593-602.
100. Bernard G, Drew K. Acute respiratory distress syndrome: Critical pathway. Vanderbilt Medical Center Pathway Development Committee. 1994.
101. Demling RH. Adult respiratory distress syndrome: Current concepts. New Horiz 1993;1:388-401.

CHAPTER 9

Hepatic Dysfunction, Hypermetabolism, and Multiple Organ Dysfunction Syndrome

Jo-ell Lohrman

The liver plays an integral role in the systemic inflammatory response syndrome (SIRS) and the multiple organ dysfunction syndrome (MODS). The liver, a vital organ performing more than four hundred functions, affects virtually every other organ system in both its healthy and pathophysiologic states. Any alteration in liver function resulting from sepsis or injury can greatly affect the overall inflammatory/immune response, because the liver contains approximately 85% of the reticuloendothelial system (RES) in the form of fixed macrophages.[1-3] The major role of the liver in total body metabolism is also greatly affected by injury, sepsis, and SIRS.

The liver plays an active role in the MODS process much earlier than has been previously suggested. Liver involvement or dysfunction may be present even before clinical markers such as elevated liver enzymes or depressed RES activity are evident.[2,4] Many clinicians believe the stages of MODS parallel liver dysfunction and failure.[5-8]

ANATOMY OF THE LIVER

The critical care practitioner must have a basic understanding of the anatomy and physiology of the liver to fully comprehend and integrate the role of the liver in MODS and its associated therapies. The liver is located in the right upper quadrant of the abdomen. It is divided into two lobes, with the right lobe being larger than the left. The liver contains 50,000 to 100,000 lobules, the functional units of the liver[9] (Fig. 9-1).

Blood supply

The liver receives a dual blood supply—from both the hepatic artery and the portal vein. The hepatic artery provides 30% of the blood supply and delivers oxygen-rich blood. The portal vein delivers the remaining 70% and contains nutrients, as well as bacteria and particulate matter from the gastrointestinal system. Blood from both vessels enters the lobule sinusoids, where numerous exchanges of oxygen, nutrients, and foreign material take place. The total blood flow from the hepatic artery and portal vein is about 1450 mL/min, or a little less than one third of the resting cardiac output.[9,10]

The blood leaves the liver lobule via the central vein. The central veins drain into the hepatic veins, which empty into the inferior vena cava. This completes the circuit of blood flow through the liver.

Portal circulation

The portal circulation terminates in the portal vein, which is responsible for draining the venous blood from most of the gastrointestinal tract. The splenic vein, the coronary (gastric) vein, the superior mesenteric vein, and the inferior mesenteric vein drain venous blood from their respective organs within the gastrointestinal system into the portal vein (Fig. 9-2).

Cell types

The two main cell types located in each liver lobule are the hepatocytes and the Kupffer cells. The hepatocytes perform most of the functions of the liver. Adjacent to the hepatocytes are the bile cana-

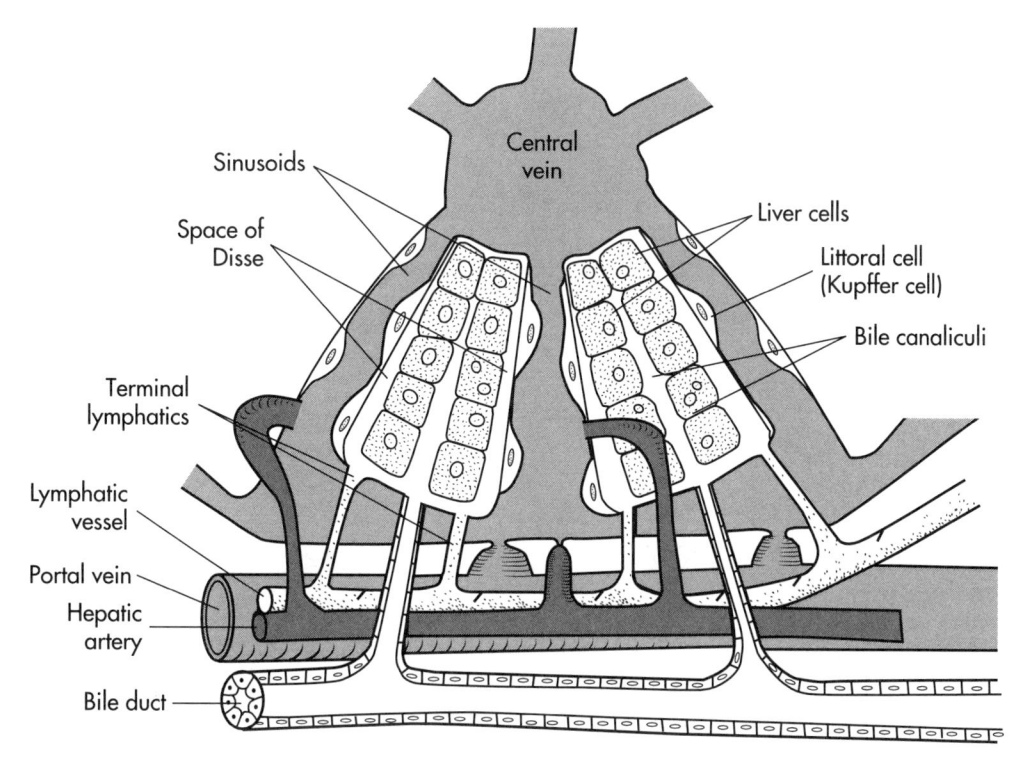

Fig. 9-1 Basic structure of a liver lobule displaying the dual blood supply, the cellular components (hepatocytes and Kupffer cells), and the bile-collecting system. (From Guyton AC. Textbook of medical physiology, 8th ed. Philadelphia: WB Saunders, 1991;772.)

liculi, which are tiny bile ducts that drain bile produced by the hepatocytes. The bile canaliculi connect to form the biliary radicles and the right and left hepatic ducts. The Kupffer cells, as tissue macrophages of the reticuloendothelial system (also known as the mononuclear phagocyte system), phagocytize bacteria and other foreign matter delivered by the portal vein.

LIVER FUNCTION AND PHYSIOLOGY
Vascular function

The major functions of the liver are classified into three categories: vascular, metabolic, and secretory.[9-11] The vascular functions include storage of blood, formation of lymph, and filtration of foreign debris. In the normal physiologic state, the liver contains approximately 450 mL, or 10%, of the total blood volume; however, the liver is capable of expanding and storing 0.5 to 1.0 L of extra blood.[9,10] Thus the liver serves as a reservoir of blood and is capable of shunting excess blood into the systemic circulation when needed. This is a valuable reserve, especially in the setting of hypovolemic shock.[11]

More than one half of the total lymphatic fluid of the body is formed in the liver. The liver sinusoids are very permeable and allow large quantities of fluid and protein to cross over into the space of Disse (space surrounding the hepatocytes) and drain into the lymphatic channels. Even slight increases in hepatic venous pressure can lead to increased movement of fluid into the space of Disse, as well as through the outer surface of the liver capsule. This accumulation of free fluid in the abdominal cavity is known as ascites.

The Kupffer cells filter foreign debris and particulate matter from the blood as the blood moves through the liver. The Kupffer cells are very efficient phagocytes and remove bacteria and foreign matter received from the intestines through the portal vein. Under physiologic conditions, fewer than

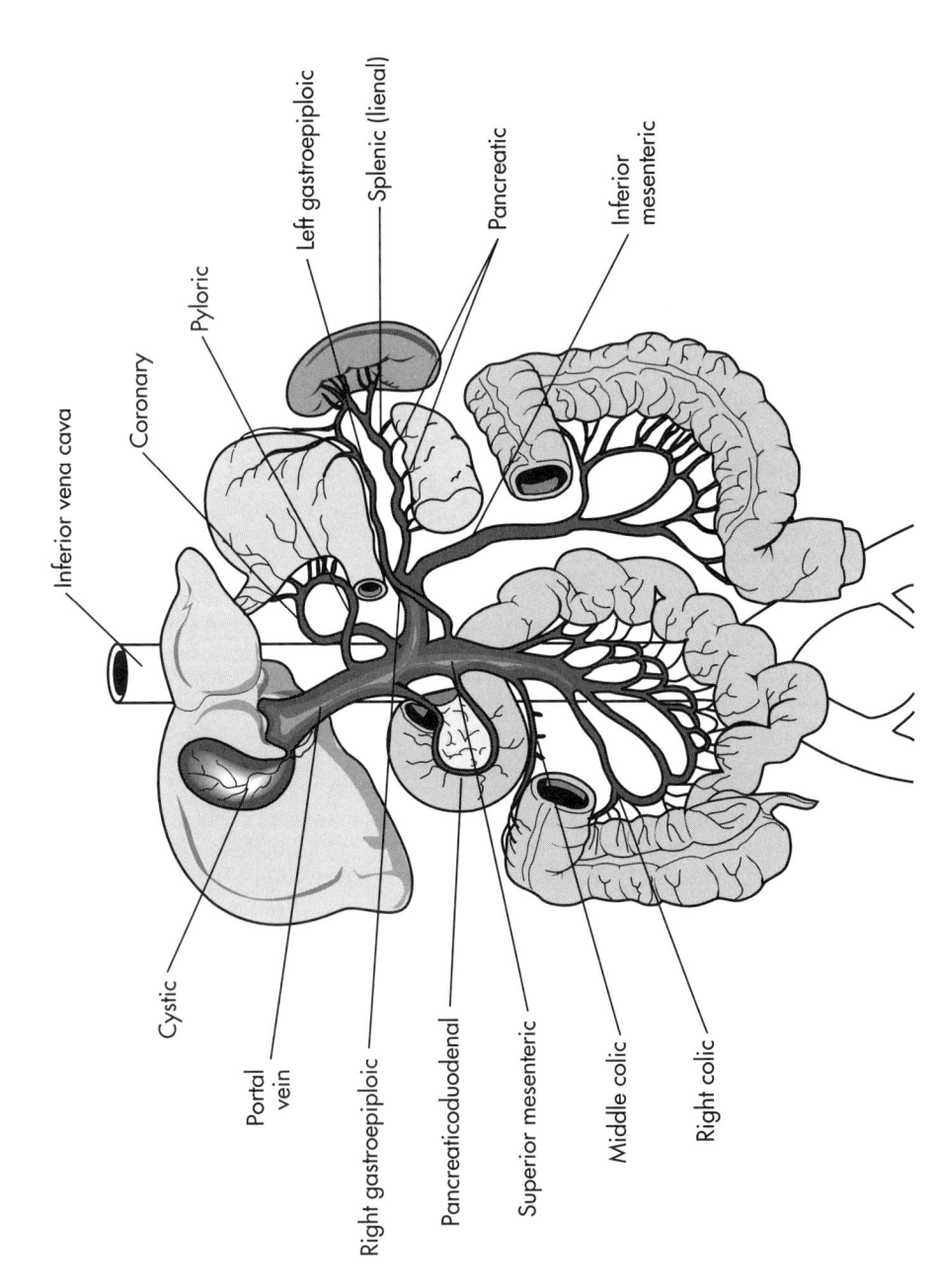

Fig. 9-2 The portal circulation. (From Thibodeau GA, Anthony CP, eds. Structure and function of the body, 8th ed. St Louis: Mosby, 1988;268.)

1% of the bacteria in the portal circulation pass into the systemic circulation.[9]

Metabolic function

Carbohydrate metabolism. The liver coordinates much of the carbohydrate, lipid, and protein metabolism of the body. In carbohydrate metabolism, the liver plays a crucial role in regulating normal serum glucose. This is achieved by the storage of simple sugars as glycogen (glycogenesis). These glycogen reserves can be reconverted to glucose (glycogenolysis) when the serum glucose concentration falls. If the glycogen stores are depleted or carbohydrate intake is inadequate, the liver is capable of converting amino acids and fats into glucose (gluconeogenesis). All of these processes work together to maintain a normal serum glucose level.

Lipid metabolism. Lipid metabolism occurs in individual body cells; however, principal aspects of lipid metabolism take place primarily in the liver. The liver breaks down the fat to provide another source of energy to meet body demands. In addition to fat catabolism, the liver converts excess carbohydrates and proteins into fat to be stored in the adipose tissue for later use.

The liver is also responsible for the synthesis of cholesterol and phospholipids. Most of the cholesterol formed is converted into bile salts and subsequently secreted into the bile. The other portion of the cholesterol, and the phospholipids generated by the liver, are used elsewhere in the body for other cellular functions. The cholesterol and phospholipids are transported by circulating lipoproteins, which are also synthesized by the liver.

Protein metabolism. Although the liver plays an important role in carbohydrate and fat metabolism, its role in protein metabolism is the most crucial for host survival. Death is imminent in a few days without proper protein metabolism by the liver.[9] The three most important functions of protein metabolism performed by the liver are deamination of amino acids, ureagenesis, and plasma protein synthesis. Deamination of amino acids refers to the removal of an amino (NH_2) group so that the amino acids can be used as an energy source. Deamination is also necessary for the amino acids to be converted into fat or carbohydrates. It is important to mention that not only does the liver deaminate amino acids, but it can also synthesize amino acids and form other compounds from these amino acids.

Ureagenesis is the process whereby the liver converts ammonia to urea. Ammonia is formed as a by-product of the deamination of amino acids and is also formed by bacteria in the gastrointestinal system. If ureagenesis is impaired, the serum ammonia level can rise, resulting in coma and ultimately death.[9,11]

The hepatocytes synthesize the majority of the plasma proteins. There are three proteins of particular importance: albumin, fibrinogen, and globulins. Albumin is found within the vascular space and is responsible for maintaining the colloid oncotic pressure. Fibrinogen is crucial for blood coagulation. Globulins function as cellular enzymes and transporters of other proteins.

The liver is responsible for the production of acute-phase reactants (also known as acute-phase proteins). These reactants are plasma proteins whose production increases selectively in the setting of tissue injury or infection. The following are the major acute-phase reactants: C-reactive protein, fibrinogen, alpha$_1$-antitrypsin, transferrin, and alpha$_2$-macroglobulin.[1] C-reactive protein receives the most attention because it is important for cellular migration and for activation of the complement system.

Miscellaneous functions. Besides the complex metabolic functions (carbohydrate, fat, and protein metabolism), the liver performs other equally important metabolic functions, including the synthesis and removal of coagulation components; detoxification of drugs, hormones, and other circulating substances; and storage of vitamins. The liver produces most of the clotting factors necessary for the coagulation cascade: fibrinogen, prothrombin (Factor II), Factors V, VII, VIII, IX, and X, and accelerator globulin. The liver also removes many of these factors after they have been activated. Detoxification of drugs, hormones, and other products further demonstrates the diverse metabolic activities of the liver. The liver breaks down these substances for excretion into the bile or urine. Some of the drugs metabolized by the liver include diazepam, acetaminophen, quinidine sulfate, and phenytoin (see the box on p. 200). In addition, the liver metabolizes and excretes numerous hormones such as estrogen, testosterone, aldosterone, cortisol, and thyroxine into the bile. It also assists in removing calcium through bile production and excretion in the stool.

COMMON DRUGS METABOLIZED BY THE LIVER

Antibiotic
Aztreonam (Azactam)
Cefoperazone (Cefobid)
Cefotaxime (Claforan)
Ceftriaxone (Rocephin)
Cephalothin (Keflin)
Chloramphenicol
Clindamycin (Cleocin)
Erythromycin
Isoniazid (INH)
Metronidazole (Flagyl)
Nafcillin (Nafcil)
Rifampin (Rifadin)
Sulfamethoxazole (Bactrim or Septra)
Tetracycline (Sumycin)
Zidovudine (Retrovir)

Analgesic
Acetaminophen (Tylenol)
Meperidine (Demerol)
Methadone
Morphine
Pentazocine (Talwin)
Propoxyphene (Darvon)

Antiepileptic
Carbamazepine (Tegretol)
Phenobarbital (Luminal)
Phenytoin (Dilantin)
Valproic acid (Depakene)

Antipyretic/antiinflammatory
Antipyrine (Auralgan)
Dexamethasone (Decadron)
Fenoprofen (Nalfon)
Ibuprofen (Motrin)
Indomethacin (Indocin)
Naproxen (Naprosyn)
Phenylbutazone (Butazolidin)
Prednisolone
Salicylic acid (Aspirin)
Sulfinpyrazone (Anturane)

Cardiovascular
Captopril (Capoten)
Digitoxin
Digoxin (Lanoxin)
Disopyramide (Norpace)
Isradipine (DynaCirc)
Labetalol (Trandate or Normodyne)

Cardiovascular—cont'd
Lidocaine
Lorcainide
Methyldopa (Aldomet)
Metoprolol (Lopressor)
Nifedipine (Procardia)
Pindolol (Visken)
Prazosin (Minipress)
Procainamide (Pronestyl)
Propranolol (Inderal)
Quinidine
Tocainide (Tonocard)
Verapamil (Calan)

Diuretic
Bumetanide (Bumex)
Furosemide (Lasix)
Spironolactone (Aldactone)
Triamterene/HCTZ (Dyazide)

Sedative/hypnotic
Amobarbital (Amytal)
Chlordiazepoxide (Librium)
Diazepam (Valium)
Flumazenil (Mazicon)
Hexobarbital
Lorazepam (Ativan)
Methohexital (Brevital)
Midazolam (Versed)
Nitrazepam
Oxazepam (Serax)
Pentobarbital (Nembutal)
Primidone (Mysoline)
Temazepam (Restoril)

Other
Alfentanil (Alfenta)
Chlorpromazine (Thorazine)
Chlormethiazole
Cimetidine (Tagamet)
Clofibrate (CPIB)
Diphenhydramine (Benadryl)
Fentanyl (Sufenta)
Ranitidine (Zantac)
Sulfisoxazole (Azo Gantrisin)
Theophylline (Theo-Dur)
Thiopental (Pentothal Sodium)
Tolbutamide (Orinase)
Warfarin (Coumadin)

SECRETORY FUNCTION
Bile production

In addition to its vascular and metabolic functions, the liver serves two important secretory functions: bile production and bilirubin metabolism. The bile is produced by the hepatocytes and consists of bile salts, bile pigments, and cholesterol. The liver produces cholesterol that is converted into bile salts, which are necessary for fat digestion in the intestines. After the bile is produced by the hepatocytes, it is drained through the bile canaliculi into the hepatic ducts. The bile then continues on to the gallbladder, where it is concentrated and stored.

Bilirubin metabolism. Bilirubin forms as a by-product of red blood cell destruction. When a red blood cell is destroyed, hemoglobin is released. After releasing its iron, the heme portion is converted to bilirubin, which combines with circulating albumin and is transported to the liver. This type of bilirubin is called free, indirect, or unconjugated bilirubin. Once in the liver, the bilirubin is combined with the other substances, forming conjugated or direct bilirubin. Conjugated bilirubin is excreted in the bile into the intestines. A small portion of conjugated bilirubin reenters the sinusoidal blood and is cleared by the kidneys and excreted in the urine.

Storage reservoir

The liver serves as a storage reservoir for blood, glucose, fat, vitamins, and minerals. Vitamins stored include vitamins A, D, and B_{12}. A large percentage of total body iron is stored as ferritin and is released when the body supply is low.

The liver performs a wide range of functions that have a tremendous impact on total body function (see the box to the right). Small derangements in liver functioning can sequentially alter the homeostatic milieu.

HYPERMETABOLISM, LIVER FUNCTION, AND THE PROGRESSION TO MODS

When the patient experiences an insult such as severe inflammation, shock, tissue injury, or ischemia, the patient mounts a metabolic response. If this response continues unabated, the patient will enter a stage of extended hypermetabolism. This often begins with the onset of pulmonary dysfunction and progresses to ARDS.[2,5,12-15]

This period of hypermetabolism and increased body requirements affects the liver significantly. Be-

---

FUNCTIONS OF THE LIVER

Vascular/immune
Storage of blood
Formation of lymph
Filtration of blood
Activity of Kupffer cells
Production of acute-phase reactants

Metabolic
Carbohydrate metabolism
Homeostasis of blood glucose
Storage of glycogenesis and glycogen
Glycogenolysis
Glyconeogenesis
Conversion of galactose and fructose to glucose
Formation of other chemical compounds from intermediates of carbohydrate metabolism

Fat metabolism
Catabolism of fat
Conversion of carbohydrates and proteins into fat for storage in the adipose tissue
Synthesis of cholesterol, phospholipids, and lipoproteins
Beta oxidation of fatty acids leading to ATP production
Formation of ketones

Protein metabolism
Deamination of amino acids
Interconversions of amino acids
Conversion of amino acids to carbohydrates or lipids
Ureagenesis
Synthesis of plasma proteins
Production of acute-phase reactants

Synthesis and removal of coagulation components
Detoxification or excretion of drugs, hormones, and calcium
Storage of vitamins
Storage of iron

Secretory/excretory
Production of bile
Metabolism of bilirubin

cause of its major role in normal metabolism, the liver plays a key role in the development and progression of the hypermetabolic state. In order to meet the increasing demands of the body, the liver increases the rate of gluconeogenesis with simultaneous increases in protein catabolism and ureagenesis.[16,17] The urinary excretion of nitrogen is subsequently increased. This process is not affected or inhibited by the exogenous administration of glucose-containing substances. There is an increase in calories obtained from amino acids, accompanied by a decrease in calories obtained from glucose and fat. The amino acids that are used for energy are the branched-chain amino acids (BCAAs) obtained from the muscle. Moyer and co-workers[18] have found that low levels or depletion of BCAAs affect liver function. They discovered that these low levels impair hepatic protein synthesis and actually produce liver dysfunction.

Hypermetabolism may last for a few days to 3 weeks. Either the condition of the patient improves or the patient deteriorates to the organ dysfunction phase. This ongoing hypermetabolism represents a change from a state of enhanced metabolic regulation into a disorganized and unregulated phase that signifies the presence of the organ dysfunction syndrome. This transition to MODS is accompanied by an increasing serum bilirubin level and evidence of hepatic failure. As a preterminal event, metabolism may become blocked or fail completely.*

A close examination of the metabolic derangements occurring in the liver as it progresses to organ failure is important (Fig. 9-3). Increased glycogenolysis and gluconeogenesis continue, and an inability to convert lactate to glucose develops; thus lactate clearance decreases as failure progresses. Eventually, the liver is unable to maintain a base-

---

*References 2, 5, 8, 13-15, 19-21.

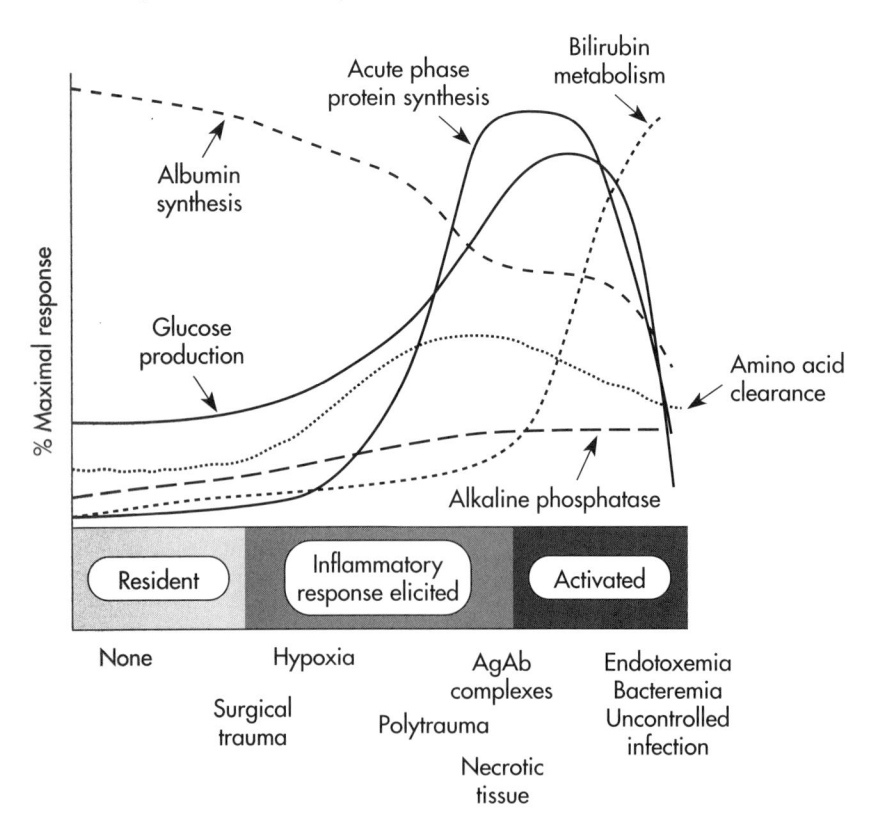

Fig. 9-3 Postulated hepatocellular dysfunction from early hypermetabolism to MODS. (From Cerra FB. Hypermetabolism-organ failure syndrome: A metabolic response to injury. Crit Care Clin 1989;5:297.)

line level of glucose, and hypoglycemia ensues.[2,16,22,23]

Lipid metabolism is altered because increased lipolysis and lipogenesis occur.[16] Feingold and Grunfeld[24] discovered that tumor necrosis factor (TNF) released by rat macrophages causes hepatocytes to increase lipogenesis. In conjunction with this increased triglyceride production there is also decreased peripheral triglyceride clearance. Serum levels indicative of lipemia are evident.

Major derangements in protein metabolism occur. The ability of the liver to extract or clear amino acids is decreased. Ureagenesis continues to increase, leading to elevated plasma urea levels, especially in the setting of renal failure. There are elevated levels of the aromatic amino acids (phenylalanine and tyrosine) but decreased levels of the BCAAs.[25,26] Some clinicians believe the accumulation of aromatic acids actually causes hepatic encephalopathy.[27-29]

Hepatic protein synthesis is also reduced, specifically that of albumin and transferrin. This reduction in albumin synthesis affects the circulating intravascular volume, because albumin plays an important role in maintaining plasma oncotic pressure. It is interesting that exogenous administration of albumin is ineffective and does not normalize the oncotic pressure. The infused albumin is quickly broken down and catabolized.[1] Keith[11] notes that an albumin level below 3.0 g/dL is associated with a poor prognosis in liver failure.

As a rule, protein synthesis is diminished; however, the production of acute-phase reactants is increased after an insult. This is believed to occur in response to infection or tissue injury and to be necessary for survival.[19] Cerra,[5] Clowes and co-workers,[30] and Pearl and co-workers[31] indicate that the inability of the liver to clear amino acids and synthesize proteins is a major determinant of mortality in MODS.

As liver failure progresses, detoxification of drugs, toxins, and hormones diminishes. Judicious use of hepatotoxic drugs is paramount. Since regulation of hormones is affected, uncontrolled increases in aldosterone and antidiuretic hormone contribute to complications such as the hepatorenal syndrome, development of ascites, and poor regulation of blood pressure.

In addition to the metabolic derangements occurring in liver failure, the immune system continues to be burdened. Kupffer cells are unable to phagocytize bacteria properly. Fibronectin is partially synthesized by the liver under homeostatic conditions and is depleted during stress or infection. Its main role is to enhance phagocytosis. Without the presence of fibronectin, the bacteria are more mobile and more difficult to phagocytize.[15,22,23]

The liver is affected by multiple factors as the body mounts a metabolic response to injury. This hypermetabolic response may continue unabated and uncontrolled, leading to MODS. All facets of carbohydrate, lipid, and protein metabolism are deranged, and normal detoxification and immune functions are impaired. All these factors combine to produce progressive liver failure. If the process continues, terminal liver failure occurs.

MECHANISMS OF LIVER DAMAGE SUSTAINED IN THE MODS PROCESS
Hypoperfusion

Differences in opinion exist among well-known clinicians concerning the mechanisms of hepatic insufficiency and damage in MODS. Baue[1] states that the role of the liver in MODS is related to changes that occur in sepsis, although the exact mechanisms are not completely understood. During sepsis there is inadequate circulation to the liver, resulting in ischemia. As a result, the Kupffer cells and hepatocytes are incapable of functioning optimally.[2] In addition, several mediators present during sepsis and SIRS have been implicated in liver damage. These include superoxides, fibrinolysin, elastase, lysosomal by-products, and permeability factors.[1]

Another consideration in hypoperfusion is the decreased substrate delivery to the liver. Without the necessary carbohydrates, proteins, and lipids, further alterations in metabolism occur. Thus Baue believes that hepatic hypoperfusion is the major factor in liver dysfunction.

Although it is obvious that low-flow states such as shock and arrest situations can lead to hepatic ischemia and tissue damage, it is less clear why decreased flow is noted during hyperdynamic states. It is suggested that after complement activation, neutrophils aggregate and release oxygen-derived free radicals and proteases. The ensuing vascular permeability, obstruction, and damage not only hinder flow but incite platelet activation and fibrin deposition. Activated platelets release thromboxane, which is a potent vasoconstrictor. The action of these inflammatory mediators, along with vascular and tissue damage, contributes to the development and progression of hepatic damage.[12,32,33]

Kupffer cell activity

Another popular theory of liver involvement in MODS is related to macrophages and their production of potent inflammatory mediators such as the cytokines TNF and interleukin-1 (IL-1). Keller and co-workers[34,35] note that hepatic failure is not always precipitated by an episode of hypoperfusion. They believe that hypoperfusion and the associated hypoxia cannot solely cause the liver damage observed in these patients. The liver dysfunction can result from a Kupffer cell–mediated response.*

This hypothesis states that the Kupffer cells are activated by endotoxin or other inflammatory stimuli from the initial insult or from secondary complications, such as shock, sepsis, and SIRS. The Kupffer cells release toxic mediators, including TNF, IL-1, oxygen-derived free radicals, lysosomal enzymes, and arachidonic acid metabolites. Since the Kupffer cells are in proximity to the hepatocytes, these mediators (specifically a cytokine such as IL-1) adversely affect the hepatocytes, but usually do not cause cell death (Fig. 9-4). This may explain why liver dysfunction is present before elevations in clinical markers such as the enzymes, serum glutamyl-oxalacetic transferase (SGOT) and serum glutamate pyruvate transaminase (SGPT), occur. (These intracellular enzymes are released after cell death.)

Hepatocellular damage, whether a result of ischemia, hypoperfusion, or Kupffer cell activation by mediators, will lead to major alterations in liver functions. Although the mechanisms involved in hepatocyte–Kupffer cell interaction have not been fully defined, Kupffer cell activity is still considered to be a major event in the pathogenesis of SIRS and MODS.[3,21,44]

If the Kupffer cell–mediated response actually occurs, two important problems surface: the ability of the liver to recover from the damage sustained and the ability of the liver to synthesize the necessary proteins and substrates for recovery.[36] Both present major challenges that the body must overcome for survival.

---

*References 2, 5, 6, 12, 20, 21, 34-43.

Ischemic reperfusion injury

A third mechanism reported in the literature which attempts to explain the development of remote organ dysfunction in the liver is described as gut ischemia/reperfusion (I/R).[45] This phenomenon is best described as tissue damage that occurs after blood flow and oxygen are returned to previously ischemic tissue. During an ischemic event, adenosine triphosphate (ATP) is not recycled and is ultimately metabolized to hypoxanthine and xanthine. Ischemia also triggers conformational changes in local enzymes, and the enzymes convert to other enzymes. Most notably, xanthine dehydrogenase is converted to xanthine oxidase. When blood flow is restored, the xanthine oxidase reacts with the arriving oxygen and the xanthine in the tissue to form oxygen-derived free radicals and uric acid (Fig. 9-5). These oxy-radicals recruit and attract circulating neutrophils, which in turn release more cytotoxic substances. In addition, the neutrophils become trapped in the local microvasculature. Thus, an environment of decreased or no blood flow is once again established in the tissues and a vicious cycle is created.[45,46]

Poggetti and co-workers[45] hypothesize that the gut I/R is responsible for simultaneous liver and lung dysfunction. They postulate that liver dysfunction occurs as a primary event rather than a sequential phenomenon of organ failure. The authors affirm that in the past the liver was thought to be part of a sequential cascade of organ failure. This belief was related to the lack of an early diagnostic marker to determine hepatic failure and the liver's substantial reserves. However, a group of researchers in Japan developed the systemic ketone body ratio (KBR) as a sensitive marker of early hepatic dysfunction in MODS.[47] By using the KBR, Pogetti's group was able to demonstrate gut I/R damage as the mechanism for liver dysfunction seen in MODS.[45] Therefore, liver dysfunction in MODS is now postulated to be a primary system event rather than the end result of sequential organ dysfunction.

Contributing factors

Not only is a perfusion deficit or ischemia implicated in hepatic damage, but persistent inflammatory foci, such as injured or necrotic tissue, may also contribute to hepatic dysfunction. Schirmer and co-workers[48] and Seibel and co-workers[49] noted that wounds associated with fractures release products

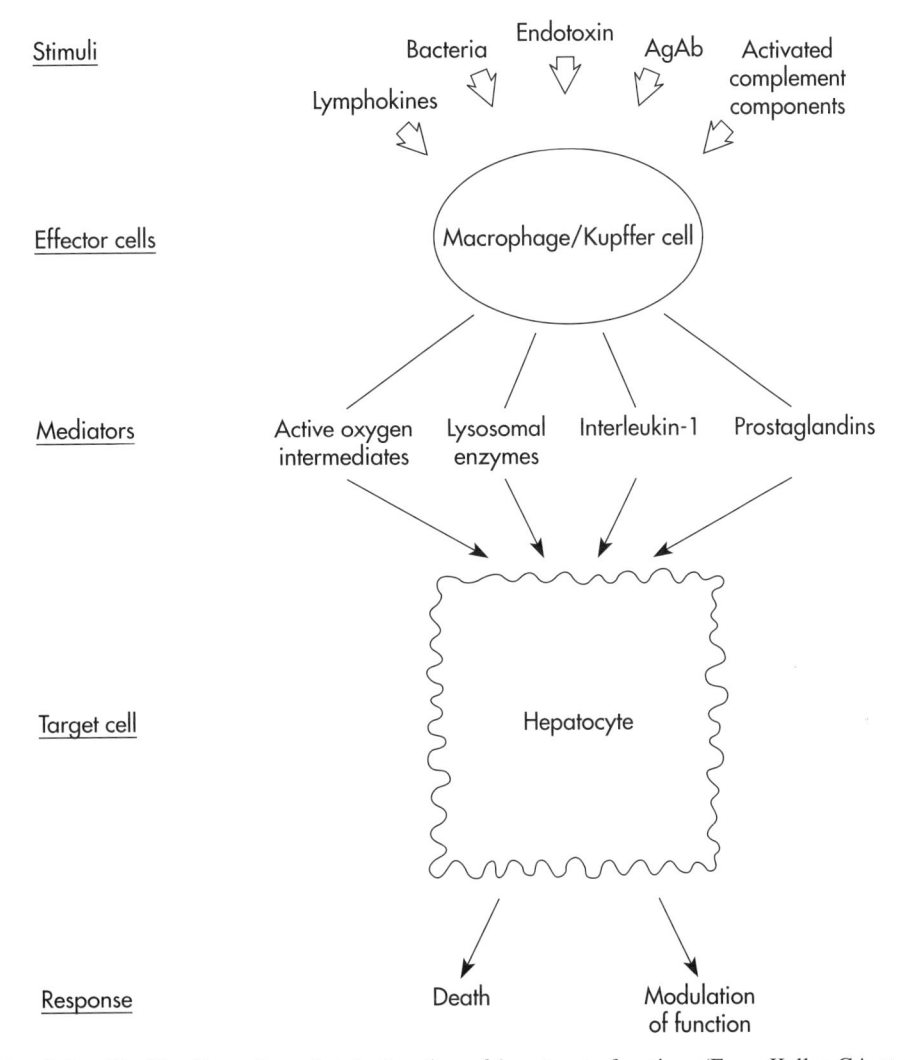

Fig. 9-4 The Kupffer cell-mediated alteration of hepatocyte function. (From Keller GA et al. Macrophage-mediated modulation of hepatic function in multiple-system failure. J Surg Res 1985;39:560.)

that alter hepatocellular function. The recent literature supports these earlier findings.[21] These findings blend with the theory that inflammation or Kupffer cell activation play a major role in the liver dysfunction in MODS.

The presence of preexisting fibrotic liver disease predisposes patients to hepatic involvement in MODS and must be considered in evaluation and treatment. These patients already suffer abnormalities in hepatocyte structure and function and are frequently malnourished. Thus any additional burden on an already compromised organ could hasten liver dysfunction and failure.

In summary, factors operating in all three theories (hypoperfusion, Kupffer cell response, and I/R injury) probably play a role in the development of liver failure in the MODS setting, along with additional contributing factors. Hypoperfusion, microcirculatory changes, Kupffer cell activation, and direct mediator damage all have the potential to greatly affect hepatic oxygen uptake, energy use, and organ function.

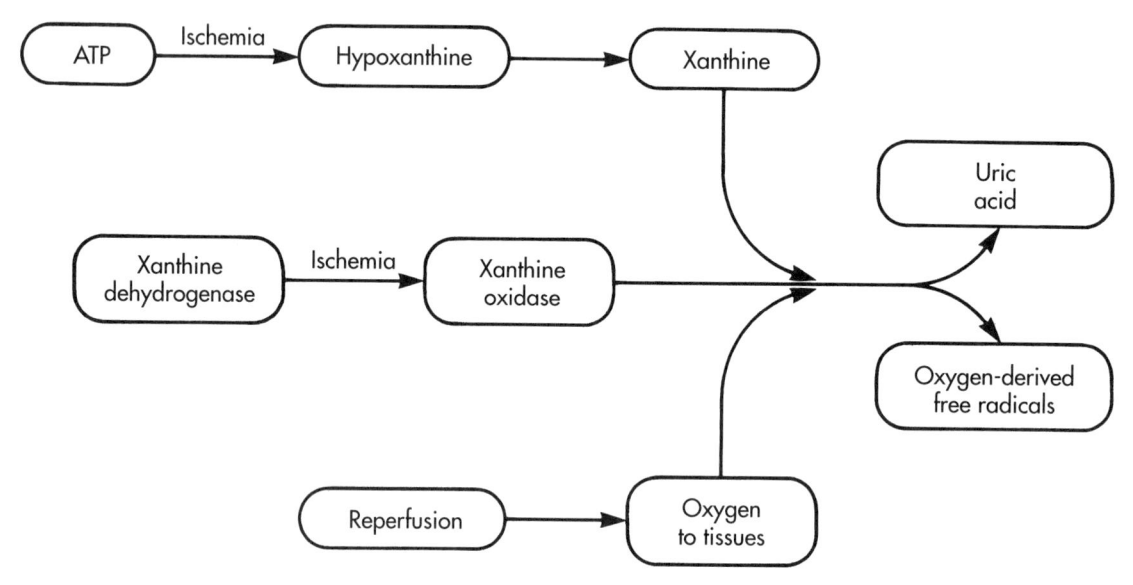

Fig. 9-5 Free radical formation in ischemia and reperfusion injury. (From Huddleston VB. Multisystem Organ Failure: A Pathophysiologic Approach: Boston, 1991, p 26.)

CLINICAL PRESENTATION AND ASSESSMENT

The American College of Chest Physicians (ACCP) and Society of Critical Care Medicine (SCCM) formulated a set of definitions to apply to patients with sepsis, inflammation, and their sequelae at the 1991 consensus conference. Although a definition of MODS was formulated, the description of, and criteria for MODS have not been determined.[50-52] Therefore, the clinical markers for liver failure in MODS have yet to be universally determined.

It is obvious that during hypermetabolism, liver involvement occurs before clinical markers appear. Hepatic dysfunction will usually be evident several days after hypermetabolism and the hyperdynamic phase are clinically evident.[53] Clinicians do not agree on a specific set or range of laboratory values or clinical markers for hepatic dysfunction, but general values commonly used are listed in the box to the right.[207]

The single clinical marker of hepatic dysfunction consistently mentioned is an elevated serum bilirubin level. Liver dysfunction is indicated by a level greater than 2 mg/dL or 3 mg/dL.* Other causes of hyperbilirubinemia, such as transfusion reaction, resorption of a large hematoma, or common bile duct blockage, must be ruled out.

Theoretically, hyperbilirubinemia can be caused by a buildup of either indirect (unconjugated) or direct (conjugated) bilirubin in the blood. In MODS, because of a possible hepatocellular excretory defect, intrahepatic cholestasis occurs. Conjugated or

---

*References 2, 12, 14, 17, 21, 52, 54.

CLINICAL MARKERS OF HEPATIC INVOLVEMENT IN MODS

Elevated serum bilirubin levels (>2 mg/dL or 3 mg/dL)
Elevated SGOT and LDH levels (two times the normal value)
Elevated plasma phenylalanine levels (>100 μmol/L)
Decreased serum albumin levels
Decreased serum transferrin levels
Jaundice
Hepatic encephalopathy
Prothrombin time >4 seconds above control values

LDH, Lactic dehydrogenase; *SGOT*, serum glutamyl-oxalacetic transferase.

direct bilirubin is absorbed back into the vascular system, causing an elevation in the plasma. Therefore the elevation in the total bilirubin level is usually reflective of an increase in the conjugated form.[53,55] In later stages of MODS, levels of both direct and indirect bilirubin are often elevated.

Elevated bilirubin levels are considered to be predictors of mortality. Sarfeh and Balint[55] state that on Day 4 after an inciting event (e.g., trauma), the bilirubin levels are lower for survivors (1.6 ± 0.3 mg/dL) than for patients who do not survive (3.6 ± 0.6 mg/dL). Cerra and co-workers[56] discovered that survivors have bilirubin levels of of 2.2 ± 0.6 mg/dL, whereas patients who die as a result of MODS or other forms of critical illness have bilirubin levels of 8.5 ± 2.2 mg/dL. Harvey reports severe liver impairment at a bilirubin level greater than 8 mg/dL, with a concomitant mortality rate exceeding 90%.[2]

Hyperbilirubinemia must not be looked at in isolation, but in conjunction with other clinical markers. Several clinicians cite the importance of measuring hepatic enzyme levels to determine liver involvement; specifically, the levels of SGOT and lactic dehydrogenase (LDH) must be double the normal value.* Furthermore, some clinicians no longer use the well-documented clinical markers of liver failure and define hepatic involvement as a prothrombin time greater than 4 seconds above control values and a bilirubin level greater than 6 mg/dL.[12]

Walvatne and Cerra[53] have emphasized increases in plasma phenylalanine levels in conjunction with an elevated bilirubin level to identify liver failure. A level greater than 100 µmol/L is considered clinically significant. Phenylalanine is an amino acid, the level of which is elevated in the plasma secondary to faulty liver metabolism. When the bilirubin is greater than 3.0 g/dL and the phenylalanine is greater than l00 µmol/L, the SGOT, SGPT, and alkaline phosphatase may only be slightly elevated or normal.[55] Thus there is a direct correlation between elevated phenylalanine, bilirubin elevation, degree of hepatic dysfunction, and mortality.[56-58]

The presence of jaundice is also considered significant, although no specific assessment guidelines are mentioned in the literature except that jaundice is seen with an elevated bilirubin level as the patient moves into MODS with liver involvement. The bilirubin level must be at least three times the normal level before jaundice is clinically observable.[9] Therefore, jaundice is often a late indicator of hepatic involvement. Dietch[21] and Rauen[54] define advanced liver failure in MODS as the presence of clinical jaundice with bilirubin level greater than or equal to 8 to 10 mg/dL.

Another clinical marker is hepatic encephalopathy. Elevated levels of certain amino acids, specifically phenylalanine and tyrosine, contribute to hepatic encephalopathy by altering cerebral neurotransmission.[25,27,28] This is difficult to evaluate in the critically ill patient because other variables that alter mental function, such as sleep deprivation and common medications are also present.

Liver involvement is present by the time the clinical markers appear. Characteristically, the excretory functions of the liver are affected before its synthetic functions. An early diagnostic marker of hepatic dysfunction would be helpful and the process may involve injecting a substance into the blood stream to be picked up by the hepatocytes and successfully excreted in the bile.[53] In the MODS setting, the substance would not be excreted properly by the hepatocyte, and would indicate cellular dysfunction. To avoid misdiagnosis, ultrasound would have to be used to rule out extrahepatic biliary obstruction, which has similar clinical findings.

In conclusion, more research is needed to develop early clinical markers of liver dysfunction. Perhaps the KBR developed by Yamamoto and co-workers[46] will be a promising tool.

IMPACT OF LIVER FAILURE ON THE MODS PROCESS

Not only is the liver damaged by the insult and the MODS process but it, in turn, affects the progression of the syndrome. MODS is not a series of isolated failures, but instead involves a constant interplay between the major organ systems. This interplay is one reason the process is so overwhelming and is associated with such a high mortality. As additional organs fail, mortality increases significantly.

Central to liver involvement are the Kupffer cells. Many of the circulating substances and inflammatory mediators in the MODS process stimulate the Kupffer cells to produce toxic products. The potent inflammatory mediators can enter the venous circu-

---

*References 1, 2, 12, 17, 21, 52.

lation directly and perpetuate the problem. The venous blood supply leaving the liver quickly enters the pulmonary circulation. These toxic products cause further damage to the pulmonary endothelium and continue to activate the pulmonary macrophages, which in turn produce their own inflammatory mediators.[2,59,60]

Matuschak discusses the role of the liver in ARDS as being unresolved and poorly understood.[61] He proposes that the pathogenesis of lung involvement in SIRS is linked to alterations in hepatic function. Specifically he states that the liver is crucial in four interrelated components of systemic host defense that can ultimately affect lung function.

1. Control of systemic endotoxemia, bacteremia, and the vasoactive by-products of sepsis and trauma
2. Production and export of inflammatory mediators
3. Metabolic inactivation of inflammatory mediators: Kupffer cell–hepatocyte interactions
4. Synthesis of acute-phase proteins essential in the control of the inflammatory response

As hepatic dysfunction continues, the normal clotting process is altered (Fig. 9-6). Simple bruising, obvious bleeding, and a prolonged prothrombin time are evident. The synthesis of clotting factors is decreased, as is the ability of the liver to remove the clotting factors once they are activated. Patients with these symptoms are predisposed to the development of disseminated intravascular coagulation (DIC),* which only compounds the severity of an already complicated and potentially fatal clinical course.

The liver also interacts closely with the gastrointestinal system. The liver receives its blood supply from the portal circulation, which may contain bacteria or bacterial products translocated from the hyperpermeable gut. Because the gastrointestinal tract is a reservoir of potentially damaging pathogens that may enter the portal circulation,[2,21,63] it is postulated that the gut continually puts the liver to the test to clear bacteria and other foreign matter. This additional bacterial load may further trigger macrophage activity and mediator production, or the bacteria may not be cleared by the dysfunctional liver.

Liver failure continues to intensify the problem of MODS treatment. It becomes a major impediment in the recovery of the patient, because the normal ability to clear and detoxify metabolites is upset. Without this ability, many general treatment methods for MODS are unsuccessful or contraindicated.

THERAPEUTIC MANAGEMENT
General therapy

In general, treatment for MODS focuses on three main goals: control of source, maintenance of oxygen transport, and nutritional support.* Whenever possible, the source of inflammation, ischemia, or infection must be removed. A persistent inflammatory focus guarantees a higher mortality.[8,14] Generic therapies to maximize oxygen delivery, such as fluid resuscitation, use of inotropes, and mechanical ventilation are used. Oxygen consumption and serum lactate levels are evaluated to determine the effectiveness of these therapies. Nutritional support is paramount since malnutrition is clearly present in the MODS patient,[8,14] and the hypermetabolic state increases fuel needs. Recent research is moving beyond the three basic modalities and examining biotechnologic modulation of mediator activity.[64,65] Refer to Chapter 18 for further description of antimediator therapies.

It is important to consider the entire clinical picture and not focus solely on treatment for an individual organ. This philosophy rests on two premises: (1) the complex interaction between organ systems is not completely understood and (2) an individual treatment for one organ system may hinder other organ systems, thus perpetuating MODS.[15,16]

Therapy for liver dysfunction

Tissue perfusion. Three areas specifically targeted for the patient suffering liver dysfunction in MODS are adequate tissue perfusion, sufficient nutritional support, and judicious use of hepatotoxic pharmacologic agents. Adequate tissue perfusion of the liver is essential to provide an environment where cell regeneration can occur. This may be assisted by administering low-dose dopamine to increase hepatic blood flow.[1,15,25] However, with in-

---

*References 22, 23, 25, 46, 62.

*References 8, 12, 14, 20, 25, 46.

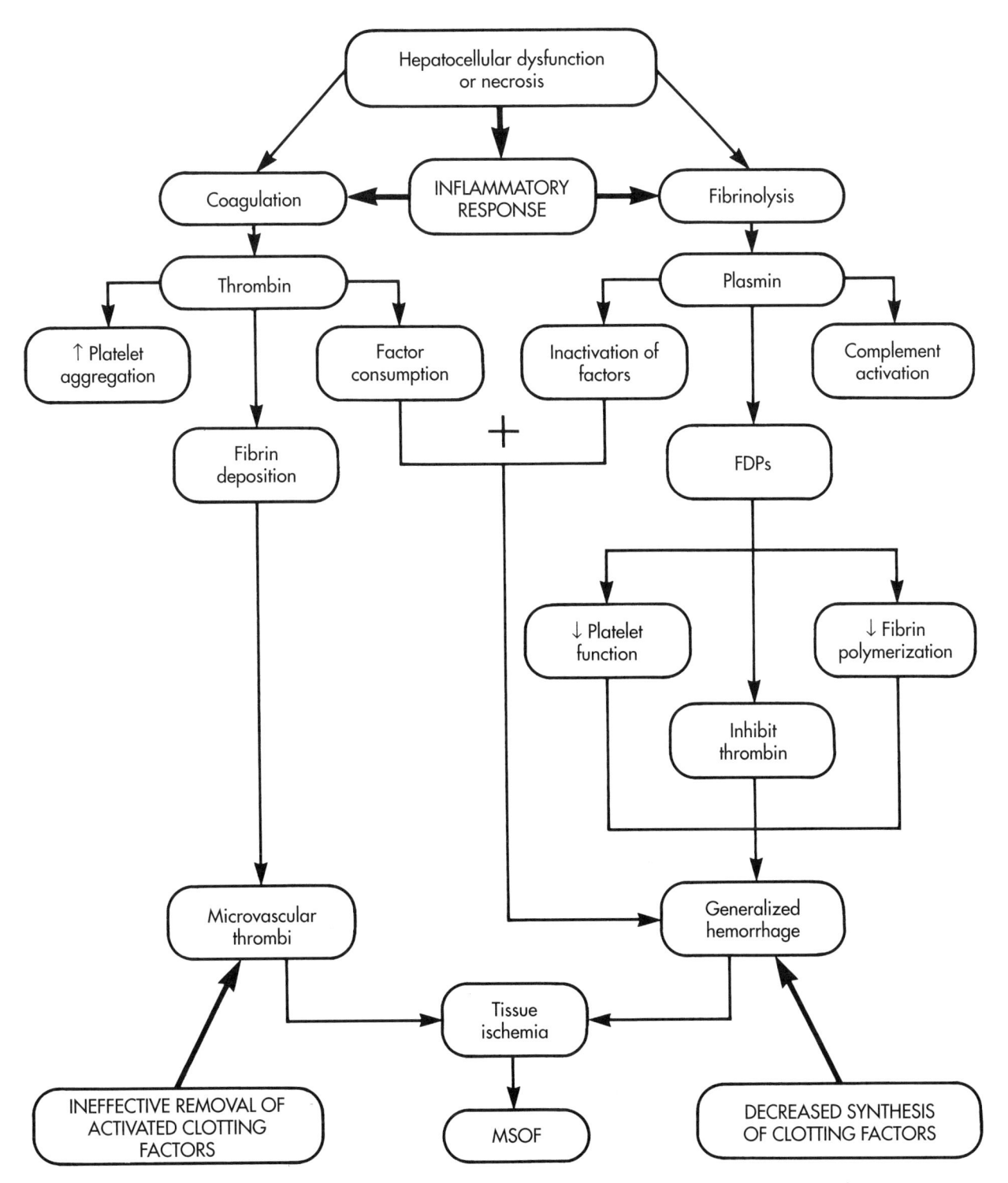

Fig. 9-6 The impact of liver dysfunction on the development and progression of DIC. Alterations occurring in hepatic damage are activation of the inflammatory response, ineffective removal of activated clotting factors, and decreased synthesis of clotting factors. *FDP,* Fibrin degradation products; *MSOF,* multisystem organ failure. (Modified from Huddleston VB. Multisystem organ failure: A pathophysiologic approach (monograph). Boston, 1991;16.)

adequate fluid resuscitation or higher doses, the vasoconstrictive properties of dopamine will decrease hepatic and splanchnic perfusion. The use of dopamine must be examined in concert with other therapies to ensure a consistent and collective treatment plan.

Another therapy under investigation is the role of dopexamine hydrochloride. Dopexamine hydrochloride is a specific splanchnic vasolidator that can improve liver blood flow in addition to improving intramucosal pH.[66-68] The improvement in intramucosal pH is thought to be related to improved oxygen delivery to the gut and a restoration of aerobic (rather than anaerobic) metabolism.

Nutritional support. Nutritional support is the mainstay of hepatic support and most of the literature focuses on its role. As previously discussed, the metabolism of carbohydrates, fats, and proteins is altered in hepatic dysfunction. The goal of nutritional support is to avoid the administration of excess carbohydrates and fats and to provide amino acids for nitrogen balance.

Specialized nutritive sources may be helpful. The BCAAs—leucine, isoleucine, and valine—are one source.* The formulas available that are high in BCAA and low in the aromatic amino acids (phenylalanine and tyrosine) include HepatAmine, FreAmine HBC, and Branchamine. These formulas supplement the low BCAA levels present in hepatic dysfunction, while simultaneously avoiding those aromatic amino acids that are already elevated and hepatotoxic.

The benefit of these formulas is threefold: They achieve nitrogen retention, support hepatic protein synthesis, and decrease ureagenesis.† Another attractive benefit is that the metabolism of these formulas occurs in peripheral muscle and not in the liver. Thus they provide energy and nutrition without depending on normal liver metabolism.[1,15,29] At present, these benefits are theoretical, and no proven difference in outcome has been demonstrated consistently among patients with MODS.[12]

This nutritional information is related to the overall prognosis of the patient. Baue[1] states that as the patient enters the late stages of liver involvement in MODS, even the initially low levels of BCAAs will rise. This suggests a poor availability of substrate for metabolism and carries a poor prognosis. Cerra and co-workers[70] also documented a higher mortality in patients who were unable to maintain protein synthesis in response to exogenous amino acid administration. Recent literature supports this premise.[12]

However, there are conflicting views in the literature regarding the BCAAs and their role in treatment. Specifically, Vente and co-workers[71] discovered that BCAA enrichment of standard total parenteral nutrition (TPN) solutions did not result in more efficient nitrogen metabolism in patients with sepsis or trauma. Kuhl and co-workers[72] conducted similar research and found no difference between standard versus BCAA-enriched TPN solutions in achieving nitrogen balance. Similar results were reported by Naylor and co-workers.[73] They reported inconclusive results with the use of BCAA solutions for hepatic encephalopathy.

Nutrition may also play a role in treatments aimed at inflammatory cells and their production of mediators. Fish oil, containing ω-3 fatty acids, is capable of entering cell membranes and altering the release of inflammatory mediators. Billiar and co-workers[74] state that Kupffer cells stimulated by endotoxin will decrease their release of TNF and IL-1 in the presence of ω-3 fatty acids. This carries important ramifications in the prevention of the postulated hepatocyte damage caused by the release of mediators by Kupffer cells.

Although aimed at patients undergoing surgery for upper gastrointestinal malignancies, Daly and co-workers[75] discovered that patients receiving enteral nutrition with supplemental arginine, RNA, and ω-3 fatty acids had significantly improved metabolic, immunologic, and clinical outcomes. Because of their positive role in enhancing immune function, it is suggested that these specific nutrient substrates may be beneficial in treatment of sepsis. In contrast, Gielen and co-workers[76] determined that diets supplemented with fish oil did not prevent multiple organ failure. Based on the conflicting findings in the literature, this remains an area for future exploration and research.[16]

Hepatotoxic agents. The third area in the treatment of liver failure and MODS is the judicious use of hepatotoxic pharmacologic agents. These agents

---
*References 1, 26, 29, 53, 69.
†References 12, 14, 20, 26, 29, 53.

should, if at all possible, be avoided in a patient with liver failure. Several factors must be evaluated for continued drug use, such as the necessity and availability of a similar nonhepatotoxic agent and the level of renal dysfunction (see the box below and Table 9-1).

Potential anti-mediator therapy. Pentoxifylline is a methylxanthine derivative used to decrease blood viscosity in chronic vascular disease.[46] It is receiving attention in the literature for its potential role in reversing the effects of TNF and IL-6. Specifically, the role of pentoxifylline in improving hepatocellular function is being investigated. In laboratory rats, pentoxifylline administrated during crystalloid resuscitation restored the depressed hepatocellular function induced by traumatic hemorrhage, and it decreased the synthesis of TNF and IL-6.[77,78,79]

A significant linear correlation existed between the levels of these cytokines and hepatocellular dysfunction. Thus, the downregulation of TNF and IL-6 may be the mechanism by which pentoxifylline restores hepatic blood flow and hepatocellular function. The use of pentoxifylline for improvement of microcirculatory abnormalities and organ function, specifically in the liver, has therefore been proposed.[46,79] At the present time, pentoxifylline has not been shown to have clinical efficacy in human trials. It is included merely to point out research efforts directed towards improving microcirculatory abnormalities and hepatocellular function.

CONCLUSION

Hepatic failure develops in 10% to 40% of patients with SIRS or sepsis. Unfortunately, there is no early, sensitive clinical marker of poor hepatic microcirculatory perfusion or hepatocellular dysfunction in MODS. Hepatic failure usually heralds the transition into true multisystem organ failure with much of MODS paralleling liver dysfunction and failure.* The more severe the liver dysfunction, the more severe the overall MODS picture. Several studies have indicated that it is the presence of liver failure, not the pulmonary or renal indices, that differentiates the survivors from the nonsurvivors. Even when oxygenation is supported, liver failure may be the common pathway leading to death in multiple organ dysfunction and failure.[33] Once liver failure occurs in the setting of MODS, mortality approaches 90% to 100%.†

Current treatment principles emphasize providing supportive care, improving tissue perfusion, providing nutritional support, and avoiding futher harm. Clinical research continues to examine therapies aimed at removing inflammatory stimuli, modulating an overzealous immune response, and finding suitable exogenous protein replacements.

DRUGS THAT SHOULD BE USED WITH CAUTION OR NOT AT ALL IN PATIENTS WITH LIVER DISEASE

Group I: Drugs capable of causing hepatic damage

Acetaminophen
Acetylsalicylic acid
Chlorpromazine
Erythromycin estolate
Methotrexate
Methyldopa

Group II: Drugs that can compromise liver functions

Anabolic and contraceptive steroids
Prednisone (in acute viral hepatitis)
Tetracycline

Group III: Drugs that make complications of liver disease worse

Cyclooxygenase inhibitors (indomethacin)
Diuretics
Meperidine and other central nervous system depressants
Morphine
Pentazocine
Phenylbutazone

From Kubisty CA, Arns PA, Wedlund PJ, Branch RA. Adjustments of medications in liver failure. In Chernow B, ed. Essentials of critical care pharmacology. 2nd ed. Baltimore: Williams & Wilkins; 1994:95-113.

*References 5, 6, 7, 8, 13, 14, 20, 31.
†References 12, 14, 17, 20, 21, 53, 54, 80.

Table 9-1 Considerations for Drug Dosage Adjustments in Liver Disease Patients

Extent of change in drug dose	Conditions or requirements to be satisfied
No change or minor change in dose	1. Mild liver disease 2. Extensive elimination of drug by kidneys and no renal dysfunction 3. Elimination by pathways of metabolism spared by liver disease 4. Drug is enzyme-limited and given acutely 5. Drug is flow/enzyme-sensitive and only given acutely by IV route 6. No alteration in drug sensitivity
Decrease in dose of <25%	1. Elimination by liver does not exceed 40% at the dose used; no renal dysfunction 2. Drug is flow-limited and given by IV route, with no large change in protein binding 3. Drug is flow/enzyme-limited and given acutely by mouth 4. Drug has a large therapeutic ratio
Decrease in dose of >25%	1. Drug metabolism is affected by liver disease; drug is administered chronically 2. Drug has a narrow therapeutic range; protein binding is altered significantly 3. Drug is flow-limited and given orally 4. Drug is eliminated by kidneys and renal function is severely affected 5. Altered sensitivity to drug as a result of liver disease

From Kubisty, CA, Arns PA, Wedlund PJ, Branch RA Adjustments of medications in liver failure In: Chernow B, ed. Essentials of critical care pharmacology. 2nd ed. Baltimore: Williams & Wilkins, 1994:95-113.
IV, Intravenous.

REFERENCES

1. Baue AE. Multiple organ failure: Patient care and prevention. St Louis: Mosby; 1990:323-329.
2. Harvey MA. Multisystem organ failure. In: Kinney MR, Packa DR, Dunbar SB, eds. AACN clinical reference for critical care nursing. St Louis: Mosby; 1993:1283-1309.
3. Ghosh S. Endotoxin—induced organ injury. Crit Care Med 1993;21:S19-S23.
4. Wang P, Hauptman JG, Chaudry IH. Hepatocellular dysfunction occurs early after hemorrhage and persists despite fluid resuscitation. J Surg Res 1990;48:464-470.
5. Cerra FB. Hypermetabolism, organ failure, and metabolic support. Surgery 1987; 101:1-14.
6. Cerra FB et al. Hepatic dysfunction in multiple systems organ failure as a manifestation of altered cell-cell interaction. Prog Clin Biol Res 1989; 308:563-573.
7. Huddleston VB. Multisystem organ failure: A pathophysiologic approach. Boston, 1991.
8. Lekander BJ, Cerra FB. The syndrome of multiple organ failure. Crit Care Nurs Clin North Am 1990; 2:331-342.
9. Guyton AC. Textbook of medical physiology. 8th ed. Philadelphia: WB Saunders, 1991:771-776.
10. Huether SE. Structure and function of the digestive system. In: McCance KL, Huether SE, eds. Pathophysiology: The biologic basis for disease in adults and children. St Louis: Mosby; 1990:1174-1211.
11. Keith JS. Hepatic failure: Etiologies, manifestations, and management. Crit Care Nurse 1985;5(2):60-86.
12. Barie PS, Jones WG. Multiple organ failure. In: Barie PS, Shires GT, eds. Surgical intensive care. Boston: Little, Brown; 1993:147-207.
13. Cerra FB. Hypermetabolism-organ failure syndrome: A metabolic response to injury. Crit Care Clin 1989;5:289-302.
14. Cerra FB. Multiple organ failure syndrome. Perspect Crit Care 1988;1:1-22.
15. Vary TC, Kearney ML. Pathophysiology of traumatic shock and multiple organ system failure. In: Cardona et al, eds. Trauma nursing—from resuscitation through rehabilitation. Philadelphia: WB Saunders; 1993:114-150.
16. Ackerman MH, Evan NJ, Ecklund MM. Systemic inflammatory response syndrome, sepsis, and nutritional support. Crit Care Nurs Clin North Am 1994; 6:321-340.
17. Fry DE. Multiple system organ failure. Surg Clin North Am 1988; 68(1):107-122.
18. Moyer E et al. Multiple systems organ failure: VII. Reduction in plasma branched-chained amino acids—correlations with liver failure and amino acid infusion. J Trauma 1981; 21:965-969.
19. Bailey PM. The metabolic response to injury: Overview and introduction to multiple system organ failure. Trauma Q 1991;7(2):1-11.
20. Barton R, Cerra FB. The hypermetabolism-multiple organ failure syndrome. Chest 1989;96:1153-1160.
21. Deitch EA. Multiple organ failure: Pathophysiology and potential future therapy. Ann Surg 1992;216:117-134.

22. DeCamp MM, Demling RH. Posttraumatic multisystem organ failure. JAMA 1988;260:530-534.
23. Kucharski SA, Fulminant hepatic failure. Crit Care Nurs Clin North Am 1993,5:141-151.
24. Feingold KR, Grunfeld C. Tumor necrosis factor-alpha stimulates hepatic lipogenesis in the rat in vivo. J Clin Invest 1987;80:184-190.
25. Collins AS. Gastrointestional complications in shock. Crit Care Nurs Clin North Am 1990;2:269-277.
26. Lehmann S. Nutritional support in the hypermetabolic patient. Crit Care Nurs Clin North Am 1993;5:97-103.
27. Fischer JE, Baldessarini RJ. False neurotransmitters and hepatic failure. Lancet 1971;2:75-79.
28. Shils M, Young VT. Modern nutrition in health and disease. Philadelphia: Lea & Febiger; 1988:1186-1188.
29. Skeie B et al. Branch-chain amino acids: Their metabolism and clinical utility. Crit Care Med 1990;18:549-571.
30. Clowes GHA et al. Survival from sepsis: The significance of altered protein metabolism regulated by proteolysis-inducing factor, the circulating cleavage product of interleukin-1. Ann Surg 1985;202:446-458.
31. Pearl RH et al. Prognosis and survival as determined by visceral amino acid clearance in severe trauma. J Trauma 1985;25:777-783.
32. Fry DE. Splanchnic perfusion and sepsis. Prog Clin Biol Res 1989;299:9-17.
33. Schwartz DB et al. Hepatic dysfunction in the adult respiratory distress syndrome. Chest 1989,95:871-875.
34. Keller GA et al. Macrophage-mediated modulation of hepatic function in multiple-system failure. J Surg Res 1985;39:555-563.
35. Keller GA et al. Modulation of hepatocyte protein synthesis by endotoxin activated Kupffer cells. Ann Surg 1985;201:87-95.
36. Carrico CM et al. Multiple-organ failure syndrome. Arch Surg 1986;121:196-208.
37. Cerra FB et al. Role of monokines in altering hepatic metabolism in sepsis. Prog Clin Biol Res 1989;286:265-277.
38. Cerra FB et al. Hypermetabolism organ failure: The role of the activated macrophage as a metabolic regulator. Prog Clin Biol Res 1988;264:27-42.
39. Mazuski JE et al. Direct effects of endotoxin on hepatocytes. Arch Surg 1988;123:340-344.
40. Meng XJ, Qui BA, Li XJ, Song XH. The role of Kupffer cells in the development of hepatic dysfunction during sepsis. Chin Med J 1992;105:34-8.
41. West MA et al. Endotoxin modulation of hepatocyte secretory and cellular protein synthesis is mediated by Kupffer cells. Arch Surg 1988;123:1400-1405.
42. West MA et al. Further characterization of Kupffer cell/macrophage-mediated alterations in hepatocyte protein synthesis. Surgery 1986;100:416-423.
43. West MA et al. Hepatocyte function in sepsis: Kupffer cells mediate a biphasic protein synthesis response in hepatocytes after exposure to endotoxin or killed *Escherichia coli*. Surgery 1985;98:388-395.
44. Border JR. Multiple systems organ failure. Ann Surg 1992;216:111-116.
45. Pogetti RS et al. Liver injury is a reversible neutrophil-mediated event following gut ischemia. Arch Surg 1992;127:175-179.
46. Secor VH. Mediators of coagulation and inflammation—relationship and clinical significance. Crit Care Nurs Clin North Am 1993;5:411-433.
47. Yamamoto Y et al. Prognostic implications of postoperative suppression of arterial ketone body ratio: time factor involved in the suppression of hepatic mitochondrial oxidation-reduction state. Surg 1990;107:289-294.
48. Schirmer WM et al. Femur fracture with associated soft-tissue injury produces hepatic ischemia. Arch Surg 1988;123:412-415.
49. Seibel R et al. Blunt multiple trauma (ISS 36), femur traction, and the pulmonary failure-septic state. Ann Surg 1985;202:283-295.
50. American College of Chest Physicians/Society of Critical Care Medicine Consensus Conference Committee. Definitions for sepsis and organ failure and guidelines for the use of innovative therapies in sepsis. Chest 1992;101:1644-1655.
51. American College of Chest Physicians/Society of Critical Care Medicine Consensus Conference Committee. Definitions for sepsis and organ failure and guidelines for the use of innovative therapies in sepsis. Crit Care Med 1992;20:864-874.
52. Hazinski MF. Epidemiology, pathophysiology, and clinical presentation of gram-negative sepsis. Heart Lung 1993;2:224-237.
53. Walvatne C, Cerra FB. Hepatic dysfunction in multiple organ failure. In: Deitch EA, ed. Multiple organ failure. New York: Thieme Medical Publishers, 1990:241-260.
54. Rauen CA. Too old to live. Too young to die. Multiple organ dysfunction syndrome in the elderly. Crit Care Nurs Clin North Am 1994;6:535-542.
55. Sarfeh IJ, Balint JA. The clinical significance of hyperbilirubinemia following trauma. J Trauma 1978;18:56-62.
56. Cerra FB et al. Multiple organ failure syndrome: Patterns and effect of current therapy. Update in Intensive Care and Emergency Medicine. Vol II. 1990.
57. Fath JJ et al. Alterations in amino acid clearance during ischemia predict hepatocellular ATP changes. Surgery 1985;98:396-404.
58. Becker W et al. Plasma amino acid clearance as an indicator of hepatic function and high-energy phosphate in hepatic ischemia. Surgery 1987;102:777-783.
59. Border JR. Hypotheses: Sepsis, multiple systems organ failure, and the macrophage (editorial). Arch Surg 1988;123:285-286.
60. Matuschak GM, Rinaldo JE. Organ interactions in the adult respiratory distress syndrome during sepsis: Role of the liver in host defense. Chest 1988;94:400-406.
61. Matuschak GM. Liver-lung interactions in critical illness. New Horiz 1994;2:488-504.
62. Shelton BK. Disorders of hemostasis in sepsis. Crit Care Nurs Clin North Am 1994;6:373-387.
63. Pinsky MR, Matuschak GM. A unifying hypothesis of multiple systems organ failure: Failure of host defense homeostasis. J Crit Care 1990;5:108-114.
64. Ackerman MH. The systemic inflammatory response, sepsis, and multiple organ dysfunction—new definitions for an old problem. Crit Care Nurs Clin North Am 1994;6:243-250.

65. Hazinski MF. Mediator-specific therapies for the systemic inflammatory response syndrome, sepsis, severe sepsis, and septic shock. Crit Care Nurs Clin North Am 1994;6:309-319.
66. Beale R, Bihari DJ. Multiple organ failure: The Pilgrim's progress. Crit Care Med 1993;21:S1-S3.
67. Maynard et al. Dopexamine and gastric intra-mucosal pH in critically-ill patients. Supplement of proceedings of the 6th European Congress on Intensive Care Medicine. Intensive Care Med 1992;18(Suppl 2):176.
68. Tighe et al. Dopexamine hydrochloride maintains portal blood flow and alternates hepatic ultrastructural changes in a porcine peritonitis model of multiple system organ failure. Circ Shock 1993;39:199-206.
69. Chiarla C et al. Inhibition of posttraumatic septic proteolysis and ureagenesis and stimulation of hepatic acute-phase protein production by branched-chain amino acid TPN. J Trauma 1988;28:1145-1172.
70. Cerra FB et al. Septic autocannibalism: A failure of exogenous nutritional support. Ann Surg 1980;192:570-580.
71. Vente JP et al. Prospective randomized double-blind trial of branched-chain amino acid enriched versus standard parenteral nutrition solutions in traumatized and septic patients. World J Surgery 1991;15:128-133.
72. Kuhl DA et al. Use of selected visceral protein measurements in the comparison of BCAAs with standard amino acids in parenteral nutrition support of injured patients. Surg 1990;107:503-510.
73. Naylor CD et al. Parenteral nutrition with BCAAs in hepatic encephalopathy. Gastroenterology 1989;97:1033-42.
74. Billiar TR et al. Fatty acid intake and Kupffer cell function: Fish oil alters eicosanoid and monokine production to endotoxin stimulation. Surgery 1988;104:343-349.
75. Daly JM et al. Enteral nutrition with supplemental arginine, RNA, and omega-3 fatty acids in patients after operation: Immunologic, metabolic, and clinical outcome. Surg 1992;112:56-67.
76. Gielen CJ et al. Do diets enriched with oil prevent multiple organ failure in mice? Eur J Surg 1993;159:609-612.
77. Flynn WJ, Cryer HG, Garrison RN. Pentoxifylline but not saralasin restores hepatic blood flow after resuscitation from hemorrhagic shock. J Surg Res 1991;50:616-621.
78. Flynn WJ, Cryer HG, Garrison RN. Pentoxifylline restores intestinal microvascular blood flow during resuscitated hemorrhagic shock. Surg 1991;110:350-356.
79. Wang P et al. Mechanism of the beneficial effects of pentoxifylline on hepatocellular function after trauma hemorrhage and resuscitation. Surg 1992;112:451-458.
80. Matuschak GM, Martin DJ. Influence of end-stage liver failure on survival during multiple systems organ failure. Transplant Proc 1987;19:40-46.

CHAPTER *10*

Gastrointestinal System: Target Organ and Source of Multiple Organ Dysfunction Syndrome

Pamela Lash O'Neill

An increasing body of evidence suggests that the gut, long thought to be quiescent in critical illness, may play a pivotal role in the multiple organ dysfunction syndrome (MODS).[1] The hypothesis that the gut may be a major mediator in MODS is not a new one. In 1923 Cannon[2] proposed that the gut was a source of profound, irreversible shock. In the 1960s Fine[3] proposed that bacteria and endotoxin escaping from the gut were the source of systemic infection. These theories, however, fell into disfavor, in part because of contradictory data published by other investigators.[4] Now, 30 years later, it is well-recognized that the gut is indeed a vital organ in the MODS syndrome.

This chapter will discuss the anatomy and physiology of the gastrointestinal (GI) system as it relates to MODS and the pathophysiologic derangements specific to the gut in MODS. Clinical evidence of failure and the impact of the GI tract on MODS will be discussed, and, finally, treatment specific to the GI tract will be presented.

ANATOMY AND PHYSIOLOGY

In addition to its role in nutrient absorption, the GI system has important metabolic, immunologic, endocrine, and barrier functions. In particular, alterations in the barrier and immunologic capabilities of the gut affect its integrity, and many of the derangements seen in MODS are the result of, or compounded by, the breakdown of these normal physiologic defense mechanisms.

General morphology

Throughout the GI tract there are four morphologic layers of the luminal walls: the mucosa, the submucosa, the muscularis, and the serosa (Fig. 10-1). The mucosal layer is of primary importance in MODS and is further subdivided into three components: the epithelium, the lamina propria, and the muscularis mucosa, which consists of a thin smooth-muscle layer. The epithelium may form glands that extend into the lamina propria or the submucosa. In other regions, the epithelium may project into the lumen as fingerlike projections (villi) or folds (rugae or plicae) that enhance the effective surface area of the gut tremendously.

The lamina propria contains abundant lymphocytes and is a major site for immunologic responses in the gut.[5] The mucosa differs considerably in different regions of the GI tract and will be addressed in greater detail when the functional anatomy of each individual site is discussed.

Vascular physiology

The GI tract receives approximately 15% to 20% of the cardiac output in a resting person. The mucosa of the hollow organs receives the highest blood flow in the GI tract, and the muscle layer receives the lowest blood flow (Fig. 10-2). This flow distribution is, in part, related to the high metabolic demands of the mucosa during digestion, absorption, and secretion. Various factors regulate the blood flow to the GI tract (Fig. 10-3). Of particular inter-

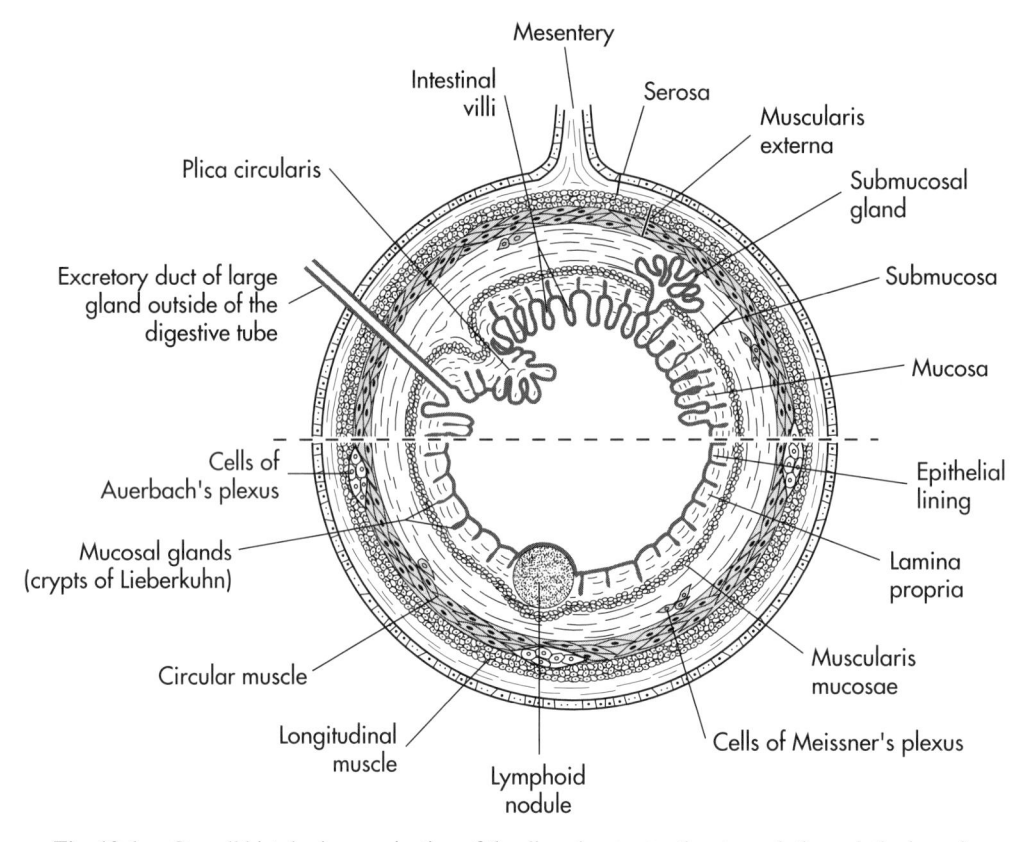

Fig. 10-1 Overall histologic organization of the digestive tract—the stomach through the large intestine. (From Bloom W, Fawcett DW. A textbook of histology. 10th ed. Philadelphia: WB Saunders. 1975; 599.)

Fig. 10-2 Detail of submucosal arteries. Note the arterial network of the mucosa. *M*, Mucosa; *ME*, muscularis externa; *MM*, muscularis mucosa; *S*, submucosa. (Modified from Barlow TE et al. Surgery, Gynecology & Obstetrics [Journal of the American College of Surgeons] 1951; 93: 668. From Larsen KR, Moody FG. In: Abramson PI, Dobrin PB, eds. Blood vessels and lymphatics in organ systems. New York: Academic Press, 1983; 412.)

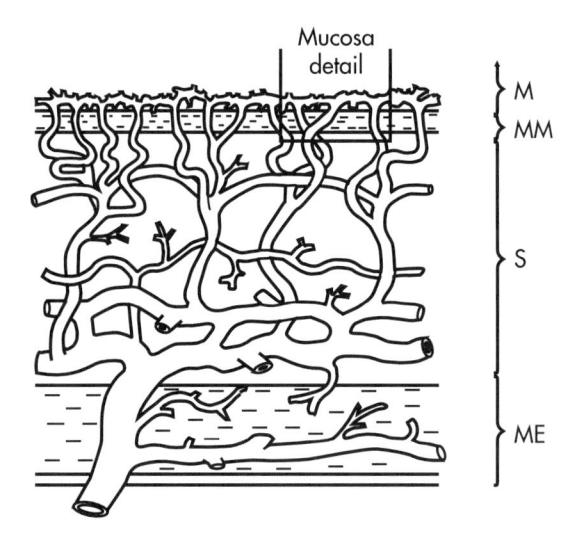

Gastrointestinal System 217

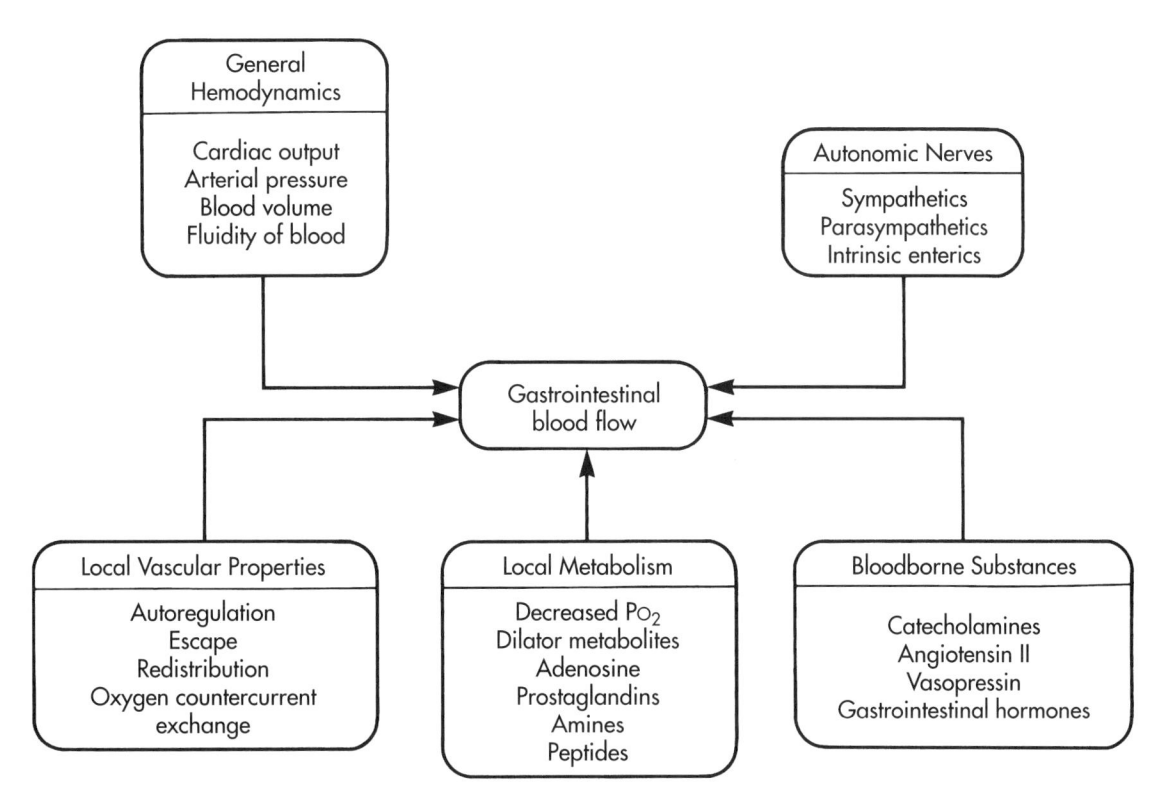

Fig. 10-3 Factors that regulate gastrointestinal blood flow. (From Jacobsen ED. In: Johnson LR, ed. Gastrointestinal physiology. 4th ed. St. Louis: Mosby, 1991; 144.)

est are the bloodborne substances and local vascular factors.

Neurohumoral substances are released from the kidney, the adrenal medulla, and other organs in response to stress, low-flow states, and other conditions associated with critical illness. Catecholamines (epinephrine and norepinephrine) and vasoactive peptides (angiotensin II) cause selective splanchnic vasoconstriction and compromise mucosal blood flow. The vasodilating metabolites, on the other hand, are released in response to increased organ function, for example, during ingestion and digestion of food. The local vascular properties of the GI tract include autoregulation, escape, redistribution, and the oxygen countercurrent exchange system.[6]

Autoregulation. Autoregulation is the ability of an organ system to maintain a steady blood flow despite fluctuations in systemic blood pressure. Organ systems that exhibit autoregulation include the brain, heart, liver, kidneys, and intestines. In general, systolic pressures from 80 to 160 mm Hg are sufficient to maintain the autoregulatory capacity within the GI tract. Any abrupt change in organ flow can cause autoregulation to fail, further compromising mucosal blood flow.

Escape. Escape is similar to autoregulation. Whereas autoregulation protects the gut from changes in systemic flow, the phenomenon of escape involves bloodborne substances, such as the catecholamines and angiotensin II, which act directly on the splanchnic resistance vessels. Although a transient fall in the blood flow through the gut occurs with this property, blood flow returns to normal within minutes because of an intrinsic escape mechanism that is not fully understood.[6]

Redistribution. Redistribution is a phenomenon that occurs secondary to stimulation of the sympathetic nervous system. In essence, blood flow is redistributed from the mucosa to the muscular layer of the gut. Although mucosal ischemia may occur, the total organ flow remains constant. By angiography, the blood flow through the superior mesenteric artery appears normal when, in fact, mucosal ischemia is present.[6]

Oxygen countercurrent exchange mechanism. An oxygen countercurrent exchange mechanism exists in the intestinal villi. Oxygen is progressively shunted from the arterial blood to the venule without going through the capillaries in the villus tip, thereby creating an oxygen gradient between the base and the tip of the villus (Fig. 10-4). Under steady-state conditions and with normal flow, the decrease in oxygen to the villus tip does not represent a significant problem. In low-flow states, however, the reduction in perfusion can lead to destruction of the luminal walls, with necrosis beginning at the villus tip and moving into the deeper layers of the gut wall.

Stomach

Functional anatomy. The stomach receives and stores ingested material, alters its composition to facilitate discharge into the duodenum, and delivers this processed substance (chyme) to the duodenum. The chyme is continually degraded until the size of the particulate matter is approximately 1 mm. It is then suspended as a liquid and moved through the pylorus.[7] In addition to their role in ingestion and digestion of food, the acidic juices of the stomach destroy ingested bacteria.

The capacity of the average stomach is 1 to 1.5 L. The stomach is divided into the cardia, the fundus, the body, the antrum, and the pylorus. The py-

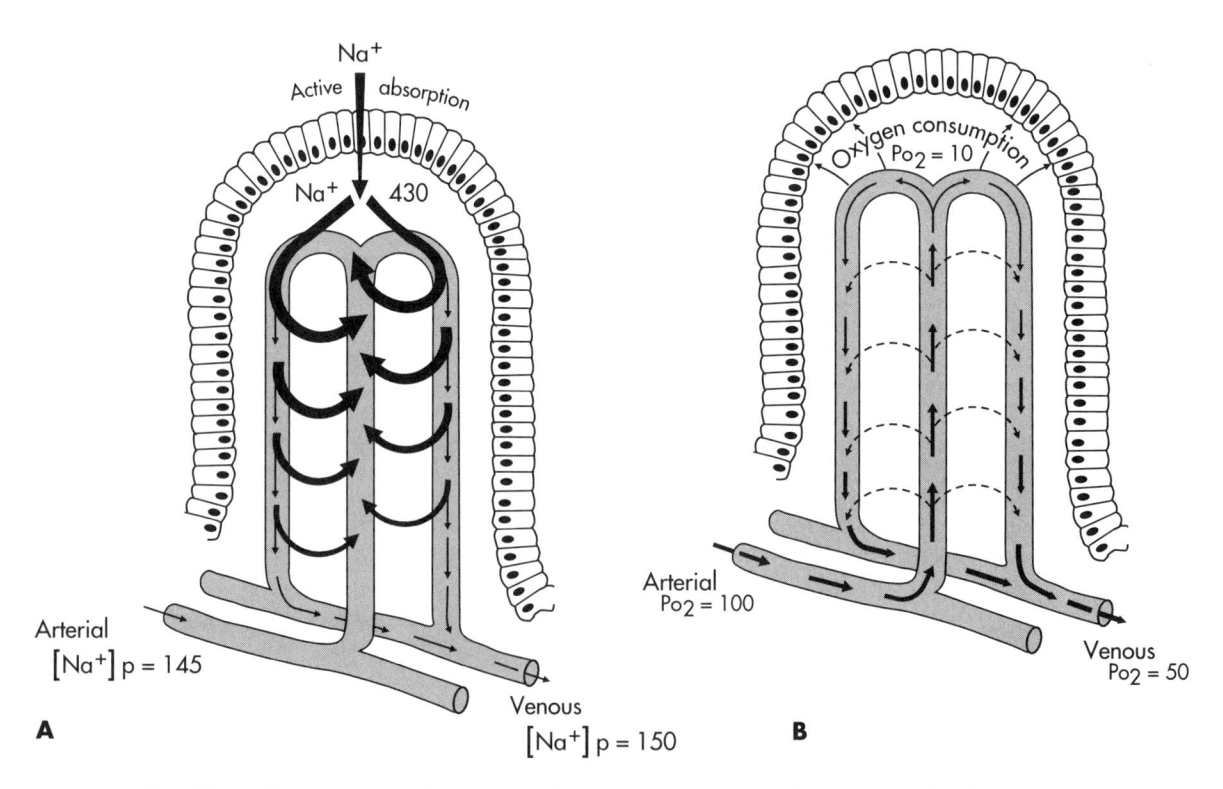

Fig. 10-4 The oxygen countercurrent exchange mechanism. **A,** sodium concentration increases at the villus tip during active absorption. **B,** a low partial pressure of oxygen at the villus tip caused by the short-circuit transfer of oxygen at the arteriole to the venule. (From Davenport H. Physiology of the digestive tract. 4th ed. St. Louis: Mosby, 1977;71.)

lorus regulates the passage of chyme into the duodenum, and the motility at the gastroduodenal junction functions as a barrier against reflux of duodenal contents into the stomach.

Blood supply. The blood supply to the stomach is derived primarily from the celiac trunk, which gives rise to the splenic, the left gastric, and the hepatic branches (Fig. 10-5). Increased blood flow to the stomach causes the rugae to fill and the mucosa to swell. Adequate flow is required for the stomach to secrete its digestive juices.

Secretory role. In the stomach, the mucosal surface is made up of columnar cells and contains individual glands that secrete pepsinogen, hydrochloric acid, or mucus. These secretory products are necessary for the digestion of ingested matter and the protection of the stomach.

Pepsinogen is converted to pepsin in the presence of hydrochloric acid. Pepsin hydrolyzes proteases and proteins to peptides. The optimal pH for pepsin activity is 1.2 to 2.4.[8] Thus the relative acidity of the stomach is necessary for effective digestive activity. Increasing the level of hydrochloric acid increases the conversion of pepsinogen to pepsin, which then converts ingested food to chyme. In addition, hydrochloric acid kills bacteria.

Mucus production in the stomach is stimulated by any irritation of the mucosa, such as the ingestion of food. The mucous layer provides lubrication and a mucosal barrier against luminal acids. This barrier function will be explored in greater detail later in this chapter as an essential defense mechanism within the GI tract. Hydrochloric acid, pepsinogen, and mucus sterilize and break down ingested material and then facilitate its transport to the duodenum for absorption.

Small intestine

Functional anatomy. The small intestine is divided into the duodenum, the jejunum, and the ileum; its primary function is to absorb nutrients. It also plays a role in the continued movement of

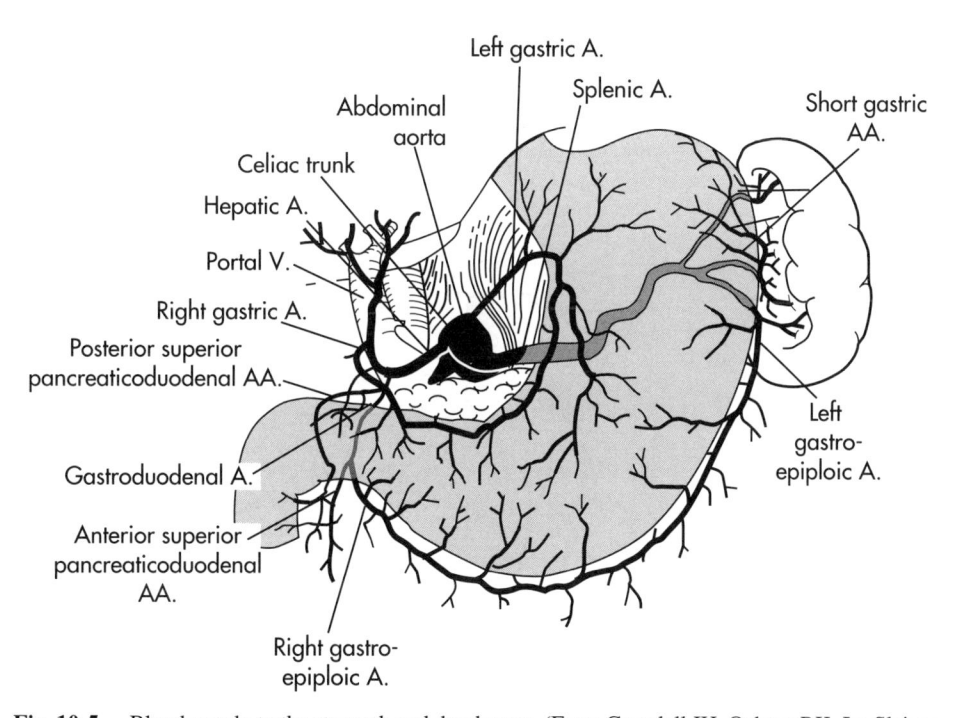

Fig. 10-5 Blood supply to the stomach and duodenum. (From Grendell JH, Ockner RK. In: Sleisenger MH, Fordtran JS, eds. Gastrointestinal disease: Pathophysiology, diagnosis, management. Vol. 2 Philadelphia: WB Saunders, 1989;1903.)

ingested substances along the intestinal tract for the purpose of elimination once absorption of nutrients has occurred.

Blood supply. The arterial supply to the small intestines is derived from the celiac artery and the superior and inferior mesenteric arteries. The celiac artery supplies blood to the mid-duodenum, and the superior mesenteric artery supplies blood from the mid-duodenum to the distal third of the transverse colon. The inferior mesenteric artery supplies blood from the distal third of the transverse colon to the anal canal (Figs. 10-5 and 10-6).

Secretory role. The digestive enzymes of the small intestine are not secreted but rather are integral parts of the brush border. The mucosal layer of the small bowel is covered with villi (Fig. 10-1) that contain glands. On the surface of the villi are hundreds of microvilli. Like the stomach, the mucosal layer of the small intestine receives the major portion of the blood supply. Because the mucosal folds and villi are less prominent in the distal part of the small intestine, almost half of the total mucosal surface is located in the first quarter of the small bowel. This is the predominant site of nutrient absorption.

Colorectum

Functional anatomy. The divisions of the colorectum include the cecum and the appendix; the ascending, the transverse, the descending, and the sigmoid colon; and the rectum. The colon functions in the absorption and final elimination of intestinal contents by reabsorbing water and secreting mucus to facilitate elimination of feces. The muscularis of the colon is divided into longitudinal bands that assist in elimination. The colon contains abundant quantities of lymphoid tissue that assist in

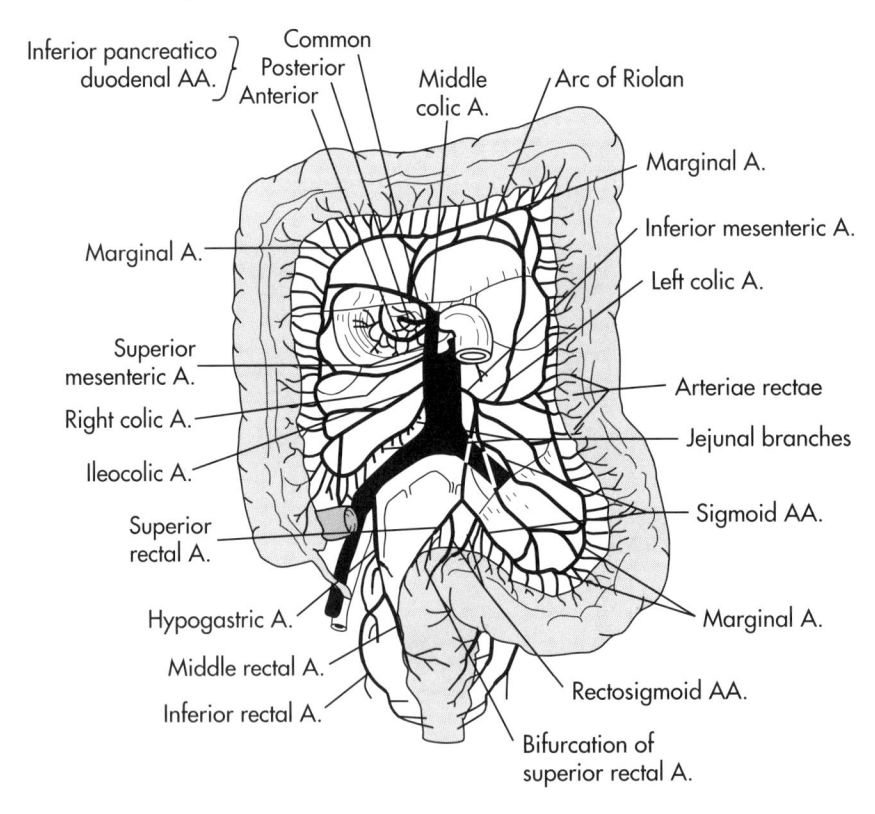

Fig. 10-6 Blood supply to the small and large intestine. (From Grendell JH, Ockner RK. In: Sleisenger MH, Fordtran JS, eds. Gastrointestinal disease: Pathophysiology, diagnosis, management. Vol. 2 Philadelphia: WB Saunders, 1989;1904.)

maintaining stability in the presence of pathogenic bacteria.

Blood supply. The superior mesenteric artery supplies the cecum, the right colon, and the transverse colon up to the splenic flexure. The inferior mesenteric artery feeds the descending colon and the proximal portion of the rectum. The hypogastric artery gives rise to the middle and rectal arteries that supply blood to the distal rectum (Fig. 10-6).

Secretory role and mucosa. The mucosa of the large intestine differs from that of the small intestine in that villi do not occur below the ileocecal valve. The colonic mucosa consists of crypts and surfaces between the crypts, which are covered by epithelial cells. The crypts and epithelial lining contain abundant mucus-producing cells. The small quantity of fluid secreted by the colon is highly alkaline and neutralizes fecal material. The outermost layer of mucus desquamates onto the fecal material, a process that facilitates fecal movement and eventual elimination from the body.[9]

GUT DEFENSES

A variety of mechanisms exist within the GI tract to preserve the overall integrity of the gut. The mucous barrier plays an essential role and protects the body by preventing translocation of the gut flora to extraintestinal sites. Motility assists in the mechanics of digestion and absorption while maintaining the flora within its proper environment. Gut immunity and acidity protect the gut against invasion by external pathogens and protect it from profound immunologic reactions against the normal gut flora. The flora present within the intestines assists in absorption and elimination. In MODS, these mechanisms are altered both by pathologic mechanisms and by therapeutic modalities that allow bacteria and their toxins access into and out of the GI lumen.

Gut barrier

Throughout the GI system, a barrier exists that is both physical and chemical. This barrier maintains GI integrity by protecting the wall of the gut from foreign or toxic substances. Potential pathogens normally found in the GI tract must be retained within the gut lumen. The barrier includes the tight junctions between the cells of the epithelial layer, the rapid turnover of the epithelial cells, and the mucous layer.

Epithelial cells. The tight junctions between the cells of the epithelium are essentially impervious to large antigenic molecules. The proliferative epithelium replaces itself at a very rapid rate, thus ensuring the integrity of the luminal walls and minimizing the adherence of the normal flora.

Mucous production. The mucous-bicarbonate barrier of the stomach protects the underlying epithelium from luminal acids. This function is accomplished by preventing hydrogen ions from diffusing backward along a gradient between the lumen and the mucosal interstitium. Secreted bicarbonate is maintained within this layer and forms a barrier of alkalinity between the epithelium and the luminal acid.[10]

Despite the efficiency of the mucous barrier, some back diffusion of acid to the mucosal layer does occur. Bicarbonate is supplied by the microvasculature to assist in the neutralization of these hydrogen ions. Increased hydrogen-ion concentration within the gastric lumen stimulates increased blood flow to the mucosa. Because bicarbonate is present in the microvascular circulation, the increased flow provides additional bicarbonate to neutralize the hydrogen ions.[11]

Mucous-producing cells are present in large numbers in the duodenum. Mucus secreted by the small intestine functions to lubricate the lumen and acts as a mechanical barrier by maintaining a neutral fluid layer along the mucosa. This mucous barrier is especially important in the duodenum, where influx of gastric acid is most likely to occur.

In the colon, the mucus is alkaline, and its production is stimulated by any irritation to the mucosa. In addition to protecting the intestinal wall from excoriation and providing the material for holding fecal matter together, the mucus protects the intestinal wall from bacterial activity within the feces. The alkalinity of the mucus provides a barrier that prevents acids formed within the feces from attacking the colonic wall.

Motility

Motility within the GI tract aids in the digestion and absorption of nutrients. In addition, it prevents bacteria in the distal small bowel and colon from migrating proximally into the sterile small intestine and stomach. The flushing action constantly keeps bacteria from adhering to the luminal wall, where penetration and translocation could occur.

In the stomach, motility maintains gut integrity by two mechanisms. If the ingested contents of the stomach are toxic, the vomiting center in the medulla is stimulated, and expulsion of gastric contents occurs. If the ingested substance is suitable for onward passage, gastric motility determines the form and speed at which the material is emptied into the duodenum. The motility at the gastroduodenal junction functions as a barrier against reflux of duodenal contents back into the stomach.

In the small intestine, contractions mix ingested food with digestive secretions, ensure contact of all intestinal contents with the mucosa, and facilitate transport to the colon. Both neural and gastrointestinal peptides control the motility of the small intestine.[12]

Colonic motility is designed for absorption and elimination of fecal matter. This is an important defense mechanism. The colon can move pathogens and potential carcinogens out of the body. In addition, normal motility ensures an even distribution of pressure along the colonic lumen and assists in protecting the integrity of the colonic wall.

Gut immunity

The gut is a reservoir of potentially pathogenic bacteria and, as such, has an extremely complicated immune system that assists in recognizing and destroying pathogens. This system also neutralizes the response of the body to the toxins that are normally present in the distal small bowel and colon.

Dispersed aggregates of nonencapsulated lymphoid tissue, known as gut-associated lymphoid tissue (GALT), are found in the submucosa of the GI tract. These lymphoid cells accumulate in the lamina propria of the intestinal wall or in Peyer's patches.[13] A large number of the B lymphocytes of the lamina propria bear surface immunoglobulin A (IgA). In addition, the Peyer's patches contain a large number of B lymphocytes that are dedicated to the synthesis of IgA antibody. Secretory IgA plays a major role in preventing the attachment of luminal bacteria to mucosal cells.[14] It predominates in the gut secretions and is extremely resistant to enzymatic degradation.

After synthesis, secretory IgA is delivered to epithelial cells in the mucous membrane where it binds to bacteria and prevents their attachment to the cells. It works in conjunction with the normal flora of the gut, which also binds to the mucous membrane cells. These resident bacteria consume nutrients and release metabolites that are toxic to pathogenic bacteria.

The bactericidal activity of the stomach includes digestion of bacteria and the secretory IgA–bacteria complex. Food ingestion stimulates secretions of the salivary glands and stomach. These secretions support the growth of commensal bacteria and assist in keeping the oropharynx and esophagus clean. Food ingestion also stimulates the growth and replication of GALT and mucus-secreting enterocytes.[15]

Although the tight junctions of the GI epithelium are essentially impervious to large antigenic molecules, ingestion of some bacterial toxins may still occur. Macrophages of the lamina propria assist in phagocytizing and removing these. Also, local synthesis of antibodies in the GALT and the evolution of a non–complement-fixing immunoglobulin isotype ensure that the reaction is minimized. Tissue-damaging immune responses are well suppressed in the mucosa.

During immunosuppressed states, it appears that an intact gut mucosa is an effective barrier against transepithelial migration of luminal contents.[16] This mucosal barrier suggests that the cell-mediated immunity of the GI tract may play a secondary role in the maintenance of overall gut integrity.

Gastric acid

In the healthy human stomach, intragastric pH varies widely, but studies have recorded a gastric pH of 1 to 2 for extended periods.[17] The acidity in the stomach is essential in protecting it from ingested bacteria and toxins. Acidity also plays an important role in intestinal defense, since it prevents bacteria or pathogens from entering the small bowel. After ingestion of food, gastric pH may rise transiently, but as digestion continues, the pH drops back to less than 4, which is generally sufficient to kill bacteria.[18] The importance of gastric acidity as a gut defense is evident in studies that have demonstrated increased gastric and jejunal colonization in patients with impaired gastric acid secretion.[19-21]

Commensal bacteria

Acid within the stomach maintains gastric sterility and also prevents migration of live organisms into the duodenum, thereby promoting sterility in the proximal small bowel; however, the distal bowel contains a normal flora that is highly complex and

Table 10-1 The Effects of Dietary Change on Bacteria in the Ileum

Dietary change	Effect
Increased dietary fiber	Increase in all organisms
Increased dietary protein	Increase in aerobic organisms
	No change in anaerobic organisms
Increased dietary fat	Increase in total anaerobes and *Bacteroides* organisms
	No effect on aerobic organisms

From Hill M. Bacterial factors. In: Losowsky MS, Heatley RV, eds. Gut defenses in clinical practice. Edinburgh: Churchill Livingstone; 1986; 148.

Table 10-2 The Composition of the Fecal Bacterial Flora

Organisms	Mean number/g feces
Bacteroides spp.	10^{11}
Gram-positive nonsporing rods	10^{11}
Bifidobacteria	
Propionibacteria	
Eubacteria	
Veillonella spp.	10^{15}
Clostridium spp.	10^6
Lactobacillus spp.	10^7
Escherichia coli and other coliform bacteria	10^7
Streptococci—total	10^7
—fecal	10^5
Bacillus spp.	10^3
Yeasts and fungi	10^3

From Hill M. Bacterial factors. In: Losowsky MS, Heatley RV, eds. Gut defenses in clinical practice. Edinburgh: Churchill Livingstone; 1986; 148.

very stable in healthy humans. Control is maintained by bacteria-bacteria and host-bacteria interactions.

The ileum contains a large number of both aerobic and anaerobic bacteria. Aerobes in the ileum include *Escherichia coli, Streptococcus faecalis,* and *Lactobacillus* and *Staphylococcus* organisms, and anaerobes include *Bacteroides, Bifidobacterium, Clostridium,* and *Veillonella* organisms.[22,23] It is of interest to note that dietary intake is a major factor influencing the bacterial population in the ileum (Table 10-1).

The bacterial flora is prolific in the large bowel and consists of a number of species (Table 10-2). The count and type of flora remain fairly constant, and fecal flora is essentially unaffected by dietary intake.[24] A symbiotic relationship exists between the mucosa and the GI flora. In fact, the bacteria found in the gut are thought to be part of the key defense of the GI system against invasion by pathogens. The normal flora competes with pathogenic species for nutrients and attachment sites and also produces inhibitory substances. Any alteration in the normal flora in the colon may actually allow overgrowth of such pathogenic organisms as *Clostridium difficile, Staphylococcus aureus,* and *Candida albicans.*[24]

PATHOPHYSIOLOGY

In ischemic and inflammatory events, the GI tract is injured and normal gut function is altered, which leads to pathophysiologic derangements. Figure 10-7 depicts the causes and effects of splanchnic ischemia. The primary events include a breakdown in the mucosal barrier, changes in the intramural pH, and alterations in the normal gut flora. These events can occur as a result of the maldistribution of circulating volume and the tissue perfusion deficits seen in MODS. The gut becomes a "victim," or a target organ in the process. However, MODS can exist in the absence of an identifiable source of infection, with symptoms mimicking intraabdominal sepsis. This phenomenon has led to the hypothesis that the gut may, in some instances, initiate MODS.[25]

Gut as a target organ in MODS

Because the GI luminal mucosa is highly vascular, it is extremely sensitive to ischemic changes. In ischemic events, the extent of destruction occurs along a time-dependent continuum: the longer the period of ischemia, the greater the mucosal damage. The effects on the gastric and the intestinal mucosa are somewhat different because of differences in their functional anatomy.

Mucosal ischemia. The stomach is susceptible to ischemic injury, such as that occurring in septic states. Increased acid production, along with increased permeability and mucosal ischemia, contributes to the development of stress ulcers. Gastric mucosal ischemia is seen in 80% of the patients

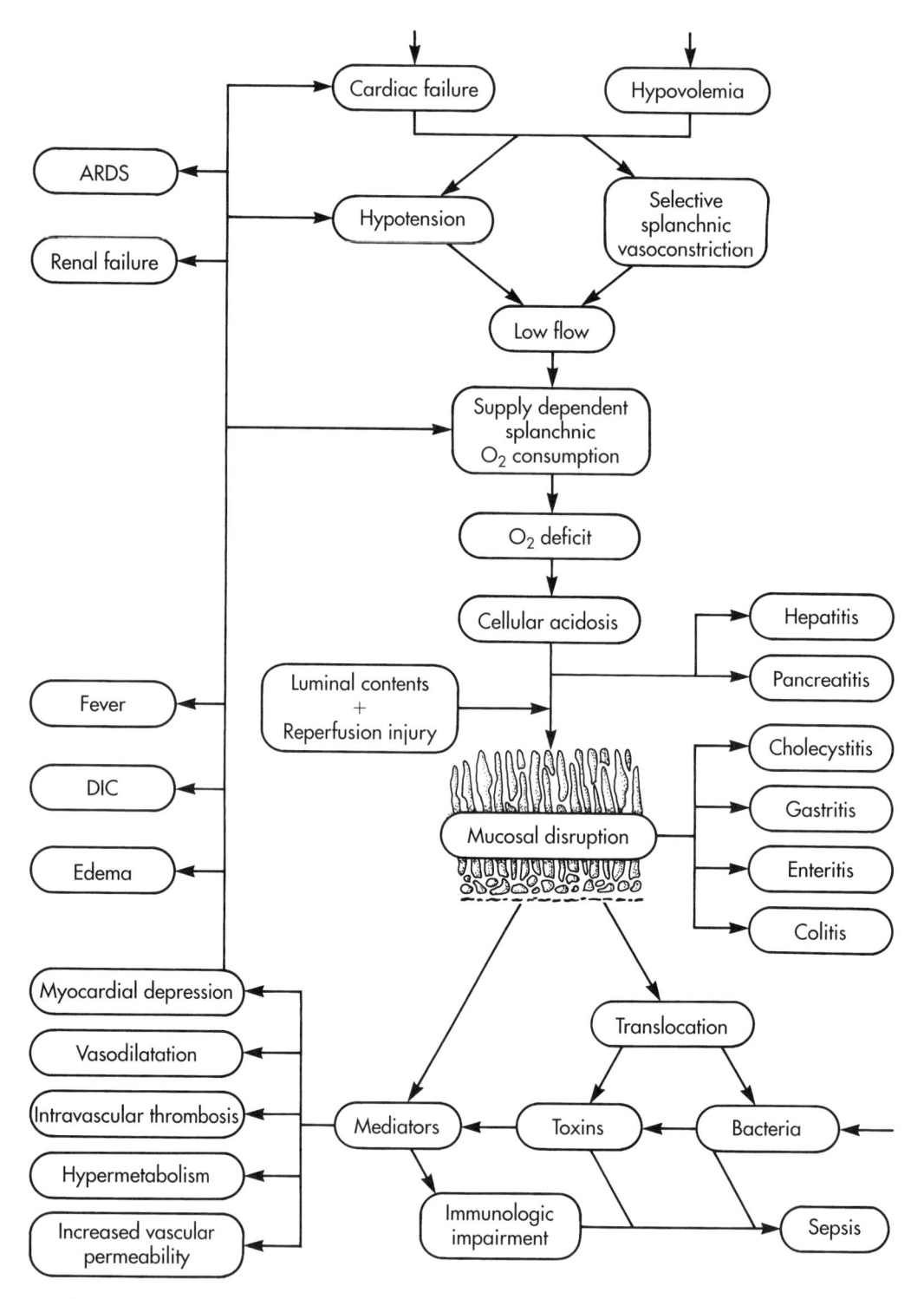

Fig. 10-7 Causes and effects of splanchnic ischemia. (From Marston A, Bulkley GB, Fiddian-Green RG, Haglund UH, eds. Splanchnic ischemia and multiple organ failure. London: Hodder and Stoughton Ltd. 1989; inside front page.)

with MODS and may be one of the earliest manifestations of core tissue perfusion in the critically ill.[26] Use of antacids to prevent stress ulceration may lead to bacterial overgrowth in the stomach and proximal small bowel. This overgrowth occurs secondary to proliferation of the nosocomial organisms residing in the pharynx or organisms from contaminated enteral feedings.[27]

The intestinal mucosa is also subject to ischemic injury.[28] Within minutes of superior mesenteric artery occlusion, ultrastructural changes are evident in the mucosal cells. In the small bowel, ischemia causes the basement membrane of the surface epithelium to detach. As the ischemic insult continues, subepithelial blebs develop. These blebs rupture, causing separation of the epithelium from the villus tips. The separation then causes an increase in capillary permeability and allows passage of plasma proteins, blood, and interstitial fluid into the intestinal lumen.

If the ischemic event is gradual, collateral circulation may develop, and infarction rarely occurs. However, rapid ischemia causes mucosal infarction within 1 to 2 hours after initiation of the ischemia, and transmural infarction occurs within 8 to 10 hours.[26] Sloughing off of intestinal mucosal cells, along with a decrease in mucus production and an increase in capillary permeability, has been demonstrated in dog models.[28,29]

Endogenous vasoconstrictors released as a consequence of sepsis and inflammation exacerbate the mucosal damage (see Chapter 3). Endogenous vasoconstrictors affecting the splanchnic circulation include angiotensin II, vasopressin, thyrotropin-releasing hormone (TRH), and prolactin. Of these mediators, angiotensin II is responsible for the selective splanchnic vasoconstriction seen in circulatory shock.[30] The vasoconstrictive effects of these destroy the luminal walls further.

Impairment of motility. Motility is also adversely affected in critical illness. Ingested food is a strong stimulus for gut motility. Total parenteral nutrition (TPN) may be initiated in the acute phase of critical illness when the patient is unable to tolerate enteral feedings. The initiation of TPN is associated with mucosal atrophy and decreased gut motility.[31-33]

Motility functions to remove gut debris. The loss of motility (ileus), coupled with colonization of bacteria throughout the GI tract, may facilitate the migration of bacteria into areas that are normally sterile, such as the proximal GI tract.

Antibiotic administration. Antibiotic use is common in critically ill patients. However, antibiotic therapy can cause overgrowth of bacteria by altering the normally stable flora within the colon.[34] Exposure of the intestinal bacteria to systemic antibiotics causes the development of a population of organisms that is resistant to these antibiotics. These highly resistant and pathogenic organisms overgrow in the GI tract rapidly when the competing, but non-resistant, organisms are killed. Translocation of these organisms may occur via the mesenteric lymph nodes.[35,36]

Reperfusion injury. It has been suggested that bowel ischemia and reperfusion may promote failure of the gut barrier and translocation of bacteria by releasing oxygen-derived free radicals, anaphylatoxins, and thromboxane. These mediators contribute to further inflammation and disruption of the gut mucosal barrier and may allow bacteria or endotoxin to leak into the systemic or portal circulations.[37] During ischemic events, hypoxic metabolism generates cytotoxic substances through xanthine oxidase pathways (see Chapter 5).

Degradation of adenine nucleotide compounds (adenosine triphosphate [ATP] and adenosine diphosphate [ADP]) produces hypoxanthine and xanthine. Upon reperfusion of the ischemic tissue, the newly delivered oxygen reacts with the hypoxanthine, xanthine, and xanthine oxidase. By-products of this reaction include uric acid and oxygen-derived free radicals. Oxygen-derived free radicals mediate lipid peroxidation within the cell during reperfusion and cause cell injury. It is the reperfusion injury with the subsequent development of arachidonate metabolites and inflammatory agents that further exacerbates splanchnic ischemia.[38]

Summary. With the breakdown of the mucosal barrier, translocation of viable organisms or bacterial products such as endotoxin across the gut mucosal barrier represents a mechanism whereby gut organisms can produce systemic infection, inflammation, and shock by triggering the release of inflammatory mediators. Substances from the GI tract move across the injured and dying gut and into the circulation. The entry of these metabolites into the circulation produces profound toxemia. Death is the end result.

These mechanisms (bacterial translocation and activation of the inflammatory response) demonstrate the effect of systemic alterations that occur within the gut secondary to MODS. In addition, there is evidence to suggest that the phenomenon of translocation may occur before the onset of MODS and may, in fact, initiate the syndrome (Fig. 10-8).

Etiologic role of the gut in MODS

Some investigators hypothesize that initiation or progression of MODS may occur secondary to the effect of inflammatory mediators released into the blood stream in response to gut mucosal ischemia. Researchers have demonstrated that gut ischemia and reperfusion induce injury in remote organs independent of endotoxin.[39] This has led to the suggestion that the gut may actually be the motor driving irreversible shock and MODS.[25]

Bacterial translocation. Bacterial translocation involves the egress of bacteria or their toxins across the mucosal barrier into the lymphatics or the portal circulation. This phenomenon has also been referred to as the gut leak syndrome or the hyperpermeable gut. Ample evidence supports the theory of translocation in animal studies, but its role in humans remains unclear.* Mechanisms associated with bacterial translocation include (1) compromised host defenses; (2) alteration in normal GI flora, especially proliferation secondary to bowel stasis; and (3) alteration in gut membrane permeability secondary to perfusion deficits, inflammatory mediators, and septic states. Although the actual mechanism for the migration of intestinal bacteria or their products to extraintestinal sites is unknown, Figure 10-9 depicts a theory of translocation.

Defense mechanisms. Host defenses, specifically the GALT, defend against invading pathogens and protect against extraluminal proliferation of bacte-

---

*References 16, 35, 36, 40-42.

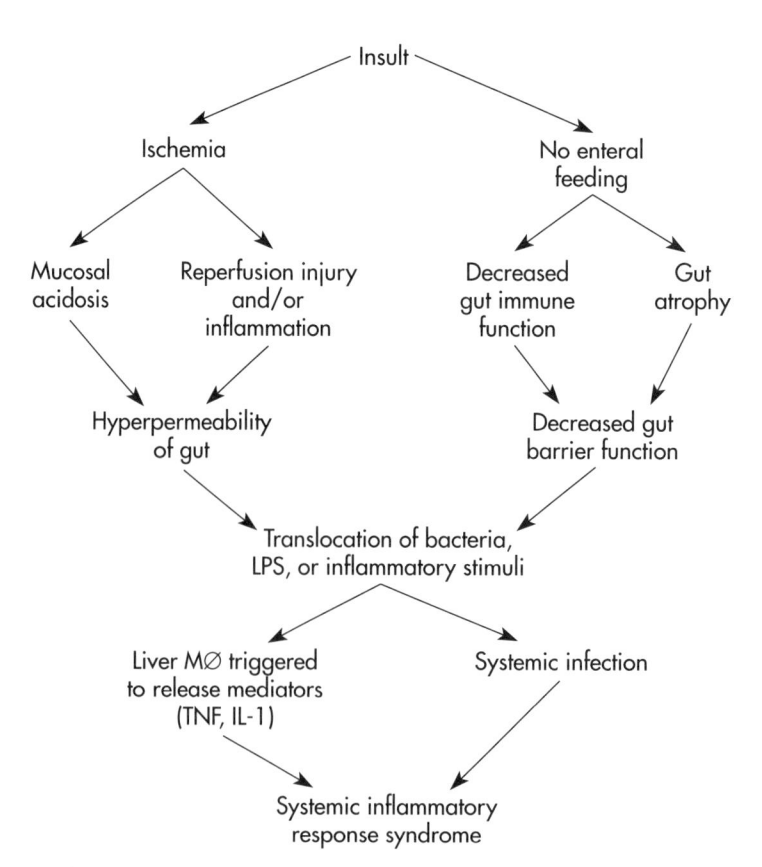

Fig. 10-8 A schematic representation of the role of the gut in the development of systemic inflammation and MODS. (Courtesy Virginia Huddleston Secor.)

ria. When these defenses are compromised, such as in immunosuppressed states, the GALT is no longer able to ward off invading pathogens. In fact, Wells and co-workers have postulated that luminal bacteria are ingested by intestinal macrophages, transported to extraintestinal sites, and then released from the dead or dying macrophages.[43] Hence, the gut macrophages may actually facilitate translocation.

Kupffer cells (liver macrophages) play an important role in the maintenance of GI integrity and bacterial containment. Impaired Kupffer cell function may facilitate translocation by allowing translocating bacteria or endotoxin to reach the systemic circulation.[41] The role of Kupffer cells is discussed in greater depth in Chapter 9.

The normal gut flora prevents the overgrowth of more pathogenic bacteria. When the gut flora is altered, as with antibiotic use, these pathogens proliferate and attach to the mucosa. This proliferation is a key factor in the translocation process.

Summary. Gut barrier integrity is maintained by an intact mucosa. This barrier protects the entire body by minimizing the entry of pathogens into the GI system and preventing egress of normal gut flora into the systemic circulation. Unfortunately, impaired gut barrier function facilitates bacterial translocation.

Translocation has been demonstrated in normal humans following ingestion of live *Candida albicans*.[44] The fact that translocation can occur in the absence of sepsis and shock supports the hypothesis that the gut plays a pivotal role in the initiation of the MODS process.

CLINICAL PRESENTATION AND ASSESSMENT

Although the indicators of gut failure are not as immediately apparent as those associated with other organ systems, the extremely high mortality associated with MODS warrants closer observation and

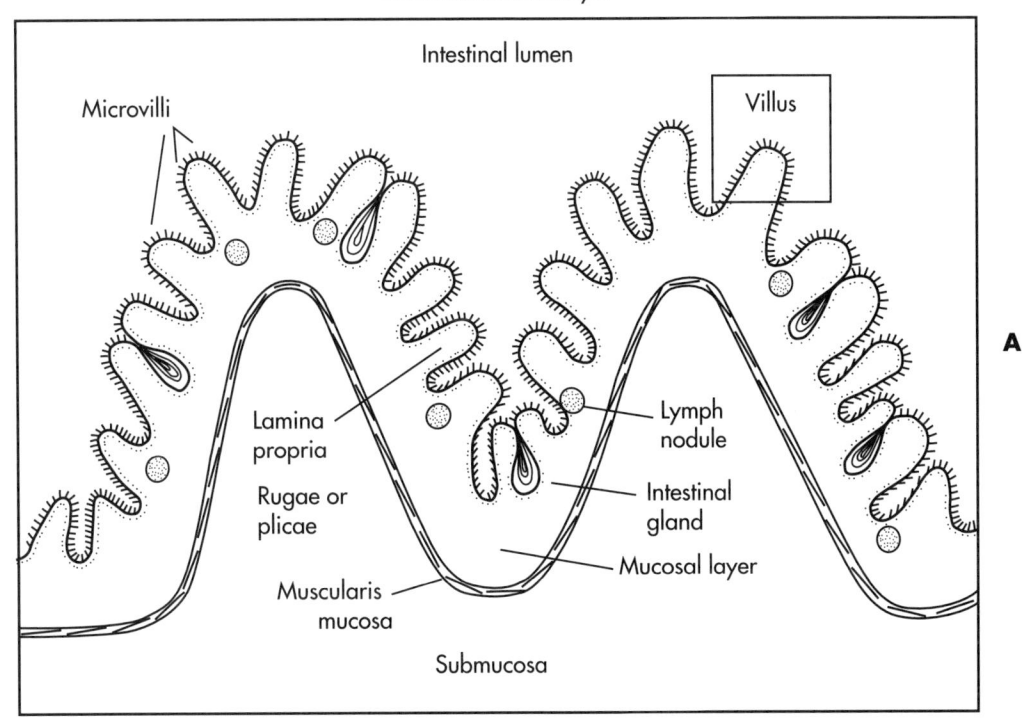

Fig. 10-9 Hypothesized mechanism of bacterial translocation from the gut. **A,** Longitudinal view of the morphologic layers of the small intestine.

Continued

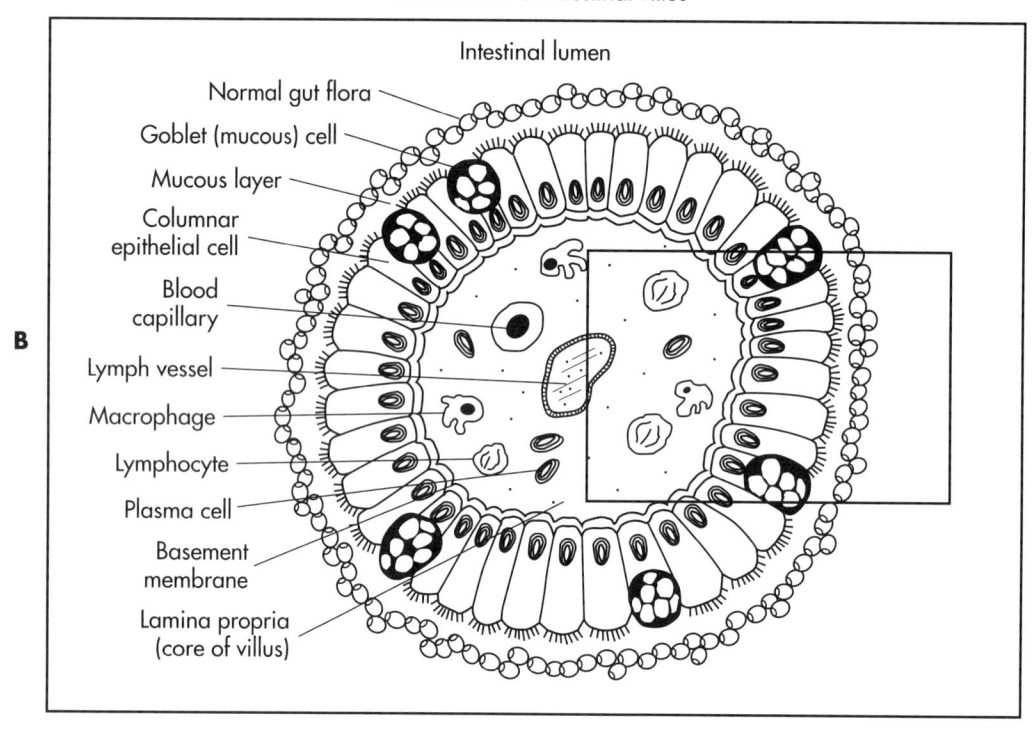

228 *Organ Involvement and Clinical Presentation*

Fig. 10-9, cont'd **B,** Cross-sectional view of the normal intestinal villus.

early intervention to improve the outcome. This is especially true for the gut.

Ileus and gastrointestinal bleeding

Development of an ileus and GI bleeding are common responses of the gut to critical illness. However, these are often late manifestations of a compromised gut that occur secondary to the breakdown of the mucous barrier and impairment of intestinal motility. Diarrhea and guaiac-positive stools may occur secondary to the breakdown of the gut barrier and result from the movement of plasma, interstitial fluid, and blood into the intestinal lumen.[45,46] These are later, nonspecific signs that may result after mucosal damage has already occurred.

Overgrowth of pathogenic bacteria

Use of antibiotics, diarrhea, and alterations in GI motility can promote bacterial overgrowth in the small and large bowel. Normal anaerobes may decrease in numbers, with a subsequent increase in coliform bacteria (*Klebsiella, Proteus,* and *Enterobacter* species). Alterations in bacterial counts on stool culture may be another indicator of gut compromise secondary to bacterial overgrowth.

Presence of enteric organisms in blood cultures

Enteric organisms are often seen in blood cultures from critically ill patients. In fact, the occurrence of enteric bacteremias with no septic focus has led to the hypothesis that the gut might initiate the MODS syndrome by releasing bacteria, yeast, or endotoxin from the GI tract into the portal and lymphatic systems.[25,47] The presence of enteric organisms in blood cultures, in the absence of a septic focus, may be an early indicator that translocation of organisms is occurring.

Elevated gastric output

Gastric output can increase for a number of reasons, including delayed emptying, increased production of gastric secretions, and reflux of material

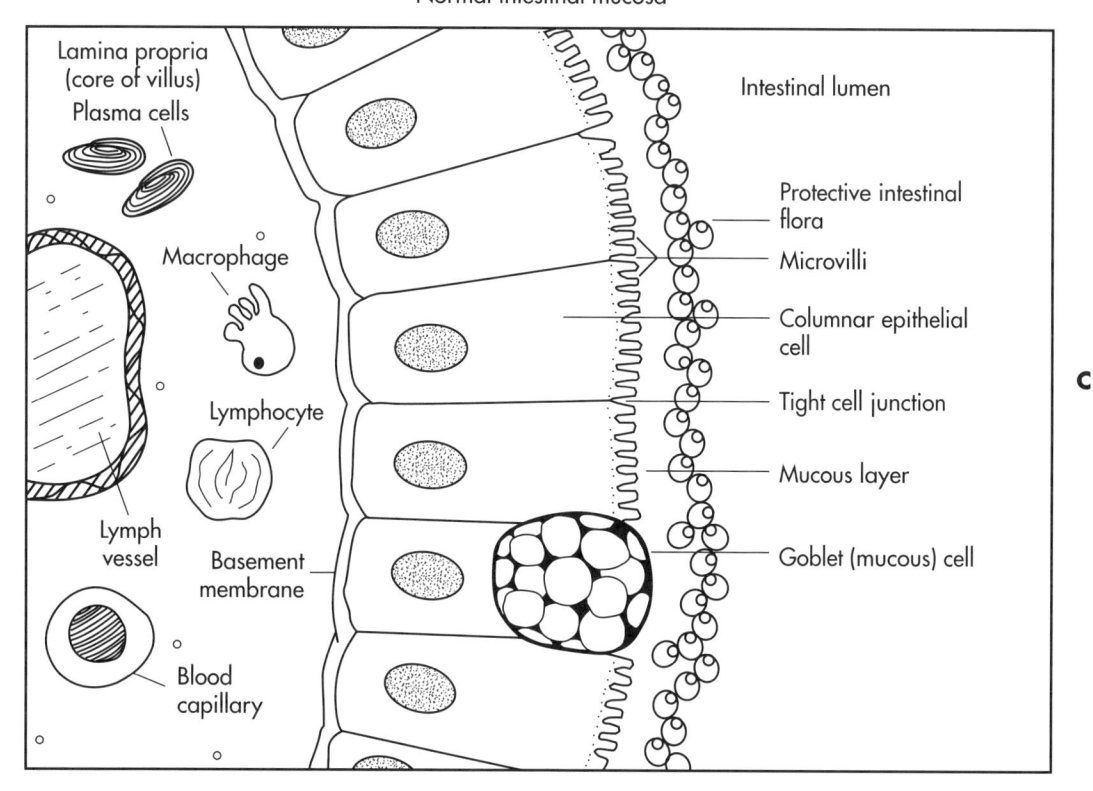

Fig. 10-9, cont'd C, Detail of normal intestinal villus. The structural and functional components of the normal villus assist in maintaining overall gut integrity. Protective intestinal flora compete with pathogenic species for nutrients and attachment sites and produce inhibitory substances. Mucous production prevents adherence of pathogens to the luminal walls. Epithelial cells of the GI tract regenerate at a rapid rate to ensure continued gut integrity of the mucous layer. Tight cell junctions are essentially impervious to large antigenic molecules, and they prevent paracellular transmission of microbes into the plasma component. A network of gut-associated lymphoid tissue, located in the lamina propria, protects the gut by preventing absorption or proliferation of anaerobes.

Continued

from the duodenum into the stomach. Although increased gastric output may be attributed to a number of factors, it may be an early indicator of a compromised gut.

Endoscopic ulcerations or erosions

Shock states have been shown to produce stress ulcers in laboratory animals. In dog models, septic shock produces bleeding gastric erosions within 2 days, and in rabbits, hemorrhagic shock causes gastric ulcers.[48,49] For this reason, ulcerative lesions seen on endoscopy can be a diagnostic indicator of mucosal compromise. Endoscopy will provide a definitive diagnosis for ulceration in approximately 90% of the cases, and this can lead to early treatment measures (such as stress ulcer prophylaxis) designed to minimize mucosal injury and maintain gut integrity.

Abdominal distention

Abdominal distention can occur secondary to alterations in motility and excess gas production. The overgrowth of bacteria causes bacterial interactions that produce gas, and the alterations in gut function and motility prevent the gas from escaping the body. Distention may also be an early indicator of gut compromise.

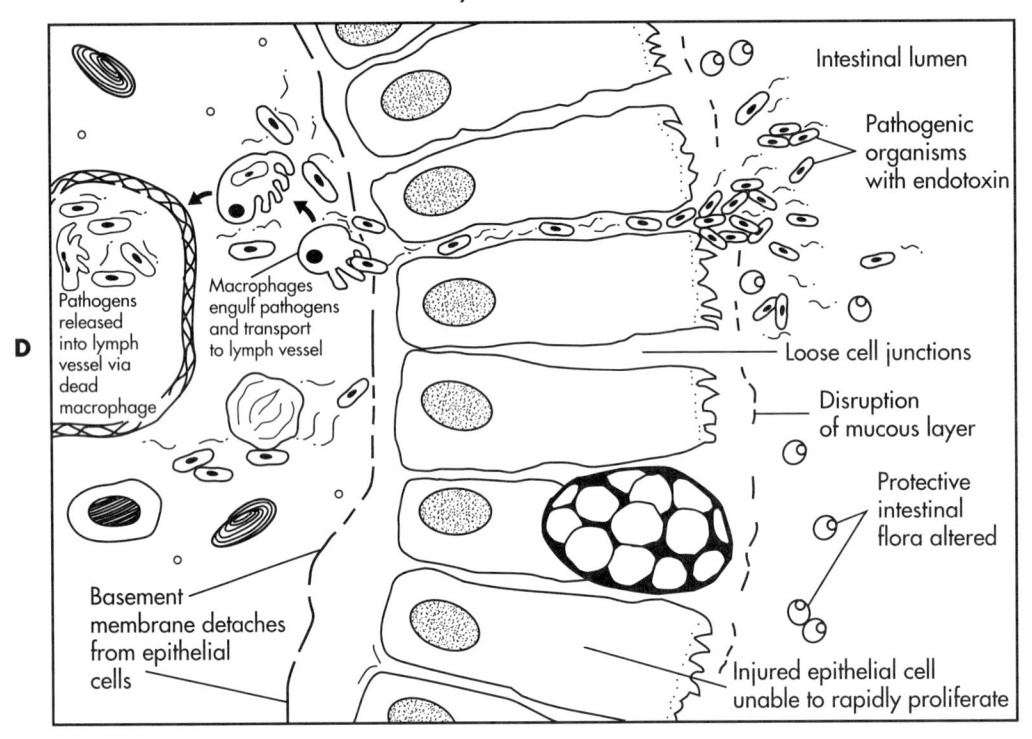

Fig. 10-9, cont'd **D,** Impaired intestinal villus. Dissolution of normal gut flora and alterations in mucous production allow pathogens to adhere to and colonize the luminal surface. Loose cell junctions and alterations in membrane integrity further compromise the mucous layer and allow transmission of bacteria or endotoxin into the lamina propria (core of the villus). Although the exact mechanism of translocation is unknown, it has been hypothesized that the intestinal bacteria are ingested by gut macrophages. From here, they are transported to extraintestinal sites via the lymph system, and liberated upon lysis of the macrophages. (Courtesy Sheila Easley, RN, Dallas, Texas.)

Mucosal pH

Routine measurement of intramucosal pH by gastric tonometry may prevent complications caused by mucosal ischemic injury (Fig. 10-10). A balloon-tipped catheter is inserted into the stomach or the sigmoid colon, and the intramural pH is calculated. Fiddian-Green and co-workers[50,51] have correlated low intramural pH values with a poor prognosis in critically ill patients. A normal pH indicates adequate perfusion, and an acidic pH is associated with tissue hypoxia. Improved methods for monitoring visceral perfusion, such as gastric tonometry, may be the hallmark for improved patient outcome.[52] Treatment can then be initiated early and effectively, with increased survival and shortened hospital stays as the ultimate goal.

In general, the symptomatology of gut compromise is nonspecific. Pathogenic bacteria in stool culture, enteric organisms in blood culture, or elevated gastric output may or may not occur with marked gut compromise. Guaiac-positive stools or nasogastric aspirates are not always present in patients with an infarcted gut.[26] A definitive diagnosis of mucosal damage is, at best, difficult. Few diagnostic tools specific to GI function are available to assist the clinician. Direct measurement of mucosal pH may be one of the best and earliest indicators of organ perfusion and gut compromise.

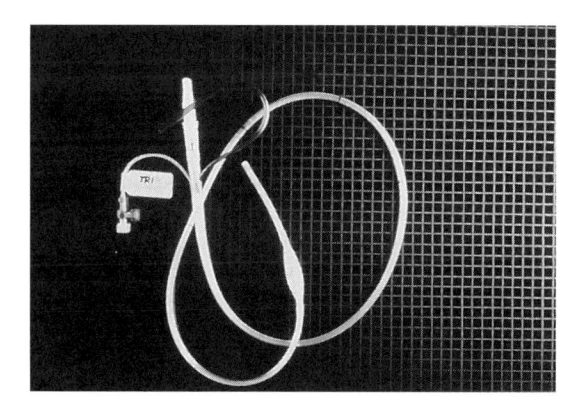

Fig. 10-10 The TRIP® nasogastric suction catheter. (Courtesy Tonometrics Division of Instrumentarium Corporation.)

THERAPEUTIC MANAGEMENT

One does not usually think of "organ-specific" therapy in relation to the GI tract. Even when nutritional support is aggressively managed, it is not so much in relation to the gut as it is to the metabolic demands of the patient. This premise, however, is beginning to change. Because it is sensitive to ischemic insult, acidosis, and the inflammatory response and because, when injured, it can trigger systemic manifestations, the gut is now becoming a focal point in managing the patient with MODS. Surgical drainage, stress ulcer prophylaxis, and enteral feedings remain the standards of therapy for managing and preventing GI pathology. Overall, the best treatment for the ischemic GI tract is restoration of flow in the microcirculation, with adequate oxygen and nutrient delivery. The assessment of systemic parameters, such as oxygen delivery and consumption, and regional measures, such as gastric tonometry, aid in guiding therapy (see Chapter 17). Various standard and investigational therapies for managing the gut in critical illness are presented below.

Surgical drainage

A common cause of MODS is intraabdominal sepsis, which has an associated mortality rate of 60% to 90%.[53,54] Abdominal exploration should be considered for any patient who exhibits persistent evidence of mucosal ischemia, such as gastrointestinal bleeding, ulcerations, and low intramural pH values. The greater the period of ischemia, the higher the incidence of complete transmural infarction of the luminal wall, and the greater the mortality.

Although various studies show that early and repeated drainage of intraabdominal abscesses does not reverse MODS in the majority of patients,[55] it is clearly a desirable therapeutic measure when compared with the alternative. In addition, there are studies that substantiate that draining purulent loculations may reverse intramucosal acidosis and therefore reduce mortality.[56] However, the use of empiric laparotomy remains controversial.

Stress ulcer prophylaxis

Antacid therapy. Traditionally, antacids were thought to protect the stomach and duodenum from erosion by maintaining a neutral pH in the presence of mucosal breakdown and increased production of luminal acids. However, indiscriminate use of antacids can result in bacterial overgrowth in the stomach and the proximal small bowel. The GI tract may also become colonized by nosocomial organisms from the pharynx.[57] In addition, undesirable side effects such as diarrhea, hypermagnesemia, or alkalemia can result from antacid therapy.[58]

Histamine antagonists. Histamine antagonists (H_2 blockers) are used as an alternative or as an adjunct to antacid therapy. Since histamine is a stimulus for acid production, H_2 blockers antagonize acid secretion. In addition, intraluminal acids may impair hemostatic mechanisms[59]; therefore, H_2 blockers have been used in treating significant gastric bleeding. However, histamine is not the only stimulus for acid secretion, and the use of H_2 blockers does not guarantee control of pH.[60] In addition,

Lunde and co-workers have demonstrated a significant decrease in mucosal blood flow after the administration of cimetidine, clearly an undesirable effect in terms of maintaining overall gut integrity.[61] H_2 blockers may also contribute to bacterial colonization of the proximal GI tract.

Sucralfate. Sucralfate is an alternative to standard stress ulcer prophylaxis in the critically ill patient. Sucralfate is a nonabsorbable aluminum salt (sucrose octasulfate) with little or no effect on gastric acid secretion. Its therapeutic actions include antibacterial properties,[62] the exertion of trophic effects on the gastric mucosa, the ability to bind pepsin and bile acids, and the ability to coat existing ulcers with a protective layer.[63] Sucralfate may also prevent stress ulcers by stimulating bicarbonate, mucus, and prostaglandin release and by stimulating mucous cell renewal.[63]

The gastric acid barrier is very important in the pathogenesis and prevention of ventilator-associated pneumonia. Maier and co-workers have demonstrated that sucralfate is as efficacious as maximum H_2 blocker therapy for prophylaxis of stress ulcers. Further, their study suggests that sucralfate may have a beneficial effect on the incidence of nosocomial pneumonia.[64] Thus sucralfate is becoming an increasingly important agent in the prophylactic management of stress ulcers.

Selective decontamination

There is considerable interest in using systemic, oral, or topical oropharyngeal antibiotics in the prophylactic treatment of bacterial translocation in critical illness. This treatment regimen is known as selective decontamination of the digestive tract (SDD). The goal of therapy is to decrease the number of aerobic and anaerobic organisms in the oropharynx and gut and yet maintain adequate numbers of obligate anaerobes in the mucous membrane. Therapy is based on the hypothesis that many infections in critically ill patients are caused by endogenous bacteria from the oropharynx and the GI tract that are either aspirated into the lungs or that translocate across the gut barrier and into the systemic circulation.

Several studies support the theory that SDD of the gut with oral nonabsorbable antibiotics reduces the incidence of translocation by reducing colonization of the oropharynx, the digestive tract, and the respiratory tract with aerobic gram-negative organisms.[65,66]

Despite the evidence in favor of SDD, concerns exist about the risk of selecting for antibiotic-resistant bacterial strains. Further, the effectiveness of SDD for long-term survival is questionable.[67,68] Continued investigation of SDD is essential before employing it as standard clinical practice in the prophylactic treatment of bacterial translocation in MODS.

Vasodilator agents

Splanchnic vasodilators, such as papaverine hydrochloride, have been employed in the clinical management of patients with nonocclusive mesenteric ischemia.[69] Studies on cat models have demonstrated that blood flow can be increased tenfold in the small and large intestines with infusions of vasodilators.[70] Other studies have demonstrated the return of normal pH in the gastric mucosa in response to low-dose dopamine.[71] This practice, however, remains controversial, and the risks may substantially outweigh the benefits.

Use of vasodilator agents is based on the theory that the therapy may override the effects of endogenous vasoconstrictors.[72] Opponents argue that many of the vasodilating drugs used exert a selective effect and may exert a "steal" syndrome, or may have opposing actions in different regions of the circulatory system.[73] In addition, some vasodilators may increase oxygen use, and the effects of individual vasodilators may be substantially different. Although many questions remain unanswered concerning the efficacy of vasodilator therapy on gut failure, better monitoring techniques, such as tonometry (which measures the adequacy of perfusion to the gut), may substantiate its validity.

Enteral feedings

Enteral feedings have been heralded as important in the treatment of the gut in MODS.[74] Enteral feeding stimulates mucosal cell turnover. In fact, the presence of food in the gut has been cited as the most important stimulus for mucosal growth.[75] In addition, the feedings stimulate hormones that have trophic effects on the gut mucosa. They also assist in the sloughing off of mucosal cells, thereby promoting new cell growth. In essence, enteral feedings prevent intestinal mucosal atrophy. Adequate enteral feedings early in the treatment of MODS appear to improve the function of the gut barrier by maintaining or promoting mucosal integrity.[76-78] Further, Nelson and co-workers suggest that the addition of dietary fiber to enterally administered diets may decrease bacterial translocation by decreasing the number of bacteria in the cecum.[79]

Glutamine

Glutamine is an important nutrient that supports cell growth and replication. Although present in small quantities in enteral feedings, it is not routinely present in TPN solutions. In fact, Alverdy and co-workers and Spaeth and co-workers[32,33] demonstrated that TPN actually promotes bacterial translocation. For this reason, glutamine is thought to play an essential role in the prevention of translocation.

In studies in which glutamine was substituted for other nonessential amino acids in TPN, mucosal thickness and protein content were significantly increased in the jejunum, ileum, and colon.[80] Glutamine-containing enteral or parenteral feedings have been associated with improved survival after gut mucosal injury.[80,81] More recently, however, Deitch noted that while fiber and glutamine had beneficial effects on the mucosa, they did not affect bacterial translocation. Thus he postulates that enteral feedings are far superior to TPN in maintaining gut barrier function.[31] Studies on the addition of specific growth factors to the diet have demonstrated increased mucosal growth as well, and the interaction of these growth factors with glutamine may maximize mucosal healing.[82] For further information on nutritional support in MODS, see Chapter 7.

Immunotherapy

Endotoxin is a constituent of the cell wall of gram-negative bacteria. Because of the detrimental effects that occur after its release from the bacterial cell wall, it has been studied extensively. Much attention has been focused on preventing endotoxemia from intestinal causes, along with endotoxemia from other sources. Studies have indicated that immunotherapy with monoclonal antibodies against endotoxin improves survival in cases where endotoxemia is a key factor leading to morbidity. Human trials have demonstrated improved survival after infusion of an antiendotoxin monoclonal antibody in patients with bacteremia and sepsis.[83,84] However, there have been questions concerning the validity of these studies.[85]

Recently, the effects of antibodies to murine interleukin-6 (IL-6) have been reviewed. IL-6 appears to play a major role in the systemic changes that occur secondary to bacterial translocation. Reducing IL-6 levels with an anti–IL-6 antibody may improve outcome.[86] More research is needed on the efficacy of treatment with antimediator antibodies and of other monoclonal antibody therapy. Although there is growing support for using immunotherapy to lessen the effects of systemic inflammation, intestinal endotoxemia, and translocation, the effects on patient outcome are much less clear.

Preventing reperfusion injury

Reperfusion injury is an important factor in the pathogenesis of GI mucosal injury. The injury occurs when ischemic tissue is reperfused and toxic oxygen metabolites, such as oxygen-derived free radicals, and other inflammatory mediators are generated. The longer the period of mucosal ischemia, the more significant a role reperfusion plays in cell injury and death. There is evidence to suggest that free radicals mediate, to some extent, the effects of endotoxin on the gut.[87] Agents such as allopurinol and superoxide dismutase (SOD) may limit mucosal damage by minimizing reperfusion injury.[39,88-90] Timely and aggressive intervention to prevent reperfusion injury may limit the extent of injury and improve survival with the gut-associated complications of MODS (see Chapters 3 and 5).

Intraluminal oxygenation

It has been suggested that intraluminal oxygenation may prevent the intestinal mucosal injury caused by intestinal ischemic events.[91] Animal studies thus far have demonstrated that intestinal mucosa deprived of its blood supply shows a decrease in endotoxin translocation and mortality when intraluminal oxygenation is utilized.[92,93]

Intraluminal oxygenation in animals has been accomplished by perfusing the gut lumen with oxygenated fluids. Fink and Fiddian-Green suggest that in humans this may be accomplished by circulating gaseous oxygen through a nasogastric tube.[69] They note that one of the problems encountered has been the difficulty of perfusing long segments of the gut

Table 10-3 Summary of Gut Responses in MODS

Gut defense	Evidence of failure	Treatment options
Barrier	Guaiac-positive stools Acid pH on tonometry Ulcerations or erosions on endoscopy	Surgical drainage Vasodilator drugs Prevent reperfusion injury: allopurinol or SOD Enteral feedings Glutamine Immunotherapy: monoclonal antibodies Intraluminal oxygenation
Motility	Ileus Distention High gastric output	Enteral feedings Glutamine
Gut immunity	Nonspecific	Support of all gut defenses
Gastric acid	Ulcerations or erosions on endoscopy GI bleeding	Stress ulcer prophylaxis Enteral feedings
Gut flora	Bacterial overgrowth on stool culture Abdominal distention Diarrhea	Selective decontamination Enteral feedings Glutamine

GI, Gastrointestinal; *SOD*, superoxide dismutase.

at a rate that would effectively oxygenate the mucosa distal to the infusion.

Although all of the experience to date has been based on animal experiments, an intraluminal membrane oxygenator has been efficacious in providing uniform oxygenation of the mucosal surface.[94] Intraluminal oxygenation may provide an answer to the problem of management of gut ischemia and maintenance of gut integrity.

CONCLUSION

The gut plays a key role in the MODS process. Table 10-3 summarizes gut defenses, clinical evidence of failure, and treatment modalities. As research continues, more information becomes available on the interaction of the gut with other organ systems and how it is affected by the process. If the gut is an etiologic factor in MODS development and progression as has been suggested, it is of the utmost importance to intervene and stop the cascade of events that culminates in MODS. As a target organ, the gut extends the damage to the whole individual and exacerbates the MODS syndrome. Improvement in monitoring and management will translate into decreased mortality and morbidity—the ultimate goal of therapy.

REFERENCES

1. Marshall JC, Christou NV, Meakins JL. The gastrointestinal tract: The undrained abscess of multiple organ failure. Ann Surg 1993;218:111-119.
2. Cannon WB. Traumatic shock. New York: Appleton; 1923.
3. Fine J. Current status of the problem of traumatic shock. Surg Gynecol Obstet 1965;120:537-544.
4. Nagler AL, Zweifach BW. Pathogenesis of experimental shock. II. Absence of endotoxic activity in blood of rabbits subjected to graded hemorrhage. J Exp Med 1961;114:195-204.
5. Padykula HA. The digestive tract. In: Weiss L, Greep RO, eds. Histology. New York: McGraw-Hill; 1977:643-700.
6. Jacobsen ED. The gastrointestinal circulation. In: Johnson LR, ed. Gastrointestinal physiology. St Louis: Mosby; 1985:140-155.
7. Meyer JH et al. Sieving of solid food by the canine stomach and sieving after gastric surgery. Gastroenterology 1979;76:804-813.
8. Smith JN. Essentials of gastroenterology. St Louis: Mosby; 1969.
9. Davenport HW. Intestinal secretion. In: Davenport HW, ed. Physiology of the digestive tract. 4th ed. St Louis: Mosby; 1977:161-165.
10. O'Brien PE. Gastric acidity: The gastric microvasculature and mucosal disease. In: Marston A, Bulkley GB, Fiddian-Green RG, Haglung UH, eds. Splanchnic ischemia and multiple organ failure. London: Hodder and Stoughton, Ltd; 1989:145-157.
11. Silen W, Merher A, Simson JN. The pathophysiology of stress ulcer disease. World J Surg 1981;5:165-174.

12. Sarna S et al. Intrinsic nervous control of migrating myoelectric complexes. Am Physiol 1981;4:G16-G23.
13. Lydyard P, Grossi C. The lymphoid system. In: Roitt I, Brostoff J, Male D, eds. Immunology. 2nd ed. London: Gower Medical Publishing; 1989:3.1-3.10.
14. Mayrhofer G. Physiology of the intestinal immune system. In: Newby TJ, Stokes CR, eds. Local immune responses of the gut. Boca Raton: CRC Press; 1984:1-96.
15. Border JR et al. The gut origin septic states in blunt multiple trauma. Ann Surg 1987;206(4):427-448.
16. Berg RD. Translocation of indigenous bacteria from the intestinal tract. In: Hentges DJ, ed. Human intestinal microflora in health and disease. Orlando: Academic Press. 1983;15:333-352.
17. Pounder RE et al. Effect of cimetidine on 24 hour intragastric acidity in normal subjects. Gut 1976;17:133-138.
18. McCloy RF, Baron JH. Intragastric pH and cimetidine, fasting and after food. Lancet 1981;1:609-610.
19. Ruddell WS et al. Gastric juice nitrite: A risk factor for cancer in the hypochlorhydric stomach. Lancet 1976;2:1037-1039.
20. Katz LA, Spiro HM. Gastrointestinal manifestations of diabetes. N Engl J Med 1966;275:1350-1361.
21. Reed PI et al. Gastric juice N-nitrosamines in health and gastroduodenal disease. Lancet 1981;2:550-552.
22. Hori S et al. The effect of dietary fibre on the bacterial flora of ileostomy fluid. J Med Microbiol 1983;16:VIII.
23. Fernandez F et al. Effect of changes in amount of dietary protein and fat on the composition of ileostomy bacterial flora. J Med Microbiol 1983;16:XV.
24. Hill M. Bacterial factors. In: Losowsky MS Heatley RV, eds. Gut defences in clinical practice. Edinburgh: Churchill Livingstone; 1986:147-154.
25. Meakins JL et al. The surgical intensive care unit: Current concepts in infection. Surg Clin North Am 1980;60:117-122.
26. Fiddian-Green RG. Splanchnic ischaemia and multiple organ failure in the critically ill. Ann R Coll Surg Engl 1988;70:128-134.
27. Driks MR et al. Nosocomial pneumonia in intubated patients given sucralfate as compared with antacids or histamine type two blockers. N Engl J Med 1987;317:1376-1382.
28. Fink MP, Antonsson JB, Wang H, Rothschild HR. Increased intestinal permeability in endotoxic pigs. Arch Surg 1991;126:211-218.
29. Gottlieb JE, Menashe PI, Cruz E. Gastrointestinal complications in critically ill patients: The intensivists' overview. Am J Gastroenterol 1986;81:227-238.
30. Reilly PM, Bulkley GB. Vasoactive mediators and splanchnic perfusion. Crit Care Med 1993;21(2suppl): S55-S66.
31. Deitch EA. Bacterial translocation: The influence of dietary variables. Gut 1994;35(1suppl): S23-S27.
32. Alverdy JC, Aoys E, Moss GS. Total parenteral nutrition promotes bacterial translocation from the gut. Surgery 1988;104:185-190.
33. Spaeth G et al. Food without fiber promotes bacterial translocation from the gut. Surgery 1990;108:240-247.
34. Marshall JC et al. The microbiology of multiple organ failure—the proximal gastrointestinal tract as an occult reservoir of pathogens. Arch Surg 1988;123:309-315.
35. Wells CL, Jechorek RP, Erlandsen SL. Evidence for the translocation of Enteroccus faecalis across the mouse intestinal tract. J Infect Dis 1990;162:82-90.
36. Jackson RJ, Smith SD, Rowe MI. Selective bowel decontamination results in gram positive translocation. J Surg Res 1990;48:444-447.
37. Zhi-Yong S, Yuan-Lin D, Xiao-Hong W. Bacterial translocation and multisystem organ failure in bowel ischemia and reperfusion. J Trauma 1992;32:148-153.
38. Longhurst JC, Benham RA, Rengig SV. Increased concentration of leukotriene B4 but not thromboxane B2 in intestinal lymph of cats during brief ischemia. Am J Physiol 1992;262:H1482-H1485.
39. Deitch EA et al. A study of the relationships among survival, gut-origin sepsis, and bacterial translocation in a model of systemic inflammation. J Trauma 1992;32:141-147.
40. Antonsson JB, Fiddian-Green RG. The role of the gut in shock and multisystem organ failure. Arch Surg 1991;157:3-12.
41. Deitch EA. The role of intestinal barrier failure and bacterial translocation in the development of systemic infection and multiple organ failure. Arch Surg 1990;125:403-404.
42. Goris RJ et al. Multiple organ failure and sepsis without bacteria: An experimental model. Arch Surg 1986;121:897-901.
43. Wells CL et al. Intestinal bacteria translocate into experimental intraabdominal abscesses. Arch Surg 1986;121:102-107.
44. Krause W, Matheis H, Wulf K. Fungaemia and funguria after oral administration of Candida albicans. Lancet 1969;2: 598-599.
45. Bounous G et al. Biosynthesis of mucin in shock: Relation to hemorrhagic enteritis and permeability to curare. Ann Surg 1966;164:13-22.
46. Bounus G. Acute necrosis of intestinal mucosa. Gastroenterology 1982;82:1457-1467.
47. Norton LW. Does drainage of intra-abdominal pus reverse multiple organ failure? Am J Surg 1985;149:347-350.
48. Menguy R, Masters YF. Mechanisms of stress ulcer. III. Effects of hemorrhagic shock on energy metabolism in the mucosa of the antrum, corpus, and fundus of the rabbit stomach. Gastroenterology 1974;66:1168-1176.
49. Odonkor P, Mowat C, Himal HS. Prevention of sepsis-induced gastric lesions in dogs by cimetidine via inhibition of gastric secretion and by prostaglandin via cytoprotection. Gastroenterology 1981;80:375-379.
50. Fiddian-Green RG, Amelin PM, Baker S. The predicted value of the pH in the wall of the stomach for complications after cardiac operations: A comparison with other forms of monitoring. Crit Care Med 1987;15:153-156.
51. Fiddian-Green RG, Gantz NM. Transient episodes of sigmoid ischemia and their relation to infection from intestinal organisms after abdominal aortic operations. Crit Care Med 1987;15:835-839.
52. Fiddian-Green RG. Associations between intramucosal acidosis in the gut and organ failure. Crit Care Med 1993;21(2suppl):103-107.
53. Fry DE et al. Multiple system organ failure. Arch Surg 1980;115:136-140.
54. Eiseman B, Beart R, Norton L. Multiple organ failure. Surg Gynecol Obstet 1977;14:323-326.

55. Norton LW. Does drainage of intraabdominal pus reverse multiple organ failure? Am J Surg 1985;149:347-350.
56. Fiddian-Green RG et al. Predictive value of intramural pH and other risk factors for massive bleeding from stress ulceration. Gastroenterology 1983;85:613-620.
57. Hillman KM et al. Colonization of gastric contents in critically ill patients. Crit Care Med 1982;10:444-447.
58. Derrida S et al. Occult gastrointestinal bleeding in high-risk intensive care unit patients receiving antacid prophylaxis: Frequency and significance. Crit Care Med 1989;17:122-125.
59. Green FW et al. Effect of acid and pepsin on blood coagulation and platelet aggregation. Gastroenterology 1978;74:38-43.
60. Noseworthy TW et al. A randomized clinical trial comparing ranitidine and antacids in critically ill patients. Crit Care Med 1987;15:817-819.
61. Lunde OC, Kvernebo K, Larsen S. Effect of pentagastrin and cimetidine on blood flow measured by laser doppler flowmetry. Scand J Gastroenterol 1988;23:151-157.
62. Tryba M, Mantey-Stiers F. Antibacterial activity of sucralfate in human gastric juice. Am J Med 1987;83(suppl 3B):125-127.
63. Tarnawski A, Hollander D, Gergely H. The mechanism of protective, therapeutic, and prophylactic actions of sucralfate. Scand J Gastroenterol 1987;22(suppl 140):7-13.
64. Maier RV, Mitchell D, Gentillelo L. Optimal therapy for stress gastritis. Ann Surg 1994;220:353-360.
65. Ulrich C et al. Selective decontamination of the digestive tract with norfloxacin in the prevention of ICU-acquired infections: A prospective randomized study. Intensive Care Med 1989;15:424-431.
66. Hartenauer U et al. Effect of selective flora suppression on colonization, infection, and mortality in critically ill patients: A one-year prospective consecutive study. Crit Care Med 1991;19:463-473.
67. Goris RJ et al. Does selective decontamination of the gastrointestinal tract prevent multiple organ failure? Arch Surg 1991;126:561-565.
68. Cerra FB et al. Selective gut decontamination reduces nosocomial infections and length of stay but not mortality or organ failure in surgical intensive care unit patients. Arch Surg 1992;127:163-169.
69. Fink MP, Fiddian-Green RG. Care of the gut in the critically ill. In: Marston A, Bulkley GB, Fiddian-Green RG, Haglung UH, eds. Splanchnic ischemia and multiple organ failure. London: Hodder and Stoughton, Ltd.; 1989:377-386.
70. Boley SJ et al. Initial results from an aggressive roentgenologic and surgical approach to acute mesenteric ischemia. Surgery 1977;82:848-855.
71. Hulten L, Lindhagen J, Lundgren O. Sympathetic nervous control of intramural blood flow in feline and human intestines. Gastroenterology 1977;72:41-48.
72. Boley SJ, Brandt LJ. Selective mesenteric vasodilators: A future role for mesenteric ischemia? Gastroenterology 1986;91:247-249.
73. Bulkley GB et al. Collateral blood flow in segmental intestinal ischemia: Effects of vasoactive agents. Surgery 1986;100:157-166.
74. Baue AE. Nutrition and metabolism in sepsis and multisystem organ failure. Surg Clin North Am 1991;71:549-565.
75. Inoue S et al. Prevention of yeast translocation across the gut by a single enteral feeding after burn injury. JPEN 1989;13:565-571.
76. Kudsk KA et al. Enteral versus parenteral feeding: Effects of septic morbidity after blunt end and penetrating abdominal trauma. Ann Surg 1992;215:503-513.
77. Epstein MD, Banducci DR, Manders EK. The role of the gastrointestinal tract in the development of burn sepsis. Plast Reconstr Surg 1992;90:524-531.
78. Bragg LE, Thompson JS, Rikkers LF. Influence of nutrient delivery on gut structure and function. Nutrition 1991;7:237-243.
79. Nelson JL et al. Influence of dietary fiber on microbial growth in vitro and bacterial translocation after burn injury in mice. Nutrition 1994;10: 32-36.
80. Jacobs DO et al. Trophic effects of glutamine-enriched parenteral nutrition on colonic mucosa. JPEN 1988;12, 1(suppl):6.
81. Alexander JW. Nutrition and translocation. JPEN 1990; 14(5suppl):170S-174S.
82. Wilmore DW et al. The gut: A central organ after surgical stress. Surgery 1988;104:917-923.
83. Ziegler EJ et al. Treatment of gram-negative bacteremia and septic shock with HA-1A human monoclonal antibody against endotoxin: A randomized double-blind, placebo-controlled trial. The HA-1A Sepsis Study Group. N Engl J Med 1991;324:429-436.
84. Greenman RL et al. Controlled clinical trial of E% murine monoclonal IgM antibody to endotoxin in the treatment of gram-negative sepsis. JAMA 1991;266:1097-1102.
85. Warren HS, Danner RL, Munford RS. Antiendotoxin monoclonal antibodies. N Engl J Med 1992;326:1153-1157.
86. Gennari R et al. Effects of antimurine interleukin-6 on bacterial translocation during gut-derived sepsis. Arch Surg 1994;129:1191-1197.
87. Deitch EA et al. Inhibition of endotoxin-induced bacterial translocation in mice. J Clin Invest 1989;84:36-42.
88. Smith SM et al. Gastric mucosal injury in the rat: Role of iron and xanthine oxidase. Gastroenterology 1987;92:950-956.
89. Sanfey H, Bulkley GB, Cameron JL. The role of oxygen-derived free radicals in the pathogenesis of acute pancreatitis. Ann Surg 1984;200:405-412.
90. Nordstrom G, Seeman T, Hasselgren PO. Beneficial effect of allopurinol in liver ischemia. Surgery 1985;97:679-683.
91. Haglund U. Therapeutic potential of intraluminal oxygenation. Crit Care Med 1993:2(2 suppl);69-71.
92. Shute K. Effect of intraluminal oxygen on experimental ischemia in the intestine. Gut 1976;17:1001-1006.
93. Shute K. Effect of intraluminal oxygen on endotoxin absorption in experimental occlusion of the superior mesenteric artery. Gut 1977;18:567-570.
94. Fiddian-Green RG et al. Early detection of intestinal ischemia in dogs by intraluminal tonometry and reversal with intraluminal membrane oxygenators. Proc Surg Res Soc S Africa, Cape Town, March 1984.

SUGGESTED READINGS

Baue AE. Gastrointestinal tract—an active metabolic organ that can fail. In: Multiple organ failure: Patient care and management. St Louis: Mosby; 1990:364-373.

Collins AS. Gastrointestinal complications in shock. Crit Care Nurs Clin North Am 1990;2:269-277.

Deitch EA. Gut failure: Its role in the multiple organ failure syndrome. In: Multiple organ failure: Pathophysiology and basic concepts of theory. New York: Thieme Medical Publishers; 1990:40-59.

Fink MP. Why the GI tract is pivotal in trauma, sepsis, and MOF. J Crit Illness 1991;6(3):253-276.

Gallavan RH, Parks DA, Jacobsen ED. Pathophysiology of intestinal circulation. In: Schultz SG, Wood JD, Rauner BB, eds. The handbook of physiology—Section 6: The gastrointestinal system. Vol 1, Part 2. Bethesda: American Physiological Society, 1989:1713-1732.

Grendell JH, Ockner RK. Vascular diseases of the bowel. In: Sleisenger MH, Fordtran JS, eds: Gastrointestinal disease: Pathophysiology/diagnosis/management. 4th ed. Vol 2. Philadelphia: WB Saunders; 1989: 1903-1932.

Marston A, Bulkley GB, Fiddian-Green RG, Haglung UH, eds. Splanchnic ischemia and multiple organ failure. London: Hodder and Stoughton, Ltd.; 1989.

Chapter 11

Acute Pancreatitis and Multiple Organ Dysfunction Syndrome

Janice McMillan Sensing

Acute pancreatitis is an inflammatory response resulting from the premature activation of pancreatic enzymes. The pathologic changes range from mild edema to extensive hemorrhage, necrosis, and abscess formation. The process is usually self-limiting; however, severe pancreatitis can occur in 25% of all cases and can affect virtually every organ system in the body.[1] Pancreatitis has an overall mortality of 10% to 20%.[2]

The pancreas plays a more causal role in multiple organ dysfunction syndrome (MODS) than do many of the other individual organs. Severe pancreatitis often leads to the development of regional and systemic inflammation, a common setting for the development of MODS. Intense activation of inflammatory mediators with concomitant changes in distribution of circulating volume, oxygen supply and demand, and metabolic alterations leads to systemic abnormalities and damage to organs distant from the site of inflammation.

ANATOMY AND PHYSIOLOGY

The pancreas is an elongated gland about 12 to 18 cm long that has both endocrine and exocrine functions.[3,4] The pancreas lies anterior to the first and second lumbar vertebrae and posterior to the stomach. It consists of three sections: the head, the body, and the tail (Fig. 11-1). The head, or right end of the pancreas, lies within the curvature of the duodenum. The left portion is the tail, which extends to the spleen. The intervening portion is the body that lies horizontally across the abdomen. Adjacent organs are easily involved in the course of acute pancreatitis because of the retroperitoneal location of the pancreas. The absence of a well-developed pancreatic capsule allows the inflammatory process to spread freely and affect such organs as the duodenum, the terminal common bile duct, the splenic artery and vein, the spleen, the mesocolon, the greater omentum, the small bowel mesentery, the celiac and the superior mesenteric ganglia, the lesser omental sac, the posterior mediastinum, the pararenal spaces, and the diaphragm.[5]

The pancreas is composed of two types of tissues: the acinar cells, which participate in exocrine function and the islets of Langerhans, which are involved in endocrine function. The endocrine role of the pancreas focuses mainly on glucagon and insulin secretion, while the exocrine role focuses on normal digestive and absorptive processes.

Endocrine function

The islets of Langerhans, also called pancreatic islets, secrete insulin and glucagon directly into the blood. The pancreas is populated by 1 to 2 million islets, which are centered around small capillaries into which the islet cells secrete their hormones.[4,6] The pancreatic islets contain three distinct types of cells: alpha cells, beta cells, and delta cells. Alpha cells, which constitute about 25% of the total islet cells, secrete glucagon. Glucagon opposes the action of insulin and protects the body from hypoglycemia by triggering the processes of glycogenolysis and gluconeogenesis and thus increasing blood glucose concentration. The beta cells comprise 60% of all islet cells and secrete insulin in response to

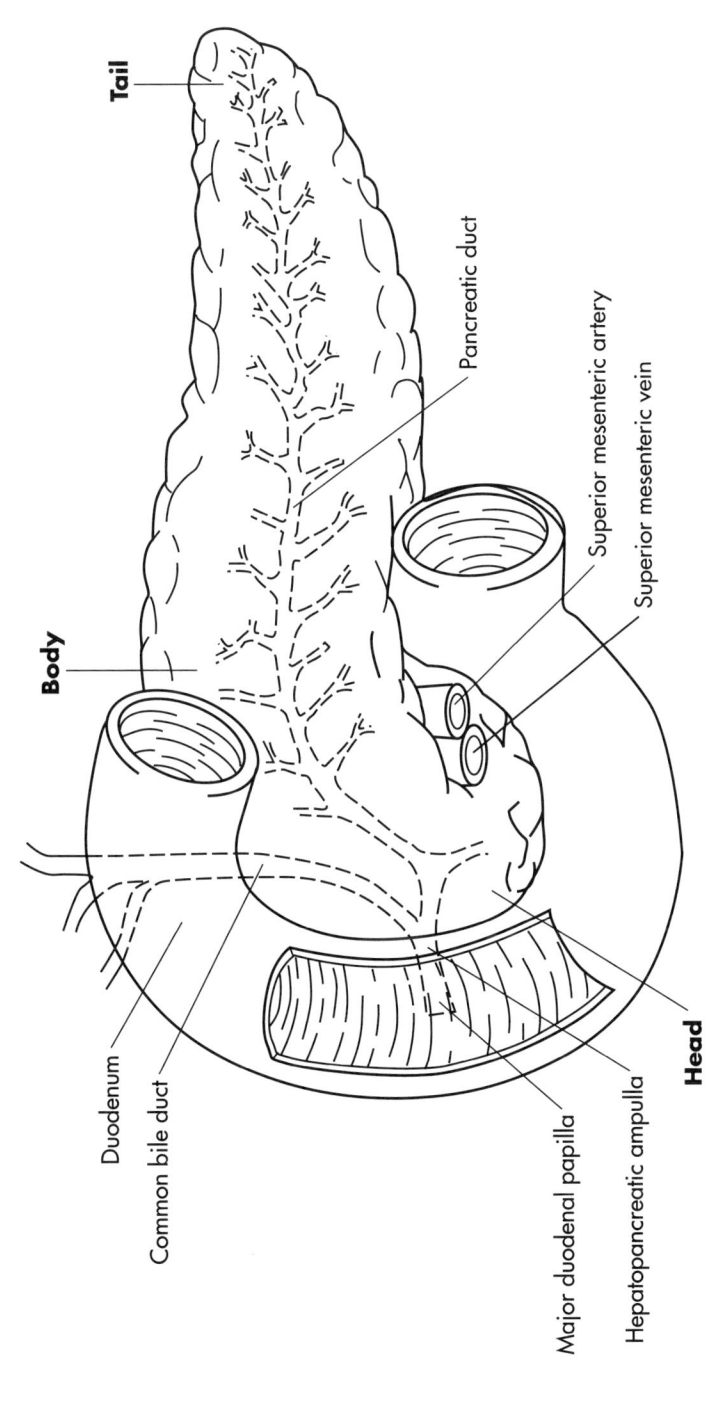

Fig. 11-1 The pancreas. (Modified from Steinberg W, Tenner S. Acute pancreatitis. N Eng J Med 1994;330(17):1198, Massachusetts Medical Society.)

rising blood glucose levels. Insulin moves glucose into cells and increases glycogen stores. The delta cells, which comprise 10% of the total islet cells, secrete somatostatin. Somatostatin depresses insulin and glucagon secretion, decreases gastrointestinal motility, and reduces gastrointestinal and pancreatic secretions.[7,8] This extends the time for assimilation of food stores into the blood and prevents rapid exhaustion of food supplies. There is at least one other type of cell, the PP cell, which secretes a hormone of uncertain function called pancreatic polypeptide.[6,9]

Exocrine function

Acinar cells are arranged in groups called acini. Acinar cells secrete 1000 to 3000 mL of pancreatic juice per day into the pancreatic duct, which drains into the duodenum.[9-11] This digestive juice contains enzymes for digesting proteins, carbohydrates, and fats. It also contains water and large quantities of bicarbonate ions that neutralize the acid chyme emptied by the stomach into the duodenum. The enzymes in pancreatic juice include proteolytic enzymes, such as trypsin, chymotrypsin, and elastases, which serve to break down proteins; pancreatic amylase, which hydrolyzes carbohydrates; and pancreatic lipase, which degrades fat (Table 11-1).

ETIOLOGY

Acute pancreatitis has a number of causes, but the most common are biliary tract disease in women and alcohol abuse in men.

Biliary tract disease

Gallstones are present in two thirds of the reported cases of pancreatitis; however, only about 5% of patients with gallstones develop pancreatitis.[12] Gallstone pancreatitis occurs two times more often in women than in men.[5] It is unclear how gallstones lead to pancreatitis, but it may be that stones impacted in the ampulla of Vater cause bile reflux, which leads to pancreatitis (Fig. 11-2). An alternative hypothesis is that gallstones cause pancreatitis by transiently obstructing the pancreatic duct without inducing bile reflux. This ultimately damages acinar cells.

Alcohol abuse

Alcohol abuse is the leading cause of pancreatitis in men. It requires many years of alcohol abuse before acute alcoholic pancreatitis develops. The patients who present with acute alcoholic pancreatitis most likely have an acute episode of pancreatitis superimposed on chronic pancreatitis. In a minority of patients, alcohol may cause acute pancreatitis in the absence of chronic disease.[13]

The pathogenesis of alcoholic pancreatitis remains unclear. One hypothesis is that protein plugs form in the pancreatic ducts and cause partial obstruction of outflow.[12,13] A second mechanism by which alcohol may cause pancreatic damage is through increased gastric acid secretion that results from alcohol ingestion. This leads to an increase in pancreatic secretion. Increased secretion leads to atony and edema of the sphincter of Oddi, which results in reflux of duodenal contents into the pancreas.[10,12,14] Alcohol also decreases the amount of trypsin inhibitor available, which makes the pancreas more susceptible to trypsin damage.[15]

Lipid abnormalities

Lipid abnormalities, specifically hypertriglyceridemia, can cause pancreatitis. These patients usu-

Table 11-1 Pancreatic Secretions

Secretion	Function
Endocrine	
Insulin	Decreases blood glucose, decreases carbohydrate metabolism, synthesizes fat and protein
Glucagon	Increases blood glucose through glycogenolysis and gluconeogenesis
Somatostatin	Depresses insulin or glucagon secretion, decreases gastrointestinal motility, reduces gastrointestinal and pancreatic secretion
Exocrine	
Trypsin	Digests protein
Chymotrypsin	Digests protein
Elastase	Digests protein
Amylase	Digests carbohydrate
Lipase	Digests fat
Bicarbonate ions	Neutralize acid chyme

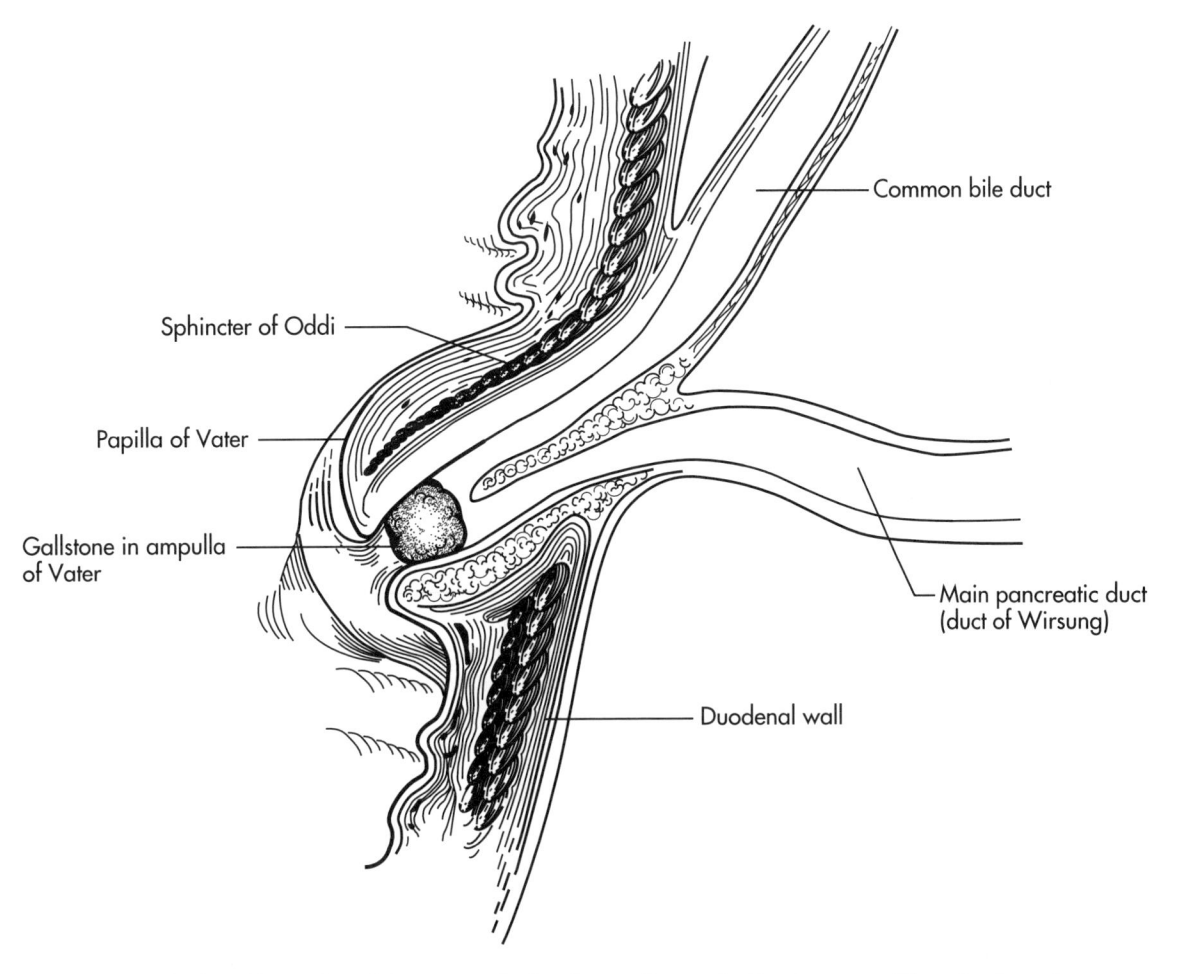

Fig. 11-2 Obstruction of the pancreatic duct by a gallstone, leading to pancreatitis and reflux of bile into the duct. (Steinberg W, Tenner S. Acute pancreatitis. N Eng J Med 1994;330(17):1198, Massachusetts Medical Society.)

ally have familial hyperlipoproteinemia of Frederickson types I, IV, or V.[5,15-17] Women taking oral contraceptives or estrogen therapy can develop type IV or V hyperlipidemia and pancreatitis.[5,15,17] The mechanism by which elevated triglycerides lead to pancreatitis is unclear; however, local lipolysis results in an excess of fatty acids that causes inflammation and damage to capillary membranes and can result in pancreatitis. Patients with lipemia-associated pancreatitis usually do not have elevated serum amylase values. Recurrences can usually be prevented by maintenance of a low-fat diet, weight reduction, and treatment with triglyceride-lowering agents.

Trauma

Physical trauma to the pancreas is the most common cause of pancreatitis in children and teenagers. Blunt trauma from compression by the steering wheel or handle bars can result in disruption of pancreatic ducts and in pancreatic contusion with resultant pseudocyst or fistula formation. Direct injury to the pancreas during abdominal surgery may also lead to pancreatitis.

Idiopathic and drug-related causes

Approximately 10% to 20% of patients with acute pancreatitis will have pancreatitis from no ascertainable cause.[1,18] Some cases of idiopathic pancreatitis may actually be related to pancreas divisum, a congenital pancreatic duct abnormality, which affects 5% to 7% of the general population.[19] In this condition, there are two separate pancreatic drainage systems. Recent studies suggest that occult biliary sludge may be the cause of perhaps two thirds of the cases of idiopathic acute pancreatitis.[20,21]

It is difficult to pinpoint whether a true connection exists between drug administration and pancreatitis or if it is an idiosyncratic reaction. Glucocorticosteroids, thiazide diuretics, furosemide, tetracycline, estrogens, methyldopa, and immunosuppressive drugs are a few of the drugs that have been associated with the development of pancreatitis.[19,22] Other causes of acute pancreatitis are listed in the box below.

PATHOPHYSIOLOGY HYPOTHESES
Autodigestion

Many immunologic and etiologic factors have been implicated in the pathogenesis of acute pancreatitis, but confusion remains over the mechanism by which these factors initiate pancreatitis. The most popular hypothesis for the development of acute pancreatitis is autodigestion. The pancreas protects itself from autodigestion by synthesizing proteolytic enzymes and phospholipase A as inactive zymogens (proenzymes) that are activated through enzymatic splitting of a peptide chain only after reaching the intestine. The other digestive enzymes (amylase, lipase, and nuclease) are synthesized in active form. The enzymes stored in zymogen granules are isolated by a phospholipid membrane in the acinar cell.

Trypsinogen, a proteolytic zymogen is activated to trypsin by enterokinase, which is secreted by the intestinal mucosa when chyme comes into contact with the mucosa. For reasons that are not clear, in acute pancreatitis trypsinogen is activated to trypsin within the pancreas. Trypsin activates all the known pancreatic zymogens that are involved in autodigestion. These activated enzymes cause proteolysis, edema, hemorrhage, coagulation necrosis, fat necrosis, parenchymal cell necrosis, and vascular damage. Thus, to prevent autodigestion of the pancreas, the proteolytic enzymes must remain as inactive zymogens until they have been secreted into the intestine.

A second safeguard against autodigestion is trypsin inhibitor. Trypsin inhibitor is a substance secreted by the same cells that secrete proteolytic enzymes into the acini of the pancreas. Because trypsin activates the other pancreatic proteolytic enzymes, trypsin inhibitor also prevents the subsequent activation of the other enzymes. If the pancreas becomes damaged or a pancreatic duct becomes blocked, secretions can back up and may pool. This increased concentration of pancreatic secretions may overpower the effect of trypsin inhibitor. The proteolytic enzymes are activated because trypsin inhibitor is ineffective. Acute pancreatitis develops as a result of the autodigestion of the pancreas.

The events that trigger the sequence of enzymatic reactions that initiate acute pancreatitis are unknown. It is probable that more than one etiologic mechanism is responsible. Although autodigestion remains the most popular hypothesis, obstruction, reflux of duodenal contents, and bile reflux have also been considered as mechanisms for initiating pancreatitis.

CAUSES OF ACUTE PANCREATITIS

Biliary tract disease (gallstones)
Alcohol
Gastric disease (duodenal ulcer)
Metabolic disorders
    Hyperlipidemia
    Hyperparathyroidism
    Renal failure
    Hypercalcemia
Drugs (thiazide diuretics, furosemide, estrogens, tetracycline, valproic acid, salicylates, corticosteroids, immunosuppressive agents, methyldopa, procainamide, pentamidine)
Hereditary pancreatitis
Infections (mumps virus; mycoplasma; coxsackie virus; hepatitis A, B, C, and D; cytomegalovirus)
Pregnancy (third trimester)
Rheumatoid arthritis
Scorpion venom
Surgery
Systemic lupus erythematosis
Trauma
Tumors

Obstruction

Some investigators hypothesize that acute pancreatitis results from obstruction to the outflow of pancreatic juice. Obstruction occurs from a biliary tract stone or from edema and inflammation caused by passage of a biliary tract stone. Pancreatic ductal hypertension occurs from continued pancreatic secretion into an obstructed ductal system and leads to pancreatic injury. Permanent decompression of a choledochocele has prevented recurrent attacks of pancreatitis in several patients, presumably by removing intermittent pancreatic outflow obstruction.[23] Evidence against obstruction as the major cause of acute pancreatitis exists, since ligation of the pancreatic duct or its occlusion by tumor generally does not result in acute pancreatitis. In addition, sphincterotomy and sphincteroplasty have been performed in patients with recurring episodes of acute pancreatitis, but with disappointing results.[5]

Duodenal reflux

Another theory is that reflux of duodenal contents leads to pancreatitis. It was hypothesized that a stone might pass through the sphincter of Oddi and stretch the muscle, making the sphincter incompetent. As a result, duodenal juices that contained activated pancreatic digestive enzymes could reflux through the incompetent sphincter into the pancreatic ductal system and trigger pancreatic inflammation. This theory, for the most part, has been discounted. Patients can develop an incompetent sphincter after undergoing a sphincterotomy without developing duodenal reflux and acute pancreatitis. In addition, the majority of patients with acute pancreatitis have been found to have a normal pressure gradient between the pancreatic duct lumen and the duodenum, which would prevent reflux. Thus, duodenal regurgitation might be a contributing factor toward development of pancreatitis in some patients, but enough evidence does not exist to support this as an applicable etiology in the majority of patients with acute pancreatitis.

Bile reflux

One of the older hypotheses is the bile reflux, or common channel hypothesis, which applies to pancreatitis associated with cholelithiasis. Opie, in 1901, discovered on autopsy that several patients who died from acute pancreatitis had a biliary stone impacted in the terminal common bile duct.[22] It was hypothesized that this impacted bile stone created behind it a common bilopancreatic channel that allowed bile to reflux into the pancreatic duct. However, several factors have suggested that the common channel theory might not be correct. In most individuals, pancreatic secretory pressure exceeds biliary secretory pressure. Thus, a stone that created a common channel would favor reflux of pancreatic juice into the biliary system rather than bile into the pancreatic ductal system. In addition, a common channel allowing bile to reflux is present in only 18% of the population.[24] This common channel is extremely short, and reflux would not occur even if an obstructing stone were present.[22] Bile reflux has not been found to cause acute pancreatitis in animals.

Summary

Many investigators hypothesize that obstruction or ligation of the pancreatic duct with associated reflux leads to pancreatic edema but not pancreatitis. Autodigestion remains the most common hypothesis explaining the development of acute pancreatitis. Although a variety of factors, such as endotoxins, exotoxins, viral infections, ischemia, anoxia, and direct trauma to the pancreas, have been considered, the exact mechanism by which autodigestion is initiated remains unclear. Figure 11-3 depicts a schematic diagram of the development of acute pancreatitis.

CLINICAL PRESENTATION AND ASSESSMENT

No single diagnostic sign or symptom of acute pancreatitis exists. Diagnosis is based upon typical clinical features and laboratory findings and remains a clinical interpretation. The clinical presentation of acute pancreatitis changes as the disease progresses. In the initial 2 to 3 hours after onset, the symptoms are suggestive of acute cholecystitis; after 6 to 8 hours, the symptoms are suggestive of a perforated ulcer; and after 2 to 3 days, the abdominal distention and ileus that develop are suggestive of intestinal obstruction. In addition, elevation of serum amylase occurs in all of these conditions.

Physical assessment

Abdominal pain is the most common symptom of acute pancreatitis. The pain may vary from mild, dull discomfort to severe, constant pain. The pain is

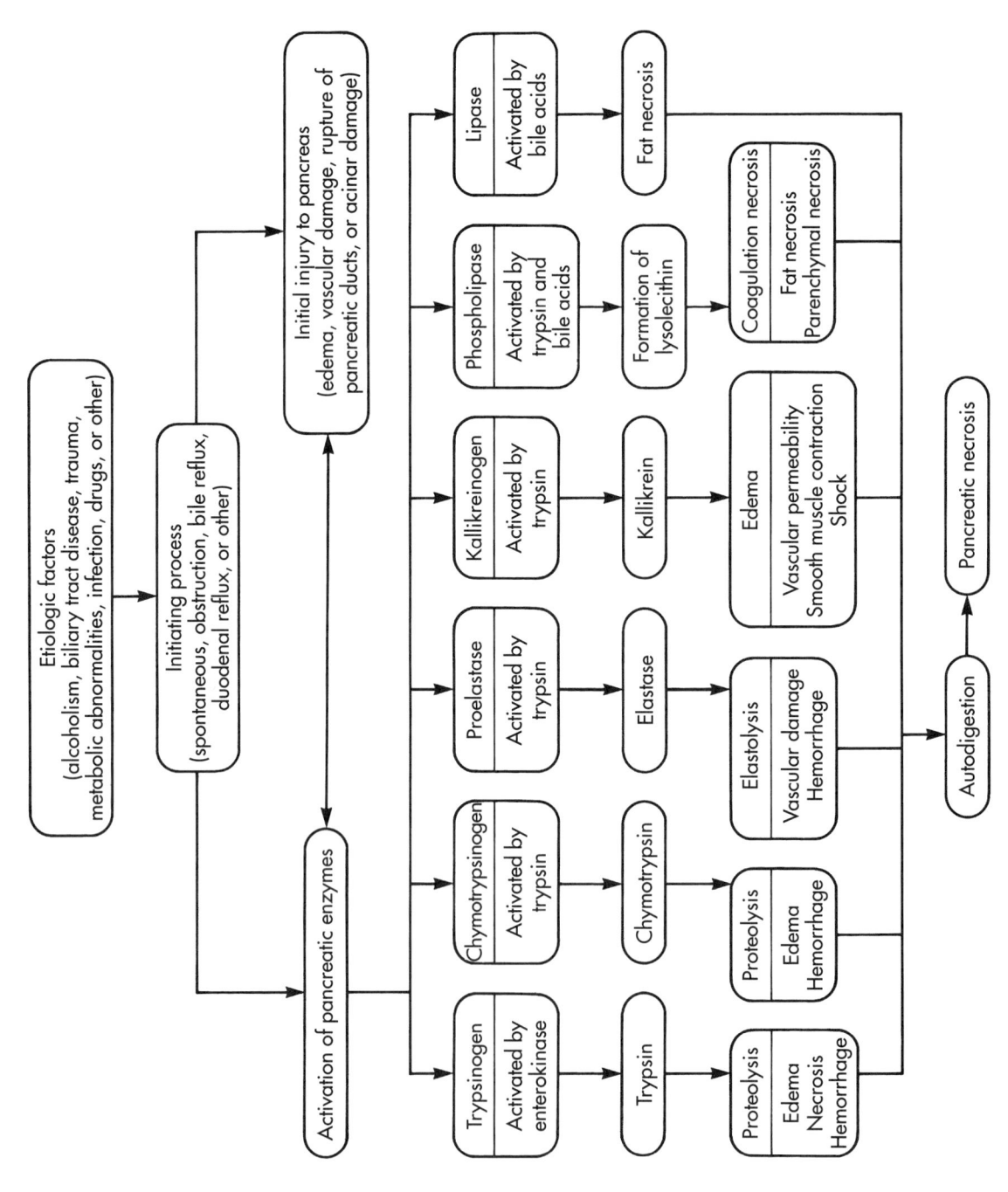

Fig. 11-3 Schematic diagram depicting the development of acute pancreatitis. (Modified from Cruetzfeldt W, Schmidt H. Scand J Gastroenterol 1970;5[suppl 6]:47-62.)

located across the midepigastrium and periumbilical region and may radiate into the back or the flanks because of the retroperitoneal location of the pancreas. The pain of pancreatitis does not have a waxing and waning pattern. It is described as having a knifelike or boring quality. The pain is worse in the supine position and is relieved by sitting with the thighs and spine flexed. Factors that cause the pain of acute pancreatitis include chemical peritonitis; extravasation of blood, inflammatory exudate, and pancreatic enzymes into the retroperitoneal space; obstruction and distention of the pancreatic ducts; edema and stretching of the pancreatic capsule; obstruction of the duodenum from edema of the head of the pancreas; and obstruction of the extrahepatic biliary tract.[25,26]

On physical examination, the abdomen is initially soft, with tenderness developing in the upper abdomen. Bowel sounds are diminished but present. During the first 2 days, abdominal distention develops because of the combined effects of the paralytic ileus and accumulation of intraperitoneal fluid. Nausea and vomiting are common and occur because of gastric and intestinal hypomotility, the ileus, and chemical peritonitis. The temperature of the patient is usually between 37.7° C (100° F) and 38.3° C (101° F) as a result of injured tissue products and inflammatory mediators entering the circulation.

Hypotension occurs in approximately 30% to 50% of patients with pancreatitis.[5,16] Shock results from a combination of factors: hypovolemia secondary to plasma exudation in the retroperitoneal space leading to a retroperitoneal burn; fluid accumulation in an atonic intestine; vomiting; hemorrhage; increased formation and release of kinin peptides that cause stimulation of smooth muscle; vasodilatation; increased vascular permeability; enhanced leukocyte migration; systemic effects of proteolytic and lipolytic enzymes released into the circulation; and impaired myocardial contractility from release of kinin peptides.[5,16] The systemic effects in pancreatitis result from absorption of activated pancreatic enzymes and the products of pancreatic digestion into the blood.

Blue-brown discoloration of the flanks (Grey Turner's sign) or in the periumbilical area (Cullen's sign) may occur as a late sign of severe pancreatitis. These signs indicate the presence of hemorrhagic pancreatitis and retroperitoneal dissection of blood into these areas. The blue-brown discoloration may not appear until after a week or two of progressive pancreatic destruction has occurred.

Laboratory findings

Diagnosis of acute pancreatitis is usually based on the clinical presentation, a history of the precipitating cause, and an elevated serum amylase concentration. Serum amylase measurement is the single most important test for the diagnosis of acute pancreatitis. Serum amylase levels are usually greater than two times the upper limit of normal levels (the normal level is 80 to 150 Somogyi units), but they do not always reflect the severity of the pancreatitis.

Relying on serum amylase values to diagnose pancreatitis has drawbacks. Amylase levels rise within a few hours of developing pancreatitis; however, amylase is rapidly metabolized and cleared by the kidneys. Serum amylase levels return to normal within 24 to 48 hours; thus, if the patient is examined several days after the onset of symptoms, the serum amylase level will be normal. Serum amylase may be falsely low in patients with hypertriglyceridemia and may be elevated in patients with renal insufficiency, cerebral trauma, intraabdominal disease, burns, or ketoacidosis. Serum amylase is more specific if isoenzymes are determined because serum amylase is composed of pancreatic and salivary isoamylase. An elevated serum amylase value along with an elevated pancreatic isoamylase value makes the diagnosis of pancreatitis likely; however, numerous intestinal disorders can lead to elevated pancreatic isoamylase levels.

Urine amylase levels are increased in patients with pancreatitis. Urinary clearance of amylase may remain elevated for 9 to 15 days after an episode of acute pancreatitis.[10] A reversible renal tubular defect is believed to be the mechanism for decreased amylase reabsorption and increased renal clearance of amylase. However, many of the conditions that can elevate serum amylase levels can also affect urine amylase levels; thus, the finding of elevated urine amylase is not specific to pancreatitis.

Other laboratory tests that may be helpful in diagnosing pancreatitis are levels of serum lipase, serum immunoreactive trypsin, serum glucose, and serum calcium, and a white blood cell count. Serum lipase levels remain elevated much longer than do amylase levels, but lipase levels can be elevated in a variety of conditions and are not specific for acute pancreatitis. An elevated level of trypsin is not specific for any one type of pancreatic disease. It can be elevated with acute pancreatitis as well as with pancreatic carcinoma. Transient hyperglycemia is often present in the early stages of acute pancreatitis because of altered pancreatic islet cell function. There is decreased release of insulin from the beta cells, increased release of glucagon from alpha cells, and increased output of glucocorticoids and catecholamines. A sustained fasting hyperglycemia with glucose levels greater than 200 mg/dL is a poor prognostic sign because it reflects pancreatic necrosis.[5] Hypocalcemia may occur 2 to 3 days after the onset of pancreatitis and can be the result of an altered response to parathyroid hormone, hypoalbuminemia, or calcium deposition in fatty necrotic areas in the abdominal cavity. Leukocytosis, with white blood cell counts of 10,000 to 25,000 cells/mm^3 is often present secondary to the inflammatory process.[5]

Recent investigations have looked at serum levels of other pancreatic enzymes such as elastase and phospholipase A as indicators for acute pancreatitis.[27-29] To date, measurement of these other pancreatic enzymes has not shown any practical advantage over the more widely available serum tests for amylase, amylase isoenzymes, and lipase.

The presence of methemalbumin may be an indicator of severe pancreatitis. Pancreatic enzymes break down retroperitoneal hemoglobin into heme, which oxidizes to hematin and combines with serum albumin to form methemalbumin.[1] However, the presence of methemalbumin is not specific to pancreatitis because it may be present with upper abdominal trauma, bleeding gastric ulcer, bone fractures, and retroperitoneal hematoma.[5]

Radiologic studies

Radiologic studies are helpful in confirming the presence of pancreatic disease, detecting complications, and establishing the presence of alternative conditions. X-ray films of the abdomen may show a sentinel loop (a distended small intestinal loop near the pancreas), a paralytic ileus, the colon cut-off sign, or evidence of other causes for the patient's abdominal pain, such as free intraperitoneal air indicating mesenteric infarction. A chest radiograph may show a pleural effusion or interstitial fluffy infiltrates similar to those seen with pulmonary edema but without associated cardiomegaly. These infiltrates are indicative of respiratory failure associated with severe pancreatitis.

The most useful radiologic techniques are abdominal ultrasonography and computed tomography (CT) of the abdomen. Ultrasonography can show gallstones, enlargement or abnormal texture of the pancreas, enlargement or distention of the common bile duct, a pancreatic mass, or an accumulation of free fluid in the abdomen. The disadvantage with the use of ultrasound is its inability to penetrate bowel gas, which means that a normal scan does not rule out acute pancreatitis. CT with contrast provides better imaging of the pancreas and is indicated if complications are suspected. CT with contrast is contraindicated if the patient is allergic to contrast medium or has compromised renal function. CT is currently used to diagnose acute pancreatitis, to assess the severity of illness and the prognosis, to detect the complications of acute pancreatitis, and to guide the aspiration and drainage of infected pancreatic necrosis, pancreatic abscesses, infected fluid collections, and pancreatic pseudocysts.[30] Specific findings of acute pancreatitis on CT scans depend on the severity of illness. In mild cases, CT scans may show only enlargement of the gland. As edema and inflammation spread to the surrounding fat, the pancreatic margins become irregular and indistinct. The pancreas may actually appear normal on CT scans in mild cases of acute pancreatitis.

Dynamic pancreatography is a technique that can be used to determine the severity of acute pancreatitis. Pancreatography is performed by rapidly injecting large volumes of contrast material (100 to 200 mL) intravenously and then rapidly obtaining a CT scan of the pancreas to determine the rate and pattern of pancreatic perfusion.[1] Some studies have shown a positive correlation between the lack of perfusion seen on dynamic pancreatography and the presence of pancreatic necrosis at the time of surgery.[1,31-32] Unfortunately, pancreatography is not helpful in detecting pancreatic abscess formation, since these patients have normal to decreased perfusion. Thus, the specificity of pancreatography is unclear.

Endoscopic retrograde cholangiopancreatography (ERCP) is indicated in two types of acute pancreatitis. In traumatic pancreatitis, ERCP is useful in establishing ductal disruption and in identifying the site of pancreatic fistula as a guide to surgery. ERCP with sphincterotomy may reduce complications in patients with biliary pancreatitis who have common duct stones.[33]

Diagnosis

The diagnosis of acute pancreatitis can usually be made when the physical examination of a patient yields abnormal findings (severe, constant abdominal pain; fever; and nausea and vomiting), abnormal laboratory values (elevated serum amylase, elevated serum lipase, and increased amylase clearance) are present, and radiologic studies show abnormalities. The severity of pancreatitis can be predicted by using Ranson's criteria. Ranson[34,35] identified 11 risk factors that aid in identifying patients who are at risk for major complications or death. Five of the factors are identifiable at the time of admission. These include the age of the patient, the WBC count, and the levels of glucose, lactic dehydrogenase (LDH), and serum glutamic-oxaloacetic transferase (SGOT). The other six factors are changes that occur during the first 48 hours after admission. These include changes in hematocrit, blood urea nitrogen (BUN), calcium, partial arterial pressure of oxygen (PaO_2), base deficit, and the amount of fluid sequestered. The major difficulty in using Ranson's criteria is that it takes 48 hours to determine whether a patient has severe pancreatitis. Ranson's risk factors and the impact of their presence on mortality are shown in the box below. To simplify the Ranson criteria, the Glasgow criteria were developed (see the box to the right); this reduced the number of criteria from 11 to 8. The Glasgow criteria also require a 48 hour period of observation. If a patient has three or more factors in the Glasgow criteria, there is a 40% chance of severe pancreatitis being present as compared to a 6% chance of severe pancreatitis with fewer than three factors.[36] The Acute Physiology and Chronic Health Evaluation (APACHE) has also been used to assess acute pancreatitis. This grading system allows severity to be calculated within hours of admission and to be recalculated daily. The system was originally developed in 1981 and considered 34 laboratory values, as well as the age and previous health status of the patient.[37] The original APACHE system was complex and difficult to use. In 1985, a modification of APACHE was developed. APACHE II examines 12 laboratory values in addition to age and previous health status.[1,16,35,37]

MODIFIED GLASGOW CRITERIA

Age >55 years
WBC >15,000/mm³
Glucose >180 mg/dL
BUN >96 mg/dL
PaO_2 <60 mmHg
Calcium <8 mg/dL
Albumin <3.2 g/dL
LDH >600 IU/L

Modified from Steinberg WM. Predictors of severity of acute pancreatitis. Gastroenterol Clin North Am 1990;19:849-860.
BUN, Blood urea nitrogen; *LDH*, lactic dehydrogenase; *PaO_2*, partial arterial pressure of oxygen; *WBC*, white blood cell.

RISK FACTORS FOR QUANTIFYING THE SEVERITY OF ACUTE PANCREATITIS AND THE IMPACT OF THEIR PRESENCE ON MORTALITY*

Risk Factors		Mortality	
At admission	*During initial 48 hours*	*Number of factors*	*Mortality (%)*
Age >55 years	Hct decreases >10 percentage points	<3	<1
WBC >16,000/mm³	BUN rises >5 mg/dL	3 to 4	15
Serum LDH >350 u/L	PaO_2 <60 mm Hg	5 to 6	40
SGOT >250 Sigma Frankel u/dL	Base deficit >4 mEq/L	7+	100
	Estimated fluid sequestration >6 L		

*References 14-16.
Modified from Ranson JHC. Risk factors in acute pancreatitis. Hosp Pract 1985;20(4):69-73.
BUN, Blood urea nitrogen; *Hct*, hematocrit; *LDH*, lactic dehydrogenase; *PaO_2*, partial arterial pressure of oxygen; *SGOT*, serum glutamic-oxaloacetic transferase; *WBC*, white blood cell.

This grading system, although modified, remains complex to use.

Progression

The initial stages of acute pancreatitis are characterized by interstitial edema. The disease can progress from acute edematous pancreatitis to necrotizing pancreatitis, which is characterized by coagulation necrosis of glandular elements and their surrounding fatty tissue. The factors determining the progression are unknown, but pancreatic elastase may mediate the thrombotic occlusion of blood vessels. Hemorrhagic pancreatitis occurs when blood collects within the pancreas or the surrounding retroperitoneal spaces from ruptured blood vessels.

Acute pancreatitis very rarely progresses to chronic pancreatitis. Chronic pancreatitis is characterized by continuing inflammation that leads to irreversible structural changes and by permanent impairment of exocrine and endocrine pancreatic function. The clinical distinction between acute and chronic pancreatitis can be difficult to make, especially in the early stages of exacerbation of chronic alcoholic pancreatitis; thus, the patient should be treated for acute pancreatitis.

COMPLICATIONS

Pancreatic necrosis, pancreatic phlegmon, pancreatic abscess, pseudocysts, or obstructive jaundice may occur secondary to acute pancreatitis. In pancreatic necrosis, there is a diffuse or focal area of nonviable pancreatic parenchyma, which, if infected, is fatal without surgical drainage. The term, pancreatic phlegmon, has been used in the past to describe a mass of inflamed pancreas, both infectious and noninfectious. Because of its ambiguity, this term has been dropped from the nomenclature.

Abscesses can occur with more severe cases of pancreatitis and are usually associated with infection within the peripancreatic collection of fluid. Gram-negative intestinal flora are the most common infecting microorganisms.[38] Abscesses are a late occurrence of pancreatitis and often may occur 4 weeks or more after the onset of pancreatitis.[39-40] Patients with abscesses have abdominal pain, high fever, leukocytosis, and vomiting. Abscesses can be detected on an abdominal CT scan, an abdominal ultrasound scan, or on an x-ray film of the abdomen that shows extraluminal gas collection. Prompt recognition and surgical intervention to drain the abscess are needed because there is a high mortality associated with undrained abscesses.

Pseudocysts are pockets of pancreatic enzymes that develop within the retroperitoneal space. These pseudocysts are frequently palpable as an upper abdominal mass and can be documented on ultrasound or abdominal CT scans or with a barium study of the upper gastrointestinal tract. Obstructive jaundice is usually secondary to edema of the head of the pancreas that causes obstruction of the extrahepatic biliary tree. In the absence of choledocholithiasis, jaundice is transient, with serum bilirubin levels returning to normal in 7 to 10 days.

MULTISYSTEM INVOLVEMENT

Patients with acute hemorrhagic or acute edematous pancreatitis develop multiple organ dysfunction. These multisystem problems begin with the lungs and the circulation and progress to other organs. They are primarily related to the intense inflammatory response that is triggered by the necrotic tissue and destructive enzymes common in pancreatitis. The systemic inflammatory response syndrome (SIRS) is the term recently coined to refer to the systemic inflammation and clinical presentation triggered by major clinical insults such as multiple trauma, sepsis, and acute pancreatitis.

Pulmonary damage

Injury to the lungs occurs from pancreatic enzymes reaching the pleural fluid by passage through pores in the diaphragm and by exudation from thoracic lymphatic channels. Alveolar capillary membrane integrity is lost, and pulmonary edema occurs. Pulmonary surfactant may be damaged by circulating free fatty acids, phospholipase A, or other vasoactive substances.[5,41] The pulmonary edema results from a reversible disruption of the alveolar capillary membrane with loss of the normal size selectivity for diffusion of plasma proteins. Therefore, both proteins and fluid move into the interstitium and the alveoli. Pleural effusions, atelactasis, pneumonia, and mediastinal abscess may develop. Adult respiratory distress syndrome (ARDS) develops in approximately 20% of patients with acute pancreatitis.[10]

Other factors associated with pancreatitis contribute to the development of pulmonary complications. Abdominal pain alters the breathing pattern, resulting in a decreased tidal volume and increased rate of breathing. Abdominal distention and inflammation under the diaphragm elevate the diaphragm and decrease expansion. Cardiovascular demands increase ventilation needs. All of these factors contribute to respiratory compromise and failure.

Circulatory abnormalities

Patients with severe pancreatitis develop a hyperdynamic circulatory state, which is characterized by decreased peripheral vascular resistance and an increase in the shunt fraction of the pulmonary circulation. This results in an elevated cardiac index and a decrease in the arteriovenous oxygen gradient.[42] A retroperitoneal burn occurs from exudation of blood and plasma protein into the retroperitoneal space and causes hypovolemia. The retroperitoneal inflammatory process demands a hyperdynamic circulation and vigorous fluid restoration. Trypsin activates the kallikrein/kinin system. The kinin peptides cause vasodilatation, increased vascular permeability, and leukocyte migration. Shock develops from the combination of hypovolemia, the effects of the kinin peptides, and the systemic effects of proteolytic and lipolytic enzymes. During the first several days, daily fluid requirements often exceed 5 to 6 L and may be as high as 10 L to maintain an adequate intravascular volume.[25]

In addition, impaired myocardial contractility can contribute to the shock state. Controversy remains concerning the presence of myocardial depression in pancreatitis. A myocardial depressant factor, which is believed to be a small peptide produced by the action of trypsin, phospholipase A, and lysosomes on compartmentalized protein, has been implicated in some of the hemodynamic alterations occurring in patients with pancreatitis.[41] It is thought that myocardial depressant factor enhances splanchnic vasoconstriction and depresses myocardial contractility. It also affects the role of calcium in myocardial contractility and electrical excitation. Although some studies have found evidence of myocardial depression, others have not.[43-46]

Disseminated intravascular coagulation

Disseminated intravascular coagulation (DIC) can occur from the release of pancreatic proteolytic enzymes into the blood. Elastase dissolves elastic fibers, which increases vascular permeability. Activation of kinin peptides also causes vasodilatation and increased vascular permeability. The severe inflammation and the endothelial damage are both potent triggers of the clotting cascade. Hypovolemia contributes to cell aggregation and the development of microthrombi. Fibrin-related antigen levels rise with a decrease in the platelet count and fibrinogen levels. Impaired clot lysis and consumption of clotting factors occur, which results in DIC.

Altered renal function

Altered renal function can develop and ranges from mild impairment to anuria. Acute renal failure results from renal tubular necrosis secondary to hypovolemia and shock. Renal artery thrombosis and renal vein thrombosis also contribute to the renal failure.

Metabolic complications

Metabolic complications include hyperglycemia, hypocalcemia, and hyperlipidemia. Hyperglycemia is usually transient and occurs because of release of excess glucagon from the alpha cells and damage to the insulin-secreting beta cells. Since the hyperglycemia is transient, diabetes mellitus usually does not develop, but it may, if the pancreatitis becomes chronic.

The cause for hypocalcemia is uncertain. Calcium deposition in areas of fat necrosis, release of glucagon, hypomagnesemia, and inadequate parathyroid function may contribute to hypocalcemia. Serum calcium levels usually remain low for 7 to 10 days, but tetany rarely occurs. Hyperlipidemia occurs in about 12% to 25% of all patients with pancreatitis,[10] although the mechanism for hyperlipidemia in pancreatitis remains unclear. Lipemia usually precedes pancreatitis, rather than lipemia being a manifestation of pancreatic inflammation. Local lipolysis with liberation of cytotoxic free fatty acids may be the factor that triggers pancreatitis.

THERAPEUTIC MANAGEMENT

Treatment of acute pancreatis focuses on halting the progression of damage to the pancreas, preventing or treating local complications, and treating systemic complications. Treatment remains symptomatic and supportive because there is no specific therapy that halts the process of autodigestion.

Suppression of pancreatic activity

In order to halt the process of pancreatic injury, attempts are made to correct the initiating factor if possible, decrease the activity of the pancreas, and inhibit the activity of damaging pancreatic enzymes. Pancreatic enzyme synthesis and pancreatic secretions are suppressed by not feeding the patient by mouth and by utilizing nasogastric suctioning. Various pharmacologic agents such as anticholinergics, antacids, cimetidine, glucagon, calcitonin, somatostatin, prostaglandin synthetase inhibitors, inhibitors of trypsin and phospholipase A_2, and infusions of fresh frozen plasma have been used in attempts to reduce pancreatic enzyme synthesis and secretion.[4,5,17] None of the pharmacologic agents has proven valuable in suppressing pancreatic secretions in clinical trials. It is also not known whether prophylactic antibiotics in acute pancreatitis are at all useful, or, if they are of use, whether they are more useful in acute pancreatitis arising from gallstones or acute pancreatitis resulting from alcohol abuse.[47]

Surgical intervention

Surgical intervention is indicated when the diagnosis of pancreatitis is uncertain, the condition of the patient worsens despite medical therapy, acute cholecystitis is present, or an abscess is suspected.[48] Peritoneal lavage and peritoneal dialysis have been performed in an attempt to remove necrotic debris and activating enzymes from the peritoneal cavity in patients with severe pancreatitis. Initially studies did not show that either of these treatments decreased mortality rates.[49-51] A recent study compared long-term (7 days) lavage with short-term (2 days) lavage and found a decrease in mortality from pancreatic abscess formation with the 7-day lavage, but the overall mortality remained the same.[52] Retroperitoneal lavage to eliminate activated pancreatic enzymes and toxins has also been used following surgical débridement of necrotizing pancreatitis. Following débridement, large catheters are left in the retroperitoneum for lavage of enzymes and debris.

CONCLUSION

Approximately 25% of all patients with pancreatitis will develop life-threatening, multisystem complications.[1] Whether pancreatitis causes SIRS and MODS or is a result of the changes and damage occurring in an existing state of MODS, the intense inflammation stimulated by the pancreatitis process and by the enzyme damage greatly increases the morbidity and mortality associated with critical illness. Because no specific therapy for acute pancreatitis is available, the major objective of therapeutic management is to support the patient until the acute phase of the disease subsides and to attempt to prevent multisystem complications.

REFERENCES

1. Steinberg WM. Predictors of severity of acute pancreatitis. Gastroenterol Clin North Am 1990;19:849-860.
2. Tran DD et al. Prevalence and prediction of multiple organ system failure and mortality in acute pancreatitis. J Crit Care 1993;8:145-153.
3. Bockman DE. Anatomy of the pancreas. In: Vay Liang W Go et al, eds. The pancreas: Biology, pathobiology, and disease. 2nd ed. New York: Raven Press; 1993:1-8.
4. Ermak TH, Grendell JH. The pancreas: Anatomy, histology, embryology, and developmental anomalies. In: Sleisenger MH, Fordtran JS, eds. Gastrointestinal disease: Pathophysiology, diagnosis, management. 5th ed, vol. 2. Philadelphia: WB Saunders; 1993:1573-1584.
5. Soergel KH. Acute pancreatitis. In: Sleisenger MH, Fordtran JS, eds. Gastrointestinal disease: Pathophysiology, diagnosis, management. 5th ed, vol. 2. Philadelphia: WB Saunders; 1993:1628-1653.
6. Guyton AC. Textbook of medical physiology. 8th ed. Philadelphia: WB Saunders; 1991.
7. Siconolfi LA. The forgotten system: Endocrine dysfunction during multiple system organ dysfunction. Crit Care Nurs Q 1994;16:16-26.
8. Toto KH. Endocrine physiology: A comprehensive review. Crit Care Nurs Clin North Am 1994;6:637-653.
9. Pandol SJ. Pancreatic physiology. In: Sleisenger MH, Fordtran JS, eds. Gastrointestinal disease: Pathophysiology, diagnosis, management. 5th ed, vol. 2. Philadelphia: WB Saunders; 1993:1585-1600.
10. Greenberger NJ. Gastrointestinal disorders: A pathophysiologic approach. 4th ed. St. Louis: Mosby;1989:253-300.
11. Spiro HM. General considerations. In: Spiro HM. Clinical gastroenterology. 4th ed. New York: McGraw-Hill; 1993: 937-948.
12. Creutzfeldt W, Lankisch PG. Acute pancreatitis: Etiology and pathogenesis. In: Berk JE, ed. Bockus gastroenterology. 4th ed. Philadelphia: WB Saunders; 1985:3971-3992.
13. Singh M, Simsek H. Ethanol and the pancreas: Current status. Gastroenterology 1990;98:1051-62.
14. Fain JA, Amato-Vealey E. Acute pancreatitis: A gastrointestinal emergency. Crit Care Nurs 1988;8:47-61.
15. Spiro HM. Inflammatory disorders. In: Spiro HM. Clinical gastroenterology. 4th ed. New York: McGraw-Hill; 1993: 959-987.
16. Marshall JB. Acute pancreatitis. Arch Intern Med 1993;153: 1185-1198.
17. Sabesin S. Countering the dangers of acute pancreatitis. Emerg Med 1987;19:70-96.
18. Steer ML. Etiology and pathophysiology of acute pancreatitis. In: Vay Liang W Go et al, eds. The pancreas: Biology, pathobiology, and disease. 2nd ed. New York: Raven Press; 1993:581-591.

19. Steinberg W, Tenner S. Acute pancreatitis. N Engl J Med 1994;330:1198-1210.
20. Lee SP, Nicholls JF, Park HZ. Biliary sludge as a cause of acute pancreatitis. N Engl J Med 1992;326:589-593.
21. Ros E et al. Occult microlithiasis in 'idiopathic' acute pancreatitis: Prevention of relapses by cholecystectomy or ursodeoxycholic acid therapy. Gastroenterology 1991;101: 1907-1709.
22. Steer ML. Acute pancreatitis. In: Taylor MB, ed. Gastrointestinal Emergencies. Baltimore: Williams & Wilkins; 1992:171-179.
23. Venu RP et al. Role of endoscopic retrograde cholangiopancreatography in the diagnosis and treatment of choledochocele. Gastroenterology 1984;87:1144-1149.
24. DiMagno EP, Shorter RG, Taylor WF. Relationships between pancreaticobiliary ductal anatomy and pancreatic ductal and parenchymal histology. Cancer 1982;49:361-368.
25. Banks PA. Medical Management of Acute Pancreatitis and Complications. In: Vay Liang W Go et al, eds. The Pancreas: Biology, Pathobiology, and Disease. 2nd ed. New York: Raven Press;1993:593-611.
26. Smith A. When the pancreas self-destructs. Am J Nurs 1991;91(8):38-48.
27. Agarwal N, Pitchumoni CS, Sivaprasad AV. Evaluating tests for acute pancreatitis. Am J Gastroenterology 1990;85:356-366.
28. Ventrucci M et al. Role of serum pancreatic enzyme assays in diagnosis of pancreatic disease. Dig Dis Sci 1989;34:39-45.
29. Gumaste VV. Diagnostic tests for acute pancreatitis. Gastroenterologist 1994;2(2):120-130.
30. Hill MC, Huntington DK. Computed tomography and acute pancreatitis. Gastroenterol Clin North Am 1990;19:811-842.
31. Bradley EL, Murphy F, Ferguson C. Prediction of pancreatic necrosis by dynamic pancreatography. Ann Surg 1989;210:495-504.
32. London NJM et al. Rapid-bolus contrast-enhanced dynamic computed tomography in acute pancreatitis: A prospective study. Br J Surg 1991;78:1452-1456.
33. Cello JP, Wilcox CM. Endoscopic therapy for pancreatitis and its complications. Sem Gastrointest Dis 1991;2(3):177-187.
34. Ranson JHC. Risk factors in acute pancreatitis. Hosp Pract 1985;20:69-73.
35. Ranson JHC. Stratification of severity for acute pancreatitis. In: Bradley EL, ed. Acute pancreatitis: Diagnosis and therapy. New York: Raven Press; 1994:13-20.
36. Blarney SL et al. Prognostic factors in acute pancreatitis. Gut 1984;25:1340-1346.
37. Wilson C, Heath DI, Imrie CW. Prediction of outcome in acute pancreatitis: A comparative study of APACHE II, clinical assessment and multiple factor scoring systems. Br J Surg 1990;77:1260-1264.
38. Collins AS. Gastrointestinal complications in shock. Crit Care Nurs Clin North Am 1990; 2:269-277.
39. Bittner R et al. Pancreatic abscess and infected pancreatic necrosis: Different local septic complications in acute pancreatitis. Dig Dis Sci 1987;32:1082-1087.
40. Bradley EL. A clinically based classification system for acute pancreatitis. Arch Surg 1993;128:586-590.
41. Baue AE. Multiple organ failure: Patient care and prevention. St. Louis: Mosby; 1990:415-417.
42. Beger HG et al. Hemodynamic data pattern in patients with acute pancreatitis. Gastroenterology 1986;90:74-79.
43. Ito K et al. Myocardial function in acute pancreatitis. Ann Surg 1981;194(1):85-88.
44. Goldfarb RD et al. Canine left ventricular function during experimental pancreatitis. J Surg Res 1985;38:125-133.
45. Altimari AF et al. Myocardial depression during acute pancreatitis: Fact or fiction? Surgery 1986;100:724-731.
46. Cobo JC et al. Sequential hemodynamic and oxygen transport abnormalities in patients with acute pancreatitis. Surgery 1984;95:324-330.
47. Bradley EL. Antibiotics in acute pancreatitis: Current status and future directions. Am J Surg 1989;158:472-477.
48. Poston GJ, Williamson RCN. Surgical management of acute pancreatitis. Br J Surg 1990;77:5-12.
49. Green JA, Pollack R, Barkin JS. Medical therapy for severe acute pancreatitis. In: Bradley EL, ed. Acute pancreatitis: Diagnosis and therapy. New York: Raven Press; 1994:77-83.
50. Mayer AD et al. Controlled clinical trial of peritoneal lavage for the treatment of severe acute pancreatitis. N Engl J Med 1985;312:399-404.
51. Stone HH, Fabian TC. Peritoneal dialysis in the treatment of acute alcoholic pancreatitis. Surg Gynecol Obstet 1980;150:878-882.
52. Ranson JHC, Berman RS. Long peritoneal lavage decreases pancreatic sepsis in acute pancreatitis. Ann Surg 1990;211: 708-716.

CHAPTER *12*

Myocardial Dysfunction in Sepsis and Multiple Organ Dysfunction Syndrome

Doris M. Gates

Cardiovascular and hemodynamic changes in sepsis, systemic inflammatory response syndrome (SIRS), and multiple organ dysfunction syndrome (MODS) are of paramount concern for the critical care practitioner. Many advanced monitoring techniques and interventions focus on supporting myocardial and hemodynamic functions to meet the increased metabolic demands of the tissues. Failure to balance supply and demand at the tissue level ultimately leads to death. Thus the performance of the cardiovascular system is of central concern in the development of MODS. Septic shock is the most common precursor to the development of MODS, and much attention has been focused on myocardial performance in this disease state.

Myocardial dysfunction in sepsis is the focus of this chapter. Many questions remain unanswered because research in this area is very difficult to conduct. Because of the severity of illness in patients, animal models have been used with varying degrees of congruence to human septic shock.[1] In addition, complex hemodynamic interactions between myocardial performance and changes in the peripheral vasculature hinder investigations exploring specific myocardial parameters. Furthermore, methods, definitions, and composition of patient groups vary among studies, often resulting in conflicting conclusions.[1,2]

HISTORICAL PERSPECTIVE

The opinions concerning the pathogenesis and relative role of the myocardium in septic shock have evolved over the last 40 years. During the 1950s and early 1960s, the hyperdynamic and hypodynamic phases of septic shock were seen as two separate clinical syndromes. Many patients had symptoms of the hypodynamic phase. Invasive monitoring was minimal, and aggressive fluid therapy was avoided because of concern about inducing pulmonary edema. Thus hypovolemia was not recognized, and hypotension with a decreased cardiac output (CO) was viewed as acute cardiac failure. This acute failure was believed to be a major component in the pathogenesis of septic shock.[3,4] With the advent of more sophisticated hemodynamic monitoring in the late 1960s and early 1970s, hypovolemia was recognized as the predominant cause for hypodynamic septic shock. Early fluid resuscitation became the standard treatment, resulting in an initial hyperdynamic state often followed by hypotension with a decreased CO. Septic shock was now seen as a continuum of shock states.[3] Many researchers hypothesized that myocardial failure was insignificant or absent in the hyperdynamic phase and instead was the mediating factor in progression to the hypodynamic phase and death. In addition, humoral myocardial depressant factors and mediators were implicated in contributing to myocardial demise.[5] Furthermore, researchers began to recognize that survival was positively correlated with maintenance of the hyperdynamic state, adequate tissue perfusion, and oxygen delivery.[3,5,6]

Intensive research on myocardial dysfunction in sepsis has continued in the 1980s and into 1990s. The definitive answer to the fundamental question of the role of the myocardium in sepsis and its progression to MODS remains elusive. However, current research indicates that the initial hyperdynamic cardiac state is the response to peripheral vasodilatation induced by alterations in tissue metabolism and mediator activity.[7,8] Significant and early myocardial depression occurs despite volume loading and increased cardiac index (CI) and hemodynamic parameters. In addition, biventricular failure is common, and myocardial systolic (contractility) and diastolic (compliance) functions are unfavorably altered.[9-12] Multiple humoral mediators and altered cellular physiology are implicated in myocardial pump dysfunction, which may lead to the ultimate demise of the patient.[3,7] Recent research has revealed significant differences between patients who recover and those who die from sepsis; patients who die 7 days or more after the onset of shock are usually victims of MODS.[2,12] Thus, despite extensive research and advances in medical technology and knowledge, the mortality rates for sepsis and MODS remain 40% to 60% and 80% to 100%, respectively.[7,13]

PATHOPHYSIOLOGY AND CLINICAL PRESENTATION
Overview

Cardiac performance in septic shock is intimately linked to the attempt of the cardiovascular system to preserve oxygen delivery to the tissues. Normally, the oxygen supply and demand balance of the tissue is maintained through peripheral vascular autoregulation and systemic compensatory mechanisms. In sepsis and SIRS, the peripheral autoregulatory mechanisms fail, leading to indiscriminate vasodilatation, maldistribution of flow, and decreased oxygen extraction. Consequently, the maintenance of tissue oxygenation is determined by the three major organ systems interacting to regulate systemic responses to oxygen requirements. The respiratory system oxygenates venous blood, the hematopoietic system contributes hemoglobin to carry oxygen, and the cardiovascular system strives to maintain tissue perfusion. The respiratory and hematopoietic systems may be limited in their ability to affect tissue requirements significantly; thus, the cardiac system performs a pivotal role in preserving oxygen supply in septic shock.[14]

Alterations occur in heart rate, preload, compliance, afterload, and contractility in an attempt to maintain cardiac function to meet the increased requirements of tissue metabolism. As various factors impinge on cardiac function and compensatory mechanisms are exhausted, oxygen transport becomes inadequate. Consequently, the combined effects of anaerobic cellular conditions, release of inflammatory mediators, and worsening cardiac function may propel the patient with sepsis into MODS. The inability to maintain hyperdynamic tissue perfusion as a result of cardiac failure has been implicated in the pathogenesis of sepsis and MODS.[7] However, the exact mechanisms of this myocardial failure are unclear, and the myocardium may be a victim and not the originator of the sequence of events leading to the ultimate demise of the patient.[2,15-17]

Septic shock and SIRS are induced by a wide variety of organisms and clinical syndromes, all of which produce the typical clinical and cardiovascular picture of hypotension, severe peripheral vasodilatation, and enhanced CO.[1] The severe decrease in systemic vascular resistance (SVR) is seen as the initiating event producing hypotension. Adequate volume loading to fill the expanded vascular space results in a compensatory increase in CO. With appropriate fluid resuscitation, 90% of patients demonstrate the hyperdynamic response.[2,7,10]

Hyperdynamic versus hypodynamic responses: misconceptions. At one time, it was a commonly held assumption that the hyperdynamic septic state was consistently followed by the hypodynamic state (hypotension, increased SVR, and decreased CO) as the condition of the patient deteriorated. With the more liberal use of volume expanders, this hypodynamic state is seen rarely and only in patients who have continually declining cardiac function.[18] Reports[10,19] demonstrate that only a minority of patients die from a progressively deteriorating CO. Unresponsive hypotension accounts for approximately 50% of the deaths, because of either a severe and persistent decrease in SVR (in 40% of the patients) or a profoundly diminished CO (in 10% of the patients). MODS is responsible for the other 50% of deaths (Fig. 12-1). Patient mortality from unresponsive hypotension usually occurs within 7 days of onset of disease, whereas deaths from MODS occur more than 7 days after onset of shock symptoms.[10,20] Thus several as yet undetermined mechanisms appear to mediate the physiologic response and outcome of sepsis and SIRS.

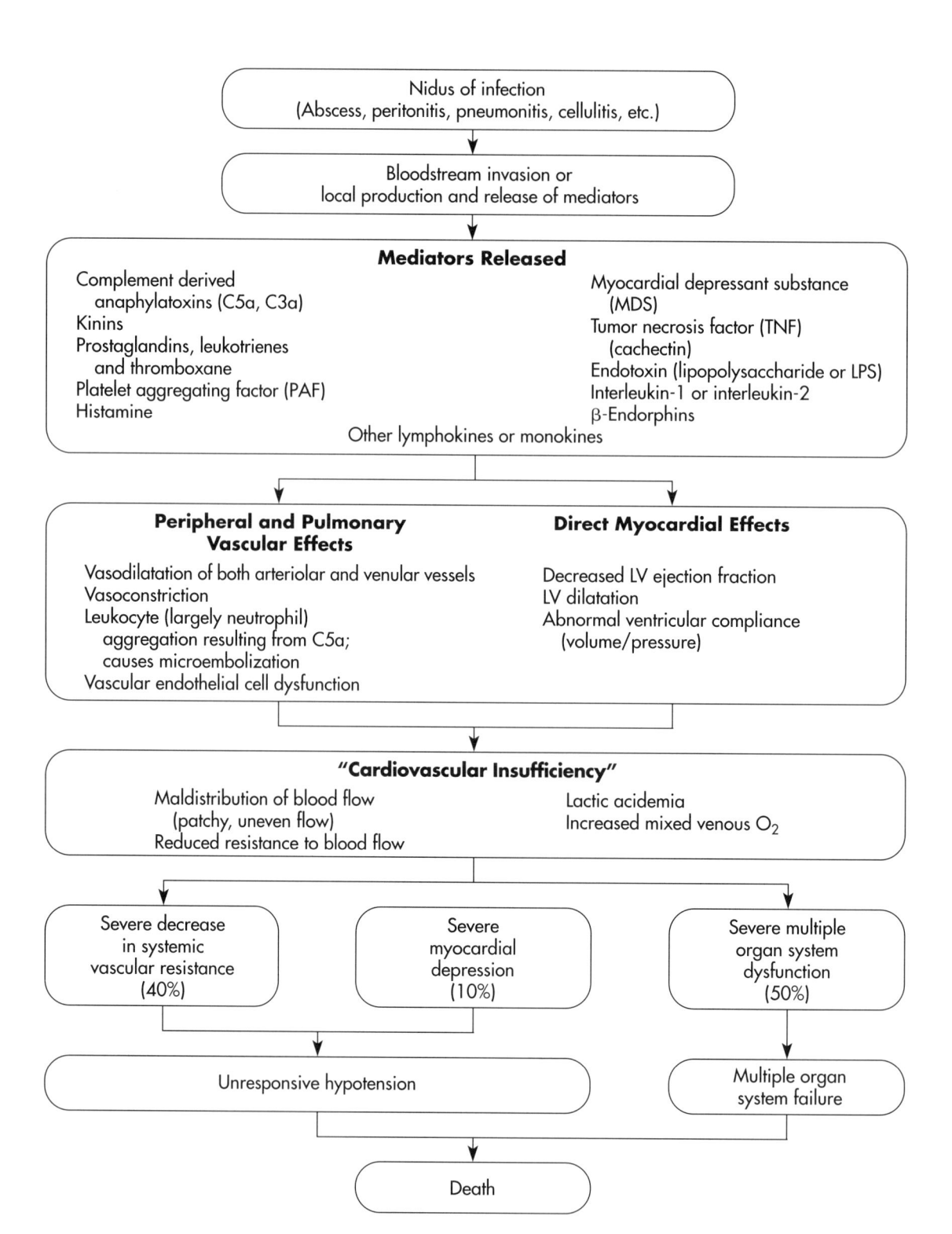

Fig. 12-1 The pathogenesis of human septic shock. (From Natanson C, Hoffman WD, Parrillo JE. Septic shock: The cardiovascular abnormality and therapy. J Cardiothor Anesth 1989:3:219.)

Whatever the etiology and progression of sepsis, myocardial dysfunction is evident early in the course of the disease. Various factors adversely affect both right- and left-ventricular performance, leading to alterations in heart rate, preload, compliance, afterload, and contractility.[2,10-12,20,21]

Alterations in hemodynamic parameters

Systemic blood pressure and mean arterial pressure (MAP) are regulated through the inverse relationship between CO and SVR. In the septic state, massive peripheral vasodilatation induces increases in CO. Since CO is determined by heart rate (HR) and stroke volume (SV) (CO = HR × SV), these two parameters are consequently altered. The HR increases, and the myocardium attempts to maintain or increase SV through alterations in the determinants of SV: preload, compliance, afterload, and contractility (Fig. 12-2).

Ventricular preload

Physiologic role. Ventricular preload is defined as the volume of blood (end-diastolic volume, [EDV]) or the amount of myocardial tension at the end of diastole.[22] The EDV determines the degree of stretch of myocardial fibers and thus, myocardial tension. According to the Frank-Starling law, the greater the myocardial fiber length or tension, the more forceful the contraction. This relationship between preload and contractile force is termed stroke work and is measured as the stroke work index (SWI). Assuming that the myocardium is healthy and will distend and stretch with added volume (compliance), increases in volume will increase the SWI. Diseased myocardial fibers are stiff and resistant to lengthening (noncompliant) and do not demonstrate significant increases in SWI with added volume (Fig. 12-3). Factors affecting preload and, thus, the SWI include fluid status, blood vol-

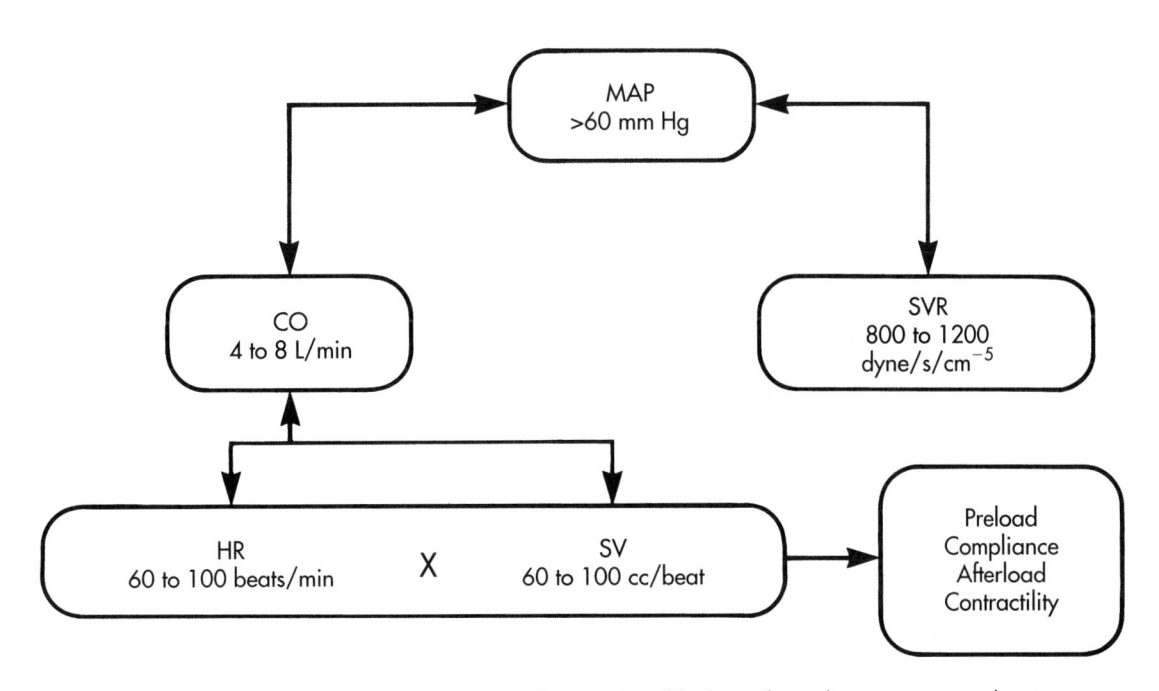

Fig. 12-2 Hemodynamic components and regulation. The hemodynamic components strive to maintain an MAP greater than 60 mm Hg. A negative change in any component of SV induces an increase in HR in order to maintain CO. If CO rises, SVR decreases. If CO falls, SVR increases. Conversely, changes in SVR induce changes in CO. If SVR falls, CO rises; if SVR rises, CO falls in order to maintain a constant MAP. *CO,* Cardiac output; *HR,* heart rate; *MAP,* mean arterial pressure; *SV,* stroke volume; *SVR,* systemic vascular resistance.

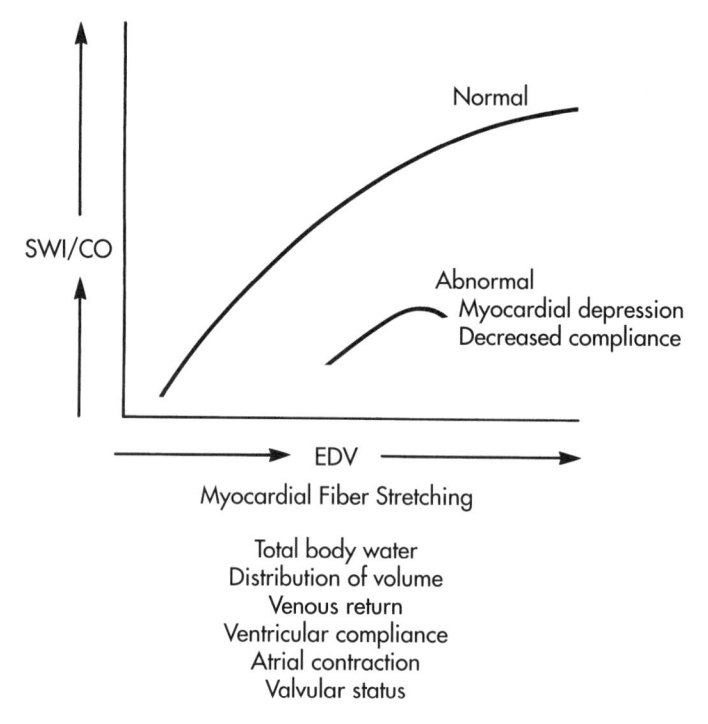

Fig. 12-3 Preload. *CO*, Cardiac output; *EDV*, end-diastolic volume; *SWI*, stroke work index.

ume distribution, venous return, ventricular compliance, atrial contraction (atrial kick), and valvular status.[22,23]

Impact of disease. In sepsis, the fluid status, the distribution of blood volume, and the venous return are the significant determinants of preload. Vasodilatation, increased peripheral capillary permeability, and maldistribution of blood volume result in a relative and actual fluid deficit in the vascular space. The expanded vasculature requires a larger volume to "fill up the tank." Various inflammatory mediators enhance capillary permeability, leading to significant interstitial edema. Therapies such as positive pressure ventilation and positive end-expiratory pressure (PEEP) reduce venous return and further displace volume into the periphery.[16] Thus preload volume and SWI are significantly depressed in the septic patient, and massive fluid resuscitation is necessary to maintain volume status and adequate myocardial stretch.

Ventricular compliance

Physiologic role. Compliance is an important factor in determining ventricular diastolic function. Ventricular compliance refers to the ability of the ventricle to stretch and dilate in response to increases in volume and is demonstrated by the end-diastolic pressure-to-volume relationship. Increases in ventricular EDV result in increases in end-diastolic pressure (EDP), commonly measured as central venous pressure (CVP) or pulmonary capillary wedge pressure (PCWP). However, this pressure-volume relationship is not linear; it is curvilinear. This relationship is illustrated in Figure 12-4. In the normal ventricle, low volume exerts a low pressure. When a fluid bolus enters an empty ventricle, only small changes in pressure occur because the ventricle is compliant and stretches, accommodating the increased volume and increasing the SWI (Fig. 12-4, point *A* to point *B*). As the ventricle fills, a point is reached wherein a fluid bolus induces a

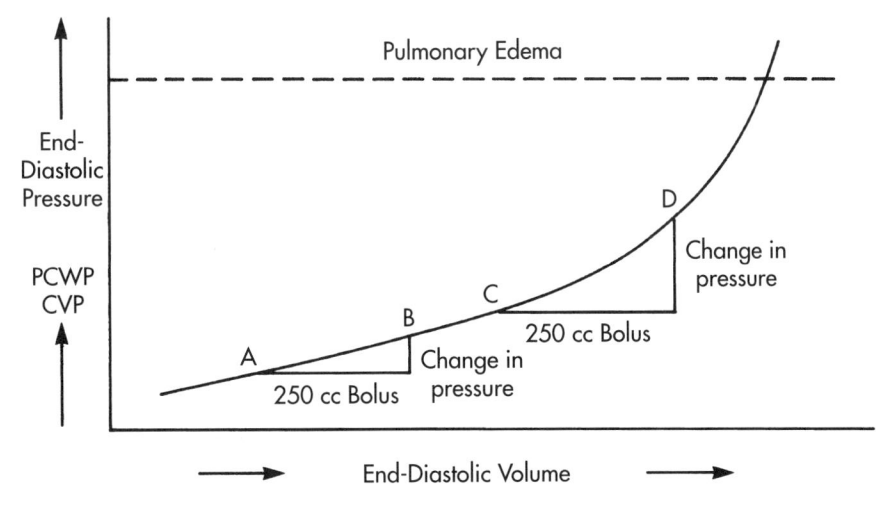

Fig. 12-4 Compliance. *CVP,* Central venous pressure; *PCWP,* pulmonary capillary wedge pressure.

larger increase in pressure (Fig. 12-4, point *C* to point *D*). On the upward curve of the relationship, additional volume does not enhance ventricular performance and SWI but merely increases pressure without any benefit to the hemodynamic status. Thus a normal ventricle becomes less compliant as it progressively fills.[19,23,24] As illustrated in Figure 12-5, noncompliant ventricles demonstrate large changes in pressure in response to volume infusions (the curve is shifted upward and to the left). Compliant, elastic ventricles exhibit smaller changes in pressure in response to volume infusions (the curve is shifted downward and to the right).

The clinical significance of the pressure-volume relationship is that CVP and PCWP do not accurately reflect ventricular volume and SWI.[25] It is an erroneous assumption that any given CVP or PCWP reflects a certain ventricular EDV and amount of myocardial stretch (Fig. 12-5). Trends and changes in these pressure readings in response to fluid therapy are clinically important and significant because they indicate the ventricular compliance at any given time and assist in directing therapy. For example, a fluid challenge of 250 mL that induces a pressure change of greater than 5 mm Hg indicates a stiff ventricle—a large pressure change occurring in response to a small volume infusion. Administration of additional fluid would result in volume overload and greatly increase the filling pressure without increasing SWI and CO. The abnormally elevated pressure would only predispose the patient to pulmonary edema. However, if several 250-mL fluid challenges are given before a pressure change of 5-mm Hg is detected, the ventricles are compliant—a larger volume of fluid is necessary to produce the same pressure change. A minimal pressure response to volume infusion indicates that the SWI and preload are not maximized and that the patient may be hypovolemic. Once volume status is optimized, other therapies are introduced as indicated by hemodynamic parameters.[19,22,26,27]

Impact of disease. The pressure-volume relationship is an important concept, especially in the septic patient. Changes in ventricular compliance occur early in the disease and affect the ultimate outcome for the patient. Several studies demonstrate that alterations in compliance occur in both ventricles during sepsis.[11,12,17,28] Survivors demonstrate increased compliance with biventricular dilatation and increased EDVs in order to maximize stroke work. The enhanced SWI maintains CI and tissue perfusion despite evidence of myocardial depression. Those who do not survive do not display this compensatory adaptation.[11,12,29]

Sepsis is often complicated by other factors that affect ventricular compliance. Adult respiratory disease syndrome (ARDS) can have a significant impact on both left- and right-ventricular compliance.

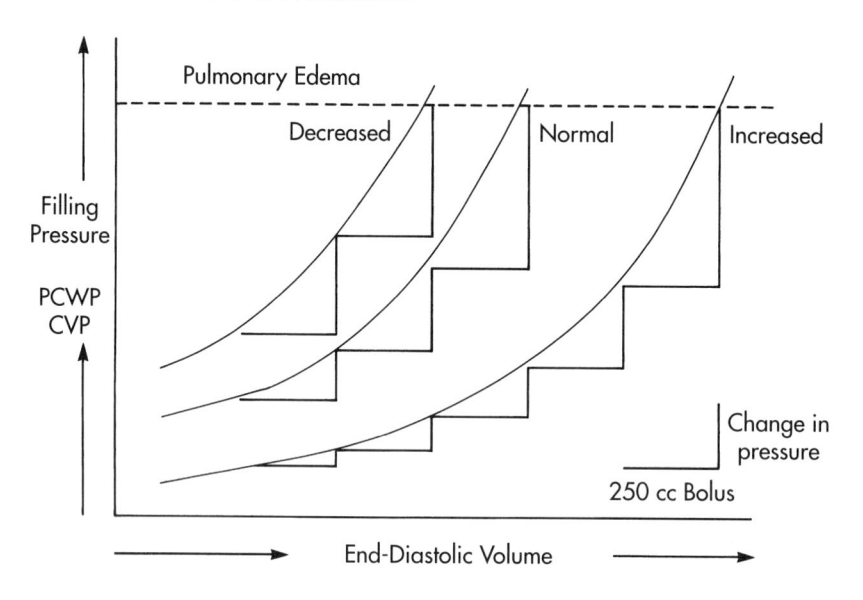

258 *Organ Involvement and Clinical Presentation*

Decreased Compliance	Increased Compliance
Progressive ventricular filling Myocardial ischemia/infarction Inotropic agents Catecholamines PEEP Cardiac tamponade ARDS Hypertension Ventricular hypertrophy	Vasodilators Calcium-channel blockers Relief of myocardial ischemia Ventricular dilatation Dilated cardiomyopathy

Fig. 12-5 Compliance and volume loading. *ARDS,* Adult respiratory distress syndrome; *CVP,* central venous pressure; *PCWP,* pulmonary capillary wedge pressure; *PEEP,* positive end expiratory pressure.

In ARDS characterized by mean pulmonary artery pressures (PAPs) of less than 30 mm Hg, the right ventricle dilates to maximize the SWI and is therefore able to maintain the forward flow to the left ventricle. However, in ARDS with mean PAPs of greater than 30 mm Hg, the right ventricle dilates, but resistance to outward flow is too great, and left-ventricular contractility diminishes.[17,28] Thus forward flow to the left ventricle is compromised, and left-ventricular preload diminishes. In addition, the extreme dilatation of the right ventricle impinges upon the left ventricle with interseptal shifts and crowding within the pericardium, further decreasing left ventricular compliance and preload. Furthermore, the use of positive pressure mechanical ventilation and PEEP exerts pressure against the pericardium, resulting in limited ventricular expansion. Other processes or therapies used in the septic state that may decrease ventricular compliance are myocardial edema, altered calcium metabolism,

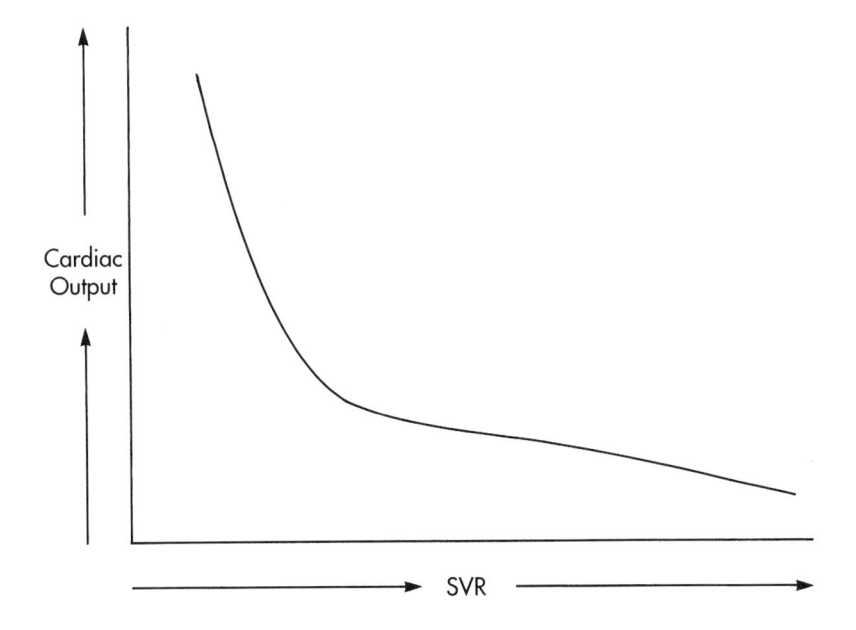

[Graph showing Cardiac Output vs SVR as an inverse relationship curve]

Decreased SVR	Increased SVR
Vasodilator agents Inflammatory mediators Increased cardiac output Hypermetabolic tissue needs	Vasopressor agents Alpha stimulators Decreased cadiac output ARDS (PVR, right ventricle) Atherosclerosis

Fig. 12-6 Afterload associated with septic shock. *ARDS*, Adult respiratory distress syndrome; *PVR*, pulmonary vascular resistance; *SVR*, systemic vascular resistance.

sympathetic stimulation, and vasopressor drugs (through direct cardiotonic actions or increases in afterload). Ventricular compliance is augmented through the use of vasodilators and calcium-channel blockers.[22] Thus it becomes evident that volume is but one determinant of ventricular pressure. Compliance plays a significant role, especially in disease states.

Ventricular afterload

Physiologic role. Ventricular afterload refers to the force or tension created in the myocardial muscle that ejects blood against a resistant vasculature. The SVR, a clinical approximation of afterload, greatly influences the quantity of blood ejected from the ventricle. High afterloads (increased resistance) obstruct the outflow of blood, whereas low afterloads (low resistance) facilitate forward flow and output. Ventricular afterload varies in response to local tissue metabolic needs, sympathetic autonomic function and stimulation, and vasoactive mediators. Right ventricular afterload is also affected by the presence of pulmonary hypertension and ARDS.[22,26] All of these factors contribute to the alterations in afterload associated with septic shock (Fig. 12-6).

Impact of disease. Massive peripheral vasodilatation in response to increased tissue metabolic demands and inflammatory mediator activity is the clinical hallmark of septic shock and requires massive fluid resuscitation to fill the expanded vascular space. The reduction in left ventricular afterload facilitates ventricular ejection, resulting in an increased CO. However, severe and persistent vasodilatation increases venous pooling and diminishes venous return. This may result in a decreased preload and CO. Perpetuation of the severe vasodilatation compounded by a failing myocardium leads to prolonged hypotension, cellular damage, and ultimately death.[11,12] Physiologic mechanisms that normally enhance vasoconstriction may be nonfunctional or ineffective. These altered mechanisms may include nonresponsive peripheral alpha-receptors and inhibition of endogenous norepinephrine release.[16,30] In addition, multiple vasoactive mediators actively enhance vasodilatation. These may involve endotoxin, tumor necrosis factor (TNF), interleukin-1 (IL-1), interleukin-2 (IL-2), complement, prostaglandins, and beta-endorphins.[19,27] Therapeutic interventions in this setting include maximum volume administration, followed by the addition of vasopressor agents to increase the SVR.

In a small number of cases, sepsis is complicated by such severe myocardial depression that a compensatory increase in SVR mimics cardiogenic shock.[20] In this setting, vasodilator therapy, along with inotropic support, is appropriate to reduce afterload, facilitate forward flow, and enhance tissue perfusion.[19]

A special consideration for right-ventricular afterload is the presence and severity of ARDS. Unlike the muscular left ventricle, the thin-walled right ventricle has minimal ability to increase contractility in response to an acutely elevated resistance or myocardial depression. Instead, the right ventricle relies on its ability to accommodate large volumes in order to maintain stroke volume. Thus changes in right ventricular preload and compliance are of primary importance in maintaining forward flow to the left ventricle in disease states such as ARDS that result in increased right ventricular afterload.[9,22]

Studies have described the impact of ARDS on right ventricular function.[17,28] In a classic study, Sibbald and co-workers[28] demonstrated an increase in right ventricular EDVs as mean PAPs increased. Significant right ventricular dilatation was seen with mean PAPs of greater than 30 mm Hg. In addition, right ventricular ejection fraction (RVEF) fell as volume increased. However, stroke volume was maintained through the Frank-Starling mechanism. Forward flow to the left ventricle was maintained; and left ventricle preload, left ventricular ejection fraction (LVEF), and contractility were unaltered in patients with ARDS without sepsis. In spite of adequate left ventricular function, left ventricular end-diastolic pressures (PCWP) were significantly higher as the mean PAPs increased. This was seen as secondary to overdistention of the right ventricle, right-to-left septal shifts, and crowding within the pericardium, which consequently decreased left ventricular compliance (a small volume exerting a large pressure in a stiff, nonexpanding left ventricle). Other studies have found similar results in septic patients, supporting the concept that right ventricular dilatation is an important compensatory mechanism in preserving right ventricular myocardial function in sepsis and MODS complicated by ARDS with an increased afterload.[9,11,17]

Ventricular contractility

Physiologic role. Ventricular contractility is defined as the ability of the myocardial fibers to shorten and effectively propel blood from the ventricular chambers independent of variations in preload or afterload.[22] Alterations in contractility are offset by changes in preload and afterload under normal conditions. Experimentally, contractility is assessed in isolated myocardial fibers by determining the velocity and strength of fiber shortening. Clinically, however, the objective determination of contractility is difficult because of the interdependence of the hemodynamic components and the effects of external factors such as circulating catecholamine levels, therapeutic measures, and intrinsic and extrinsic myocardial depressant factors (Fig. 12-7). Various derived measures of flow, volume, and pressure are used to infer contractile force.* These include CO, CI, ejection fraction, SWI, and end-systolic volume (Table 12-1).

The CO and CI are measures of the flow of blood from the heart to the periphery. As a measure of flow only, CI does not take into account the work generated by the myocardium to produce the flow. CI is very dependent upon multiple variables, such as preload, afterload, heart rate, and contractility that change substantially during the course of the

---

*References 4, 10, 19, 22, 29.

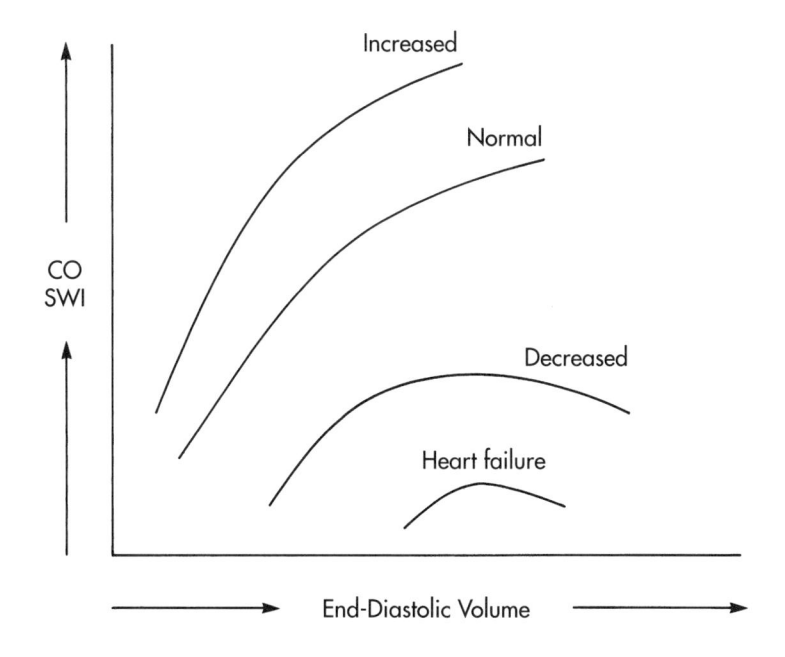

Increased Contractility	Decreased Contractility
Catecholamines Inotropic agents Increased end-diastolic volume	Decreased sympathetic stimulation Decreased compliance Decreased end-diastolic volume Myocardial edema Loss of myocardial tissue Hypoxia Acidosis Inflammatory mediators Depressant factors Beta blockers Calcium-channel blockers

Fig. 12-7 Contractility. *CO,* Cardiac output; *SWI,* stroke work index.

disease. As in the case of sepsis, a depressed myocardium that is stimulated by endogenous or exogenous catecholamines has an increased EDV, and faces a low resistance to flow will usually exhibit a normal or increased CI. Thus clinically the CI is a reliable indicator of the delivery of blood to the tissues but not of the contractile force necessary to sustain that delivery of flow.[19,22]

Ejection fraction (EF) is the percentage of the end-diastolic volume ejected from the ventricle. EF is a better indicator than CI of baseline ventricular function; however, it is also affected by preload, afterload, and compliance.[1] In general, EF falls because the myocardial contractile force is insufficient to propel blood from the ventricles. The heart attempts to maintain stroke volume and flow through

Table 12-1 Calculated Hemodynamic Variables

Parameter	Calculation	Normal range
Flow		
MAP	$\frac{S-D}{3} + D$	60-105 mm Hg
CI	$\frac{CO}{BSA}$	2.5-4.0 L/min
CO	$HR \times SV$	4.0-8.0 L/min
Volume		
SV	$\frac{CO \times 1000}{HR}$	60-100 mL/beat
SVI	$\frac{CI}{HR}$	33-47 mL/beat/m^2
PCWP		8-12 mm Hg
CVP	cm H$_2$O = mm Hg $\times$ 1.34	2-6 mm Hg
Resistance		
SVR	$\frac{MAP - CVP}{CO} \times 80$	800-1200 dyne/s/cm^{-5}
SVRI	$\frac{MAP - CVP}{CI} \times 80$	1760-2600 dyne/s/cm^{-5}/m^2
PVR	$\frac{mPAP - PCWP}{CO} \times 80$	37-250 dyne/s/cm^{-5}
PVRI	$\frac{mPAP - PCWP}{CI} \times 80$	45-225 dyne/s/cm^{-5}/m^2
Contractility		
LVSWI	SVI (MAP − PCWP) × 0.0136	38-85 g·m/m^2/beat
RVSWI	SVI (mPAP − PAD) × 0.0136	7-12 g·m/m^2/beat

BSA, Body surface area; *CI*, cardiac index; *CO*, cardiac output; *CVP*, central venous pressure; *D*, diastolic; *HR*, heart rate; *LVSWI*, left-ventricular stroke work index; *MAP*, mean arterial pressure; *mPAP*, mean pulmonary artery pressure; *PAD*, pulmonary artery diastolic pressure; *PCWP*, pulmonary capillary wedge pressure; *PVR*, pulmonary vascular resistance; *PVRI*, pulmonary vascular resistance index; *RVSWI*, right-ventricular stroke work index; *S*, systolic; *SV*, stroke volume; *SVI*, stroke volume index; *SVR*, systemic vascular resistance; *SVRI*, systemic vascular resistance index.

the use of preload reserve (ventricular dilatation). If the compensatory increase in compliance with larger preload volumes is inadequate to maintain forward flow, afterload increases, further restricting EF. In sepsis, an initially low EF is, paradoxically, associated with increased survival.[2,29] This phenomenon is explained by compensatory ventricular dilatation in response to myocardial depression that results in larger end-diastolic volumes to maintain stroke volume. Ventricular size, preload, and EF return to normal as the sepsis and myocardial depression subside (Fig. 12-8). Conversely, the EF in patients who do not survive is usually normal throughout the duration of the disease until death. For unknown reasons, compensatory ventricular dilatation does not occur (perhaps because of decreased compliance), and the lower peripheral resistance in those who do not survive is seen as facilitating the maintenance of EF.[11,27,31] These changes in EF have been demonstrated in both the right and left ventricles. In addition, the changes occur together in the majority of cases, thus indicating a biventricular contractile dysfunction.[11,27]

Stroke work index (SWI) is a composite variable used to assess ventricular contractility. It is a measure of the relationship between myocardial fiber

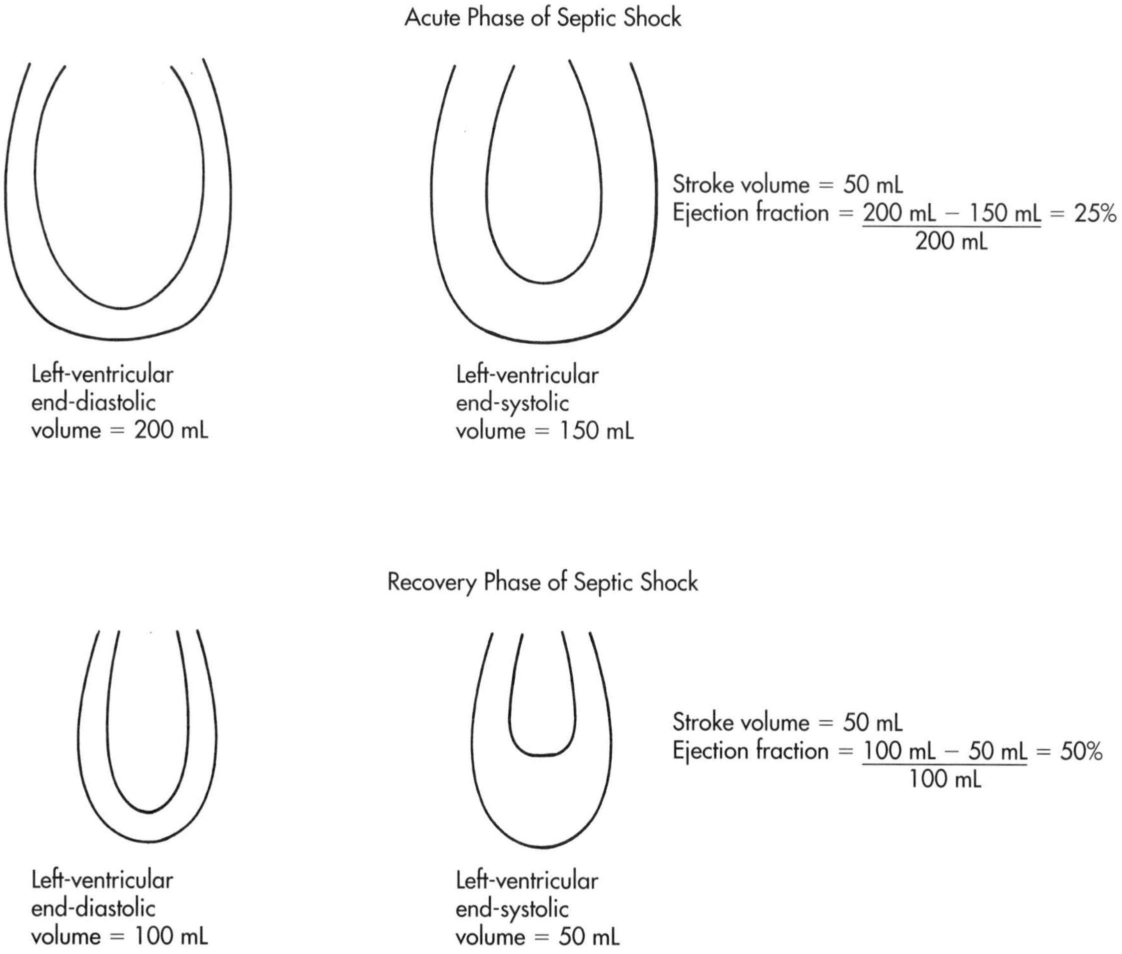

Acute Phase of Septic Shock

Left-ventricular end-diastolic volume = 200 mL

Left-ventricular end-systolic volume = 150 mL

Stroke volume = 50 mL
Ejection fraction = $\frac{200\ mL - 150\ mL}{200\ mL} = 25\%$

Recovery Phase of Septic Shock

Left-ventricular end-diastolic volume = 100 mL

Left-ventricular end-systolic volume = 50 mL

Stroke volume = 50 mL
Ejection fraction = $\frac{100\ mL - 50\ mL}{100\ mL} = 50\%$

Fig. 12-8 Ventricular changes in septic shock. A schematic representation of the reversible myocardial depression seen in the survivors of septic shock. (From Parker MM et al. Profound but reversible myocardial depression in patients with septic shock. Ann Intern Med 1984:100:488).

tension (contractile force) and preload volume (i.e., the Frank-Starling law). Given a set volume infusion, normal myocardial tissues exhibit greater increases in contractile force (or SWI) than do depressed myocardial tissues (Fig. 12-3). In other words, larger volumes and greater stretch are necessary to maintain contractile force and output in the depressed myocardium. Biventricular myocardial depression, indicated by low SWI, has been consistently demonstrated in survivors and nonsurvivors of sepsis. Decreases in SWI are noted early in sepsis, and survivors demonstrate a return to normal SWI while the SWI continues to decline in patients who ultimately die.[11]

End-systolic volume (ESV) is another useful measure in evaluating contractility. As contractile ability declines, less blood is propelled from the heart (falling EF) resulting in more blood remaining at the end of systole (increased ESV). In addition, alterations in afterload affect ESV. Increased resistance impedes outflow, resulting in an increased ESV; conversely, decreased resistance facilitates ventricular ejection, leading to smaller ESV. In sepsis, studies have demonstrated increased left ventricular ESV (LVESV) despite lower resistance, signifying a decrease in left ventricular contractility.[4,12] Right ventricular ESV (RVESV) has also been shown to rise regardless of the presence of an elevated afterload (as in ARDS), thus leading researchers to conclude that right ventricular myocardial depression is also apparent during sepsis.[3,9,11,27]

Impact of disease. In summary, biventricular diastolic and systolic dysfunction is evident in early sepsis. In response to myocardial depressant stimuli, diastolic components (preload and compliance) are altered to compensate for declining systolic function (contractility).[21] In addition, as illustrated in Table 12-2 and Table 12-3, these changes follow distinct patterns in survivors and nonsurvivors of septic shock. Regardless of the final outcome, the symptoms in most of the patients (in more than 90%) include an elevated CI, low systemic vascular resistance index (SVRI), and hypotension. By 2 to 5 days after the onset of hypotension, survivors show evidence of significant myocardial depression. Despite a normal or elevated CI, these patients display a dilated left ventricle, increased left ventricular end diastolic volume (LVEDV), low LVEF, a low left

Table 12-2 Initial and Final Hemodynamic Changes in Survivors and Nonsurvivors of Septic Shock

Parameters	Survivors (n = 22) Initial	Final	p*	Nonsurvivors (n = 17) Initial	Final	p
Heart rate, beats/min	105	95	NS†	111	129	0.006
Mean arterial pressure, mm Hg	77	85	0.017	74	74	NS
Pulmonary artery wedge pressure, mm Hg	13.7	9.6	0.047	14	13.4	NS
Central venous pressure, mm Hg	9.5	4.4	0.016	9.8	10.7	NS
Cardiac index, L/min/m^2	4.1	4.1	NS	4.9	4.8	NS
Stroke volume index, mL/m^2	39.9	42	NS	45.5	38.6	NS
Systemic vascular resistance index, dynes/s/cm^{-5}/m^2	1470	1691	NS	1262	1176	NS
Pulmonary artery mean pressure, mm Hg	22	17	0.036	22	24	NS
Pulmonary vascular resistance index, dynes/s/cm^{-5}/m^2	204	150	NS	144	193	NS
Left ventricular stroke work index, g·m/m/m^2	34	41	NS	37	34	NS
Right ventricular stroke work index, g·m/m/m^2	5.4	7.3	.03	7.2	6.3	NS

*Paired sample *t* test.
†NS indicates not statistically significant.
From Parker MM et al. Right ventricular dysfunction and dilation, similar to left ventricular changes, characterize the cardiac depression of septic shock in humans. Chest 1990;97:126-131.

Table 12-3 Initial and Final Ejection Fraction and End Diastolic Volume Index in Survivors and Nonsurvivors of Septic Shock

Parameters	Survivors (n = 22) Initial	Final	p*	Nonsurvivors (n = 17) Initial	Final	p
Left ventricular ejection fraction	.31	.47	.001	.40	.43	NS†
Left ventricular end diastolic volume index, mL/m^2	145	106	.012	124	102	NS
Right ventricular ejection fraction	.35	.51	.001	.41	.39	NS
Right ventricular end diastolic volume index, mL/m^2	124	88	.03	120	114	NS

*Paired sample *t* test.
†NS indicates not statistically significant.
From Parker MM et al. Right ventricular dysfunction and dilatation, similar to left ventricular changes, characterize the cardiac depression of septic shock in humans. Chest 1990;97:126-131.

ventricular stroke work index (LVSWI), and a normal or low SVRI. They tolerate large volumes of fluid before maximum filling pressure is reached (PCWP at 12 to 15 mm Hg) and may require only transient inotropic and vasopressor support, because hemodynamic parameters typically return to normal within 7 to 10 days. Symptoms of right ventricular dysfunction closely parallel those described in left ventricular dysfunction, indicating a severe but reversible biventricular abnormality.[2,10-12]

Conversely, nonsurvivors do not demonstrate adequate compensatory changes in diastolic function to offset systolic abnormalities. Significant increases in left ventricular dilatation and LVEDV do not occur in response to myocardial depression. Their stiff ventricles render these patients intolerant to massive fluid resuscitation, and other therapies (inotropes, vasopressors) are necessary to support hemodynamics. Despite persistent hypotension, nonsurvivors typically maintain a hyperdynamic profile with a normal or elevated ejection fraction, stroke volume, and CI until death. They exhibit a more severe vasodilatory response to sepsis than do survivors, which perhaps enables the depressed myocardium to continue to propel blood through the tissues. In addition, the higher heart rate of nonsurvivors aids in maintaining CI in the event stroke volume index (SVI) falls (CO = HR × SV). Considerable cardiac reserve is necessary to support such abnormal demands, and eventually irreversible failure ensues. Thus the ability of the ventricles to dilate and use preload reserve in response to myocardial depression is correlated positively with survival. Stiff, noncompliant ventricles are associated with higher mortality rates.[1,2,10-12]

ETIOLOGY OF MYOCARDIAL DYSFUNCTION

Although most authors and researchers agree that myocardial depression is evident early in the course of sepsis, the pathogenesis of this altered performance is ill defined and controversial. However, several conditions and multiple mediators have been implicated in the development of myocardial dysfunction in sepsis and overwhelming inflammation.

Coronary blood flow

Global perfusion. Reduction in coronary blood flow producing global myocardial ischemia has been postulated as a precursor to myocardial failure in septic shock.[2] However, several studies demonstrate significant increases in coronary blood flow without parallel increases in myocardial demands.[32-35] Under physiologic conditions, coronary perfusion is directly determined by myocardial metabolic demands. The myocardium maintains an almost complete (70% to 75%) extraction of arterial oxygen. Increases in oxygen demand that cannot be met by enhanced extraction are met by changes in coronary blood flow. Through autoregulatory mechanisms, the coronary vasculature precisely maintains perfusion to match myocardial requirements. Abrupt changes do not disturb this delicate balance even over a wide range of perfusion pressures (from 60 mm Hg to 140 mm Hg).[32,33,36]

Loss of autoregulation. In sepsis, this autoregulatory ability to match perfusion with myocardial requirements is lost. Although myocardial requirements do not increase in sepsis, excessive vasodilatation, high coronary blood flow, and reduced oxygen extraction are apparent. The net production of lactate is not increased, indicating the absence of global myocardial hypoxia and ischemia.[32-35] A global measure of myocardial metabolism, however, may not detect local ischemia resulting from possible maldistribution of flow within the myocardium. Several authors have described microcirculatory disturbances and scattered necrosis in the septic heart, but the role of these symptoms in the pathogenesis of myocardial failure has not been resolved.[37,38]

Maldistribution of coronary blood flow. The changes in coronary circulation are similar to the alterations of high CO, low SVR, and reduced oxygen extraction described in the systemic circulation. Factors precipitating myocardial circulatory changes are unclear but may result from the release of vasoactive mediators such as epinephrine, histamine, kinins, and prostacyclin.[33] The vasodilatation may also be a compensatory mechanism to counteract the negative effects of decreased oxygen extraction.[32] In addition, alterations in myocardial energy metabolism may contribute to coronary vasodilatation and myocardial dysfunction. Dhainaut and co-workers[33] described alterations in myocardial substrate extraction that were associated with poor cardiac performance in patients with sepsis. Patients with sepsis relied primarily on lactate and endogenous cardiac reserves for metabolism and did not use exogenous glucose, fatty acids, and ketone bodies appropriately for energy production. The decrease in exogenous substrate use was more pronounced in patients who did not survive, indicating a greater metabolic derangement. The precise relationship between altered myocardial circulation, energy metabolism, and myocardial depression remains to be defined through further research.[32-34]

Calcium metabolism, coronary artery disease, and myocardial edema. Altered calcium metabolism[39] and the presence of preexisting coronary artery disease[40] have been shown to decrease ventricular compliance and thus reduce the available preload reserve necessary to compensate for decreased intrinsic contractility. In addition, myocardial edema has been implicated in contributing to both systolic and diastolic myocardial dysfunction.[41] Edematous myocardial tissues do not contract or relax adequately; thus contractile force and compliance are diminished. Myocardial edema may be more pronounced in nonsurvivors, contributing to the inability of the myocardium to dilate in response to acute contractile depression. Furthermore, edema may interfere with myocardial microperfusion by compressing the coronary circulation and increasing diffusion distance.[14] Thus the presence of myocardial edema may be a critical determinant of early cardiac dysfunction.[21,27]

Sympathetic nervous system responsiveness

Alterations in sympathetic nervous system responsiveness may contribute to diminished ventricular performance in septic shock. Contractility and CO are enhanced through sympathetic nervous system stimulation of myocardial beta receptors. In shock states, such stimulation is a vital compensatory mechanism that maintains ventricular performance and may, in fact, obscure any underlying primary cardiac dysfunction. Increased circulating catecholamine levels and enhanced beta-adrenergic stimulation have been demonstrated in early sepsis (preshock).[30,42] However, after the initial compensatory period and as sepsis progresses, the myocardium becomes less sensitive to circulating catecholamines and contractility declines. Contractile reserves are reduced through the down-regulation of beta-adrenergic receptors, contributing to biventricular depression that is increasingly refractory to elevated plasma levels of endogenous epinephrine, norepinephrine, and other administered catecholamines.[16,30]

Mediator activity

Myocardial depressant factor. Circulating cardiodepressant and vasoactive mediators have been described in the pathogenesis of sepsis. The existence of myocardial depressant factor (MDF) and its potential role in myocardial dysfunction in shock states have been intensely researched and debated for nearly 20 years, and general consensus has yet to be achieved.[2] However, studies have demonstrated a direct effect of MDF or other humoral factors on myocardial function. An early study by Parrillo and co-workers[43] demonstrated that serum from patients with sepsis who exhibited acute myocardial dysfunction (low LVEF) produced a 25% to 34% decrease in contractility of rat myocytes. As the patients with sepsis recovered and the LVEF returned to normal, their sera no longer contained MDF or affected the rat myocyte contractility. In addition, the degree of LVEF reduction in patients paralleled the extent of rat myocyte depression. Furthermore, increased levels of MDF were associated with substantially elevated LV filling pressures, ventricular dilatation, and mean peak lactate concentrations. Reilly and co-workers[44] described similar hemodynamic alterations, ventricular dilatation, and reversible myocardial depression in septic shock patients with circulating MDF.

Strong evidence exists that supports the presence of a circulating myocardial depressant factor in septic shock; however, this factor has yet to be isolated and its precise mechanism of action determined.[2,45] In addition, conflicting evidence exists as to its site of origin. It is hypothesized that the pancreas, stimulated by hypoperfusion and ischemia, produces MDF through a series of cellular autolytic reactions. MDF is then released into the blood stream, from where it is transported to the heart. However, removal of the pancreas does not necessarily prevent myocardial depression in septic animals. Therefore the presence, actions, and relative importance of humoral depressant factors require further research.[46]

Endotoxin. Endotoxin appears to exert a direct cardiodepressant effect. Studies in dogs have shown a direct depressant effect that is dose-dependent.[2] In healthy volunteers, small doses of endotoxin resulted in the classic septic hemodynamic response of high CO, left ventricular dilatation, decreased LVEF, and systemic vasodilatation.[47] In patients with septic shock, detectable serum levels of endotoxin were found in only 43% of patients and its presence was intermittent during the 24-hour study period. However, the presence of endotoxin was associated with a higher mortality, myocardial depression, renal failure, ARDS, and MODS.[48] These studies suggest that endotoxin plays a role in the cardiovascular changes and myocardial depression in septic shock, but the mechanism for its action is not clear. The effects may be the result of direct myocardial depression, or endotoxin may stimulate the release of other humoral mediators that reduce cardiac contractility.[48]

Tumor necrosis factor. Tumor necrosis factor, a cytokine produced primarily by macrophages, has been detected in animal[49] and human[47] experimental models after exposure to endotoxin. In healthy volunteers, peak levels of TNF coincided with the onset of the hyperdynamic cardiovascular state. As the septic event progressed to the stage of myocardial depression and ventricular dilatation, TNF was no longer detectable in the serum of the subjects.[47] Animal studies[49,50] have shown similar results, leading researchers to postulate that TNF stimulates a cascade of mediators that produce the classic symptoms of septic shock and systemic inflammation. In fact, TNF has been found in patients with severe sepsis and patients in septic shock and is often correlated with increased mortality.[27,49] TNF is generated in response to endotoxin and may either have a delayed effect on myocardial contractility or may itself initiate the release of other mediators with direct cardiodepressant effects.[27,47]

Other mediators. The by-products of infectious microorganisms and injured tissue activate macrophages and other inflammatory cells resulting in a cascade of events including the release of various cytokines and mediators. These mediators produce and exacerbate the hemodynamic effects characteristic of septic shock. IL-1[51] and IL-2[52] have been associated with the heart failure and hemodynamic changes seen in septic shock. Complement has been associated with the severe vasodilatation and hypotension.[53] Thromboxane A_2 may act as an intermediary by generating plasma myocardial depressant substances.[54] Prostaglandin F_2[54] has been shown to produce myocardial depression. Platelet activating factor also decreases myocardial contractility and has been shown to induce arrhythmias, increase capillary leakage, and contribute to myocardial edema.[55] High levels of nitric oxide have been shown to produce massive vasodilation[56,57] and may potentiate the myocardial depressant effects of TNF.[58] Therefore many endogenous mediators may be involved directly or indirectly in the production of cardiac dysfunction.

In conclusion, myocardial depression is the result of numerous physiologic derangements and humoral mediators. The precise interaction and roles of these factors and mediators are unknown. Research continues in this area to identify and clarify the mechanisms producing the abnormal cardiovascular sequelae described in the syndromes of sepsis and SIRS.

ROLE OF MONITORING

Patients in septic shock typically present with hypotension, warm and flushed skin, bounding pulses, fever, tachypnea, and alterations in mental status. Other associated clinical symptoms include leukocytosis, respiratory alkalosis, and evidence of end-organ insufficiency (i.e., elevated creatinine, jaundice, hyperbilirubinemia, and elevated lactate).[59] If the patient is not already in the critical care unit, he or she must be admitted. Analysis of survival rates in sepsis has demonstrated a decrease in mortality rates for patients admitted to critical care units staffed by full-time critical care physicians and nurses with the knowledge and capabilities for hemodynamic monitoring and support.[2]

Arterial access

Invasive monitoring in the intensive care unit begins with an arterial line for continuous monitoring of blood pressure because cuff pressures are often inaccurate in shock states. An adequate systolic pressure (≥ 90 mm Hg) is often indicative of flow; however, when coupled with a very low diastolic pressure as is often seen in septic shock, perfusion to some vascular beds can be impaired. Thus, the mean arterial pressure (MAP) is the best indicator of perfusion because it takes into account both systolic and diastolic values. An MAP greater than 60 mm Hg is necessary to maintain perfusion to the vital organs. In addition to blood pressure monitoring, arterial lines allow frequent blood sampling for various parameters such as arterial blood gases, electrolytes, lactate, and metabolites that can change rapidly during the course of the disease.[4,19] Common metabolic derangements in sepsis such as acidosis, hypoxia, hypophosphatemia, and hypocalcemia are known cardiac depressants and must be avoided in order to optimize CO.[27]

Pulmonary artery catheter

A pulmonary artery catheter allows for the initial differential diagnosis of the cause of shock (Table 12-4). Ongoing cardiac status and fluid balance are evaluated through serial analysis of cardiac filling pressures (PCWP and CVP), cardiac flow (CO and CI), cardiac contractility (SV, SVI, and SWI), and afterload (SVR). Measurement of mixed venous blood gases and arterial oxygen saturations allows for calculations of total body oxygen consumption. Correct assessment and interpretation of these parameters is important in choosing the appropriate treatments, determining the response to interventions, and monitoring the progress of the patient.[4,8]

Venous access and cardiac monitoring

A central line (single or multiple infusion) and two or more peripheral lines are often required to allow for simultaneous administration of resuscitation fluids, antibiotics, vasoactive infusions, and blood products. In addition, continuous cardiac monitoring is necessary. Atrial arrhythmias (atrial fibrillation, atrial flutter, or supraventricular tachycardia) are more common than are ventricular arrhythmias in patients with sepsis. Atrial arrhythmias can significantly diminish CO and exacerbate the hypotension and abnormal organ flow. Conversion to normal sinus rhythm can be accomplished with medications or synchronized cardioversion. The use of cardioversion may necessitate concurrent administration of sedatives and analgesics that can further lower blood pressure; therefore, the use of such agents must be considered on an individual basis. Pharmacologic agents such as verapamil, procainamide, or quinidine may also be useful in slowing tachyarrhythmias or holding a conversion rhythm. Again, the side effects of hypotension and direct myocardial depression must be weighed against the overall condition of the patient.[60] The guiding principle when using these therapies is to begin at the lowest dose or watt-seconds and titrate up until the desired effect is achieved.

THERAPEUTIC MANAGEMENT

Sepsis and MODS are complex disease states that require prompt and knowledgeable interventions in order to maximize the probability of survival for the patient. The high mortality rate associated with these disease states reflects our inability to reverse the underlying pathologic process that results in persistent hypotension, maldistribution of flow, and eventual end-organ demise. The use of antimediator therapy is promising but requires further investigation before it can be applied effectively. Thus, maintenance of cardiac and end-organ function is the cornerstone of therapy while the injurious processes run their course and the infection, if present, is treated.[61] Much research has focused on identifying the overall hemodynamic goals that would facilitate patient survival. These key goals[8,14,18,53] are outlined in Table 12-5.

Table 12-4 Hemodynamic Parameters in Shock States

Shock state	MAP	CO	SVR	PCWP	CVP	Treatments
Distributive						
Septic	↓	↑	↓	↓	↓	Fluid
Neurogenic						Vasopressors
Anaphylactic						Inotropes
Cardiogenic	↓	↓	↑	↑	↑	Fluid
						Inotropes
						Vasodilators
Hypovolemic	↓	↓	↑	↓	↓	Fluid/blood
Obstructive						
Cardiac tamponade	↓	↓	↑	↑	↑	Pericardiocentesis
						Reentry sternotomy

CO, Cardiac output; *CVP*, central venous pressure; *MAP*, mean arterial pressure; *PCWP*, pulmonary capillary wedge pressure; *SVR*, systemic vascular resistance.

Almost all (90%) septic shock patients present in the hyperdynamic state after initial volume infusion. In the early stages, maximizing the hyperdynamic state via volume infusion, inotropes, and vasopressor drugs may reduce mortality by enhancing oxygen delivery and consumption.[8,18,62-64] However, once the inflammatory response becomes systemic as a result of tissue hypoxia, injury, or infection, the hyperdynamic state alone has not proven to increase survival. The majority of patients are able to maintain the hyperdynamic state either spontaneously or artificially until they begin to recover or until death occurs. A minority of patients progress to the hypodynamic state, and their treatment includes volume infusion, inotropes, and vasodilating drugs if the SVR increases above 1000 to 1200 dynes/sec/cm^5.[18]

Volume infusion

Goal. Increasing preload through volume infusion is the best initial hemodynamic therapy to treat hypotension. Initially, preload and cardiac filling pressures (CVP and PCWP) are significantly reduced as a result of vasodilatation. Ongoing preload reduction results from increased capillary leakage, displacement of volume, and maldistribution of blood flow. Fluid infusion increases ventricular volume, maximizes myocardial stretch (Frank-Starling mechanism), and maintains CO. Although CO is often elevated in septic shock, MAP and SVR are reduced. The goal of fluid resuscitation is to increase CO to supranormal levels and to keep MAP greater than 60 mm Hg to preserve adequate perfusion and oxygen transport to the hypermetabolic organs.[7,8]

Response. Response to volume infusion is determined through serial measures of filling pressures (PCWP), ventricular performance parameters (CO, CI, SVR, SVI, and SWI), and end-organ function. Trends and magnitude of changes in PCWP during volume infusion are interpreted, since isolated PCWP values do not accurately reflect end-diastolic volume (preload) and are influenced by ventricular compliance. Fluid challenges of 250 to 500 mL are administered when the PCWP is less than 10 to 12 mm Hg. If the PCWP increases by 3 to 5 mm Hg, the ventricle is compliant and can accommodate more fluid to maximize stretch. Fluid challenge continues as long as the PCWP changes no more than 3 to 5 mm Hg with subsequent boluses. However, when the PCWP increases by more than 5 to 7 mm Hg in response to a fluid bolus, maximal preload volume and stretch have been achieved, and further fluid administration will only increase filling pressure and put the patient at risk for developing pulmonary edema[22] (Fig. 12-5). Measures of ventricular performance are assessed along with PCWP to give the total picture of response to fluid therapy. Stroke volume, SWI (a measure that considers both ventricular volume and pressure), and CO should increase as preload is augmented. As optimal fluid status is achieved, further increases in these measures of ventricular function will be absent or minimal with additional volume infusion. If maximum volume infusion fails to alleviate hypotension, inotropic agents and vasopressor therapy are added.[7]

In general, PCWP is maintained between 12 and 15 mm Hg in patients with sepsis. However, decreases in ventricular compliance as a result of either intrinsic changes in myocardial muscle fibers (myocardial edema) or extrinsic causes (ARDS, PEEP) may require pressures between 15 and 18 mm Hg to maintain stroke volume. Patients with a PCWP greater than 20 mm Hg often develop pulmonary edema.[7,27]

Crystalloids versus colloids. Because of myocardial and peripheral vascular abnormalities, large quantities of fluid are necessary to maintain blood pressure and organ perfusion. The use of colloids or crystalloids continues to be researched, but neither has consistently proven to be superior over the other

Table 12-5 Key Therapeutic Goals in Septic Shock[8,14,18,53]

Clinical parameter	Goal/endpoint
Mean arterial pressure (MAP)	≥60 mm Hg
Cardiac index (CI)	≥4.5 L/min/m^2
Systolic blood pressure (SBP)	≥90 mmHg
Systemic vascular resistance (SVR)	700-800 dyne/sec/cm^{-5}
Pulmonary capillary wedge pressure (PCWP)	12-18 mmHg
Oxygen delivery (Do$_2$)	>600 mL/min/m^2
Oxygen consumption (Vo$_2$)	>170 mL/min/m^2
Arterial oxygen saturation (Sao$_2$)	≥90 mmHg
Hematocrit (Hct)	30%-35%
Hemoglobin (Hg)	10 g/dL
Albumin	>2.5 g/dL

in terms of cardiovascular performance or ultimate mortality.[7,18] Crystalloids (normal saline and lactated Ringer's solutions) are inexpensive and have relatively few, if any, side effects but may decrease oxygen consumption secondary to interstitial edema formation.[8] Colloids (albumin, protein solutions, and blood products) and synthetic colloids (hetastarch and dextran) are more expensive and have increased side effects, but they remain in the vascular space longer and may decrease the incidence of pulmonary and systemic edema.[7] In addition, studies have illustrated an increase in oxygen delivery and consumption when colloids are used during resuscitation.[65] However, opponents of colloid use argue that the colloids leak into the interstitial space in the presence of increased vascular permeability and exacerbate vascular fluid loss and peripheral edema.[4] Assessment of the needs of individual patients is the best guide to fluid therapy. If the patient is anemic (hematocrit ≤30% to 35%), blood is usually administered to maintain not only volume status but also oxygen-carrying capacity.[7,14] If the patient is hypoalbuminemic (albumin level ≤2.5 g/dL), albumin solutions (50 to 100 g albumin given as a 25% solution) are appropriate.[18] With an acceptable hematocrit and albumin level, crystalloid solutions may be indicated.[8,18]

Survivors versus nonsurvivors. Studies demonstrate that preload requirements change as the sepsis evolves and are different in survivors and nonsurvivors.[4,10-12] Survivors demonstrate acute ventricular dilatation (more fluid must be infused before maximum PCWP and ventricular performance are attained), decreased ejection fraction, high CO, tachycardia, and low SVR that return to normal within 7 to 10 days. Thus fluid requirements decrease as the patient progresses toward recovery. Patients who do not survive typically maintain an elevated CO, severe vasodilatation, tachycardia, and hypotension without ventricular dilatation and decreased ejection fraction. Decreased ventricular compliance renders patients less tolerant to fluid resuscitation measures, and they exhibit higher filling pressures with less volume. If the patient develops ARDS, further decreases in left ventricular compliance and size occur as a result of right ventricular dilatation, interventricular shifts, and PEEP therapy and are reflected in even higher filling pressures. These higher filling pressures (15 to 18 mm Hg) are necessary to maintain stroke volume, and the persistence of the peripheral vascular abnormalities and capillary leakage require continued fluid support.[4,10-12,31]

Inotropic and vasopressor therapy

Goal. Inotropic or vasopressor agents are indicated if maximum volume infusion (up to a PCWP of 15 to 18 mm Hg) does not normalize blood pressure, attain key therapeutic goals (Table 12-5), and improve organ perfusion as judged by decreased lactate levels, adequate urine output, and normal organ function studies. Persistent hypotension is usually secondary to profound vasodilatation. Inotropes or vasopressors are necessary to increase cardiac output, to induce vasoconstriction, or to do both. The inotropic or vasopressor effects of most of these drugs are dose dependent, and they vary in their influence on the heart and peripheral vasculature (Table 12-6).[66,67] In addition, their prolonged use in

Table 12-6 Commonly Used Vasopressor Agents: Relative Potency*

		Cardiac		Peripheral vasculature		
Agent	Dose	Heart rate	Contractility	Vasoconstriction	Vasodilatation	Dopaminergic
Dopamine	1-10 μg/kg/min	2+	2+	0	2+	4+
	>10 μg/kg/min	2+	2+	2-3+	0	0
Levarterenol (norepinephrine)	2-8 μg/min	2+	2+	4+	0	0
Dobutamine	1-10 μg/kg/min	1+	4+	1+	2+	0
Isoproterenol	1-4 μg/min	4+	4+	0	4+	0
Epinephrine	1-8 μg/min	4+	4+	4+	3+	0
Phenylephrine	20-200 μg/min	0	0	4+	0	0

*The 1 to 4+ scoring system represents an arbitrary quantitative scoring system to allow a judgment of comparative potency among these vasopressor agents.
From Parrillo JE. Septic shock: Clinical manifestations, pathogenesis, hemodynamics, and management in a critical care unit. In Parrillo JE, Ayres SM. Major issues in critical care medicine. Baltimore: Williams & Wilkins Co; 1984:111-125.

profound septic shock and MODS may require increasingly larger doses to maintain hemodynamic stability. This phenomenon may be caused by the decreased responsiveness of the alpha and beta receptors, circulating mediators, and continued losses of intravascular volume through capillary leakage and maldistribution of flow (sympathomimetics are ineffective in the presence of hypovolemia) seen in the septic shock.[7,18,68] As responsiveness to the vasopressors decreases, maintenance of vascular tone and blood pressure becomes more difficult.[1]

Debate in the literature continues concerning which drug protocol optimally achieves therapeutic goals after fluid resuscitation in septic shock patients. Edwards and co-workers[64], advocated the use of dobutamine and norepinephrine as first-line drugs, with dopamine being added only if endpoints were not achieved. Tuschschmidt and colleagues[62] described increased survival when colloids, dopamine, and dobutamine were administered. Moran and co-workers[69] successfully managed patients using epinephrine alone. Schoemaker and co-workers[8] reported end-point attainment after administering colloids, dobutamine, and vasodilators. Vasopressors were used only as a last resort to maintain hemodynamic stability. Gregory and colleagues[70] described successful management with colloid, phenylephrine, dobutamine, and low-dose dopamine. It is therefore evident that further research in this area is necessary. Each drug has its advantages and disadvantages and its effect on any particular patient may be variable. Thus, the fluid, inotrope, vasopressor, vasodilator, or combination of drugs that achieves the therapeutic goals should be used as long as the clinical status of the patient continues to improve.[8,64]

Dopamine. Dopamine has inotropic, chronotropic, and vascular effects because it stimulates alpha, beta, and dopaminergic receptors. Low-dose dopamine (1 to 5 µg/kg/min) may be the initial inotrope of choice in the hypotensive patient because of its ability to improve cardiac function and blood pressure and yet preserve renal function and improve flow to the liver and gut.[7] Dopamine in the dosage range of 1 to 5 µg/kg/min (and up to 10 µg/kg/min in some patients because of considerable interpatient variability) stimulates cardiac and peripheral beta receptors to produce moderate inotropic, chronotropic, and peripheral vasodilatory effects that increase stroke volume, heart rate, CO, and blood pressure. This dose also stimulates dopaminergic receptors of the renal and splanchnic vasculature, resulting in renal vasodilatation that protects the kidneys from the detrimental effects of shock and improved flow to the gut. If hypotension persists within the low-dose range, dopamine can be titrated up to a maximum of 20 µg/kg/min to keep the MAP greater than 60 mm Hg and to optimize hemodynamic and organ function parameters. At dosage ranges of 10 to 20 µg/kg/min, dopamine continues to have positive inotropic and chronotropic effects; however, renal and splanchnic vasodilatation is lost, and peripheral vasoconstriction occurs in all vascular beds as a result of alpha-receptor stimulation. When dopamine begins to exert its vasoconstrictive effect, maldistribution of flow in the microcirculation is worsened and oxygen delivery and consumption are decreased. It is at this point that dobutamine may be a better choice of inotrope.[8] At dosages greater than 20 µg/kg/min, dopamine is an unreliable vasoconstrictor, and adverse effects (extreme tachycardia, atrial dysrhythmia, ventricular dysrhythmia) are more common.[27,67] Some patients exhibit tachycardias and decreased oxygenation parameters at even low doses of dopamine. In these patients, the use of dopamine may not be beneficial.[7,8,27]

Dobutamine. Dobutamine is a synthetic beta receptor agonist that produces a significant increase in myocardial contractility and moderate peripheral vasodilatation.[67] In the past, the use of dobutamine in septic shock was limited to the minority of patients exhibiting profound cardiac depression and vasoconstriction[71] because its vasodilatory effects were difficult to control.[60] Recently, however, the use of dobutamine in septic shock has been reevaluated by several researchers,[8,62,64,72-74] and it has been found to have favorable inotropic effects in septic shock and MODS. In dosages of 2 to 20 µg/kg/min, dobutamine is used to overcome the myocardial depression of septic shock and increases CI, LVSWI, RVSWI, oxygen delivery, oxygen consumption, and at higher doses, the heart rate. MAP and PCWP have shown no appreciable changes, and SVR decreases. It is postulated that the effects on oxygen delivery and consumption result from a greater blood flow through previously constricted arterial beds. When compared to dopamine, dobutamine provides significantly greater tissue perfusion and has less effect on the heart rate.[8]

The disparity between recent and earlier studies in the use of dobutamine may be attributed to the volume status of the patients.[64] Aggressive fluid therapy is now the norm in the treatment of septic shock and MODS, and it has been shown that the volume status significantly influences the cardiovascular effects of catecholamines.[68,75] Thus, the vasodilatory effects of dobutamine may be controlled with adequate volume or the addition of other inotropes or vasopressors.[8,64,76]

Norepinephrine. Norepinephrine is predominantly an alpha receptor agonist that produces powerful vasoconstriction, mild increases in myocardial contractility, and no effect on the heart rate.[77] Its use in hyperdynamic septic shock is aimed at inducing an adequate SVR and MAP when volume infusion and inotropes (dopamine or dobutamine) fail. Norepinephrine is infused at a rate of 1 to 10 µg/min until the MAP is greater than 60 mm Hg and the SVR is within the lower end of the normal range. Elevating the MAP is necessary to maintain tissue perfusion pressure. However, excessive norepinephrine-induced vasoconstriction could potentially worsen the shock syndrome by vasoconstricting vascular beds and aggravating abnormalities of flow. This excessive vasoconstriction results in organ tissue damage, especially in the kidneys. In addition, if vasoconstriction produces too high an afterload, myocardial contractility and CO are reduced. Therefore the minimal effective dose of norepinephrine is administered to guard against its powerful vasoconstrictive side effects.[67,78]

Concern for the preservation of renal function has led researchers to attempt to define the parameters for norepinephrine use. Most researchers[77-80] agree that norepinephrine should be used only in the presence of refractory hypotension that has not responded to volume resuscitation and administration of dopamine or dobutamine. When used in patients with a hyperdynamic hemodynamic profile with abnormally low SVR[78,80] and normal lactate levels,[79] urine output was improved and no deleterious renal effects were noted. In addition, oxygen delivery and consumption were enhanced.[75,77] Several studies also support the use of low-dose dopamine in conjunction with norepinephrine infusions[77,78,80] to protect the renal and mesenteric circulations. By following serial hemodynamic and renal function studies, the combination therapy can be adjusted to maximize the status of the patient.

Phenylephrine. Phenylephrine is a pure alpha receptor agonist. It therefore produces powerful vasoconstriction without direct cardiac effects. If the patient responds adversely to dopamine or norepinephrine, phenylephrine can be used effectively in dosages ranging from 20 to 200 µg/min or more. Phenylephrine has been shown to have effects similar to those of norepinephrine in refractory hyperdynamic shock. CI, oxygen delivery, and oxygen consumption were increased,[70,81] especially when phenylephrine was administered with dobutamine.[70] Higher doses than normal are often necessary, further supporting the belief that the prolonged vasodilatation is partially due to the down-regulation of α-adrenergic receptors in the septic shock state.[70]

Epinephrine. Epinephrine is an alpha receptor and beta receptor agonist that has dose-dependent effects. At low doses, effects on beta receptors predominate while effects on alpha receptors are seen at higher doses.[67] In one study,[69] therapeutic endpoints were attained successfully through the use of epinephrine alone in septic shock patients. Dosage ranged from 3 to 27 µg/min. Furthermore, in patients who are hypotensive because of profound myocardial depression (cardiogenic shock superimposed on septic shock) and who are refractory to other therapies, epinephrine administration may result in stabilization and survival.[3,4] The major disadvantage of epinephrine is its tendency to produce arrhythmias and tachycardias and increase myocardial oxygen needs.[67]

Vasodilator therapy

Goal. Patients who maintain a high CO and low systemic resistance during the course of their disease rarely require vasodilating therapy; in fact, such therapy could compound the hypotension and provide no clinical benefit. However, sepsis and MODS can progress to a hypodynamic state in which the patient demonstrates profound cardiac failure characterized by a low CO and stroke volume, high left ventricular filling pressure, and increased SVR.[18] The intense vasoconstriction is deleterious to cardiac function and must be treated. This picture of cardiogenic shock results from severe biventricular myocardial depression, and perhaps is more pronounced in patients with overt or occult cardiac disease.[40] The status of this patient population is also often complicated by the presence of ARDS and MODS. The goal of vasodilator therapy in this setting is to reduce the obstruction to flow (afterload), enhance ventricular performance (contractility), decrease filling pressures, increase CO, and sustain tissue perfusion and oxygen delivery.

Nitroprusside. Sodium nitroprusside is usually the vasodilator of choice because of its balanced effect on arterial resistance and venous capacitance. Nitroprusside simultaneously reduces SVR and venous return (preload) and is especially useful in the presence of pulmonary edema. Its afterload-reducing effects enhance contractility and allow a higher ejection of blood. The decreased venous return coupled with enhanced ejection reduces myocardial and pulmonary congestion, and filling pressures (CVP and PCWP) are reduced.[19,82] Nitroprusside infusion is begun at a dosage of 0.5 µg/kg/min and is increased in small increments every 5 to 10 minutes until the MAP falls 5 to 10 mm Hg below previous levels but the systolic pressure remains above 95 to 90 mm Hg. The normal therapeutic range of nitroprusside administration is 0.5 to 8.0 µg/kg/min. Hemodynamic, oxygenation, and organ function parameters are repeated and assessed for improvement in the status of the patient, and therapy is adjusted appropriately.[82]

Combination therapy. Combination therapy with an inotrope and a vasodilator is the most common form of unloading therapy used in the treatment of sepsis-induced cardiogenic shock. The inotrope maintains the MAP and enhances contractility, whereas the vasodilator reduces afterload and PCWP. The combined effects result in a greater increase in CO than does either medication alone. Patients who require such massive hemodynamic support have a poor prognosis.[19]

Mechanical support

Other therapies for cardiac augmentation are the mechanical support devices: the intraaortic balloon pump (IABP) and ventricular assist devices (VAD). Both devices have been effective when used in the population of patients with primary cardiac disease. Their use in the patient with septic shock and MODS is not supported by the literature.[83,84]

CONCLUSION

Myocardial dysfunction in septic shock is a complex phenomenon that results from numerous physiologic derangements and humoral mediators. The biventricular systolic and diastolic alterations lead to critical changes in hemodynamic parameters that vary significantly between survivors and nonsurvivors. The ability of the ventricles to dilate and use preload reserve in response to the declining pump function appears to be a key determinant in survival. In addition, early and aggressive interventions by a knowledgeable health-care team are essential. The goal of therapy is to increase and maintain perfusion, often at supranormal levels, in order to meet the demands of the hypermetabolic organs. Initial treatment includes volume resuscitation to achieve an MAP greater than 60 mm Hg, a PCWP of 12 to 15 mm Hg, and end-organ perfusion. If volume resuscitation is ineffective, inotropes and vasopressor agents are added to the treatment regimen. Systemic vasodilators are indicated only in the minority of patients who demonstrate a clinical picture that is consistent with cardiogenic shock. Mechanical support is sometimes attempted in patients with severe myocardial depression, but such support rarely improves the final outcome. Antimediator therapy[49] has been the focus of intense research and some studies with these drugs have shown promise in reducing mortality. Future treatment modalities will most likely include a combination of antibiotics, antimediator drugs, and cardiovascular drugs that will support the patient through the systemic inflammatory response.

Despite advances in critical care technology and science, the mortality of patients with septic shock remains at 40% to 60%; mortality from MODS remains at 60% to 100%. However, research in this area continues in order to identify, clarify, and inhibit the mechanisms producing the abnormal cardiovascular sequelae characteristic of sepsis and the MODS syndrome.

REFERENCES

1. D'Orio V et al. Accuracy in early prediction of prognosis of patients with septic shock by analysis of simple indices: Prospective study. Crit Care Med 1990;18:1339-1345.
2. Parrillo JE. Pathogenic mechanisms of septic shock. N Engl J Med 1993;20:1471-1477.
3. Cunnion RE, Parrillo JE. Myocardial dysfunction in sepsis. Crit Care Clin 1989;5:99-118.
4. Natanson C, Hoffman WD, Parrillo JE. Septic shock: The cardiovascular abnormality and therapy. J Cardiothor Anesth 1989;3:215-227.
5. Hess ML, Hastillo A, Greenfield LJ. Spectrum of cardiovascular function during gram-negative sepsis. Prog Cardiovasc Dis 1981;23:279-298.
6. Rackow EC et al. Hemodynamic response to fluid repletion in patients with septic shock: Evidence of early depression of cardiac performance. Circ Shock 1987:22:11-22.

7. Rackow EC, Astiz ME. Pathophysiology and treatment of septic shock. JAMA 1991:266:548-553.
8. Shoemaker WC, Appel PL, Kram HB. Oxygen transport measurements to evaluate tissue perfusion and titrate therapy: Dobutamine and dopamine effects. Crit Care Med 1991:19:672-688.
9. Dhainaut JF et al. Right ventricular dysfunction in patients with septic shock. Intensive Care Med 1988:14:488-491.
10. Ognibene FP et al. Depressed left ventricular performance: Response to volume infusion in patients with sepsis and septic shock. Chest 1988:93:903-910.
11. Parker MM et al. Right ventricular dysfunction and dilatation, similar to left ventricular changes, characterize the cardiac depression of septic shock in humans. Chest 1990:97:126-131.
12. Parker MM et al. Profound but reversible myocardial depression in patients with septic shock. Ann Intern Med 1984:100:483-490.
13. Knaus WA, Wagner DP. Multiple systems organ failure: Epidemiology and prognosis. Crit Care Clin 1989:5:221-232.
14. Tuchschmidt J, Oblitas D, Fried JC. Oxygen consumption in sepsis and septic shock. Crit Care Med 1991:19:664-671.
15. Adams HR, Parker JL, Laughlin MH. Intrinsic myocardial dysfunction during endotoxemia: Dependent or independent of myocardial ischemia? Circ Shock 1990:30:63-76.
16. Bersten MB, Sibbald WJ. Circulatory disturbances in multiple systems organ failure. Crit Care Clin 1989:5:233-254.
17. Russell JA et al. Oxygen delivery and consumption and ventricular preload are greater in survivors than in nonsurvivors of the adult respiratory distress syndrome. Am Rev Respir Dis 1990:141:659-665.
18. Demling RH, Lalonde C, Ikegami K. Physiologic support of the septic patient. Surg Clin North Am 1994:74:637-658.
19. Parrillo JE. Septic shock in humans: Clinical evaluation, pathogenesis, and therapeutic approach. In: Shoemaker WC, Ayres S, Grenvik A, Holbrook PR, Thompson WL, eds. Textbook of critical care. Philadelphia: WB Saunders; 1989:1006-1024.
20. Parrillo JE. Cardiovascular dysfunction in human septic shock. Prog Clin Biol Res 1989:308:191-199.
21. Jafri R et al. Left ventricular diastolic function in sepsis. Crit Care Med 1990:18:709-714.
22. Calvin JE, Sibbald WJ. Applied cardiovascular physiology in the critically ill with special reference to diastole and ventricular interaction. In: Shoemaker WC et al, ed. Textbook of critical care. Philadelphia: WB Saunders; 1989:312-326.
23. Braunwald E, Sonnenblick EH, Ross J. Mechanisms of cardiac contraction and relaxation. In: Braunwald E, ed. Heart disease: A textbook of cardiovascular medicine, Volume 1. Philadelphia: WB Saunders; 1988:383-414.
24. Raper R, Sibbald WJ. Misled by the wedge? The Swan-Ganz catheter and left ventricular preload. Chest 1986:89:427-434.
25. Law W et al. Left ventricular diastolic compliance changes during septic shock. Crit Care Med 1993:21:S134.
26. Weil MH, von Planta M, Rackow EC. Acute circulatory failure (shock). In: Braunwald E, ed. Heart disease: A textbook of cardiovascular medicine, Volume 1. Philadelphia: WB Saunders; 1988:561-578.
27. Zenaide MN, Quezado MD, Natanson C. Systemic hemodynamic abnormalities and vasopressor therapy in sepsis and septic shock. Am J Kidney Dis 1992:20:214-222.
28. Sibbald WJ et al. Biventricular function in the adult respiratory distress syndrome: Hemodynamic and radionuclide assessment, with special emphasis on right ventricular function. Chest 1983:84:126-134.
29. Parker MM, Ognibene FP, Parrillo JE. Reversible depression of myocardial function in septic shock (SS) confirmed by load-independent measure of ventricular performance. Clin Res 1990:38:340A.
30. Silverman HJ et al. Impaired beta-adrenergic receptor stimulation of cyclic adenosine monophosphate in human septic shock: Association with myocardial hyporesponsiveness to catecholamines. Crit Care Med 1993:21:31-39.
31. Parker MM et al. Responses of left ventricular function in survivors and nonsurvivors of septic shock. J Crit Care 1989:4:19-25.
32. Cunnion RE et al. The coronary circulation in human septic shock. Circulation 1986:73:637-644.
33. Dhainaut JF et al. Coronary hemodynamics and myocardial metabolism of lactate, free fatty acids, glucose, and ketones in patients with septic shock. Circulation 1987:75:533-541.
34. Shapiro R et al. Sepsis induced coronary vasodilatation (Abstract). Circ Shock 1985:16:79-80.
35. Solomon MA et al. Myocardial cytosolic phosphorylation potential in a canine sepsis model. Clin Res 1991:39:164A.
36. Braunwald E, Sobel BE. Coronary blood flow and myocardial ischemia. In: Braunwald E, ed. Heart disease: A textbook of cardiovascular medicine, Volume 2. Philadelphia: WB Saunders; 1988:1191-1203.
37. Hersch M et al. Histopathological evidence of tissue ischemia in a hyperdynamic and nonhypotensive septic animal model (Abstract). Crit Care Med 1988:16:421.
38. Solomon, MA et al. Ultrastructural and histologic changes associated with myocardial depression in a canine model of septic shock. Clin Res 1991:39:321A.
39. Archer LT. Myocardial dysfunction in endotoxin- and E coli-induced shock: Pathophysiological mechanisms. Circ Shock 1985:15:261-280.
40. Raper RF, Sibbald WJ. The effects of coronary artery disease on cardiac function in nonhypotensive sepsis. Chest 1988:94:507-511.
41. Yu P et al. Myocardial collagen damage in rats with hyperdynamic sepsis at 24 and 48 hours. Crit Care Med 1993:21:S277.
42. Raymond RM. When does the heart fail during shock? Circ Shock 1990:30:27-41.
43. Parrillo JE et al. A circulating myocardial depressant substance in humans with septic shock: Septic shock patients with a reduced ejection fraction have a circulating factor that depresses in vitro myocardial cell performance. J Clin Invest 1985:76:1539-1553.
44. Reilly JM et al. A circulating myocardial depressant substance is associated with cardiac dysfunction and peripheral hypoperfusion (lactic acidemia) in patients with septic shock. Chest 1989:95:1072-1080.
45. Ognibene PF, Cunnion RE. Mechanisms of myocardial depression in sepsis. Crit Care Med 1993:21:6-8.
46. Parker JL, Jones CE. The heart in shock. In: Hardaway RM. Shock: The reversible stage of dying. Littleton: PSG Publishing Company; 1988:348-363.
47. Suffredini AF et al. The cardiovascular response of normal humans to the administration of endotoxin. N Engl J Med 1989:321:280-287.

48. Danner RL. Mediators and endotoxin inhibitors. In: Parrillo JE, moderator. Septic shock in humans: Advances in the understanding of pathogenesis, cardiovascular dysfunction, and therapy. Ann Intern Med 1990:113:227-242.
49. St. John RC, Dorinsky PM. Immunologic therapy for ARDS, septic shock, and multiple-organ failure. Chest 1993: 103:932-943.
50. Kumar A et al. Tumor necrosis factor produces a concentration-dependent depression of myocardial cell contraction *in vitro*. Clin Res 1991:39:321A.
51. Ohlsson K et al. Interleukin-1 receptor antagonist reduces mortality from endotoxin shock. Nature 1990:348:550-552.
52. Ognibene FP et al. Interleukin-2 administration causes reversible hemodynamic changes and left ventricular dysfunction similar to those seen in septic shock. Chest 1988:94:750-754.
53. Hazinski MF et al. Epidemiology, pathophysiology, and clinical presentation of gram-negative sepsis. Am J Crit Care 1993:2:224-237.
54. Hechtman HB et al. Prostaglandin and thromboxane mediation of cardiopulmonary failure. Surg Clin North Am 1983:63:263-283.
55. Anderson BO, Bensard DD, Harken AH. The role of platelet activating factor and its antagonists in shock, sepsis and multiple organ failure. Surg Gynecol Obstet 1991:172:415-424.
56. Nava E, Palmer RMJ, Moncada S. Inhibition of nitric oxide synthesis in septic shock: How much is beneficial? Lancet 1991:338:1555-1557.
57. Petros A, Bennet D, Vallance P. Effect of nitric oxide synthase inhibitors on hypotension in patients with septic shock. Lancet 1991:338:1557-1558.
58. Kumar A et al. Tumor necrosis factor-induced myocardial cell depression in-vitro is mediated by nitric oxide generation. Crit Care Med 1993:21:S278.
59. Bone RC et al. Definitions for sepsis and organ failure and guidelines for the use of innovative therapies in sepsis. Chest 1992:101:1644-1655.
60. Parker MM, Parrillo JE. Septic shock and other forms of distributive shock. In: Parrillo JE, ed. Current therapy in critical care medicine. Philadelphia: BC Decker, 1987:44-55.
61. Parrillo JE. Management of septic shock: Present and future. Ann Intern Med 1991:115:491-492.
62. Tuchschmidt J et al. Elevation of cardiac output and oxygen delivery improves outcome in septic shock. Chest 1992: 102:216-220.
63. Shoemaker WC, Appel PL, Kram HB. Role of oxygen debt in the development of organ failure sepsis, and death in high-risk surgical patients. Chest 1992:102:208-215.
64. Edwards JD et al. Use of survivors' cardiorespiratory values as therapeutic goals in septic shock. Crit Care Med 1989:17:1098-1103.
65. Shoemaker WC, Kram HB. Effects of crystalloids and colloids on hemodynamics, oxygen transport, and outcome in high risk surgical patients. In: Simmons RC, Udekuo AS, eds. Debates in Clinical Surgery. Chicago: Mosby; 1990:263-316.
66. Parrillo JE. Septic shock: Clinical manifestations, pathogenesis, hemodynamics, and management in a critical care unit. In: Parrillo JE, Ayres SM, ed. Major issues in critical care medicine. Baltimore: Williams & Wilkins; 1984:111-125.
67. Lollgen H, Drexler H. Use of inotropes in the critical care setting. Crit Care Med 1990:18:S56-S60.
68. Natanson et al. Fluid loading eliminates differences in cardiovascular responses to dopamine and norepinephrine in awake dogs. Clin Res 1990:38:340A.
69. Moran JL et al. Epinephrine as an inotropic agent in septic shock: A dose-profile analysis. Crit Care Med 1993:21:70-77.
70. Gregory JS et al. Experience with phenylephrine as a component of the pharmacologic support of septic shock. Crit Care Med 1991:19:1395-1400.
71. Schremmer B, Dhainaut JF. Heart failure in septic shock: Effects of inotropic support. Crit Care Med 1990:18:S49-S55.
72. Knox J et al. Effect of dobutamine on oxygen consumption and fluid and protein losses after endotoxemia. Crit Care Med 1991:19:525-531.
73. DeBacker D et al. Relationship between oxygen uptake and oxygen delivery in septic patients: Effects of prostacyclin versus dobutamine. Crit Care Med 1993:21:1658-1664.
74. Vincent JL, Roman A, Kahn RJ. Dobutamine administration in septic shock: Addition to standard protocol. Crit Care Med 1990:18:689-693.
75. Specht M et al. Effects of dobutamine vs norepinephrine therapy on oxygen supply and oxygen consumption in septic patients. Crit Care Med 1993:21:S276.
76. Edwards JD. Oxygen transport in cardiogenic and septic shock. Crit Care Med 1991:19:658-663.
77. Hesselvik JF, Brodin B. Low dose norepinephrine in patients with septic shock and oliguria: Effects on afterload, urine flow, and oxygen transport. Crit Care Med 1989:17:179-180.
78. Martin C et al. Renal effects of norepinephrine used to treat septic shock patients. Crit Care Med 1990:18:282-285.
79. Fukuoka T et al. Effects of norepinephrine on renal function in septic patients with normal and elevated serum lactate levels. Crit Care Med 1989:17:1104-1107.
80. Desjars P et al. Norepinephrine therapy has no deleterious renal effects in human septic shock. Crit Care Med 1989:17:426-429.
81. Lindner K et al. Effects of norepinephrine versus phenylephrine on oxygen consumption in septic shock. Crit Care Med 1993:21:S126.
82. Sibbald WJ et al. Concepts in the pharmacologic and non-pharmacologic support of cardiovascular function in critically ill surgical patients. Surg Clin North Am 1983:63:455-482.
83. Kormos RL, Griffith BP. Ventricular assist devices. In: Shoemaker WC et al, eds. Textbook of critical care. Philadelphia: WB Saunders; 1989:428-438.
84. Reemtsma K et al. Mechanical circulatory support: Advances in intra-aortic balloon pumping. In: Shoemaker WC et al, eds. Textbook of critical care. Philadelphia: WB Saunders; 1989:420-428.

CHAPTER 13

The Kidney in Multiple Organ Dysfunction Syndrome

Kathleen H. Toto

Acute renal failure (ARF) is a potentially fatal complication of critical illness, traumatic injury, and certain therapeutic regimens. The introduction of dialysis in 1952 reduced the mortality rate of acute renal failure from 80% to 90% to approximately 50%.[1] Despite scientific advances in the management of ARF, mortality remains at 50%.[2] Although the incidence of ARF associated with obstetrics, hemodialysis, and elective surgery has decreased, ARF in older patients with complex problems, who often have multiple organ dysfunction and septicemia has actually increased.[3] That overall mortality in acute renal failure has not changed in over forty years can most likely be attributed to two major factors: (1) improved resuscitation techniques eliminating mild forms of acute renal failure and (2) the increased incidence of critically ill patients with a severe primary insult and multiple organ dysfunction who, in the past, would have died before ever developing acute renal failure.[4-6]

Thirty-six years ago, the leading cause of death in 72% of patients with ARF was infection.[7] Although infection (pulmonary, urinary tract, and wound infections, and septicemia) continues to be a leading cause of mortality associated with ARF,[8] multiple organ dysfunction syndrome (MODS) is also a major cause of death in critically ill patients with ARF.[6]

BASIC PHYSIOLOGIC CONCEPTS

A brief review of renal anatomy and physiology is essential before the discussion of the alterations in renal function in MODS. Some basic concepts are explained below and serve as a foundation for the remainder of this chapter.

Nephron

The functional unit of the kidney is the nephron; therefore overall renal function may be explained in terms of the function of individual neurons. There are approximately 500,000 to 1,000,000 nephrons in each adult kidney. Each nephron consists of a vascular component and a tubular component (Fig. 13-1). Blood from the aorta flows into the renal arteries, which branch into progressively smaller arteries and arterioles before finally terminating in the afferent arterioles. Each afferent arteriole then divides into a capillary tuft called the glomerulus. The glomerular capillaries rejoin to form the efferent arteriole, which branches into the peritubular capillaries and the vasa recta. The peritubular capillaries and the vasa recta are extensively and intimately associated with the renal tubules, allowing for constant movement of solutes and water (i.e., reabsorption and secretion) between the filtrate of the renal tubules and the plasma of the peritubular capillaries and the vasa recta[9,10] (Fig. 13-1).

Glomerular filtration

The kidneys receive 20% to 25% of the cardiac output each minute for a total of 1200 mL/min. The glomerular capillary bed is a highly permeable area. As a result, fluid continuously filters from the glomerular capillary bed into Bowman's capsule (a lower pressure area as compared to the higher pressure area in the glomerulus) at an average rate of

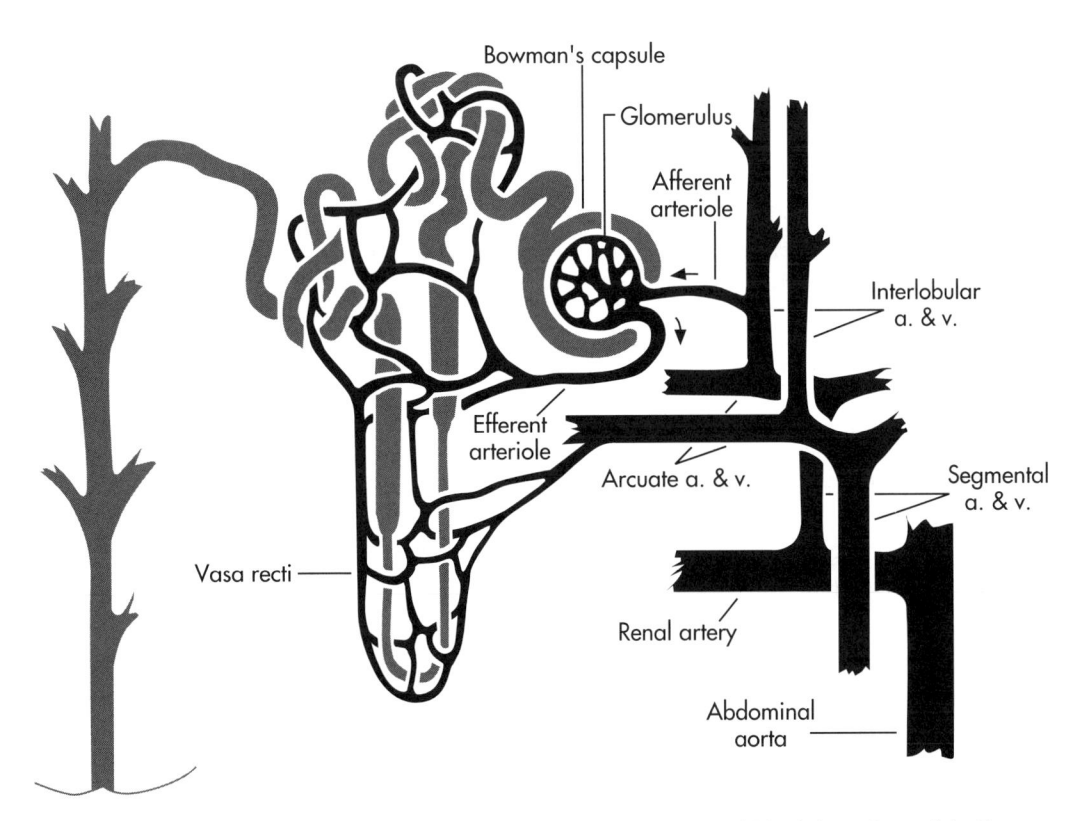

Fig. 13-1 Renal vasculature. *a*, Artery; *v*, vein. (From Toto KH: Renal Physiology: Beyond the Basics. Lewisville, Texas, Barbara Clark Mims Associates, 1995.)

125 mL/min.[9,10] The kidney has the ability to autoregulate to maintain the glomerular filtration rate (GFR) within normal limits despite wide variations in arterial blood pressure. For example, a change in arterial blood pressure from 70 mm Hg to 160 mm Hg has almost no effect on the GFR.[9] Mechanisms responsible for autoregulation are explained in the next section. Based on an average GFR of 125 mL/min, approximately 180 L is filtered from the glomeruli into Bowman's space every 24 hours. 98% to 99% of this filtrate is then reabsorbed, leaving a urine output of about 1.5 to 2 L per day. However, the kidneys can make significant changes in the urine output depending on the state of hydration. In conditions of fluid deficit, maximal amounts of tubular filtrate are reabsorbed, and a small amount of concentrated urine is excreted. Conversely, in conditions of fluid excess, tubular reabsorption decreases, and a large amount of dilute urine is excreted.

Autoregulation and tubuloglomerular feedback

Renal autoregulation refers to the maintenance of constant GFR and renal blood flow despite fluctuations in renal perfusion pressure. Tubuloglomerular feedback, the renal autoregulation process, is controlled by the juxtaglomerular apparatus (JGA). The JGA consists of specialized cells located at the point at which the distal convoluted tubule of each nephron loops and comes into contact with the angle of the afferent and efferent arterioles of that nephron.[9,10] The anatomic structure of the JGA allows for a feedback system between the distal tubule and the afferent and efferent arterioles. The cells of the distal tubule located at this junction are called the macula densa. The macula densa provides input to the JGA in response to tubular fluid composition. The macula densa cells sense changes in tubular fluid volume and electrolytes (primarily sodium and chloride).[11] If tubular flow rates are sluggish and there is a reduction in salt and water delivery to the distal tubule, the macula densa communicates with the JGA to stimulate afferent arteriolar dilatation and increase GFR. As the afferent arteriole dilates, blood flow and hydrostatic pressure in the glomerular capillary bed increase, thus maintaining the glomerular capillary pressure and GFR.[9] Conversely, an increase in sodium and chloride at the macula densa causes afferent arteriole constriction, decreased glomerular blood flow, and a reduction in GFR. In this manner, a "tubular sensor" adjusts glomerular filtration rate.

A decrease in sodium and chloride delivery at the macula densa also causes renin release from the juxtaglomerular cells. Through several physiologic reactions (Fig. 13-2), renin catalyzes the conversion of angiotensinogen to angiotensin I, which is then converted to angiotensin II, causing efferent arteriolar constriction. Efferent arteriolar constriction also helps maintain the hydrostatic pressure in the glomerular capillary bed and helps the GFR remain normal.[9]

To summarize, autoregulation maintains renal blood flow and GFR within a narrow range despite wide fluctuations in arterial blood pressure. However, once the mean arterial pressure (MAP) falls below 50 to 70 mm Hg, the renal autoregulatory processes are no longer able to maintain adequate renal blood flow and GFR. As a result, in states of prolonged hypotension and renal hypoperfusion, drastic changes occur in renal function. MODS is one of those conditions typically characterized by prolonged hypotension, renal hypoperfusion, and ischemia. Renal responses to hypoperfusion, ischemia, and toxic mediators of MODS are discussed later in this chapter.

Renal response to hypotension

The blood flow to the kidneys is high (1200 mL/m) and far exceeds renal oxygen requirements. However, when the kidneys are hypoperfused, they are very susceptible to injury. Renal hypoperfusion activates the renin-angiotensin system (RAS), resulting in systemic vasoconstriction and aldosterone-mediated renal sodium and water retention (Fig. 13-2). Stimulation of the sympathetic nervous system (SNS) and circulating catecholamines will also initiate the release of renin. The combined effect of catecholamines and high angiotensin II levels results in systemic vasoconstriction as well as intrarenal vasoconstriction. Activation of the RAS and the SNS also stimulates the kidneys to synthesize and release vasodilating prostaglandins (PGs) (PGE_2 and PGI_2). The end result is that much of the vasoconstrictive action of norepinephrine and angiotensin II on the renal vasculature is opposed by the local vasodilator action of these PGs. Therefore, renal resistance changes much less and renal perfusion is protected (Fig. 13-3).

For example, a patient in hemorrhagic shock is confronted by three factors that reduce renal blood flow: hypotension, SNS stimulation, and angiotensin II activity. Simultaneously, two factors act to protect renal blood flow: autoregulation (as long as the MAP is ≥50 to 60 mm Hg) and the renal vasodilating prostaglandins.

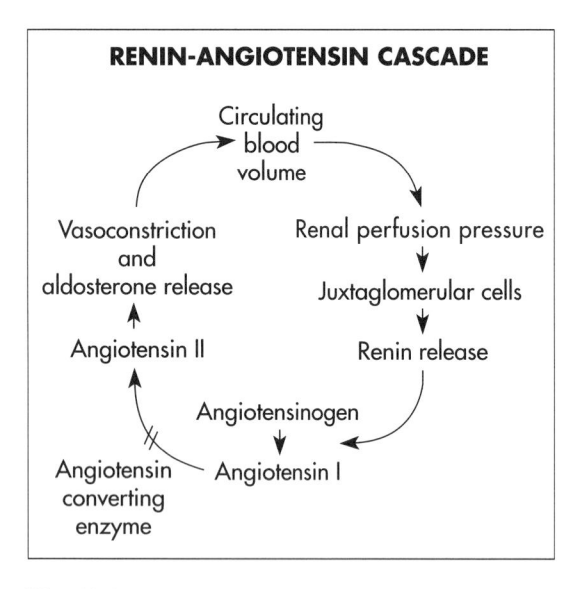

Fig. 13-2 Renin-angiotensin cascade. A decrease in blood volume or blood pressure that results in a fall in renal perfusion pressure is sensed by the juxtaglomerular cells (functioning as a baroreceptor) and stimulates the release of renin. Renin converts angiotensinogen to angiotensin I, which is then converted to angiotensin II by a converting enzyme arising from vascular endothelial cells. Angiotensin II stimulates intense systemic vasoconstriction and aldosterone release that stimulates renal sodium and water retention; the end result is an improvement in circulating blood volume and renal perfusion pressure. (From Toto KH: Renal Physiology: Beyond the Basics. Lewisville, Texas, Barbara Clark Mims Associates, 1995.)

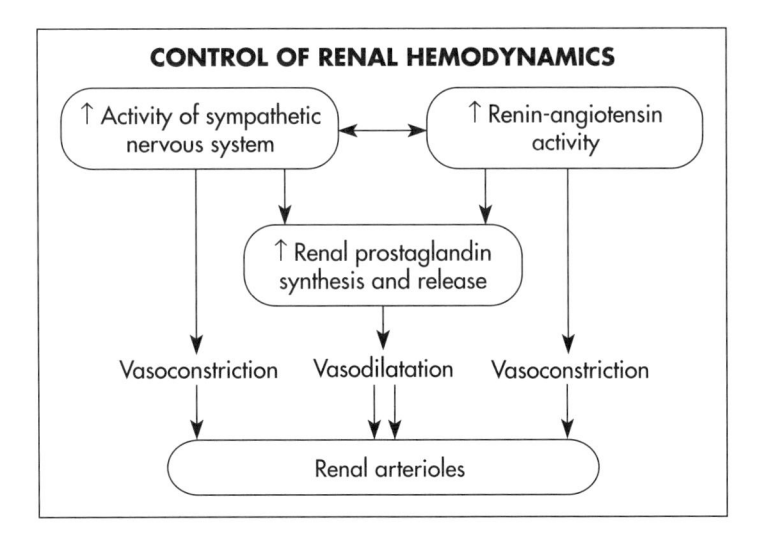

Fig. 13-3 Control of renal hemodynamics. Stimulation of the renal sympathetic nerves (SNS) and activation of the renin-angiotensin system (RAS) and increased angiotensin II levels result in systemic and renal vasoconstriction. However, an increase in sympathetic activity and angiotensin II levels initiates the synthesis and release of renal vasodilating prostaglandins that locally counteract SNS and RAS-mediated vasoconstriction. The renal vasodilating prostaglandins act to protect renal blood flow in states of renal hypoperfusion.

Elimination of metabolic waste products

Elimination of metabolic waste products is an important physiologic function of the kidney. The primary metabolic waste products excreted by the kidney include urea, creatinine, uric acid, bilirubin, and metabolic acid. Urea is of particular interest because it serves as a surrogate marker for uremia in the catabolic patient with ARF.

Urea is the end product of protein metabolism resulting from amino acid metabolism and ammonia breakdown in the liver. Plasma urea levels are influenced by renal excretion, hepatic function, protein metabolism, dietary protein intake, and volume status. The critically ill patient has many variables affecting the level of blood urea nitrogen (BUN). BUN may be elevated because of increased synthesis (high protein parenteral nutrition, a catabolic state, a gastrointestinal bleed, or steroid therapy) and depressed excretion (volume depletion or renal failure). It may be low in states of decreased synthesis (malnutrition and liver failure) and volume expansion. Therefore, when evaluating the BUN in the critically ill patient, many variables must be considered in order to identify the etiology of altered BUN levels accurately.

Creatinine, like urea, is the end product of protein metabolism but unlike urea, it is produced by muscle. Muscles release small amounts of creatinine into the extracellular fluid compartment at relatively constant rates, and with normal renal function, creatinine is completely filtered and excreted by the kidney. Therefore, the level of creatinine is a more reliable index of renal function and is less likely to be affected by many of the variables that affect BUN levels. However, the serum creatinine can be elevated after muscle injury (trauma, crush or burns) and may be low in cases of chronic malnutrition and muscle wasting. Both the BUN and creatinine levels should be taken into consideration when evaluating renal function. The normal BUN/creatinine ratio is 10:1 to 15:1.

Overview of renal function

An extensive discussion of normal renal physiology is beyond the scope of this chapter; however, to orient the reader a brief summary of essential renal functions not previously discussed is presented. The kidneys are responsible for the following functions:

1. Maintenance of intravascular volume through the processes of glomerular filtration and tubular reabsorption of sodium and water and the effects of aldosterone, antidiuretic hormone, and natriuretic hormone
2. Regulation of water balance and plasma osmolality in response to antidiuretic hormone
3. Regulation of electrolyte balance via the processes of glomerular filtration and selective tubular reabsorption and secretion that are under the influence of various hormones, such as aldosterone and parathyroid hormone
4. Regulation of acid-base balance, along with the buffer and respiratory systems, through glomerular filtration and tubular reabsorption of bicarbonate and excretion of acid
5. Excretion of end products of metabolism (uremic toxins) and certain exogenously administered substances, such as drugs
6. Regulation of red blood cell production by erythropoietin production
7. Metabolism of weak vitamin D precursors to the active, potent form (1,25-dihydroxycholecalciferol [1,25-DHCC])
8. Regulation of blood pressure regulation through renin production by the JGA

DEFINITION AND CLASSIFICATION OF ACUTE RENAL FAILURE

Acute renal failure can be defined as an abrupt deterioration in renal function characterized by progressive azotemia (high blood concentrations of nitrogen waste products, e.g., BUN and creatinine). ARF is usually associated with a fall in GFR manifested as a decline in urine output. The etiology of ARF may be attributed to prerenal, postrenal, or intrarenal causes (Fig. 13-4). ARF from postrenal causes, also termed obstructive renal failure, accounts for less than 10% of all cases of ARF,[12] and is uncommon in the intensive care setting. The discussion on the classification and differentiation of ARF will focus on prerenal and intrarenal causes. Prerenal and especially intrarenal failure are the most common forms of ARF in the patient with MODS.

In the clinical setting, the terms acute renal failure and acute tubular necrosis (ATN) have become synonomous. Mortality rates of ARF quoted in the

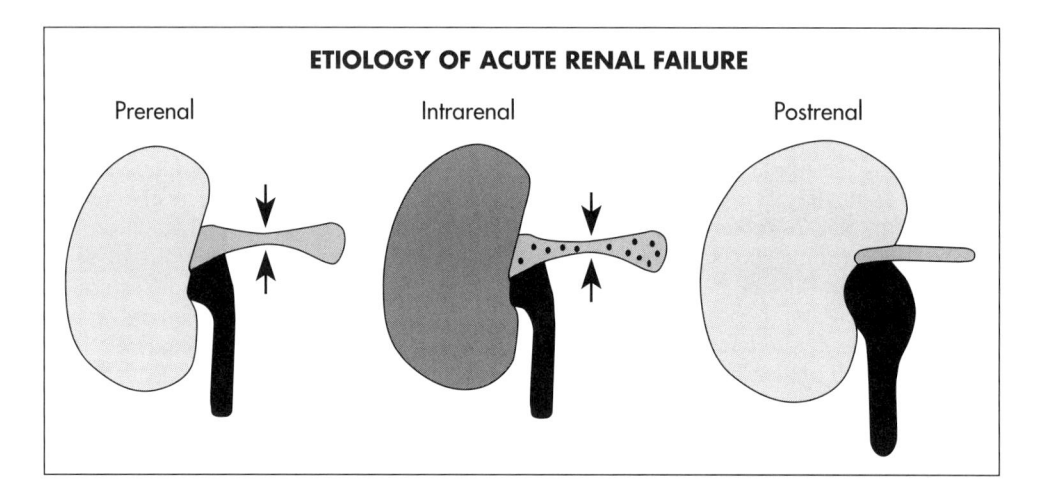

Fig. 13-4 Etiology of acute renal failure. Prerenal causes of ARF can be attributed to a reduction in renal blood flow (demonstrated by renal vasoconstriction) and a kidney that is structurally and functionally intact. Intrarenal failure (ATN) occurs when there is structural and functional damage to the nephrons of the kidney. It may be caused by renal hypoperfusion or exposure to a nephrotoxin (represented by black dots in renal artery). Postrenal failure is due to a disruption of the flow of urine from the urinary tract (dilated renal pelvis and hydronephrosis) and is rarely associated with intrarenal damage. (From Toto KH: Renal Physiology: Beyond the Basics. Lewisville, Texas: Barbara Clark Mims Associates, 1995.)

vast majority of the literature actually refer to mortality rates of acute tubular necrosis. For the purpose of this chapter, acute renal failure and acute tubular necrosis will be used interchangeably unless otherwise specified, for example, acute renal failure resulting from prerenal or postrenal causes.

Prerenal failure

Prerenal failure is a rapidly reversible form of ARF responsible for 50% of the cases of ARF in hospitalized patients.[13] Prerenal failure is due to renal hypoperfusion, and the attendant prerenal azotemia can be acute, chronic, severe, or mild. As illustrated in Table 13-1, renal hypoperfusion is precipitated by a variety of conditions.

In prerenal failure, the glomeruli are unable to filter blood because of hemodynamic compromise. In this setting both the glomeruli and the tubules are functionally and structurally intact. With restoration of adequate blood flow, the kidney in prerenal failure can resume normal function. However, prolonged or severe prerenal azotemia can lead to the development of ischemic acute tubular necrosis. Therefore, recognition and prompt treatment of prerenal failure is extremely important.

Prerenal failure is diagnosed by the evaluation of blood and urine chemistries. The serum BUN/creatinine ratio is substantially increased in the prerenal state from the normal ratio of 10:1 to a ratio greater than 20:1. Both creatinine and BUN are elevated secondary to a reduction in the GFR. However, BUN is elevated more dramatically because of increased urea reabsorption in the renal tubules secondary to slow tubular flow rates. The BUN/creatinine ratio can also increase in catabolic states and with steroid therapy, sepsis, burns, surgery, high fever, or gastrointestinal bleeding.[13]

Chemical and microscopic analysis of the urine is also extremely helpful in distinguishing prerenal failure from other types of renal failure. The urine sodium level is low because the hypoperfused kidneys avidly hold on to sodium and water to restore what is perceived as a decrease in blood volume. The renal reabsorption of water also results in urine that is concentrated, with high osmolality and specific gravity. Laboratory values in prerenal failure are outlined in Table 13-2.

Treatment of prerenal failure depends on the cause. Initial management should be directed toward restoring a normal hemodynamic status. Failure to correct the hemodynamic alteration may result in the development of ischemic ATN, a form of intrarenal failure.

Acute tubular necrosis

Acute tubular necrosis is the most common form of ARF and accounts for the majority of cases of hospital-acquired ARF. ATN is characterized by renal tubular cell damage caused by either a nephrotoxic or an ischemic insult. The hallmark of ATN is the acute onset or worsening of azotemia that is not immediately reversed by the removal of the

Table 13-1 Hemodynamic Classification of Prerenal Failure

Impaired cardiac performance	Vasodilation	Vasoconstriction	Intravascular volume depletion

Congestive heart failure
Myocardial infarction
Cardiogenic shock
Pericardial tamponade
Arrhythmias
Acute pulmonary embolism
	Sepsis
	Anaphylaxis
	Drugs
		Catecholamines
		  Endogenous
		  Exogenous
		Anesthesia
		Surgery
			Volume depletion
			  Hemorrhage
			  GI losses
			    Diarrhea
			    Vomiting
			  Renal losses
			    Osmotic diuresis
			    Diuretic drugs
			Volume shifts
			  Burns
			  Peritonitis
			  Pancreatitis
			  Ileus
			  Sepsis
			Inadequate volume replacement

Table 13-2 Laboratory Values Differentiating Prerenal Failure and Acute Tubular Necrosis*

Laboratory values	Prerenal	ATN
BUN/creatinine ratio	20:1-40:1	10:1-15:1
Urine sodium level	<20 mEq/L	>20 mEq/L
Urine concentration	Concentrated	Dilute
Osmolality	High (>500)	Low (<300)
Specific gravity	High (>1.020)	Low (<1.010)
Urinary sediment	Normal (hyaline casts)	Abnormal (cellular casts and debris)
Fractional excretion of sodium (FE_{Na})	≤1%	>1%

*Pediatric values are the same as adult values; neonatal values vary.

causative agent or correction of hemodynamic alterations.[13]

Ischemic acute tubular necrosis. Ischemic ATN accounts for about half of all cases of ATN.[13] It occurs when perfusion to the kidneys is obliterated or severely reduced. Below the critical systemic MAP of 50 to 60 mm Hg, the autoregulatory properties of the afferent and efferent arterioles regulating glomerular filtration are lost. Sympathetic stimulation and angiotensin II cause further vasoconstriction in the renal vascular bed, worsening the ischemia. The final outcome of prolonged tubular ischemia is cell swelling, cell necrosis, and damage of the tubular basement membrane (Fig. 13-5). The mechanisms responsible for renal tubular dysfunction in ischemic ATN are multifactorial and include accumulation of cellular debris in the tubular lumen, tubular cell swelling, and a reduction in renal cell adenosine triphosphate (ATP).

Accumulation of cellular debris in the tubular lumen is a common finding in ATN. Examination of the urine in patients with ATN has revealed the presence of both necrosed and viable renal tubular epithelial cells with 30% to 50% of the exfoliated renal tubular epithelial cells being viable.[14] This has resulted in the reevaluation of cell necrosis as the sole mechanism of tubular cell sloughing in ATN. Exfoliation of viable tubular cells is thought to result from the loss of cell attachments to adjacent cells and underlying substrate.[15] Renal tubular cells are anchored to their basement membrane by a variety of adhesion molecules. For example, integrins are a family of protein adhesion molecules localized in the basolateral membrane of these tubular cells. Integrins on the tubular cells bind to receptors in the extracellular matrix, thus holding the cell in place. Ischemic injury causes integrin molecules to retract from their receptors in the extracellular matrix causing the cell to lose its adherence to the basement membrane and slough off into the tubular lumen. The tubular cells can then bind to each other, forming tubular casts resulting in intratubular obstruction. This results in an increase in tubular pressure, a fall in glomerular filtration rate, and ultimately a reduction in urine output.

Secondly, swelling of the tubular cells mechanically obstructs the renal capillaries (this is worse in the renal medulla), which decreases capillary blood flow, increases ischemia and cell injury, and contributes to further renal tubular dysfunction. In addition, a reduction of renal cell ATP causes cell dysfunction resulting in accumulation of intracellular calcium and production of oxygen-derived free radicals, both of which further contribute to tubular cell injury.

Nephrotoxic acute tubular necrosis. A number of nephrotoxic agents, both endogenous and exogenous, can cause ATN (Table 13-3). Toxic insult to the renal tubules causes swelling and necrosis of tubular cells, similar to that seen with ischemic ATN. However, the basement membrane of the renal tubular cells may not be injured as severely as with ischemic ATN (Fig. 13-5). Therefore, the healing process with nephrotoxic ATN is more rapid. Additionally, the underlying disease is not usually as severe with nephrotoxic ATN as it is with ischemic ATN. Patients with uncomplicated nephrotoxic injury usually have a good chance for full recovery of renal function. The toxic effect of most nephrotoxins is enhanced in states of volume depletion and renal hypoperfusion that result in sluggish renal tubular flow rates and prolonged toxic exposure of the renal tubules to the nephrotoxin.

Table 13-3 Causes of Acute Tubular Necrosis

Ischemic	Nephrotoxic
All causes of pre-renal failure (see Table 13-1)	Endogenous Pigments
Decreased cardiac output	Hemoglobin Myoglobin
Surgery	Crystals
Thoracic	Uric acid
Abdominal	Calcium phosphate
Vascular	Exogenous
Cardiopulmonary bypass	Antibiotics Aminoglycosides
Hypotension	Cephalosporins
Sepsis	Amphotericin B
Hypovolemia	Nonsteroidal antiinflammatory drugs
Catecholamines	Radiographic contrast media
Volume shifts	Chemotherapeutic agents
	Organic solvents
	Ethylene glycol

Ischemic and nephrotoxic ATN can occur simultaneously in a patient with an ischemic event, who has also been exposed to a nephrotoxin. Approximately 70% of patients will have more than one possible cause for the ATN.[16] For example, a patient suffering a traumatic crush injury releases myoglobin (an endogenous nephrotoxin) from injured muscle and is also at risk for ischemic ATN if hypovolemic shock develops. Additionally, a patient in septic shock who receives aminoglycoside antibiotics will also be at risk for both ischemic and nephrotoxic ATN. Clinically, ischemic ATN may be impossible to differentiate from nephrotoxic ATN. Once azotemia develops, a thorough search for a potential exposure to nephrotoxins should be undertaken in addition to identification of any events that may have resulted in renal hypoperfusion and ischemia.

Laboratory values in ATN

Laboratory studies on serum and urine are very helpful in distinguishing a prerenal state from ATN. However, if the patient has received diuretics before urine is obtained for laboratory evaluation, the results will be difficult, if not impossible, to evaluate for differentiating the etiology of ARF. For this reason, urine electrolytes should be obtained before the administration of diuretics.

In ATN, the BUN/creatinine ratio is usually normal (10:1 to 15:1) with both BUN and creatinine levels being elevated. For example, the BUN level is 60 mg/dL, the creatinine level is 5.8 mg/dL. The BUN/creatinine ratio is not a reliable parameter in ATN in patients with increased urea production rates, such as catabolic states, gastrointestinal bleeding, or increased dietary protein intake.

In ATN, the urine sodium level is usually >20 mEq/L as compared to prerenal failure in which the urine sodium is low, <20 mEq/L. The functioning prerenal kidney avidly reabsorbs sodium. In contrast, in ATN, the dysfunctional renal tubules cannot retain the sodium. However, the values can overlap, and with a urine sodium level between 20 to 40 mEq/L either prerenal failure or ATN can be seen and additional evaluation, including calculation of the fractional excretion of sodium (FE_{Na}), may be helpful.

The fractional excretion of sodium is a very useful calculation that assesses renal tubular function. The FE_{Na} is the ratio of the amount of sodium excreted to the amount of sodium filtered by the kidney. The normal FE_{Na} is ≤1%. In prerenal states, renal tubular function is not impaired and therefore FE_{Na} is normal (≤1%). In ATN, there is renal tubular dysfunction and the FE_{Na} is abnormal (>1%).

To determine the FE_{Na}, a spot urine sample and a serum sample are obtained simultaneously for sodium and creatinine determination. The FE_{Na} is calculated as follows:

$$FE_{Na} = \frac{U_{Na} \times P_{Cr}}{U_{Cr} \times P_{Na}} \times 100$$

where U_{Na} = urine sodium concentration, P_{Na} = plasma sodium concentration, U_{Cr} = urine creatinine concentration, and P_{Cr} = plasma creatinine concentration.

Urine osmolality and specific gravity reflect the concentrating and diluting abilities of the kidney. These measures are also helpful in distinguishing between prerenal and intrarenal failure. Early in the course of ATN, the kidneys lose the ability to concentrate the urine. This is often seen even before a rise in the serum creatinine occurs. In ATN, the renal tubules cannot concentrate the urine normally, therefore the urine is dilute and has an osmolality similar to that of plasma (isoosmolar urine): urine osmolality <300 mOsm/kg and specific gravity <1.010. The kidney in prerenal failure is able to

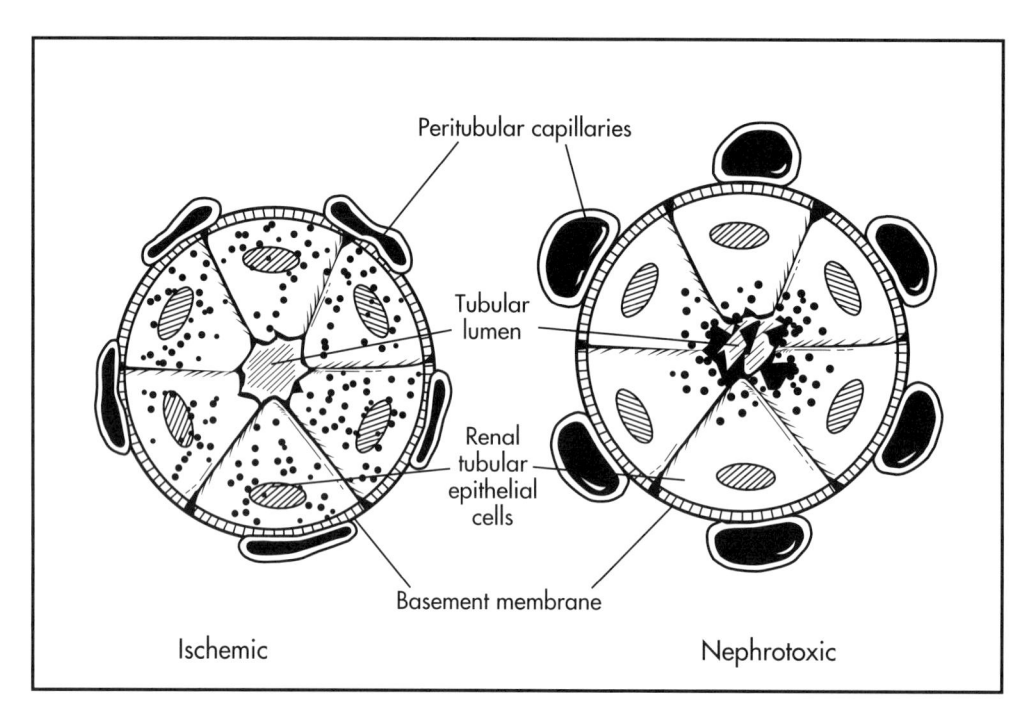

Fig. 13-5 Pathogenesis of ischemic versus nephrotoxic ATN. This diagram depicts the cross-section of two renal tubules, one that has suffered an ischemic event and the other that has been exposed to a nephrotoxin. The renal tubule is made up of a single layer of renal tubular epithelial cells emerging from the basement membrane. The cells receive oxygen and nutrients from the peritubular capillaries (depicted as cross-sectional view around tubules). In ischemic ATN, there is a decrease in renal blood flow (demonstrated by small peritubular capillaries) and a reduction in oxygen delivery resulting in renal tubular cell ischemia, swelling, necrosis, and eventually sloughing. Depending upon the degree and severity of renal hypoperfusion, nephron function may or may not resolve. In nephrotoxic ATN, the renal tubular cells are exposed to a toxin (demonstrated by triangles in the tubular lumen) resulting in tubular cell swelling and necrosis. Most nephrotoxins exert their toxic effect on the intraluminal aspect of the tubule, which is likely to preserve basement membrane function. If the basement membrane is not affected (even if tubular cell necrosis and sloughing occurs), it will regenerate a new renal tubular cell, and full recovery of renal function is typical. (From Toto KH: Renal Physiology: Beyond the Basics. Lewisville, Texas: Barbara Clark Mims Associates, 1995.)

concentrate the urine and the urine osmolality is usually >500 mOsm/kg and the specific gravity >1.020.

The composition of urinary sediment (cells and casts) also gives clues to the etiology of ATN. Casts are cylindrical molds of the tubular lumen and consist of protein and cellular elements. Their presence usually implies intrinsic renal disease of the glomeruli, renal tubules, or renal interstitium. Urinary sediment is usually normal in prerenal failure. In intrarenal failure the sediment is abnormal, and cells, tubular debris, and casts become prominent. Granular and renal tubular epithelial cell casts are commonly seen in ATN. Table 13-2 summarizes the laboratory differentiation of prerenal failure from acute tubular necrosis.

Clinical course of ATN

The clinical course of ATN, originally described many decades ago, has traditionally been divided into three phases: the oliguric, the diuretic, and the recovery phases. However, these classic phases are rarely seen in modern times. In the initial phase of ATN, only 50% of patients are oliguric and the remaining 50% are nonoliguric. Oliguria is defined as a urine output of <400 mL/24 hours and nonoliguria as >400 mL/24 hours. The urine output in ARF in the critically ill patient should be evaluated with a Foley catheter in place. Nonoliguric ATN is most often associated with nephrotoxins, and oliguric ATN, with ischemic events. The development and introduction of new pharmacologic agents (e.g., aminoglycoside antibiotics, cephalosporins, contrast media) is the most likely reason for the increased incidence of nephrotoxic ATN and an alteration in the first phase of ATN with an increase in patients with nonoliguria versus those with oliguria.

The diuretic phase of ATN is rarely seen today. This can be attributed to earlier and more efficient dialysis techniques that keep excess fluid volume and azotemia to a minimum. The diuretic phase described in the past resulted from the excretion of excess fluid and metabolic waste products that accumulated during the oliguric phase and were not dialyzed out early as they are today. The diuretic phase of ATN may still be seen in situations where dialysis is initiated late or the patient is underdialyzed, for example, in developing countries with inadequate medical care, in patients who present to the hospital late in their clinical course, or with dialysis that is inefficient.

Currently, the clinical course of ATN is more likely to present in the following pattern: initiating phase, maintenance phase, and recovery phase.[13]

Initiating phase. Patients in this early phase of ATN usually present as oliguric (50% of the patients) or nonoliguric (50% of the patients) and rarely as anuric (urine output <100 mL/24 hours). This phase lasts from the onset of decreased renal function to that of established ARF.[13] It can be reversed by correcting the underlying ischemic event or removing the offending nephrotoxin. Both morbidity and mortality rates are lower in patients with nonoliguric ATN as compared with rates in patients with oliguric ATN.[3]

Maintenance phase. In this phase, ATN is not reversible and may last from a few hours to several weeks depending on the cause and severity of renal tubular cell injury. In oliguric patients, renal function usually improves spontaneously after 10 to 16 days and in nonoliguric patients, after 5 to 8 days.[13] The systemic manifestations of ARF, which contribute to morbidity and mortality in the oliguric patient, include volume overload, electrolyte imbalances, metabolic acidosis, uremia, hematologic abnormalities, and infection (see Table 13-4).

Recovery phase. The recovery phase is heralded by a reduction in BUN and creatinine levels independent of dialysis. Both oliguric and nonoliguric patients will increase their urine output. Although the BUN and creatinine gradually return to normal, in a few patients, they may never return to normal. At the onset of recovery, there is an initial, relatively, rapid return in renal function lasting about 1 to 2 weeks, followed by a period of slower improvement.[17] Of the patients surviving ATN, approximately 62% will recover normal renal function, 33% will be left with some degree of residual renal insufficiency (but not require dialysis), and at least 5% will require long-term hemodialysis.[5,18]

ACUTE RENAL FAILURE—SEPSIS—MODS

Acute renal failure is frequently seen in the context of multiple organ dysfunction and failure, with sepsis or systemic inflammation as major causative factors. Many variables put the septic patient at risk for developing ARF, including hemodynamic, humoral, and cellular alterations, as well as the potential for exposure to both endogenous and exogenous nephrotoxins.

Acute renal failure and sepsis

Sepsis (systemic bacterial infection) is a major factor in the etiology of ARF in the critically ill patient. Sepsis in the intensive care setting is most often caused by infection from gram-negative bacteria. The release of endotoxin from the cell wall of these bacteria and the activation of numerous host mediators are the initiating events of the systemic inflammatory response syndrome (SIRS), sepsis, and eventually septic shock. Sepsis-induced cardiovascular and pulmonary failure often precede ARF. Cardiopulmonary failure can result in severe and persistent renal hypoperfusion and a transition from prerenal failure to ATN. However, restoration of renal blood flow does not always reverse the renal failure. Acute renal failure in the septic patient is not solely due to hemodynamic changes; humoral and cellular mediators have also been shown to affect renal function adversely.[19]

Hemodynamic factors. Renal hypoperfusion is a common finding in septic shock, which is characterized by decreased renal blood flow and a reduc-

Table 13-4 Systemic Manifestations of Acute Renal Failure

Problem	Clinical manifestations	Etiology	Management
Volume overload	Pulmonary edema Congestive heart failure Hypertension Edema (peripheral, sacral, periorbital) Weight gain Hyponatremia (dilutional)	Prerenal—physiologic response to reduction in renal blood flow ATN—tubular obstruction, tubular backleak of water	Fluid restriction Diuretics Ultrafiltration Dialysis
Electrolyte imbalances *Hyperkalemia*	*Cardiac* Mild—tall, peaked T waves Moderate—flattening P wave with prolonged PR interval Severe—complete heart block, widened QRS, asystole, ventricular tachycardia, ventricular fibrillation *Neuromuscular* Mild/moderate—muscle cramps, twitching Severe—paresthesias, paralysis *Gastrointestinal* Mild/moderate—abdominal cramps, diarrhea Severe—ileus	↓ Renal excretion of potassium Metabolic acidosis Catabolism Dietary intake GI bleeding Blood transfusions	Limit potassium intake Treat catabolism (nutrition) Hypertonic glucose and insulin (IV) Sodium bicarbonate (IV) Calcium gluconate (IV) Albuterol (inhaled) Kayexalate (PO, PR) Dialysis
Hypocalcemia/hyperphosphatemia	*Neurologic* Paresthesias, anxiety *Musculoskeletal* Cramps, tetany, Trousseau's and Chvostek's signs, seizures, laryngospasm Metastatic calcifications	↓ Renal excretion of phosphate Secondary hyperparathyroidism ↓ Renal synthesis of Vitamin D If calcium/phosphorus product (Ca × PO$_4$) > 70, causes CaPO$_4$ deposits in soft tissues (metastatic calcifications)	Limit phosphorus intake Hypertonic glucose and insulin (IV) Phosphate binding medications (given PO with meals)—Amphojel, Basaljel, Calcium Carbonate Vitamin D supplements Calcium supplements (if phosphate <6 mg/dL) Dialysis

Hypermagnesemia	*Neuromuscular* ↓ Deep tendon reflexes Respiratory depression Respiratory arrest *Cardiovascular* Flushing Arrhythmias: bradycardia, AV block, asystole Hypotension	↓ Renal magnesium excretion Inadvertent magnesium administration (Maalox, magnesium citrate, magnesium added to parenteral nutrition)	Calcium gluconate (IV) Hypertonic glucose and insulin (IV) Dialysis
Metabolic acidosis	↑ Minute ventilation Altered mental status Hyperkalemia If pH <7.20: CV effects—→ ↓ CO, ↓ BP, arrhythmias	↓ Renal H⁺ excretion ↓ Renal HCO₃⁻ reabsorption ↓ Renal ammonia synthesis and ammonium excretion Catabolism	Shohl's solution (PO) Sodium bicarbonate (IV) Dialysis
Uremia	*Neurologic* Lethargy, confusion Asterixis Unusual behavior Seizures Stupor and coma	Effect of uremic toxins on nervous system	Dialysis to keep BUN <100 mg/dL and patient asymptomatic
	Gastrointestinal Anorexia Nausea and vomiting Gastritis and GI bleeding Diarrhea Stomatitis	Mucous membrane inflammation due to uremic toxins and GI degradation of urea to ammonia causing irritation	Dialysis as above
	Cardiovascular Hypervolemia, hypotension Congestive heart failure Pericarditis (cardiac tamponade)	↑ BUN causes ↑ in serum osmolality and ECF volume expansion Inflammation of pericardial membrane from uremic toxins and potential for bleeding and effusion into pericardial cavity	Dialysis as above

Continued.

Table 13-4 Systemic Manifestations of Acute Renal Failure—cont'd

Problem	Clinical manifestations	Etiology	Management
Uremia—cont'd	**Hematologic** Anemia Potential for bleeding	Shortened RBC life span due to uremic toxins Direct effect of uremia on capillary integrity and inhibition of platelet aggregation	Dialysis as above
	General Decreased resistance to infection Discoloration of skin Dry skin, pruritus	→ Macrophage activity because of uremic toxins Hypothermic effect of urea Deposition of uremic toxins in skin and irritation of peripheral nerves	Dialysis as above
Hematologic abnormalities	Anemia	↓ Renal erythropoietin production Hemodilution Shortened RBC life span Blood loss with hemodialysis GI blood loss	PRBC transfusion for symptomatic anemia Minimize collection of blood for laboratory work-up
Infection	Temperature elevation (may be subtle) Pneumonia Urinary tract infections Wounds	Altered immune response (↓ macrophage activity and ↓ temp due to uremia) Disruption of normal anatomic barriers (IV lines, access for RRT, endotracheal tube)	Culture for specific microorganisms and treatment with appropriate antibiotics Minimize use of invasive lines and catheters Utilize strict aseptic technique

Modified from Toto K: Renal physiology: Beyond the basics. Lewisville, TX: Barbara Clark Mims Associates, 1995, and Lancaster L: Renal response to shock. Crit Care Nurs Clin North Am 1990;2:228-229.

ATN, Acute tubular necrosis; *AV*, atrioventricular; *BP*, blood pressure; *BUN*, blood urea nitrogen; *Ca*, calcium; *CO*, cardiac output; *CV*, cardiovascular; *ECF*, extracellular fluid volume; *GI*, gastrointestinal; H^+, hydrogen; HCO_3, bicarbonate; PO_4, phosphorus; *PRBC*, packed red blood cells; *RBC*, red blood cell; *RRT*, renal replacement therapy.

tion in oxygen delivery to tissues and organs. The renal response to shock is variable and depends on the duration and severity of hypoperfusion. Figure 13-6 depicts the hemodynamic alterations and the pathophysiology of renal cell injury occurring in shock.

As discussed previously, hypotension and shock lead to activation of the SNS and the RAS and the attendant intense renal vasoconstriction. Renal vasodilating prostaglandins (PG) (PGE$_2$ and prostacyclin), along with intrarenally released endothelial-derived relaxant factor (also called nitric oxide

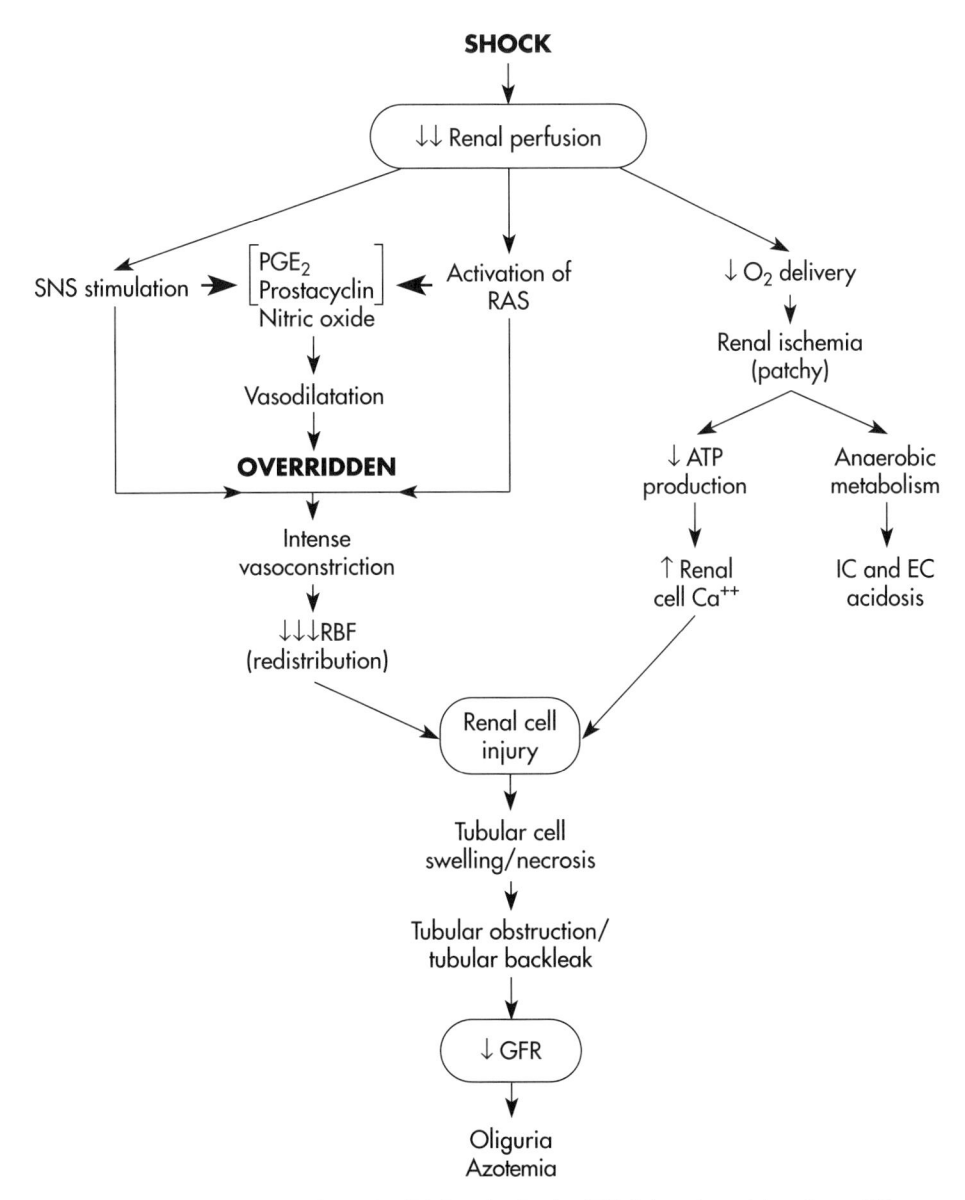

Fig. 13-6 Pathophysiology of renal cell injury in shock. *ATP,* Adenosine triphosphate; *EC,* extracellular; *GFR,* glomerular filtration rate; *IC,* intracellular; *RAS,* renin-angiotensin system; *RBF,* renal blood flow; *SNS,* sympathetic nervous system. (From Toto KH: Renal Physiology: Beyond the Basics. Lewisville, Texas: Barbara Clark Mims Associates, 1995.)

[(NO)] act locally on the renal vasculature to counteract these vasoconstrictive effects. With minor to moderate decreases in renal perfusion, PGE_2, prostacyclin, and NO help in maintaining renal perfusion via their local renal vasodilatory effects. However, in the setting of severe hypoperfusion (shock), this protective vasodilatory effect is overwhelmed and a severe reduction in renal blood flow occurs. Furthermore, redistribution of renal blood flow from the cortex (outer portion of kidney) to the medulla (inner portion of kidney) takes place, thereby aggravating ischemic injury to the glomeruli and the majority of tubular components that are located in the cortex.

The decrease in oxygen delivery to the kidney that occurs in renal hypoperfusion causes patchy renal ischemia because certain segments of the renal tubules (the proximal tubule and the thick ascending limb) consume more oxygen and are therefore more susceptible to ischemic injury. Clinically this is manifested by dilute urine (urine osmolality <300 mOsm/kg) and a urine sodium >20 mEq/L. The precise mechanism of renal cell injury from oxygen deprivation is the subject of intense experimental investigation. A decrease in oxygen delivery decreases the mitochondrial production of ATP. This results in an alteration in renal cell concentrations of sodium (increased), chloride (increased), magnesium (decreased), potassium (decreased), phosphate (decreased), and calcium (increased).[3] The increase in intracellular calcium is thought to be a primary mediator of renal cell injury. Furthermore, oxygen deprivation converts cell metabolism from aerobic to anaerobic and results in both intracellular and extracellular acidosis because of lactate production. There are conflicting data regarding the effect of acidosis on renal cell injury. Some data suggest acidosis is detrimental to renal function and other, more recent studies, propose that acidosis may actually protect the renal tubular cells from ischemic injury by decreasing energy expenditure.[21,22]

Renal cell injury causes swelling and necrosis resulting in tubular obstruction from sloughed cells and cast formation. Tubular backleak also occurs because of ischemic damage to the basement membrane, which increases the permeability of the tubules. Most of the filtrate presented to the tubules leaks back into the interstitium and the peritubular capillaries, rather than being excreted as urine. Tubular obstruction combined with tubular backleak results in a reduction in the GFR and is clinically manifested as oliguria and azotemia.[3]

Renal reperfusion injury. Prolonged renal hypoperfusion occurring in shock clearly results in renal cell injury. During reperfusion, the oxygen and substrate delivered to the tissues may not be entirely beneficial to the cells. Several studies have demonstrated that during reperfusion and reoxygenation after shock, additional cell injury occurs. Figure 13-7 depicts the mechanisms of renal reperfusion injury.

When renal blood flow is restored after an ischemic event, additional renal cell injury occurs from (1) increased calcium delivery and intracellular calcium flux, (2) correction of cellular acidosis, and (3) increased oxygen delivery and production of oxygen-derived free radicals.

Reperfusion is also accompanied by an increase in the delivery of calcium to the cells. Because cell membrane damage has already occurred, an increased permeability to extracellular calcium exists and calcium moves into the cell. This increase in intracellular calcium activates phospholipases present in the cell membrane, which results in structural damage to the cell membrane and a persistent increased permeability of the cells to calcium.[3] There is a great deal of interest in the protective effects that calcium-channel blockers may have in preventing renal reperfusion injury by reducing intracellular calcium influx and concentration.

Correction of intracellular acidosis and an optimal cellular pH restore enzyme activity previously hindered by the acidosis. These enzymatic reactions contribute to phospholipase activation and cell membrane damage. Additionally, it is thought that the normalization of the intracellular pH coupled with increased oxygen delivery provides adequate conditions for the formation of oxygen-derived free radicals.[23]

The formation of oxygen-derived free radicals most likely occurs during reperfusion after total ischemia. Oxygen-derived free radicals are highly cytotoxic and cause cell destruction. Experimental data have demonstrated a protective effect afforded by agents that block the production of oxygen-derived free radicals.[24]

In addition to the hemodynamic changes that contribute to ARF in septic shock, there are also humoral and cellular mediators that play an important role. These humoral and cellular factors interact extensively to alter systemic and renal hemodynamics further.

Humoral and cellular mediators

In sepsis caused by gram-negative organisms such as *Escherichia coli, Pseudomonas* spp., *Enter-*

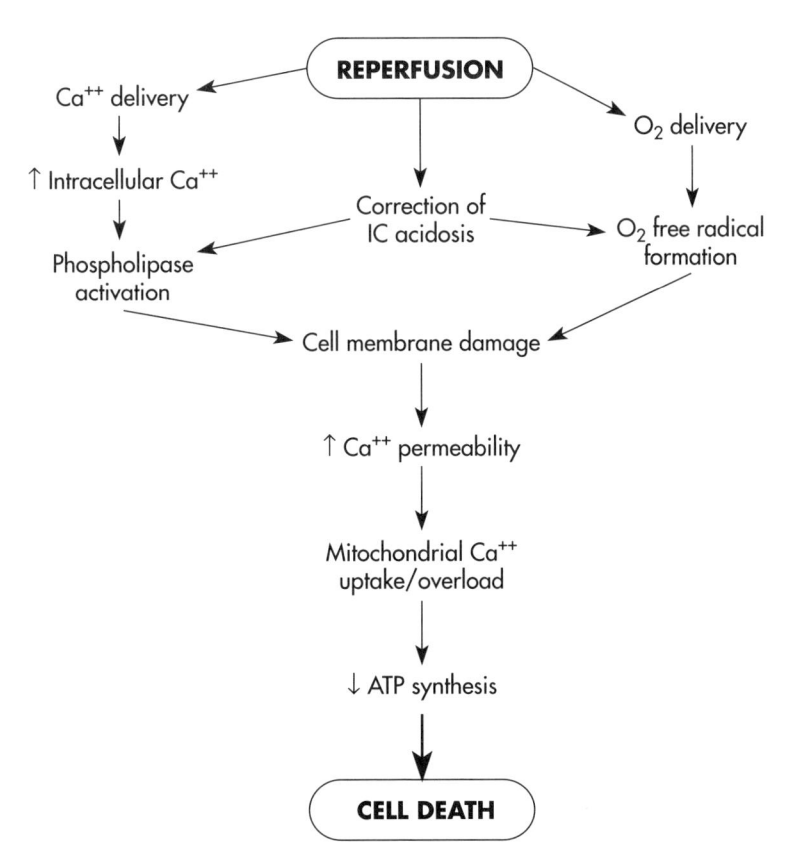

Fig. 13-7 Renal reperfusion injury. *ATP,* Adenosine triphosphate; *IC,* intracellular. (Modified from: Burke TJ et al. Renal Response to Shock. Ann Emerg Med 1986; 15:1398.)

ococcus spp., and others, endotoxin is released from bacteria in the blood stream. Endotoxin is a constituent of the gram-negative bacterial wall released upon the death of the bacteria. Endotoxin initiates a variety of systemic responses seen in septic shock that are depicted in Figure 13-8.

Cytokine release induced by circulating endotoxin includes tumor necrosis factor (TNF), interleukin-1 (IL-1), and platelet-activating factor (PAF), which play a major role in the renal changes in septic shock. Along with their own numerous individual effects, these cytokines, together with bacteria, activate the complement system, which triggers the release and activation of vasoactive and chemotactic factors, as well as the coagulation and fibrinolysis cascades.[19] (See Chapter 3.)

Endotoxin causes endothelial damage that activates Hageman factor (factor XII) and initiates the intrinsic coagulation pathway, which ultimately results in microthrombi formation and possibly disseminated intravascular coagulation (DIC). In the kidney, DIC causes renal capillary thrombosis, reducing the glomerular filtration rate and potentiating renal cell injury through ischemia. Endotoxin also activates mediators that cause systemic vasodilatation and hypotension. Hypotension stimulates the SNS and activates the RAS, both of which cause renal vasoconstriction and a fall in the GFR. Furthermore, evidence suggests that endotoxin may have a direct vasoconstrictive effect on renal vasculature, contributing to renal ischemia.[25]

Tumor necrosis factor is released from macrophages activated by endotoxin, other pathogens, and foreign debris. TNF has a variety of actions including endothelial damage, which results in ischemia and renal cell injury. TNF is a procoagulant

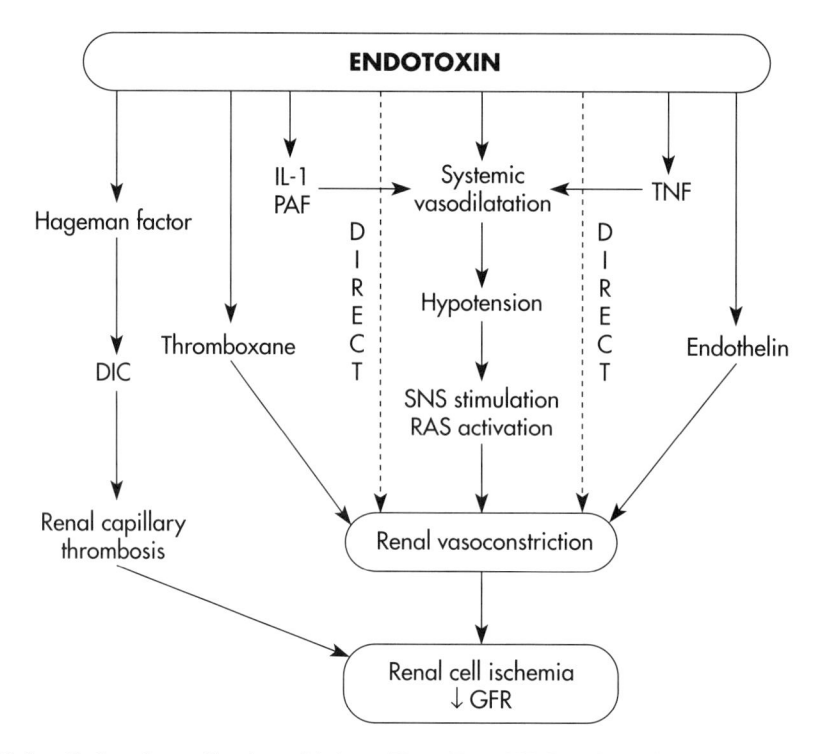

Fig. 13-8 Endotoxin-mediated renal injury. (From Toto KH: Renal Physiology: Beyond the Basics. Lewisville, Texas: Barbara Clark Mims Associates, 1995.)

mediator that potentiates the formation and deposition of microthrombi in the microcirculation. Additionally, production of TNF indirectly causes vasodilatation and hypotension secondary to its effect on increased NO synthesis.[25] NO, produced in endothelial cells, causes systemic vasodilatation, inhibits platelet aggregation, and inhibits neutrophil adhesion, plugging, and migration into sites of inflammation.[20] In the septic patient, NO may have detrimental systemic effects related to decreased systemic vascular resistance and hypotension, but in the kidney, NO is necessary to maintain organ perfusion and prevent vascular thrombosis.[20] In experimental models, blocking NO production induces a profound reduction in splanchnic and renal blood flow.[19]

Interleukin-1 acts synergistically with TNF in sepsis. IL-1 acts directly on blood vessels inducing vasodilatation via production of PAF and NO.[25] PAF causes hypotension and capillary leak syndrome.[26] Both IL-1 and PAF contribute to reducing renal blood flow by causing systemic vasodilatation and hypotension. Endothelin is another mediator released in endotoxemia that causes intense vasoconstriction to which the kidney appears to be very sensitive.[19,27]

Renal prostaglandins released in sepsis and endotoxemia secondary to renal hypoperfusion have both protective and deleterious effects. The vasodilating prostaglandins, as previously discussed, protect renal blood flow; the vasoconstricting prostaglandins, predominantly thromboxane, reduce renal blood flow. Drugs that block prostaglandin synthesis such as nonsteroidal antiinflammatory drugs (such as aspirin, ibuprofen, and indocin) have not been beneficial in treating shock-induced renal vasoconstriction by blocking thromboxane synthesis because these drugs also block the protective vasodilating prostaglandins (PGE_2, prostacyclin). The physiologic factors activated by endotoxins and other inflammatory stimuli that lead to a reduction in renal blood flow, as well as opposing factors acting to protect renal blood flow are listed in Table 13-5.

Given all the variables listed in Table 13-5, it may be difficult to predict renal blood flow in the patient with septic shock, based on hemodynamic values alone. Although severe and prolonged renal hypoperfusion is important, it certainly is not the sole factor contributing to the development of ARF during septic shock and endotoxemia.[19] Aside from the humoral and cellular factors previously discussed, additional factors affecting renal function include exposure to nephrotoxins and dysfunction in other systems (cardiac, pulmonary, gastrointestinal, and hepatic) that may be affected by SIRS, sepsis, and MODS.

Nephrotoxins and Sepsis

Gram-negative bacterial infections are commonly treated with aminoglycoside antibiotics such as gentamicin, tobramycin, amikacin, netelmycin, and sisomycin. Although the aminoglycosides are efficacious in the treatment of gram-negative bacterial infections, 10% to 26% of patients treated with aminoglycosides develop nephrotoxicity.[13] Risk factors for aminoglycoside-induced nephrotoxicity include advanced age, prolonged therapy, preexisting renal insufficiency, volume depletion, liver disease, and electrolyte disorders (hypercalcemia, hypokalemia, hypomagnesemia, and metabolic acidosis).[24] The nephrotoxicity of aminoglycosides correlates better with the total cumulative dose than with plasma levels and is usually apparent with the onset of azotemia after 5 to 10 days of therapy.[13] In the septic patient, there are additional factors that potentiate the nephrotoxic effect of aminoglycosides, including fever, endotoxemia, and renal hypoperfusion.[24] In the presence of septicemia, aminoglycoside-induced nephrotoxicity is enhanced and may result from release of endotoxin after antibiotic-mediated bacteriolysis.[25]

Cephalosporins may also be used in the treatment of gram-negative bacterial infections and although they are less nephrotoxic than are the aminoglycosides, they can also cause nephrotoxic ATN. Vancomycin, used to treat staphylococcal infections, has only mild nephrotoxic effects. However, its primary route of elimination is renal, and in the presence of reduced or absent renal function, excretion is greatly delayed.[28] Additionally, removal of vancomycin by hemodialysis is limited. Vancomycin-

Table 13-5 Endotoxin-Mediated Factors Affecting Renal Blood Flow

Physiologic factors activated by endotoxin	Renal effect
Factors reducing renal blood flow	
Endotoxin	Renal vasoconstriction, systemic vasodilatation and ↓ BP → ↓ renal blood flow
SNS and release of norepinephrine	Renal and systemic vasoconstriction
RAS and release of angiotensin II	Renal and systemic vasoconstriction
Thromboxane	Renal vasoconstriction
Tumor necrosis factor	Systemic vasodilatation and ↓ BP → ↓ renal blood flow, microthrombi formation, and renal capillary thrombosis
Platelet activating factor	Systemic vasodilatation, ↓ BP and cellular leakiness → ↓ renal blood flow
Hageman factor and DIC	Microthrombi formation, renal capillary thrombosis, ↓ GFR, and ischemic renal cell injury
Endothelin	Renal vasoconstriction
Factors protecting renal blood flow	
Vasodilating prostaglandins (PGE$_2$, prostacyclin)	Renal vasodilatation
Nitric oxide	↑ renal blood flow, ↓ vascular thrombosis
Renal autoregulation (if MAP >50 mmHg)	Renal vasodilatation

BP, Blood pressure; *DIC*, disseminated intravascular coagulation; *GFR*, glomerular filtration rate; *MAP*, mean arterial pressure; *RAS*, renin-angiotensin system; *SNS*, sympathetic nervous system.

Table 13-6 Mortality Rates Associated with Acute Renal Failure

ARF + additional organ failure	Mortality rate (%)
ARF alone with no complications	8
ARF + uncontrolled sepsis	65
ARF + liver failure	65
ARF + pulmonary failure	71
ARF + circulatory failure	76

ARF, Acute renal failure.
From EDTA-European Renal Association Registry data presented at association meeting in Brussels, June 1985 as cited in Hays SR: Ischemic acute renal failure. Internal Medicine Grand Rounds, University of Texas Southwestern Medical Center, Dallas, Texas, September 5, 1991.

Table 13-7 Mortality from Acute Renal Failure in Association with Multiorgan Failure

No. of other organs failed*	Mortality rate (%)
0	38
1	56
2	70
3	81
4	100

*Failure of other organ systems included circulatory failure (SBP ≤100), respiratory failure (mechanical ventilation), congestive heart failure, sepsis, or GI dysfunction (bleeding ileus or obstruction).
As cited in Hays SR. Ischemic acute renal failure. Internal Medicine Grand Rounds, University of Texas Southwestern Medical Center, Dallas, Texas, September 5, 1991.

associated hearing loss can be seen in patients with renal insufficiency and vancomycin levels greater than 80 to 100 mU/mL.[28]

Acute renal failure and MODS

Acute renal failure is frequently seen in the context of MODS. When the kidney is the only organ to fail, mortality is only 8%. However, when ARF is associated with either uncontrolled sepsis or pulmonary, liver, or heart failure, the mortality rate dramatically increases (Table 13-6).

Spiegel and co-workers[29] reported that adult respiratory distress syndrome, ventilatory failure, and the need for ventilatory support were powerful predictors of mortality in ARF. In a large prospective study, Liano and co-workers[30] reported that neurologic, respiratory, or cardiovascular failure was most predictive of a poor outcome in ARF. Many studies have documented that as the number of failing organs increases, mortality increases.[29,31] Table 13-7 demonstrates the mortality from ARF as a function of the number of additional organ systems that have failed.

Although the actual number of organs failed clearly affects mortality, organ-organ interaction may be an equally important determinant of outcome in ARF in the setting of MODS.[6] Considering the poor prognosis of ARF in MODS, it is apparent that the initiation of dialysis in such patients presents ethical issues. Dialysis in the patient with multiple organ failure, particularly when it includes acute respiratory failure requiring ventilatory support, is most likely a procedure that will merely prolong the patient's death despite correction of fluid and electrolyte imbalances and uremia.[30,32]

PREVENTION AND TREATMENT OF ACUTE RENAL FAILURE
Diuretics

The initial treatment of ARF is aimed at correcting hypotension or any fluid deficits that may exist. If the patient is normotensive and euvolemic but still remains oliguric, a diuretic may be needed. The loop diuretics and mannitol are often used in the early stages of ARF. Beneficial effects of diuretics include the following: (1) prophylaxis to prevent ARF in high-risk clinical situations, (2) halting progression of ARF, and (3) accelerating the rate of recovery in established ARF.[17] Levinsky and Bernard[33] studied patients early in the course of ARF and were able to demonstrate that in patients with oliguric ARF who responded to diuretics the mortality rate was 24% as compared to a 42% mortality rate in diuretic-resistant patients.

The loop diuretics (furosemide, bumetanide, and torsemide) are the most potent diuretics. When given for ARF, high doses are often required because the dose must be increased in proportion to the reduction in GFR. The loop diuretics can be administered via intermittent intravenous bolus or continuous intravenous infusion. In addition to their effect on the loop of Henle in enhancing salt and water excretion, these agents also increase renal blood flow and GFR by enhancing synthesis of renal PGs.[16] Adverse effects include ototoxicity and hearing loss that is usually reversible.

Dopamine

Renal-dose dopamine is a commonly used drug for the treatment of oliguric ARF in the critically ill patient. Renal-dose dopamine (1 to 3 µg/kg/min) has been shown to enhance renal blood flow, improve renal perfusion, and increase urine output in euvolemic subjects with normal renal function.[34] Renal-dose dopamine has also been shown to increase urine output in patients with congestive heart failure. Additionally, when given with a diuretic, renal-dose dopamine increases urine output in patients previously unresponsive to diuretics.[35] Activation of dopaminergic receptors results in renal and mesenteric vasodilatation that decreases afterload and thereby, increases cardiac output and renal perfusion.[36] Additionally, activation of β-adrenergic receptors (even at a dose of 2 to 5 µg/kg/min) increases cardiac output. However, the effect of renal-dose dopamine on renal function in critically ill patients with ARF has not been clearly established.

There are limited studies supporting the benefit of renal-dose dopamine in combination with a diuretic (usually a loop diuretic) to increase urine output in the oliguric patient with ARF[37]; however, these studies are small and lack adequate control groups. In patients with sepsis, multiple organ dysfunction, and ARF, studies demonstrating a benefit from renal-dose dopamine in preserving or improving renal function and reducing mortality in these patients do not exist. Additionally, any benefit dopamine may have in increasing renal blood flow and urine output diminishes with prolonged infusions. Therefore, it should be discontinued if the patient remains oliguric.[37] Clearly there is a need for large, controlled studies evaluating the benefit of renal-dose dopamine in oliguric critically ill patients with ARF.

Renal replacement therapy

If the patient in ARF does not respond to conservative management (volume maintenance, diuretics, and renal-dose dopamine), a renal placement therapy such as ultrafiltration or dialysis may be required. Table 13-8 reviews all currently available forms of renal replacement therapy.

Ultrafiltration. Ultrafiltration is indicated for the volume overloaded, diuretic-resistant patient. Ultrafiltration is defined as the bulk flow of solutes and water through a semipermeable membrane in the direction of a hydrostatic pressure difference (from area of high pressure to area of low pressure). Ultrafiltration primarily removes water and small molecules such as electrolytes, urea, and creatinine. Solutes removed with ultrafiltration are swept along with water that is removed, a process called "solvent drag." However, because there is no dialysate infused through the dialyzer, the principle of diffusion is not utilized and therefore rapid clearance of urea and other metabolic waste products is not possible. Ultrafiltration techniques include intermittent hemofiltration (IHF), continuous arteriovenous hemofiltration (CAVH), and continuous venovenous hemofiltration (CVVH). (See Table 13-8.)

Dialysis. The most common indications for acute dialysis are volume overload, hyperkalemia, metabolic acidosis, uremia, and prophylactic dialysis to maintain the BUN <100 mg/dL.[38] Dialysis is the process of diffusion of a solute down its concentration gradient across a semipermeable membrane. During clinical dialysis, both diffusion and ultrafiltration take place simultaneously. Dialysis techniques include intermittent hemodialysis (the most commonly used form of renal replacement therapy in ARF), continuous arteriovenous hemodialysis (CAVHD), continuous venovenous hemodialysis (CVVHD), and peritoneal dialysis (the oldest and least commonly used form of renal replacement therapy in ARF).

Nutritional support

In patients with ARF and MODS, nutritional intervention must consider multiple metabolic consequences related to the loss of renal function. There are several factors accelerating catabolism during the course of ATN in the septic patient; these include metabolic acidosis and stress hyperglycemia (elevated catecholamines and glucagon, insulin resistance, and glucose intolerance).[39]

The catabolic stress of infection is very common in critically ill patients and often results in malnutrition. Malnutrition and an untreated catabolic response can lead to immunosuppression, poor wound healing, and musculoskeletal weakness, all of which can contribute to an increase in morbidity and mortality.[40] Appropriate nutritional support slows the development of these conditions and may improve survival in patients with ARF. However, nutritional support is more difficult when the patient is oliguric because fluid management may be a major problem.

Renal replacement therapy may need to be initiated to administer adequate quantities of nutritional

Table 13-8 Renal Replacement Therapy

Mode	Principles involved	Access	Pump assisted	Indications
Ultrafiltration				
IHF (Intermittent hemofiltration)	Ultrafiltration Solvent drag	Venovenous	Yes	Diuretic resistant, volume overloaded patient who can tolerate rapid fluid removal and is hemodynamically stable
CAVH (Continuous arteriovenous hemofiltration)	Ultrafiltration Solvent drag	Arteriovenous	No	Diuretic resistant, volume overloaded, hemodynamically unstable patient who cannot tolerate rapid fluid shifts; Parenteral or enteral alimentation in volume overloaded patient; IHF unavailable
CVVH (Continuous venovenous hemofiltration)	Ultrafiltration Solvent drag	Venovenous	Yes	Diuretic resistant, hemodynamically unstable, volume overloaded patient who cannot tolerate rapid fluid shfts; Parenteral or enteral alimentation in volume overloaded patient; Solute clearance (as efficient as CAVHD)
Dialysis				
IHD (Intermittent hemodialysis)	Ultrafiltration Diffusion	Venovenous	Yes	Emergent, catabolic, fluid overloaded states; Life-threatening electrolyte imbalances ($\uparrow K$, $\uparrow PO_4$, $\uparrow Mg$, $\downarrow Ca$); Metabolic acidosis; Uremia
CAVHD (Continuous arteriovenous hemofiltration dialysis)	Ultrafiltration Diffusion	Arteriovenous	No	Volume overloaded hemodynamically unstable patient with azotemia or uremia; Catabolic acute renal failure; Electrolyte imbalances and acidosis; Parenteral and enteral alimentation in volume overloaded, catabolic patient; IHD unavailable

Advantages	Complications/disadvantages
Rapid, efficient fluid removal	May not be well tolerated in hemodynamically unstable patients Some anticoagulation required Poor control of azotemia, may need intermittent dialysis for waste product removal Rebound hyperkalemia Hypotension Requires dialysis nurse to run machine
Continuous, gradual, treatment (fewer high and low extremes) High rate of fluid removal/replacement allows flexibility in fluid balance Requires less technical support and equipment than IHF	Prolonged arterial cannulation required Ideally, need MAP of $\cong 60$ mmHg to drive extracorporeal circuit Anticoagulation, bleeding Hypotension Access complications (bleeding, clotting, infection) Requires strict monitoring of fluid and electrolyte replacement to avoid deficits or overload Poor control of azotemia, may need intermittent dialysis for waste product removal Poor emergent treatment of hyperkalemia/acidosis Air embolism Loss of limb (distal arterial ischemia) ICU setting only Requires 1:1 nurse/patient ratio
Precise fluid control Can be done in patient with low MAP Less hemodynamic instability than IHF Ease of initiation Large volume of parenteral nutrition may be administered No arterial cannulation Better solute clearance than CAVH Requires less technical support and equipment than IHF	Same as above (CAVH) except MAP of 60 mmHg not needed Waste product removal not as efficient as CVVHD or IHD but better than CAVH Requires special pump to augment blood flow through extracorporeal circuit Requires training of ICU nurses in use of pump
Rapid and efficient Cost effective	Hemodynamic instability (hypotension arrhythmias, ischemia) Hypoxemia Fluid, electrolyte, and osmolar shifts Access complications (clotting, bleeding, infections) Systemic bleeding from anticoagulation Disequilibrium syndrome Requires dialysis nurse to run machine
Requires less technical support and equipment than hemodialysis Precise fluid control Ease of initiation Less hemodynamic instability than with IHD Large volume of parenteral nutrition may be administered	Anticoagulation, bleeding Access complications (bleeding, clotting, infection) Prolonged arterial cannulation required Air embolism Requires strict monitoring of fluid and electrolyte replacement to avoid deficits or overload ICU setting only Usually requires 1:1 nurse/patient ratio Disequilibrium syndrome (unlikely—due to slow BUN removal) Not as efficient as CVVHD or IHD

Continued.

Table 13-8 Renal Replacement Therapy—cont'd

Mode	Principles involved	Access	Pump assisted	Indications
CVVHD (Continuous venovenous hemodialysis)	Ultrafiltration Diffusion	Venovenous	Yes	Volume overloaded hemodynamically unstable patient with azotemia or uremia Catabolic acute renal failure Electrolyte imbalances and metabolic acidosis Parenteral and enteral alimentation in volume overloaded, catabolic patient IHD unavailable
PD (Peritoneal dialysis)	Ultrafiltration Diffusion	Peritoneal catheter (nonvascular)	No	Hemodynamically unstable or bleeding patient when vascular access is difficult or when hemodialysis is unavailable

From Toto KH. Renal physiology: Beyond the basics. Lewisville, Texas: Barbara Clark Mims Associates, 1995.
BUN, Blood urea nitrogen; *Ca,* calcium; *ICU,* intensive care unit; *K,* potassium, *MAP,* mean arterial pressure; *PO₄,* phosphorus.

support. The continuous renal replacement therapies may have an advantage over intermittent therapies in that fluid can be removed "around-the-clock" and the likelihood of developing volume overload because of nutritional support is less likely. Protein and energy requirements in critically ill patients with ARF are the same as in any other patient in the intensive care unit and are approximately 30 to 40 kcal/kg/day.[40] Protein is usually given in the range of 1.0 to 1.5 g/kg/day depending on the degree of azotemia.[40] If too much protein is given, the BUN can increase because of high-intake protein metabolism. However, if dietary protein is not adequate, catabolism worsens, which also causes the BUN to rise. Hyperkalemia and metabolic acidosis can also be exacerbated in the catabolic patient with ARF.

During parenteral nutrition, potassium, phosphate, and magnesium levels must be closely monitored and alterations corrected. Although levels of these electrolytes are usually elevated in ARF, the initiation of high glucose feedings and the increase in insulin (endogenous or exogenous) levels can lower serum electrolyte values. Insulin transports potassium, phosphorus, and magnesium intracellularly. Therefore, the plasma levels of these electrolytes may decrease with the initiation of high glucose feedings and increase if they are added to the feeding. Daily evaluation of plasma electrolytes and consideration of the constituents of parenteral nutrition are essential.

FUTURE TRENDS IN MANAGEMENT AND PREVENTION OF ACUTE TUBULAR NECROSIS

Current treatment for ATN is limited to conservative medical treatment including volume correction, diuretics, renal-dose dopamine, and renal replacement therapy while passively awaiting recovery of nephron function and renal tubular regeneration. The majority of the current research in ATN is directed at finding drugs that prevent renal cell damage or promote recovery of function after

Advantages	Complications/disadvantages
No arterial cannulation	Anticoagulation, bleeding
Requires less technical support and equipment than IHD	Access complications (bleeding, clotting, infection)
	Air embolism
Precise fluid control	Requires strict monitoring of fluid and electrolyte replacement to avoid deficits or overload
Ease of initiation	
Less hemodynamic instability than with HD	ICU setting only
	Requires 1:1 nurse/patient ratio
Large volume of parenteral nutrition may be administered	Disequilibrium syndrome (unlikely—due to slow BUN removal)
	Not as efficient as IHD
Better solute clearance than CAVHD	Requires special pump to augment blood flow through extracorporeal circuit
Can be done in patient with low MAP	
	Requires training of ICU nurses in use of pump
Requires less technical support and equipment than any of the other renal replacement therapies	Peritoneal drainage failure, fluid retention
	Less predictable fluid removal
	Access complications (peritonitis, catheter infection)
No anticoagulation required	Reduced diaphragmatic compliance, decreased ventilation
Nonvascular access	Hyperglycemia, hyperosmolarity (due to hypertonic glucose in dialysate)
	Slower waste product removal than other modes of dialysis
	Inefficient in emergency
	Therapy may be contraindicated by abdominal surgery (adhesions), abdominal drains, wounds

an ischemic event or exposure to a nephrotoxin. Numerous research studies have evaluated the effects of a variety of agents used in the treatment of ATN in both humans and animal models.

Atrial natriuretic peptide

Atrial natriuretic peptide (ANP) is a naturally occurring hormone released from cardiac myocytes in the right atrium (and to a lesser extent in the left atrium). Recent studies[41,42] in animals have demonstrated that ANP reduces the severity of and enhances recovery from ischemic and nephrotoxic ATN. The mechanisms of action relate to the following effects of ANP: (1) increased glomerular filtration rate secondary to afferent arteriolar vasodilatation combined with efferent vasoconstriction; (2) dramatic increase in sodium and water excretion; and (3) systemic vasodilatation opposing norepinephrine-induced vasoconstriction.[43] In a small clinical study, Rahman and co-workers[44] demonstrated that intravenous ANP increases the GFR and reduces the need for dialysis in patients with established ATN. Larger, randomized, placebo-controlled human studies are currently under way. ANP has also been shown to be effective in reducing the risk of nephrotoxic ATN when given intravenously during cardiac catheterization and exposure to radiographic contrast media.[45] Side effects of intravenous ANP administration include hypotension and bradycardia.

Urodilatin. The kidney produces a natriuretic peptide, urodilatin, which is structurally similar to ANP. Actions of urodilatin are also similar to the actions of ANP. However, in comparison to ANP, systemic urodilatin administration in humans displays a minimal hypotensive effect, but exceeds ANP in increasing the GFR.[46] Experimental ATN (in rats) of either ischemic or nephrotoxic origin may be attenuated by exogenous urodilatin administration combined with low-dose dopamine.[46] Additional studies are needed to evaluate the clinical usefulness of urodilatin in human models of ARF.

Growth factors

Growth factors are produced by a variety of cells in the body and act at a local level to enhance cell division and growth. Growth factors are produced by the liver, kidneys, endothelium, and hematologic cells and include insulin-like growth factor (IGF-1), epidermal growth factor (EGF), transforming growth factor β (TGF-β). There are over 20 known growth factors.

The use of growth factors as therapeutic agents has been proposed for both acute and chronic renal failure.[47] In animal studies of ATN, the administration of EGF and IGF-1 accelerated the recovery of renal function and reduced mortality.[47] The proposed mechanisms by which growth factors act in acute tubular necrosis are as follows: (1) stimulation of renal hypertrophy and promotion of anabolism, (2) reduction of the catabolic response in ARF, (3) enhancement of tubular regeneration, and (4) maintenance of glomerular filtration.[48] IGF-1 has been used safely in humans with chronic renal failure and has been shown to enhance GFR and renal blood flow.[47] Human studies are currently under way to establish the role of IGF-1 as a therapeutic agent in ATN.[48]

The importance of growth factors is that they may improve renal function after the ischemic event rather than acting in a protective manner. Growth factors are promising agents that may hasten recovery from ischemic ATN.

MgCl$_2$-ATP

After ischemia, cellular ATP levels fall rapidly, which potentiates cell damage. MgCl$_2$-ATP (an exogenous adenine nucleotide) infusions given up to 48 hours after ischemia have been found to improve renal clearance significantly in a rat model. It is thought that the MgCl$_2$-ATP infusion stabilizes the cell membrane during anoxia and after reperfusion by providing the precursors for rapid ATP formation.[49]

Calcium-channel blocking agents

Both animal and human studies have shown that calcium-channel blockers provide a beneficial effect on renal function in ischemic ARF. The beneficial effect of these agents is thought to be caused by the lessening of the increase in intracellular calcium accumulation that occurs in ischemic acute renal failure (both during ischemia and during reperfusion).[35] Any beneficial impact of calcium-channel blockers requires that they be given *before* the ischemic event, thereby serving as protective agents.[17] There is little beneficial effect when these agents are given after the ischemic event. Calcium-channel blockers (verapamil and diltiazem) are currently being used in renal transplant patients and have demonstrated a significant reduction in posttransplant ATN.[22] Calcium-channel blockers may also be beneficial in the prevention of radiocontrast nephrotoxicity when administered before the contrast media.[50] However, there are no studies demonstrating that calcium-channel blocking agents prevent ischemic ATN or attenuate the course of established ARF.

Antioxidants

Oxygen-derived free radicals such as superoxide anion (O_2^-) and hydroxyl radical (OH) are mediators of renal cell injury in endotoxin-mediated ARF, ischemic ATN, and renal reperfusion injury.[24,51] Endotoxin has been shown to activate the release of oxidants by activated white blood cells in the microvasculature and in the lungs.[51] The genesis of oxidants with a reperfusion injury has been previously reviewed in the section on renal reperfusion injury. Free oxygen radicals are highly reactive substances that induce cell injury in a variety of disease states. Several animals studies have demonstrated that xanthine oxidase inhibitors such as allopurinol or superoxide dismutase may prevent ARF or attenuate its course when given *before* the ischemic event.[35] Additionally administration of the hydroxyl scavenger dimethylthiourea, also improved renal function in the same model.[35] However, antioxidants and oxygen-derived free radical scavengers have not been shown to improve renal function in the postischemic period.[24]

Zurorsky and Gispaan[51] performed animal studies that demonstrated that the antioxidants dimethylthiourea and superoxide dismutase had a beneficial effect in halting progressive renal damage associated with endotoxemia. Antioxidant therapy has also been applied to renal injury (animal and in vitro studies) induced by nephrotoxins such as gentamicin, cyclosporin, cis-platinum, and contrast media, with mixed results.[35] Additional studies are needed to evaluate the clinical usefulness of antioxidant strategies in human models of endotoxin-mediated ARF, ischemic ATN, and renal reperfusion injury.

Antiendothelin strategies

Endothelin is a potent vasoconstrictor released from a variety of cell types (endothelial cells, fibroblasts, and renal tubular epithelial cells). Hypoxia, mechanical stress or trauma to the cell surface, growth factors, thrombosis, and hormones such as epinephrine stimulate the release of endothelin.[35] Endothelin is important in the pathogenesis of renal injury in a variety of insults, most notably septic shock. Animal studies have shown the use of antiendothelin antiserum in the postischemic model increases the GFR and glomerular plasma flow rates.[35] This may be yet another beneficial area of research in treating ATN associated with ischemia and sepsis.

In summary, the current management of ARF focuses primarily on prevention of ischemic and nephrotoxic insults, attention to fluid and electrolyte balance, diuretics, adequate nutrition to prevent catabolism, and the initiation of a renal replacement therapy. The efficacy of several of the investigational strategies discussed above raises the possibility that in the near future interventions may be undertaken to prevent and, most importantly, interrupt pathways of tissue injury, as well as enhance recovery after the injury has already occurred.[35]

CONCLUSION

The mortality rate for ARF associated with multiple organ dysfunction is extremely high. However, although these patients may die *in* ARF, they rarely die *from* ARF. The ability to predict outcome in ARF remains somewhat elusive. There is no exact method to identify patients who will have a poor outcome; there are only associated conditions that increase the probability of death.[29] The decision of whether or not to initiate dialysis in these critically ill patients remains an ethical issue best determined by a team consisting of the patient, the family, the nurse, the primary physician, the nephrologist, the social worker, and the chaplain.

On a more positive note, the majority of patients who survive ARF and MODS, recover renal function and discontinue dialysis.[5,18] Therapeutic regimens including ANP, growth factors, and antioxidants are currently being evaluated in both laboratory and clinical studies. These agents may attenuate ischemic injury, enhance recovery of renal function, and improve survival in patients with ARF and MODS.

REFERENCES

1. Bartlett RH et al. Acute renal failure revisited: The full circle in ARF mortality. Trans Am Soc Artif Intern Organs 1984;30:700-702.
2. O'Meara YM, Bernard DB. Clinical presentation, complications, and prognosis of acute renal failure. In: Jacobson HR, Striker GE, Klahr S, eds. The principles and practice of nephrology. St. Louis: Mosby; 1995.
3. Conger JD, Briner VA, Schrier RW. Acute renal failure: Pathogenesis, diagnosis, and management. In: Schrier RW, ed. Renal and electrolyte disorders. 4th ed. Boston: Little Brown; 1992.
4. Tran DD et al. Factors related to multiple organ system failure and mortality in a surgical intensive care unit. Nephrol Dial Transplant 1994;9:172-178.
5. Bonomini V et al. Long-term follow-up of acute renal failure. Nephrol Dial Transplant 1994;9:224-228.
6. Cosentino F, Chaff C, Piedmonte M. Risk factors influencing survival in ICU acute renal failure. Nephrol Dial Transplant 1994;9:179-182.
7. Bluemle LW, Webster GD, Elkinton JR. Acute tubular necrosis: Analysis of one hundred cases with respect to mortality, complications, and treatment with and without dialysis. Arch Intern Med 1959;104:180-197.
8. Coratelli P et al. Acute renal failure after septic shock. Adv Exp Med Biol 1986;212:233-241.
9. Guyton AC. Textbook of medical physiology. 9th ed. Philadelphia: WB Saunders; 1995;273-353.
10. Lancaster LE. Renal and endocrine regulation of water and electrolyte balance. Nurs Clin North Am 1987;22:761-772.
11. Conlin PR, Dluhy RG, Williams PR. Disorders of renin-angiotensin-aldosterone system. In: Schrier RW. Renal and electrolyte disorders. Boston: Little Brown Co.; 1992;405-446.
12. Anderson RJ, Schrier RW. Acute tubular necrosis. In: Schrier RW and Gottschalk CW, eds. Diseases of the kidney. Boston: Little, Brown; 1988;1413-1446.
13. Tisher CC, Wilcox CS, eds. Nephrology for the house office. 2nd ed. Baltimore: Williams and Wilkins; 1993.
14. Lake EW, Humes HD. Acute renal failure: Directed therapy to enhance renal tubular regeneration. Semin Nephrol 1994;14:83-97.
15. Goligorsky MS et al. Integrin receptors in renal tubular epithelium: New insights into pathophysiology of acute renal failure. Am J Physiol 1993;264:F1-F8.
16. Tisher CC, Wilcox CS, eds. Nephrology for the house officer. Baltimore: Williams and Wilkins; 1989.
17. Hays SR. Ischemic acute renal failure. Internal medicine grand rounds. Dallas: University of Texas Southwestern Medical Center; 1991.
18. Kjellstrand CM, Ebben J, Davin T. Time of death, recovery of renal function, development of chronic renal failure and need for chronic hemodialysis in patients with acute tubular necrosis. Trans Am Soc Artif Intern Organs 1981;27:45.
19. Groenveld ABJ. Pathogenesis of acute renal failure during sepsis. Nephrol Dial Transplant 1994;9:47-51.
20. Star R. Nitric oxide: Friend and foe. Internal medicine grand rounds. Dallas: University of Texas Southwestern Medical Center; 1995.
21. Schrier RW, Burke TJ. New aspects in pathogenesis of acute renal failure. Nephrol Dial Transplant 1994;9:9-14.
22. Bonaventure JV. Mechanisms of ischemic acute renal failure. Kid Int 1993;43:1160-1178.
23. Burke TJ et al. Renal response to shock. Ann Emerg Med 1986;15:1397-1400.

24. Zager RA. Endotoxemia, renal hypoperfusion, and fever: Interactive risk factors for aminoglycoside and sepsis-associated acute renal failure. Am J Kidney Dis 1992;20:223-230.
25. Wiecek A, Zeier M, Ritz E. Role of infection in the genesis of acute renal failure. Nephrol Dial Transplant 1994;9:40-44.
26. Tracey KJ, Lowry SF. The role of cytokine mediators in septic shock. Adv Surg 1990;23:21-56.
27. Wardle EN. Acute renal failure and multiorgan failure. Nephrol Dial Transplant 1994;9:104-107.
28. Thompson JR, Henrich WL. Nephrotoxic agents and their effects. In: Jacobson HR, Striker G, Klahr S. The principles and practice of nephrology. St. Louis: Mosby; 1995:788-796.
29. Spiegel DM et al. Determinants of survival and recovery in acute renal failure patients dialyzed in intensive care units. Am J Nephrol 1991;11:44-47.
30. Liaño F et al. Prognosis of acute tubular necrosis: An extended prospectively contrasted study. Nephron 1992;63:21-31.
31. Maher ER et al. Prognosis of critically ill patients with acute renal failure: APACHE II score and other predictive factors. Q J Med 1989;72:857-866.
32. Bone R. Multiple system organ failure and the sepsis syndrome. Hosp Prac 1991;26:101-126.
33. Levinsky NG, Bernard DB. Mannitol and loop diuretics in acute renal failure. In: Brenner B, Lazarus J, eds. Acute renal failure. New York: Churchill-Livingstone; 1988:841-856.
34. Ter Wee PM et al. Effect of intravenous infusion of low-dose dopamine on renal function in normal individuals and in patients with renal disease. Am J Nephrol 1986;6:42-46.
35. Fischereder M, Trick W, Nath KA. Therapeutic strategies in the prevention of acute renal failure. Semin Nephrol 1994;14:41-52.
36. Beregovich J et al. Dose-related hemodynamic and renal effects of dopamine in congestive heart failure. Am Heart J 1974;87:550-557.
37. Szerlip HM. Renal-dose dopamine: Fact or fiction. Ann Intern Med 1991;115:153-154.
38. Daugirdas JT, Ing TS. Handbook of dialysis. 2nd ed. Boston: Little, Brown; 1994.
39. Cambi V, David S. Basic therapeutic requirements in the treatment of sepsis in acute renal failure. Nephrol Dial Transplant 1994;9:183-186.
40. Seidner DL, Matarese LE, Steiger E. Nutritional care of the critically ill patient with renal failure. Semin Nephrol 1994;14:53-63.
41. Conger JD, Falx SA, Hammond WS. Atrial natriuretic peptide and dopamine in established acute renal failure in the rat. Kid Int 1991;40:21-28.
42. Shaw SG, Weidmann P, Zimmerman A. Urodilation, not nitroprusside, combined with dopamine reverses ischemic acute renal failure. Kidney Int 1992;42:1153-1159.
43. Lieberthal W, Sheridan AM, Valeri CR. Protective effect of atrial natriuretic factor and mannitol following renal ischemia. Am J Physiol 1990;27:F1266.
44. Rahman SH et al. Effects of atrial natriuretic peptide in clinical acute renal failure. Kidney Int 1994;45:1731-1738.
45. Weisberg LS, Kurnik PB, Kurnik BR. Risk of radiocontrast nephropathy in patients with and without diabetes. Kidney Int 1994;45:259-65.
46. Shaw SG et al. Atrial natriuretic peptide protects against acute ischemic renal failure in the rat. J Clin Invest 1987;80:1232-1237.
47. Hammerman MR, Miller SB. Therapeutic use of growth factors in renal failure. J Am Soc Nephrol 1994;5:1-11.
48. Ding H, Kopple JD, Cohen A, Hirschberg R. Recombinant human insulin-like growth factor-I accelerates recovery and reduces catabolism in rats with ischemic acute renal failure. J Clin Invest 1993;91:2281-2287.
49. Gaudio KM et al. Accelerated recovery of single nephron function by the postischemic infusion of ATP-MgCL$_2$. Kidney Int 1982;22.
50. Russo D et al. Randomised prospective study on renal effects of two different constrast media in humans: Protective role of calcium-channel blockers. Nephron 1990;55:254-257.
51. Zurovsky Y, Gispaan I. Antioxidants attenuate endotoxin-induced acute renal failure in rats. Am J Kidney Dis 1995;25:51-57.

SUGGESTED READINGS

Bagshaw ONT, Anaes FRC, Hutchinson A. Continuous arteriovenous haemofiltration and respiratory function in multiple organ systems failure. Intensive Care Med 1992;18:334-338.

Bellomo R et al. Acute renal failure in critical illness: Conventional dialysis versus acute continuous hemodiafiltration. ASAIO Journal 1992;M654-M657.

Bellomo R, Parkin G, Boyce N. Acute renal failure in the critically ill: Management by continuous veno-venous hemodiafiltration. J Crit Care 1993;8:140-144.

Chima CS et al. Protein catabolic rate in patients with acute renal failure on continuous arteriovenous hemofiltration and total parenteral nutrition. J Am Soc Nephrol 1992;3:1516-1521.

Cummings AD. Sepsis and acute renal failure. Renal Failure 1994;16:169-178.

Druml W. Nutritional considerations in the treatment of acute renal failure in septic patients. Nephrol Dial Transplant 1994;9(Suppl 4):219-223.

Duke GJ et al. Renal support in critically ill patients: Low-dose dopamine or low-dose dobutamine? Crit Care Med 1994;22:1919-1925.

Dyson EH et al. Volumetric control of continuous haemodialysis in multiorgan failure. Artificial Organs 1991;15:439-442.

Faedda R et al. Superoxide radicals (SR) in the pathophysiology of ischemic acute renal failure (ARF). In: Amerio A, Coratelli P, eds. Adv Exp Med Biol 1986;212:69-73.

Fish EM, Molitoris BA. Alterations in epithelial polarity and the pathogenesis of disease states. N Engl J Med 1994;330:1580-1588.

Goligorsky MS, DiBona GF. Pathogenic role of Arg-Gly-Asp-recognizing integrins in acute renal failure. Proc Natl Acad Sci 1993;90:5700-5704.

Halstenberg WK, Goormastic M, Paganini E. Utility of risk models for renal failure and critically ill patients. Semin Nephrol 1994;14:23-32.

Hoitsma AJ, Wetzels FM, Koene RAP. Drug-induced nephrotoxicity: Aetiology, clinical features and management. Drug Safety 1991;6:131-147.

Jochimsen F, Schäfer J, Maurer A, Distler A. Impairment of renal function in medical intensive care: Predictability of acute renal failure. Crit Care Med 1990;18:480-485.

Martin C et al. Assessment of creatinine clearance in intensive care patients. Crit Care Med 1990;18:1224-1226.

Martin SJ, Danziger LH. Continuous infusion of loop diuretics in the critically ill: A review of the literature. Crit Care Med 1994;22:1323-1329.

Norman J et al. Epidermal growth factor accelerates functional recovery from ischaemic acute tubular necrosis in the rat: Role of the epidermal growth factor receptor. Clin Science 1990;78:445.

Price CA. Acute renal failure: A sequelae of sepsis. Crit Care Nurs Clin North Am 1994;6:359-372.

Schaer GL et al. Renal hemodynamics and prostaglandin E_2 excretion in a nonhuman primate model of septic shock. Crit Care Med 1990;18:52-59.

Schrier RW ed. Renal and electrolyte disorders. 4th ed. Boston: Little Brown; 1992.

Sieberth HG, Mann H, Stummvoll HK, eds. Continuous hemofiltration. Contributions to Nephrology 1990;93:1-271.

Simon EE. Potential role of integrins in acute renal failure. Nephrol Dial Transplant 1994;9(Suppl 4):26-33.

Spurney RF, Fulkerson WJ, Schwab SJ. Acute renal failure in critically ill patients: Prognosis for recovery of kidney function after prolonged dialysis support. Crit Care Med 1991;19:8-11.

Toback FG. Regeneration after acute tubular necrosis. Kid Int 1992;41:226-246.

Toto KH. Acute renal failure: A question of location. Am J Nurs 1992;92:44-53.

Verstrepen WA, Nouwen EJ, De Broe ME. Renal epidermal growth factor and insulin-like growth factor-I in acute renal failure. Nephrol Dial Transplant 1994;9:57-68.

Wolfson RG, Millar CGM, Neila GH. Ischaemia and reperfusion injury in the kidney: Current status and future direction. Nephrol Dial Transplant 1994;9(Suppl 4):1529-1531.

Yates NA et al. Renal actions of atrial natriuretic factor: Modulation of effect by changes in sodium status and aldosterone. AJP 1990;258:F684-F689.

Zorzanello MM. Preventing acute renal failure in patients with chronic renal insufficiency: Nursing implications. ANNA 1989;16:443-436.

CHAPTER *14*

Central Nervous System Dysfunction in Multiple Organ Dysfunction Syndrome

Tess L. Briones

Infection, tissue injury, and ischemia evoke a systemic inflammatory response syndrome (SIRS) brought about by the defense mechanisms of the body.[1,2] This inappropriately intense systemic inflammatory response results from the release of inflammatory mediators such as cytokines, complement activation products, vasoactive amines, arachidonic acid metabolites, and proteases. Inflammatory mediators are produced by activated macrophages, monocytes, neutrophils, lymphocytes, and endothelial cells. SIRS often leads to multiple organ dysfunction and failure and eventually death.[3]

The central nervous system (CNS) is one of the first organ systems to manifest the alteration in function brought about by the effects of SIRS.[3] Functional alterations of the CNS can be manifested by a variety of symptoms ranging from disorientation and confusion to coma. The exact etiology of the CNS dysfunction associated with SIRS is not clear, but two hypotheses that have been postulated are formation of brain microabscesses and occurrence of cerebral ischemia.[4,5]

ETIOLOGY AND PATHOPHYSIOLOGY

Multiple organ dysfunction syndrome (MODS) secondary to the systemic inflammatory response is a major problem in intensive care. Presently, the etiologic factors affecting CNS dysfunction in MODS remain unclear; however, several mechanisms have been proposed. First, neuropathologic findings on these patients have consistently shown that multiple brain microabscesses are present in about two thirds of the fatal cases.[4,6] Second, inadequate and maldistributed blood flow associated with SIRS has been reported to cause a reduction in cerebral blood flow (CBF). The decrease in CBF associated with SIRS can be due to a direct insult to the brain or the result of secondary mechanisms triggered by a primary systemic inflammatory response.[5,7,8] Thus, the pathogenesis of cerebral ischemia in SIRS may be classified as primary or secondary.

Brain microabscesses

The presence of brain microabscesses in patients with septic encephalopathy was first reported by Jackson and colleagues in 1985.[9] Subsequent studies, however, reported that brain microabscesses were only present among patients with severe encephalopathy secondary to MODS.[10-12] The occurrence of these abscesses was not related to the use of antimicrobial agents. The causative microorganisms most commonly identified in the brain microabscesses were *Staphylococcus aureus* and *Candida albicans*.[12] Neuropathologic studies have reported that brain microabscesses are frequently found in the cerebellum and the basal ganglia.[13,14] Microscopic examination of brain microabscesses shows a collection of polymorphonuclear (PMN) leukocytes, macrophages, and microglia.

Given the report by Anker and Stroun[15] that systemic microorganisms have a direct effect on the brain and that subsequent clinical and neuropathologic findings report the presence of brain microabscesses in severe sepsis, it is possible that SIRS, triggered by infection, may cause alterations in CNS function. Although the incidence of brain microabscesses is relatively low and the exact mechanism by which they disrupt the integrity of the CNS remains unclear, this phenomenon is now widely accepted. Therefore, the possibility of brain microabscesses in SIRS should be considered a potential cause of the changes in CNS function.

Cerebral ischemia

Measurements of cerebral hemodynamics in laboratory and clinical studies have provided valuable insight into the pathophysiology of cerebral ischemia. The incidence of cerebral ischemia is a function of the relationship between CBF and cerebral metabolic needs, that is, the adequacy of CBF to match brain metabolism. Thus, a clear understanding of the two components of cerebral hemodynamics, CBF and cerebral metabolism, is essential to gaining a thorough knowledge of cerebral ischemia.

Cerebral blood flow. Cerebral blood flow is expressed as the volume of blood delivered to a defined mass of tissue per unit of time. Resting CBF is approximately 50 mL per 100 g of brain tissue per minute.[16] Although in normal conditions, total CBF is relatively stable over variations in body activity, cardiac output, and blood pressure, focal CBF is closely coupled to cerebral metabolism and increases significantly when cortical regions become active. Reductions in CBF can cause either global or focal ischemia. Global cerebral ischemia such as that seen in traumatic brain injury (TBI), cardiac arrest, or SIRS, is caused by a reduction of the total blood flow to the brain, whereas, focal cerebral ischemia is caused by decreased blood flow to a certain brain region.

Cerebral metabolism. Cerebral metabolism reflects the energy state of the brain and is usually expressed as the amount of nutrients required by a defined mass of tissue per unit of time. Cerebral metabolic rate depends on the amount of oxygen and glucose delivered via blood flow. Under normal resting conditions, the cerebral metabolic rate of oxygen ($CMRO_2$) is 165 mol per 100 g of brain tissue per minute and the cerebral metabolic rate of glucose (CMRGlu) is 30 μmol per 100 g of brain tissue per minute.[16] Approximately one third of the oxygen and one tenth of the glucose delivered to the brain are used. The normal $CMRO_2$/CMRGlu molar ratio is 5.5 instead of 6, because the glucose is not completely oxidized. Thus, the brain normally produces a small amount of lactate via glycolysis.[16] The energy needs of the brain are usually divided into three components: synaptic transmission (30%), ion transport (30%), and other unidentified processes (40%).[16]

Ischemic threshold. Normal resting CBF in humans was first quantified by Kety and Schmidt in 1946.[17] Subsequently, clinical and laboratory studies demonstrated that reductions in blood flow without a corresponding decrease in metabolism lead to functional loss in the brain, thus establishing the concept of the ischemic threshold[16-19] (Fig. 14-1). Changes in CNS function start to occur when CBF is reduced by 50%. At flows less than 20 mL/100 g/min, evoked potentials cannot be elicited and at 18 mL/100 g/min, the electroencephalogram (EEG) becomes isoelectric. In addition, CBF less than 15 mL/100 g/min results in increased ionic fluxes giving rise to metabolic acidosis; and blood flow less than 10 mL/100 g/min leads to neuronal death. Between the thresholds of electric failure (20 mL/100 g/min) and metabolic failure (15 mL/100 g/min) is a small circumscribed range of CBF at which, despite loss of neuronal function, cell membrane homeostasis and structural integrity are maintained. This circumscribed range of CBF is known as the *ischemic penumbra.*[18] The concept of ischemic penumbra can best be explained by the clinical phe-

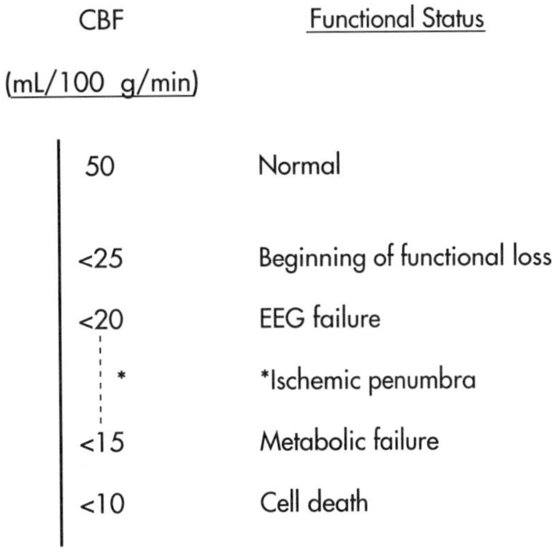

CBF (mL/100 g/min)	Functional Status
50	Normal
<25	Beginning of functional loss
<20	EEG failure
*	*Ischemic penumbra
<15	Metabolic failure
<10	Cell death

Fig. 14-1 CNS dysfunction at specified levels of cerebral blood flow. *CBF,* Cerebral blood flow; *EEG,* electroencephalogram.

nomenon of reversible ischemic neurologic deficit (RIND). In RIND, patients develop neurologic impairments such as confusion, disorientation, or decreased level of consciousness, and when the CBF and cerebral metabolic rate ratio return to normal or near-normal levels, total recovery of neurologic function follows.

Until recently, clinical findings of cerebral ischemia were rare because documentation of CBF in critical care was on an intermittent basis and usually done once patients were fairly stable. The lack of continuous monitoring and delay in CBF measurements were due largely to technological limitations. Because of these limitations, changes in CBF occurring in the early course of the disease remained clinically obscure. Additionally, intermittent measurements of CBF were unable to detect short-lived episodes of cerebral ischemia resulting from transient drops in blood pressure. However, despite these limitations several hypotheses have been proposed regarding the pathogenesis of cerebral ischemia resulting from both primary and secondary causes.

Primary mechanisms in the pathogenesis of cerebral ischemia. Severe TBI is an event that often initiates cerebral ischemia directly. The annual incidence of TBI is reported to be 2.1 million cases in the Unites States alone.[20] In addition, the cost of this health problem is staggering and has been estimated at twenty-five billion dollars per year attributed to hospitalization, rehabilitation expenses, and lost wages.[20] In terms of human suffering, impact on social relationships, and economic burden, the costs of TBI are incalculable.

The outcome after TBI depends largely on whether or not the damage to the brain is accompanied by hypotension, hypoxia, or a secondary head injury. Cerebral ischemia is an important component of the neuronal damage that occurs with TBI. Recently, it was reported that ischemic brain damage was found on neuropathologic examination in 88% of head-injured patients.[21] Several hypotheses exist regarding the pathologic cascade in cerebral ischemia. More than 15 years ago, it was suggested that the pathologic cascade triggered during the ischemic episode and during reperfusion results in the formation of free radicals.[22-25] These free radicals were thought to aggravate the original brain insult by causing peroxidative damage to membrane lipids.[22-25] Later, it was postulated that the release of excitatory amino acids (EAAs), namely, the neurotransmitters glutamate and aspartate, was the major factor in the ischemic cascade that caused neurometabolic derangements leading to acidosis.[26-30] More recently, it has been suggested that neither free radicals nor excitatory neurotransmitters alone can produce the biochemical and cellular changes that occur in cerebral ischemia. This recent hypothesis suggests that the biochemical and cellular changes associated with ischemia are the result of the interaction between free radical formation and EAA release.[31,32]

Oxygen-derived free radical hypothesis. The pathologic cascade involving oxygen-derived free radical formation during cerebral ischemia is similar to the mechanisms seen in SIRS. Oxygen-derived free radicals are normal by-products of cerebral metabolism, and they are generated from free fatty acid metabolism, ischemia-reperfusion injury, and during the respiratory burst of neutrophils. During normal cerebral metabolism, free radicals are bound to the process of oxygen reduction and, thus, are not harmful.[22] However, in cerebral ischemia, the depletion in adenosine triphosphate (ATP) causes biochemical alterations that allow the release of free radicals. These free radicals activate phospholipase activity and the breakdown of phospholipids in the cell membrane, causing the release of free fatty acids, namely, arachidonic acid, and its products such as the prostaglandins.[24,25] Arachidonic acid is metabolized via the lipoxygenase and the cyclooxygenase pathways. Leukotrienes are produced from the lipoxygenase pathway, and endoperoxides, thromboxanes, and prostaglandins are formed via the cyclooxygenase pathway[22-25] (Fig. 14-2). Thromboxanes and leukotrienes have been implicated in intravascular coagulation, producing vascular occlusion and cerebral vasospasm.[23] Endoperoxides are unstable precursors produced early in the cyclooxygenase pathway that are usually metabolized to the more stable prostaglandins; however, endoperoxides can also be utilized in the production of toxic oxygen-derived free radicals such as singlet oxygen, hydroxyl radicals, superoxide radicals, and hydrogen peroxide. These toxic oxygen-derived free radicals have been implicated in vascular paralysis.[25] During the period of reperfusion, progression of ischemic damage can occur as a result of increased prostaglandin synthesis from arachidonic acid accumulated during the initial ischemic injury[24] (Fig. 14-2).

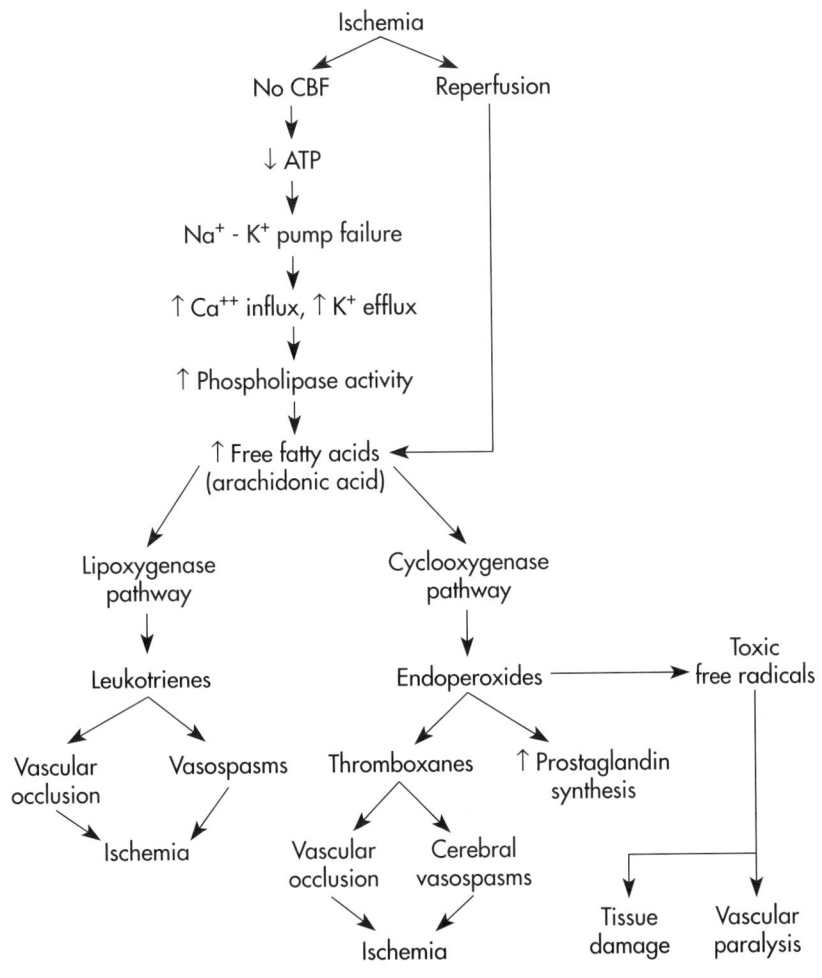

Fig. 14-2 Processes triggered in ischemia leading to the production of toxic oxygen free radicals and arachidonic acid metabolites.

Although the role of free radicals in the pathologic changes occurring during cerebral ischemia is now widely accepted, it has not been well documented. One reason for this is the indirect methodology used by investigators. Because free radicals are unstable and difficult to measure, investigators have measured levels of free-radical scavengers. These investigators believe that decreased levels of free-radical scavengers indicate increased levels of free radicals because the scavengers are consumed as they break down the excess free radicals. Although these conclusions based on levels of free radical scavengers may have an explanatory value, some skepticism justifiably still exists.

Excitatory amino acids hypothesis. During the 1960s, reports on neuronal death in the retina and brain after systemic administration of monosodium glutamate were met with great skepticism.[26,27] Although these findings were replicated many times, the excitotoxic hypothesis of ischemic damage did not flourish until the 1980s. Both laboratory and clinical studies have since produced evidence supporting the role of EAAs, specifically glutamate, in inducing neuronal damage.[26-30] Glutamate is an

EAA neurotransmitter, released from primary afferent neurons, that binds to calcium-mediated, voltage-dependent receptors. The most studied calcium-mediated receptor to which glutamate binds is the N-methyl-D-aspartate (NMDA) receptor. In normal neuronal depolarization, the majority of these receptors are blocked by magnesium, preventing their binding by EAAs.[33] However, an increase in calcium influx displaces magnesium, opening the NMDA receptors and allowing glutamate binding. When excessive amounts of EAAs such as glutamate are present and bind to NMDA receptors, neuronal injury usually occurs.[33]

The mechanism by which EAAs cause neuronal injury involves prolonged depolarization and persistent stimulation of neurons which, in turn, results in increased brain electric activity and depletion of ATP[27-29] (Fig. 14-3). The massive amounts of glutamate released as a result of primary insult to the brain cause this EAA to bind to NMDA receptors. Binding of glutamate to NMDA receptors aggravates the injury-induced ionic fluxes (increased influx of sodium and calcium and increased efflux of potassium) by further increasing intracellular calcium levels and prolonging depolarization. During prolonged depolarization, energy expenditure in-

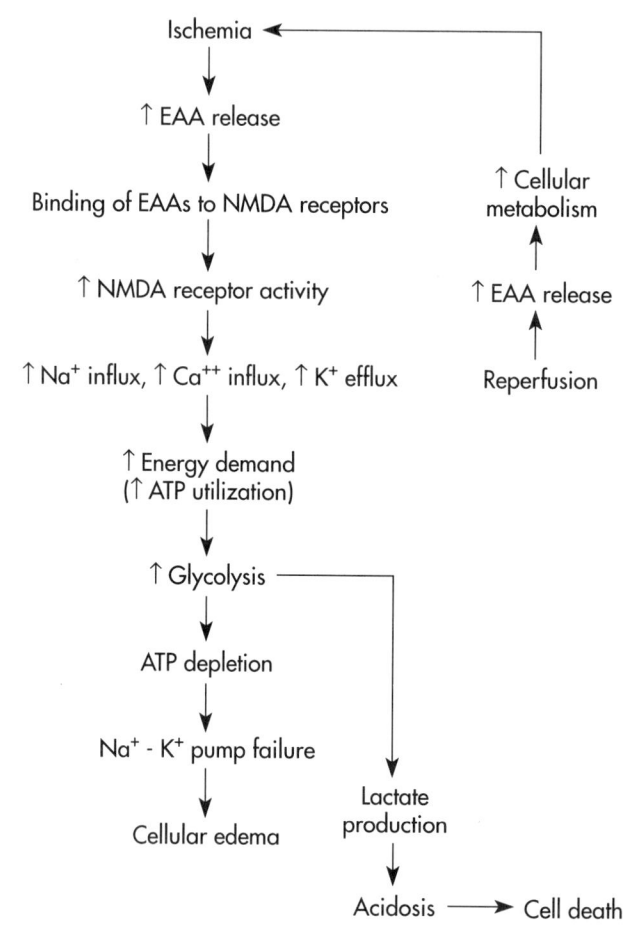

Fig. 14-3 Processes triggered by increased levels of excitatory neurotransmitters released in ischemia. Once ATP is depleted, increased release of excitatory amino acids occurs even into the period of reperfusion. *ATP*, Adenosine triphosphate; *EAA*, excitatory amino acid; *NMDA*, N-methyl-D-aspartate.

creases, and increased synthesis of ATP is needed to maintain the sodium-potassium pump and reestablish ionic balance. Depletion of ATP leads to sodium-potassium pump failure with resultant accumulation of intracellular sodium, causing cellular edema. In addition, the increased glycolysis needed to meet energy demand leads to acidosis and eventually, cell death.

Oxygen-derived free radical and EAA interaction hypothesis. Recently, investigators proposed that the neuronal damage seen in cerebral ischemia might be caused by interrelated events involving free radical formation and the excitotoxic effects of EAAs[31,32] (Fig. 14-4). This proposed mechanism is not hierarchical, but instead is interactive. Free radicals have been shown to lead to leakage of EAA neurotransmitters and by the same token, EAAs have been reported to increase the production of the hydroxyl radical, a toxic free radical.[32] Although this mechanism of neuronal damage proposes the interaction between free radicals and EAA, it is possible that neuronal dysfunction, but not necessarily cell death, can occur in any part of the cycle.[31]

Free radicals have been shown not only to cause formation of free fatty acids but also to promote the release of EAAs, which in turn exert their toxic effects by binding to NMDA receptors. Stimulation of NMDA receptors enhances influx of calcium, thereby increasing intracellular calcium concentrations. The increased calcium influx then activates intracellular phospholipases, proteases, and endonucleases. The triggering of these calcium-mediated processes can lead to neuronal death or the possibility of starting another destructive cycle. Based on this hypothesized mechanism, free-radical scavengers are being developed as neuroprotective agents to prevent the radical-induced neuronal morphologic impairment and glutamate excitotoxicity seen in cerebral ischemia.[32]

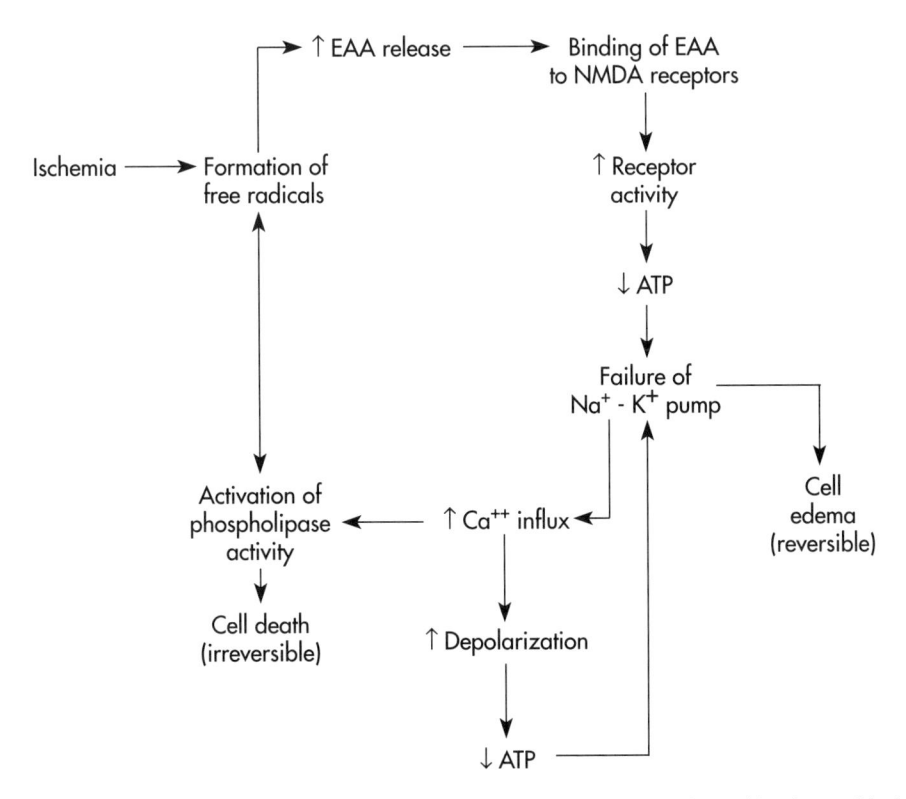

Fig. 14-4 Interactive processes between free radicals and excitatory amino acids triggered in ischemia. *ATP,* Adenosine triphosphate; *EAA,* excitatory amino acid; *NMDA,* N-methyl-D-aspartate.

Secondary mechanisms in the pathogenesis of cerebral ischemia. In SIRS most clinicians are concerned with assessment of systemic blood flow and systemic vascular resistance. However, assessment of these parameters alone cannot provide adequate information on CBF and metabolism; thus, there is a dearth of reports on cerebral ischemia secondary to SIRS. SIRS-induced cerebral ischemia can be caused by the disruption or malfunction in the communication between the CNS, the neuroendocrine system, and the immune systems or by the action of inflammatory mediators on the CNS.[34,35]

Central nervous system-neuroendocrine system-immune system. Flow of information between the CNS and the neuroendocrine and immune systems comprises an important homeostatic mechanism in the body. Cytokines and other inflammatory mediators play a crucial role in this communication and exert powerful effects on neurons in the CNS[35] (Fig. 14-5). During the inflammatory response, the CNS is involved in both the perception and the regulation of tissue activity.[34] Signals from higher centers in the brain are sent to the thymus, a primary lymphoid organ. Lymphocytes from the thymus then migrate to the spleen and other peripheral lymphoid organs, via the circulating blood and lymphatics.

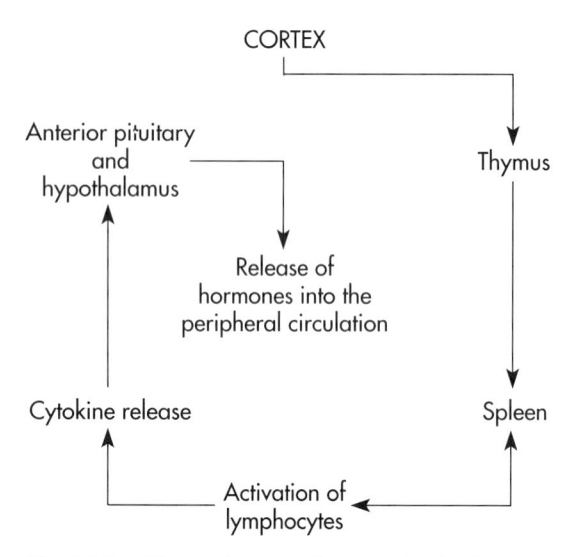

Fig. 14-5 The mechanism of communication between the central nervous system, neuroendocrine system, and immune system. Communication aids in the maintenance of a homeostatic environment and predominantly occurs via the anterior pituitary and hypothalamus.

When the lymphocytes and other cells of the inflammatory/immune response come in contact with antigens, they produce mediators to invoke the inflammatory/immune response. These mediators, through their action on the hypothalamus and the anterior pituitary, trigger the release of neuroendocrine hormones such as epinephrine, norepinephrine, and corticosteroids. These neuroendocrine responses lead to sodium and water retention in order to maintain intravascular volume.

In the presence of SIRS, however, a state of increased capillary permeability exists secondary to mediator activity and endothelial damage. The increase in capillary permeability seen in SIRS results in fluid shifts from the intravascular to the extravascular space. Thus, hemodynamic alterations may persist despite the compensatory neuroendocrine response because of intravascular fluid depletion. The common hemodynamic alterations seen in SIRS are hypovolemia, systemic hypotension, acid-base imbalances, and inadequate tissue oxygenation.[36] Therefore, it is not surprising that cerebral ischemia occurs in SIRS.

Actions of inflammatory mediators. The concept that the brain is insulated from the effects of the immune system, has changed dramatically during the past few years. This is due to the discovery that astrocytes are capable of mediating an immune response in the brain and that some cytokines affect brain activity. Cytokines are a family of protein messengers of the inflammatory/immune response that also possess neurotransmitter and hormonelike properties. They are synthesized by a large number of cells, most notably immune cells, epithelial cells, astrocytes, and glial cells. Cytokines primarily provide feedback to alter the function of their cell of origin (autocrine effect) or bind to nearby cells and alter their function (paracrine effect). Cytokines can also enter the circulation and produce systemic effects (endocrine effect). In addition, studies have shown that cytokines produced systemically can reach areas of the brain not protected by the blood-brain barrier, such as the arcuate nucleus, the hypothalamus, the tuber cinereum, and the pineal gland[33,37,38] (Table 14-1). Some researchers believe it is possible that the systemically produced cytokines can also reach areas of the CNS where the blood-brain barrier has been made more permeable by pathologic conditions such as SIRS.[39] Others hypothesize that systemically produced cytokines,

Table 14-1 Physiologic Anatomy of Selected Brain Structures

Structure	Location	Function
Arcuate nucleus	Middle hypothalamic region	Major source of dopamine Regulates the release of growth hormone Plays a role in opiate analgesia
Basolateral amygdala	Limbic system	Plays a role in attaching emotional significance to a stimulus
Cerebellar Purkinje cells	Cerebellum	Participate in learning of motor tasks (onset and offset as well as timing in performing motor tasks)
Hippocampus	Limbic system	Plays a major role in the processing of memory Believed to play a role in the retrieval of memories
Hypothalamus	Diencephalon	Regulates cardiovascular parameters (heart rate and arterial blood pressure) Regulates body temperature Regulates body water
Pineal gland	Diencephalon	Secretes melatonin (a hormone thought to influence circadian rhythmicity)
Serotonin-containing region or raphe nucleus	Midline of lower pons and medulla	Releases serotonin to promote normal sleep (inhibitory property of serotonin)
Thalamic nuclei	Diencephalon	Serve as synaptic relay station and important integrating center for most of the input to the cortex Thought to provide input to the cortex regarding rhythmicity of EEG wave
Tuber cinereum	Hypothalamus	Regulates anterior pituitary function through peptide neurohormones

which are large protein molecules, do not pass through the blood-brain barrier but exert their effect by acting on glial cells that then trigger the increased production of resident cytokines in the CNS.[40,41] Still others suggest that systemically produced cytokines affect the CNS through endothelial cell– or glial cell–derived second messengers such as prostaglandins.[42,43]

Cytokines that have been found to be synthesized in the CNS (Table 14-2) include interleukin-1 (IL-1), interleukin-6 (IL-6), neuronal interferon-γ (IFN-γ), tumor necrosis factor-α (TNF-α), and transforming growth factor-$β_1$ (TGF-$β_1$).[37-43] Recent evidence has also shown that a high density of cytokine immunoreactive fibers are present in the hypothalamus, the hippocampus, and the dentate gyrus indicating that these areas are the most likely to be influenced by cytokine activities.[38,39] Furthermore, receptors for cytokines have been identified in the cerebellar Purkinje cells, the CA3 region of the hippocampus, the dorsal thalamic nucleus (both anterior and medial), the basolateral amygdala, and the serotonin-containing region of the raphe nucleus[33,38] (Table 14-1).

Cytokines have also been reported to stimulate neurotransmitter release. CNS neurotransmitters affected by cytokine activity include norepinephrine, serotonin (5-HT), γ-aminobutyric acid (GABA), and acetylcholine (Ach).[42] In addition, increased release of several neuropeptides such as opioids and neurosubstance P, have also been reported to be influenced by cytokines.[41] Similarly, a number of second messenger systems in neurons such as release of arachidonic acid, calcium flux, and activation of cAMP, are affected by cytokines.[40] However, despite the compelling evidence that a variety of cytokines affect neuronal function, their exact mechanism of influence is unclear.

Given that the inflammatory/immune response is intensified in SIRS, it is reasonable to postulate that

Table 14-2 Cytokines Commonly Found in the CNS

Cytokine	Cellular source	CNS effects
Interleukin-1 (IL-1)	Monocytes/macrophages Endothelial cells Astrocytes Some B cells	Modulates pain Stimulates hypothalamic hormone release (↑ HR, ↑ BP) Decreases appetite Induces sleep Releases neuropeptides Causes EEG changes Induces fever
Interleukin-2 (IL-2)	T lymphocytes	Induces sleep Causes confusion Causes stupor and coma Causes convulsions Causes EEG changes Induces fever Activates hypothalamic-pituitary-adrenal (HPA) axis
Interleukin-6 (IL-6)	T cells Monocytes/macrophage Some B cells	Induces fever Suppresses appetite Releases neuropeptides Activates HPA axis
Interferon-γ (IFN-γ)	T cells Monocytes/macrophages	Induces fever Performs immunoregulatory functions primarily (participates in CNS immune response)
Tumor necrosis factor (TNF-α)	Monocytes/macrophages Glial cells	Activates HPA axis Other effects similar to those of IL-1
Transforming growth factor-β$_1$ (TGF-β$_1$)	Astrocytes Macrophages Microglial cells T cells Platelets	Deactivates macrophage activities and suppresses microglial cytotoxicity Has neurotrophic properties (promotes cell growth), thus, this cytokine can influence axonal growth following ischemia or injury

SIRS-induced cerebral ischemia can be caused indirectly by the increased brain metabolism brought on by excessive cytokine activity. Thus, during SIRS, CBF may not be sufficient to meet cerebral metabolic needs.

CLINICAL MANIFESTATIONS

The CNS is highly vulnerable to the pathologic effects of SIRS, and the neurologic impairments observed are varied. However, the most common CNS manifestations exhibited by patients with SIRS are fever, confusion, disorientation, decreased level of consciousness, seizures, and EEG abnormalities.[3,37-39] The exact etiology of CNS dysfunction in SIRS is not clear but it is possible that cerebral ischemia and cytokine activity in the brain could explain the symptomatology seen in these patients.

Fever

Febrile responses seen in patients with SIRS are not always a result of sepsis. This is evident in the 25% to 50% of patients with SIRS with negative culture reports.[44] Fever in SIRS may be attributed to the effect of inflammatory mediators in the brain. The large numbers of macrophages, T cells, and neutrophils activated in SIRS are a rich source of inflammatory mediators such as cytokines. Cytokines such as IL-1, TNF-α, and IL-6 produced in SIRS have all been documented to be endogenous pyrogens.[38] Though as yet unspecified, peripherally produced IL-6 affects the preoptic area of the anterior hypothalamus that contains sites of thermoregulation.

Other studies have also shown that IL-1 is a pyrogenic cytokine.[37-39] In these studies, however, brain levels of IL-1 correlated directly with the febrile response but elevated levels of systemic IL-1 did not. Studies implicating IL-1 in the febrile response postulate that the organum vasculosum laminae terminalis (OVLT) facilitates the synthesis of IL-1 upon the OVLT's interactions with inflammatory stimuli such as endotoxin. Thus the OVLT is thought to be the interface in the translation of circulating pyrogens into fever.[39,40] The OVLT is a circumventral organ located in the anterior wall of the third ventricle that provides input to the hypothalamus for neurohormone release.[33] In addition, the OVLT contains reticuloendothelial cells including macrophages; thus, it is possibly the site of inflammatory mediator synthesis.

Another cytokine, similar to IL-1, that has pyrogenic properties is TNF-α. A rise in plasma concentrations of TNF-α seen in conditions such as SIRS can result in temperature elevation.[39] However, in contrast to other cytokines identified as endogenous pyrogens, TNF-α also possesses cryogenic (fever-reducing) properties. It has been documented that TNF-α produces a ceiling effect on body temperature, that is, it prevents body temperature from becoming too high.[39] This cryogenic action of TNF-α is not clear but it is hypothesized that the drop in body temperature could be due to a direct effect by TNF-α on the thermoregulatory system or to an indirect effect via another endogenous cryogen such as arginine vasopressin.

Confusion and disorientation

Cerebral ischemia is an important component of the CNS dysfunction that occurs in SIRS. The most common clinical manifestation of transient global cerebral ischemia is memory impairment usually exhibited as confusion and disorientation.[45] Memory impairment occurs because the areas involved in memory contain populations of neurons that are "selectively vulnerable" to ischemia.[46-48] That is, these regions of the brain are more susceptible than others to ischemic insult.

The brain region most vulnerable to cerebral ischemia is the hippocampus[46-48] (Fig. 14-6, A). The hippocampus is a brain structure involved primarily in the processing of memory as shown by numerous laboratory and clinical studies.[49-53] Within the hippocampus, the neurons in the CA1 region are most selectively vulnerable to cerebral ischemia.[46-48] The selective damage to the CA1 pyramidal neurons may be caused by the ischemia-induced increased release of EAAs.[28] When excessive glutamate is released, it binds to NMDA receptors and produces neurotoxicity. Thus, the high concentration of NMDA receptors on the dendritic trees of the CA1 pyramidal neurons of the hippocampus very likely explains the vulnerability of this hippocampal subfield to ischemic brain damage.[33]

The flow of information within the hippocampus (Fig. 14-6, B) for memory processing is unidirectional.[33] Information is transmitted from the entorhinal cortex to the dentate gyrus (which projects to the hippocampus) via the perforant path. From the dentate gyrus, information flows to the CA3 subfield via the mossy fiber pathway and ends in the CA1 subfield through the Schaffer collaterals (projections from CA3). Information flows out of the hippocampus through the subiculum, which projects to the entorhinal cortex. The fact that the CA1 pyramidal neurons comprise an essential link in the chain of information flow in the hippocampus is likely to account for the memory deficits that are seen after cerebral ischemia.

Decreased level of consciousness

One of the early clinical manifestations of CNS dysfunction in SIRS is changes in the level of consciousness (LOC). These changes in LOC can vary from increasing drowsiness to coma, and it is possible that the degree of change in the LOC correlates directly with the severity of the illness. The exact mechanism of changes in LOC in SIRS is not known but it can be postulated that decreased LOC may be a result of cytokine action, namely that of IL-1 and IL-2, in the CNS.[37]

Recent evidence has shown that IL-1 and IL-2 in the brain produce dose-dependent soporific (sleep-inducing) effects.[37-39] Any action of IL-1 is assumed to involve IL-1 receptors and one of the sites identified as expressing IL-1 receptors is the serotonin-containing region of the dorsal raphe complex.[38] Given that this area directly correlates with the general behavioral state, relating more to the sleep-wake cycle, it is possible that the decreased LOC seen in SIRS, is related to excessive levels of IL-1 binding to its designated receptors in the dorsal raphe complex.

Similarly, IL-2 has been shown to affect the locus coeruleus, a small area located bilaterally and posteriorly at the junction between the pons and the mesencephalon.[33] Because the locus coeruleus is

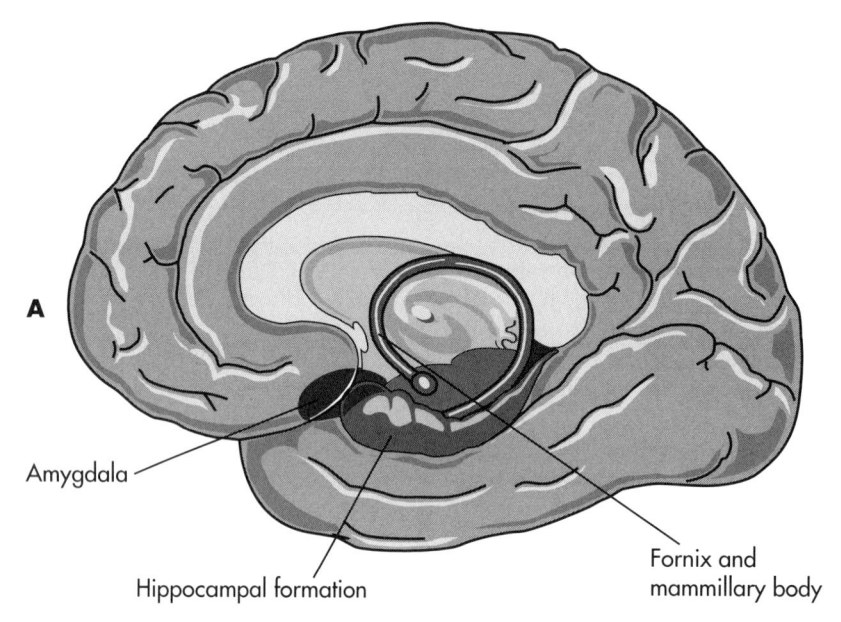

Fig. 14-6 **A,** Sagittal section of the brain illustrating the location of the hippocampus in the limbic system. Components of the hippocampal formation include subiculum, hippocampus proper or Ammon's horn, and dentate gyrus. (From Martin, JH. Neuroanatomy. Text and Atlas. Norwalk: Appleton and Lange; 1989, p. 18.)

also primarily involved in the sleep-wake cycle, the IL-2–induced inhibition of cells firing in this area of the brain might be one reason to explain the changes in the LOC seen in patients with SIRS.

Seizures and EEG Abnormalities

Although uncommon, seizures and EEG abnormalities can be manifested by patients with SIRS. Like most of the CNS effects of SIRS, the exact mechanism in the development of seizures and EEG abnormalities is not known. However, it is possible that these clinical manifestations are caused by the effects on the CNS of increased levels of EAA or cytokines (specifically IL-2) induced by cerebral ischemia.[28,37] Laboratory studies have reported that high doses of IL-2 produce EEG changes.[37,38] These EEG changes have been shown to be preceded by spiking in cortical recordings, sometimes associated with episodes of "wet-dog shakes."[38] Thus, the increased synthesis of IL-2 seen in SIRS may precipitate the development of seizures in these patients.

In addition, previous studies have reported that a characteristic consequence of excessive circulating EAAs is increased brain electric activity.[26-29] Given that high levels of EAAs are present in cerebral ischemia, it seems reasonable to assume that the clinical manifestation of seizures may also be caused by repetitive stimulation of the neuronal afferents.

THERAPEUTIC MANAGEMENT

Resuscitative efforts in the management of patients with MODS must not only be aimed at restoring the systemic circulation but should also be brain-oriented. A rational approach to the therapeutic management of CNS dysfunction in SIRS depends largely on an understanding of the mechanisms of ischemic neuronal injury. However, the scarcity of information on the incidence of cerebral ischemia in SIRS has not led to the development of empirically based therapeutic management strategies. Thus, most of the strategies discussed here have been extrapolated from research on acute head injury. Although these strategies are within the context of head injury, the mechanisms of cerebral ischemia, whether resulting from TBI or SIRS, are similar. In essence, the two guiding principles in

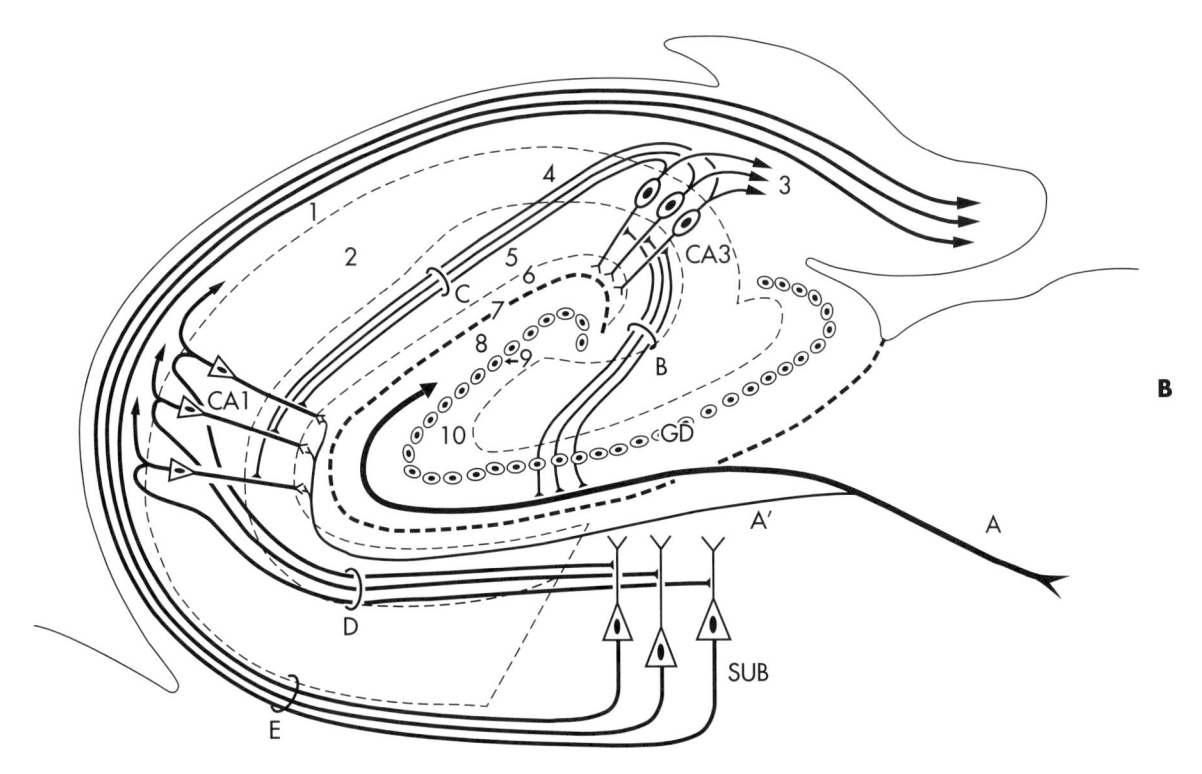

Fig. 14-6, cont'd **B,** The flow of information in the hippocampus (the trisynaptic circuit). *A, B, C, D, E* are parts of the neuronal chain forming the principal pathways. *SUB,* subiculum; *1,* alveus; *2,* stratum pyramidale; *3,* axon of pyramidal neurons in CA3 region; *4,* Schaffer collaterals; *5,* stratum radiatum and lacunosum; *6* and *8,* stratum moleculare; *7,* hippocampal sulcus; *9,* stratum granulosum; *10,* polymorphic layer; *GD,* dentate gyrus; *CA1* and *CA3,* subfields or regions of the hippocampus. (From Duvernoy, HM. The Human Hippocampus. An Atlas of Applied Anatomy. New York: Springer-Verlag; 1988.)

CNS management of patients with MODS are (1) prevention of further injury and (2) resuscitation of salvageable brain tissues. Strategies such as patient positioning, use of hyperventilation, fever management, and environmental management should be utilized to maximize CBF.

Similarly, techniques for salvaging reversibly injured brain tissue should also be aimed at maximizing CBF. The goal of maximizing CBF can be accomplished by optimizing systemic circulation, decreasing brain oxygen requirements, and blocking the "no-reflow phenomenon." The "no-reflow phenomenon" is a term used to describe persistent hypoperfusion in which the CBF is 40% to 50% lower than preischemic values for a period of several hours after the restoration of normal blood flow.[54] Thus, to prevent further ischemic insult to the neurons, close monitoring of CBF and cerebral metabolism is of prime importance.

Patient monitoring

The concept of monitoring brain function in SIRS and in the intensive care unit in general, has lagged significantly behind the monitoring of other organ systems such as the heart and the kidneys. In part, this is because of the complex, recalcitrant, and often concealed nature of events in the cranial vault. Ideally, brain monitoring methods should give information on oxygen delivery requirements, which can be evaluated through blood flow to the tissues, and the metabolic rate of the tissue. In essence, these data will be most useful in patients at risk for cerebral ischemia because they provide information on the adequacy of blood flow to meet metabolic needs.

Routine or continuous measurements of CBF and $CMRO_2$ in the critical care unit are technically difficult. However, CBF and $CMRO_2$ information can be obtained indirectly by calculating the difference between arterial oxygen content of systemic blood and the venous oxygen content of the jugular bulb, the arteriovenous oxygen difference ($AVDO_2$).[55] Theoretically, CBF is the ratio of $CMRO_2$ to the amount of oxygen extracted by the brain from the circulating blood (the $AVDO_2$); thus, obtaining $AVDO_2$ values can provide information on the coupling between blood flow and metabolism (Table 14-3). The range of normal $AVDO_2$ values is 5 to 7.5 vol%.[54] High $AVDO_2$ values (>7.5 vol%) denote increased oxygen extraction by the brain almost always indicating inadequate CBF or cerebral ischemia.[55] When $AVDO_2$ values are low (<5 vol%), they denote decreased oxygen extraction by the brain and may indicate that blood flow is excessive for metabolic needs. However, this is not true in most cases of low $AVDO_2$. In most clinical situations, low $AVDO_2$ usually indicates that there is "compensated hypoperfusion," that is, decreased CBF to brain tissues is compensated by increased oxygen extraction.[56] In this setting, it is unclear as to why the $AVDO_2$ is paradoxically low when the extraction is high, but it could be related to the increase in extracerebral blood present in the jugular bulb when CBF is low.[55]

Presently, it is possible to monitor $AVDO_2$ continuously through jugular venous oximetry. The principle applied in jugular venous oximetry is similar to that used in critically ill patients with a fiberoptic pulmonary artery catheter for measuring systemic mixed venous oxygen saturation (SVO_2). With jugular venous oximetry, the fiberoptic catheter is inserted in a retrograde fashion until the tip of the catheter is sitting in the jugular bulb (Fig. 14-7). Data obtained from this monitoring technique provide clinicians with information on CBF and $CMRO_2$, allowing early identification of patients at risk for cerebral ischemia. In addition, this information may be used to implement early treatment strategies to prevent secondary brain injury.

Although $AVDO_2$ monitoring is by far the most informative monitoring technique available in evaluating and preventing cerebral ischemia, it is not without limitations (Table 14-4). Further, because of the invasive nature of this technique, it should be used judiciously. Additionally, nurses taking care of patients with jugular venous oximetry must be familiar with the limitations of the technique and its potential hazards and have a clear understanding of cerebral hemodynamics (Table 14-5).

Intracerebral microdialysis

Another monitoring technique still experimental at this time is intracerebral microdialysis. Intracerebral microdialysis is a method that continuously measures the metabolic state of the brain. Through intracerebral microdialysis, endogenous substances such as lactate, EAAs, phosphocreatinine, and pyruvate, which result from increased cerebral metabolism, can be removed from brain extracellular fluid without extracting extracellular water.[57] The probe for intracerebral microdialysis (Fig. 14-8) is usually inserted in the ventricle along with an intraventricular intracranial pressure (ICP)–monitoring device. Given that intracerebral microdialysis reflects the energy state of the brain, continuous patient monitoring using this method would be valuable in the management of cerebral ischemia.

Patient positioning

One of the fundamental responsibilities of nurses in critical care is maintaining an optimal position for acutely ill patients. Most often, critically ill patients are maintained in the supine, head elevated, position. In patients with increased ICP, this position is usually standard therapy. Nurses face a dilemma when caring for patients with SIRS-induced hypovolemia who, at the same time, have increased ICP. On the one hand, putting the patient flat in bed on a horizontal plane helps eliminate gravitational factors, thereby enhancing systemic circulation. On the other

Table 14-3 The Relationship Between Cerebral Blood Flow, Cerebral Metabolism, and the Arteriovenous Oxygen Difference

$$CBF^* = \frac{CMRO_2}{AVDO_2} \qquad AVDO_2 = \frac{CMRO_2}{CBF}$$

*CBF is regulated by the relationship between cerebral perfusion pressure (CPP) and cerebrovascular resistance (CVR):

$$CBF = \frac{CPP}{CVR}$$

$AVDO_2$, Arteriovenous oxygen difference; *CBF*, cerebral blood flow; $CMRO_2$, cerebral metabolism.

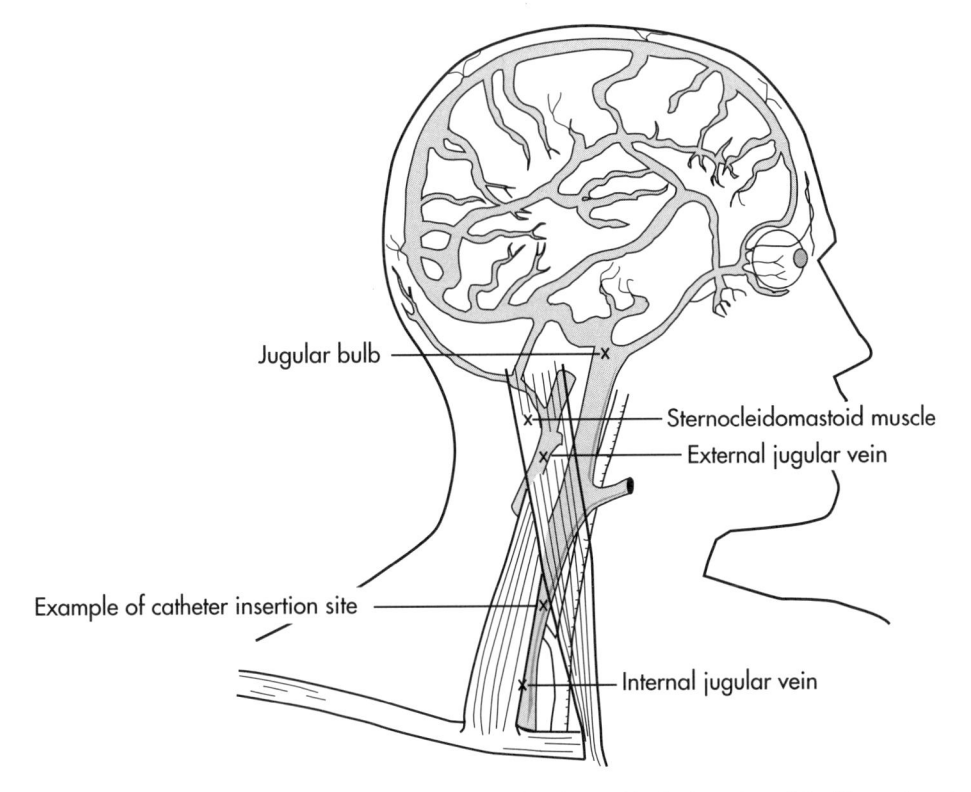

Central Nervous System Dysfunction in Multiple Organ Dysfunction Syndrome 317

Fig. 14-7 Location of the jugular bulb and landmarks used in the insertion of the fiberoptic catheter necessary for AVDo$_2$ monitoring. (From Kerr ME, Lovasik D, Darby J. AACN Clinical issues: advanced practice in acute and crit care, p. 6, Vol. 9 No. 1.)

Table 14-4 Limitations of AVDo$_2$ Monitoring

Limitations	Reasons
Ineffective for monitoring focal cerebral ischemia	Decreased sensitivity in detecting regional changes in CBF/CMRo$_2$ ratio. Because jugular bulb oximetry is unable to detect regional CBF changes, values projected in the monitor may be falsely high.
Bohr effect	In the presence of alkalemia, the oxyhemoglobin dissociation curve shifts to the left. Under these conditions, increased oxygen affinity for hemoglobin exists, making it difficult for oxygen to be released at the tissue level. Because of this, the jugular bulb oxygen saturation will be falsely high.
Ineffective for monitoring intratentorial blood flow	Decreased sensitivity in detecting CBF changes at the level of the brain stem and the cerebellum. Jugular bulb oximetry only assesses global blood flow at the cerebral level; thus, it is not useful for patients whose primary injury is at the level of the brain stem or cerebellum.

Table 14-5 Nursing Responsibilities in the Care of Patients Being Monitored for AVDo$_2$

- Perform in vitro calibration of continuous jugular bulb oximetry apparatus prior to insertion
- Perform in vivo calibration of continuous jugular bulb oximetry apparatus at least every 12 hours
- Monitor patients for complications such as sepsis, coagulopathies, and arteriovenous fistula formation
- Troubleshoot for problems if desaturation occurs
- Do not administer any medication through the jugular bulb catheter
- Flush the jugular bulb catheter ONLY when necessary
- Maintain alignment of the patient's head and neck for accuracy of monitoring

hand, keeping the patient on a horizontal plane may further increase ICP. However, the practice of elevating the head to help decrease ICP is currently being challenged by contradictory findings reported in studies on patients with increased ICP in whom both cerebral perfusion pressure (CPP) and CBF were measured during position changes.[58-61] Some investigators have reported that elevating the head of the bed lowered the ICP but did not significantly change CPP or CBF.[58,59] Others however, reported that although ICP decreased, both CPP and CBF also decreased.[60,61] This latter finding, if confirmed, is cause for alarm in patients with cerebral ischemia in whom the CBF is already compromised, because elevating the head of the bed in these patients will cause further decreases in CBF.

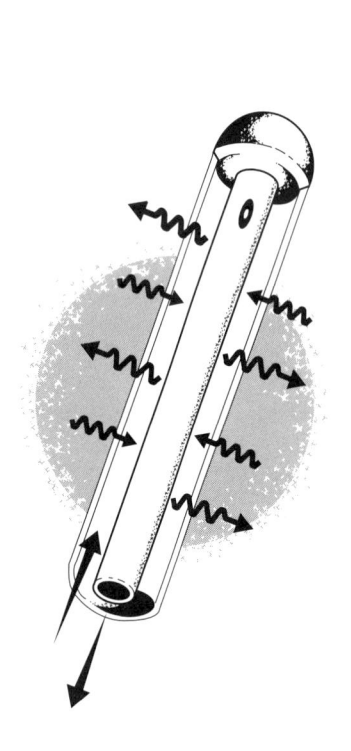

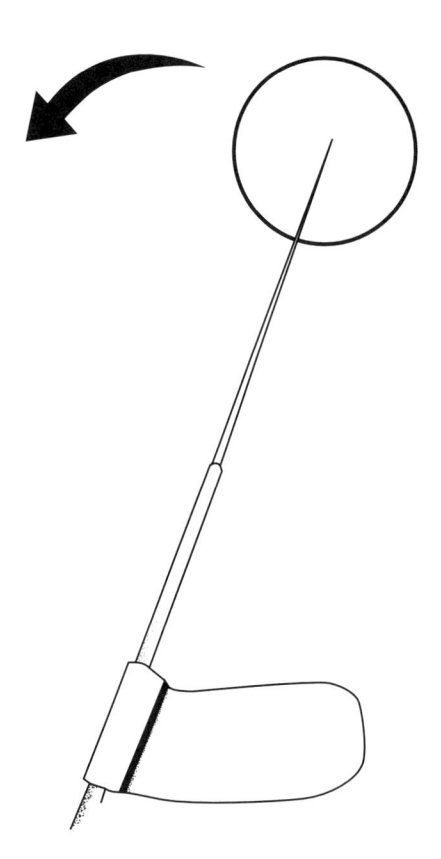

Fig. 14-8 The microdialysis probe. The probe is a specially designed cannula with a semipermeable membrane at the tip. The probe mimics the function of a blood vessel, and once it is implanted into the tissue, endogenous substances from the extracellular fluid filter into the tip by diffusion. (Courtesy CMA Microdialysis, Stockholm, Sweden.)

Additionally, in SIRS-induced cerebral ischemia, elevating the head of the bed without restoring systemic intravascular volume is dangerous.[36] Because these patients are hypovolemic, elevating the head of the bed will cause a further drop in both CPP and CBF. Furthermore, nurses must be cautious in relying on measurement of systemic blood pressure or CPP alone to position patients because of instances of false autoregulation. *False autoregulation* refers to a state wherein systemic blood pressure and CPP are high but CBF is low, thereby contraindicating head elevation in such patients.

At present, it is suggested that in patients with cerebral ischemia, the head of the bed must be maintained flat to maximize CBF and cerebral perfusion.[60,61] This departure from usual protocols provides evidence of our evolving knowledge in the care of patients with cerebral ischemia. Thus, to provide optimal patient care, nurses must gauge the efficacy of existing therapies with the present knowledge in the field.

Use of hyperventilation

Hyperventilation to a partial arterial pressure of carbon dioxide ($PaCO_2$) of 27 to 30 mm Hg is an established and effective method of lowering ICP and decreasing CBF. However, hyperventilation can be detrimental to the metabolic activities of the brain and may also induce or potentiate cerebral ischemia.[62,63] In addition, it appears that the effectiveness of continuous hyperventilation in diminishing cerebral blood volume decreases significantly over time.[64,65] Thus, it is now recommended that this therapy be implemented only during the early stages of intracranial hypertension and be used judiciously after 4 days.[66]

The knowledge that cerebral ischemia is a common phenomenon in critically ill patients has resulted in the present recommendations that include the avoidance of profound hyperventilation. The practice of hyperventilation/hyperoxygenation during endotracheal suctioning should also be used with caution. Furthermore, if hyperventilation is used, this therapy must be guided by information on CBF and $CMRO_2$. Thus, jugular bulb oximetry should be used in conjunction with hyperventilation.

Fever management

Body temperature usually varies within a 24-hour period according to the circadian rhythm. Fever is usually defined as a body temperature that rises above the upper limit of normal, which is 38° C (100° F) in healthy adults. Fever is a common occurrence in patients with SIRS. The etiology for this temperature elevation can vary from the presence of infection to the effects of IL-1, TNF-α, and IL-6.[12,37] In the clinical setting there is a tendency to assume that the febrile response has adverse effects on the patient, and thus, every attempt is made to lower the patient's body temperature. However, most of the documented adverse effects of fever such as tachycardia, increased metabolic rate, and patient discomfort are not that severe with the exception of seizures, which can be caused by extremely high temperatures (>106° F or >42° C).[66] In fact, the presence of fever in a septic patient suggests that the patient's defense mechanism is intact. Furthermore, studies have shown improved outcomes in septic patients with fever but not in those who are hypothermic.[66,67] In the critical care setting, however, fever is usually treated because of the desire by the physician or the nurse to have the patient maintain a "normal" body temperature.

In SIRS-induced fever, arbitrary treatment of the febrile response without compelling evidence to justify the reduction of an elevated temperature *must be avoided*. Fever must be treated only if there is reason to believe that the patient will suffer deleterious effects from the febrile response. In patients whose SIRS-induced fever must be treated, physical cooling methods such as sponging with cool or tap water and using cooling blankets must be treated with caution. Because physical cooling methods are usually aimed at normalizing peripheral body temperature, these methods lower body temperature but the hypothalamic set-point remains elevated. When the hypothalamus senses the systemic hypothermia, shivering occurs in an attempt to raise body temperature to match the elevated set-point. Shivering not only increases body temperature, but also increases oxygen demands in the body, thereby contravening the initial reason for lowering the temperature (i.e., to decrease oxygen demands). In this case, the use of physical cooling methods for fever management is not only futile but counterproductive.[67] Thus, pharmacologic means are recommended for treatment of SIRS-induced fever. Pharmacologic agents recommended for the treatment of SIRS-induced fever are aspirin and ibuprofen, because they inhibit the synthesis of prostaglandins by blocking the cyclooxygenase pathway.[68]

In summary, given the benefits of fever and the fact that most patients tolerate elevations in temperature and its minor side effects, the practice of routine treatment of the febrile response should be avoided. However, if the febrile response must be treated, the most effective treatment strategy must be used for optimal patient care.

Environmental management

Managing the environment of the patient has been clearly within the domain of nursing since the time of Florence Nightingale.[69] Indeed, every conceptual framework describing the science of nursing emphasizes the importance of the environment to health.[69-72] Numerous studies have examined the effects of the environment such as conversation, music, touch, and family visitation, on critically ill patients.[73-76] The consistent finding reported from these studies is that environmental factors did not have a deleterious effect on overall patient outcome. However, despite these results, critical care nurses tend to maintain patients in a quiet environment at all times in the belief that these sick patients need rest to facilitate recovery. Though a restful environment helps in patient recovery, therapeutic sensory stimulation is also needed by these patients.[75]

Sensory stimulation has been reported to be beneficial in rehabilitation medicine.[76] Although no studies have examined the use of a formalized sensory stimulation program in critical care, it is possible that this therapy will also help critically ill patients. Use of sensory stimulation is based on the premise of neuronal plasticity (the capacity of neurons to recover from a direct insult), which has been documented to be active early in life and present throughout the life span. Neuronal plasticity after ischemia and injury has been attributed to the release of neurotrophic factors (molecules that promote neuronal growth) such as TGF-β_1 within the first 24 hours of insult.[77] These factors facilitate increased dendritic branching and spine density, and thus, may promote neuronal survival. Given that sensory stimulation has been found useful in rehabilitating neurologic patients and that high levels of neurotrophic factors have been documented in the CNS within 24 hours of injury and ischemia, it seems reasonable to assume that implementing an *early* formalized sensory stimulation program for critical care patients may enhance neuronal plasticity. Such a program could improve patient outcomes by speeding recovery and possibly decreasing morbidity.

Family interactions are another important environmental factor in critical care. Most of the research conducted on families in critical care has been on visitation hours and the knowledge needs of family members. Rarely has the focus been on patient recovery despite the suggestion that social support and family may have positive effects, including enhancement of the patient's immune system.[78] Thus, it is conceivable that strengthening the patient's family and social support of a patient may have an impact on the recovery of the patient. Presently, little is known about the effects of environmental therapy on the immune system in patients with SIRS. Therefore, the effects of the environment in managing critically ill patients is a rich area for future nursing research.

Cerebral resuscitation

The complete repertoire of brain-oriented resuscitative efforts consists of improving CBF by restoring fluid volume, decreasing oxygen requirements, blocking the "no reflow phenomenon," and preventing secondary brain tissue damage potentially caused by free-radical formation and excessive EAAs[79-82] (Table 14-6). Through these measures, recovery of salvageable brain tissue is optimized because the problems induced by cerebral ischemia are corrected.

Hypovolemia, commonly seen in patients with SIRS, produces hypotension and has serious consequences in patients with cerebral ischemia.[36] Clinical studies have shown that episodes of hypotension increase the morbidity and mortality in patients with cerebral ischemia.[55,79,82] Thus, hypovolemia often requires volume resuscitation to expand both the vascular and the interstitial compartments, which could eventually optimize CBF. The fluids used for volume resuscitation often contain dextrose. In patients with cerebral ischemia, this is dangerous because dextrose infusion can increase the production of lactic acid, thereby, potentiating the cerebral ischemic insult. The ability of carbohydrates to promote cerebral ischemic damage is not a new finding, but it is frequently forgotten or overlooked.[83] In the presence of cerebral ischemia, the infusion of dextrose-containing fluids can promote anaerobic glycolysis that results in the production of large

Table 14-6 Guidelines in Cerebral Resuscitation

Goal	Recommended therapies
↑ Cerebral blood flow	Use fluid resuscitation to expand vascular volume*
	Maintain position that will optimize CBF
	Avoid hyperventilation
	Induce hypertension
↓ Oxygen requirements	Use neuromuscular blocking agents
	Use hypothermia judiciously
Block "no-reflow phenomenon"	Maintain normovolemic hemodilution (Hct >26% but <30%)
	Use dextran if not contraindicated
	Use calcium channel blockers
Prevent secondary tissue damage	Use calcium channel blockers

*Avoid glucose-containing intravenous fluids.

quantities of lactic acid. Thus, although the prelude to improving CBF is maintaining normovolemia, use of dextrose-containing fluids for volume resuscitation or routine infusion should be avoided in patients with cerebral ischemia.

Another component of cerebral resuscitation is decreasing the oxygen requirements, which may be helpful in the presence of low CBF. Current techniques used to lower metabolic requirements include, but are not limited to, hypothermia, barbiturate therapy, and paralysis.[80,84-86] The use of hypothermia and barbiturates is controversial. Although it is widely accepted that hypothermia can protect the brain from neuronal ischemic damage, recent studies have shown that the effectiveness of this therapy is time-dependent, in that it is effective only before cerebral ischemia occurs.[84,85] In addition, mild hypothermia seems to have more benefits than deep hypothermia.[85] Similarly, the effectiveness of barbiturate therapy in cerebral ischemia is being questioned. Although this therapy can lower ICP, it can also cause significant hypotension that would be detrimental to patients with SIRS-induced cerebral ischemia.[86]

The third component of cerebral resuscitation efforts is blocking the "no-reflow phenomenon" by correcting microcirculatory alterations. Microcirculatory alterations can lead to cerebral ischemia and, unfortunately, are common in SIRS.[2] If the ischemic insult is mild, there will typically be no postischemic hypoperfusion once normal vascular volume is restored.[80,81] If the ischemic insult is severe, however, the "no-reflow phenomenon" can occur.[80-82] The "no-reflow phenomenon" is usually attributed to capillary sludging, platelet aggregation, endothelial damage, and vascular spasms.[2,79-82] Table 14-6 provides some examples of therapy instituted to block the "no-reflow phenomenon."

The fourth component of cerebral resuscitation efforts is preventing further brain tissue damage. Cerebral vasospasm is likely to cause secondary brain injury because it is believed to induce postischemic hypoperfusion.[79] It has also frequently been shown to coexist with blood clots, and its occurrence is closely related to elevated levels of free radicals.[78-80] Cerebral vasospasms are thought to be a result of increased calcium influx. Unlike vascular smooth muscle cells in the extracerebral circuits, cerebrovascular smooth muscle has a relatively small intracellular calcium pool.[79] Thus, increased influx of extracellular calcium serves as a major mechanism in the spastic contraction of the cerebrovascular smooth muscles. Therefore, administration of calcium antagonists may prevent cerebral vasospasm and lead to the improvement of CBF.

FUTURE DIRECTIONS

Presently, studies to determine the best agents to protect the brain from secondary injuries after the initial ischemic insult are being performed.[87-90] Pharmacologic agents such as superoxide dismutase, tirilazad (aminosteroid), and ibuprofen are being tested for their neuroprotective effects as free-radical scavengers or as inhibitors of prostaglandin synthesis.[87,88] Similarly, dextromethorphan, a widely used antitussive agent, is being tested for its neuroprotective properties as an NMDA antagonist.[89] Similarly, adenosine is being examined for its ability to antagonize the excessive release of EAAs.[90] Although some of these pharmacologic agents show some promise, we are still a long way off from determining the best pharmacologic agents to use in blocking the complex biochemical and cellular changes that occur in cerebral ischemia.

CONCLUSION

Dysfunction of the CNS is an early manifestation in MODS. The etiology of the CNS dysfunction in these patients, brought about by SIRS, can be brain microabscesses or cerebral ischemia. These patients exhibit a broad spectrum of symptoms that are usually caused by cerebral ischemia or the actions of inflammatory mediators released in SIRS. Because of our increasing knowledge in recognizing the mechanisms of SIRS and cerebral ischemia, new therapeutic strategies are suggested for the care of these patients. These new therapies, made possible by the technologic advancements and sophisticated research methods of today, bring into serious question the efficacy of current treatments. Finally, because of these advances, nurses need to be willing to question their practice and change their paradigms as necessary in delivering care for the patients with SIRS and MODS.

REFERENCES

1. Korthuis RJ, Anderson DC, Granger DN. Role of neutrophil-endothelial cell adhesion in inflammatory disorders. J Crit Care 1994;9:47-71.
2. Hollenberg SM, Cunnion RE. Endothelial and vascular smooth muscle function in sepsis. J Crit Care 1994;9:262-280.
3. Siesjö BK, Katsura K, Kristián T. The biochemical basis of cerebral ischemia. J Neurosurg Anesthesiol 1995;7:47-52.
4. Young GB et al. The electroencephalogram in sepsis-associated encephalopathy. J Clin Neurophysiol 1992;9:154-152.
5. Bowton DL et al. Cerebral blood flow is reduced in patients with sepsis syndrome. Crit Care Med 1989;17:399-403.
6. Young GB et al. The encephalopathy associated with septic illness. Clin Invest Med 1990;13:297-304.
7. Phillis JW. A radical view of cerebral ischemic injury. Prog Neurobiol 1994;42:441-448.
8. Wahl M et al. Mediators of vascular and parenchymal mechanisms in secondary brain damage. Acta Neurochir (Suppl) 1993;57:64-72.
9. Jackson AC et al. The encephalopathy of sepsis. Can J Neurol Sci 1985;12:303-307.
10. Heard SO, Fink MP. Multiple organ failure syndrome—part 1: Epidemiology, prognosis, and pathophysiology. Intensive Care Med 1991;6:279-294.
11. Maher J, Young GB. Septic encephalopathy. J Intensive Care Med 1993;8:177-187.
12. Bone CR et al. Sepsis syndrome: A valid clinical entity. Crit Care Med 1989;17:389-393.
13. Pendlebury WW et al. Disseminated microabscesses of the central nervous system. (Abstr). Neurology (Suppl 2) 1983;33:223.
14. Pendlebury WW, Perl DP, Muòoz DG. Multiple microabscesses in the central nervous system. A clinicopathologic study. J Neuropathol Exp Neurol 1989;48:290-300.
15. Anker P, Stroun M. Bacterial ribonucleic acid in the frog brain after a bacterial peritoneal infection. Science 1971;178:621-623.
16. Powers WJ. Hemodynamics and metabolism in ischemic cerebrovascular disease. Neurol Clin 1992;10:31-48.
17. Kety SS, Schmidt CF. The effect of active and passive hyperventilation on the cerebral blood flow, cerebral oxygen consumption, cardiac output, and blood pressure of normal young men. J Clin Invest 1946;25:107-119.
18. Astrup J, Siesjö BK, Symon L. Thresholds in cerebral ischemia—the ischemic penumbra. Stroke 1981;12:723-725.
19. Obrist WD et al. Relation of cerebral blood flow to neurological status and outcome in head-injured patients. J Neurosurg 1979;51:292-300.
20. Committee on Life Science and Health/Subcommittee on Brain and Behavioral Sciences. Decade of the Brain. 1900-2000. National Institute of Health 1990. Publication No. PB91-133769.
21. Graham DI et al. Ischemic brain damage is still common in fatal non-missile head injury. J Neurol Neurosurg Psychiatry 1989;52:346-350.
22. Siesjö BK, Agardh CD, Bengstsson F. Free radicals and brain damage. Cerebrovasc Brain Metab Rev 1989;1:165-211.
23. Ikeda Y, Long DM. The molecular basis of brain injury and brain edema: The role of oxygen free radicals. Neurosurgery 1990;27:1-11.
24. Hall ED, Andrus PK, Yonkers PA. Brain hydroxyl radical generation in acute experimental head injury. J Neurochem 1993;60:588-594.
25. Beckman JS et al. Apparent hydroxyl radical production of peroxynitrite: implications for endothelial injury from nitric oxide and superoxide. Proc Natl Acad Sci U S A 1990;87:1620-1624.
26. Meldrum B et al. Ischemic brain damage: the role of excitatory activity and of calcium entry. Br J Anesth 1985;57:44-46.
27. Kawamata T et al. Administration of excitatory amino acid antagonists via microdialysis attenuates the increase in glucose utilization seen following concussive brain injury. J Cereb Blood Flow Metab 1992;12:12-24.
28. Ginsberg MD. Neuroprotection in brain ischemia: An update. Part I. The Neuroscientist 1995;1:95-103.
29. Benveniste H. The excitotoxin hypothesis in relation to cerebral ischemia. Cerebrovasc Brain Metab Rev 1991;3:213-245.
30. Rothman SM. Excitotoxins: Possible mechanisms of action. Ann N Y Acad Sci 1992;648:132-139.
31. Pellegrini-Giampietro DE et al. Excitatory amino acid release and free radical formation may cooperate in the genesis of ischemia-induced neuronal damage. J Neurosci 1990;10:1035-1041.

32. Boisvert DPJ, Schreiber C. Interrelationship of excitotoxic and free radical mechanisms. In: Krieglstein J, Oberpichler-Schwenk P, eds. Pharmacology of cerebral ischemia. Stuttgart, Germany: Wissenschaftliche Verlkagsgesellschaft; 1992:311-320.
33. Guyton AC. Basic neuroscience. Anatomy and physiology. 2nd ed. Philadelphia: W.B. Saunders Co; 1991.
34. Hopkins SJ, Rothwell NJ. Cytokines and the nervous system I: Expression and recognition. TINS 1995;18:83-88.
35. Rothwell NJ, Hopkins SJ. Cytokines and the nervous system II: Actions and mechanisms of action. TINS 1995;18:130-136.
36. Michelson D, Gold PW, Sternberg EM. The stress response in critical illness. New Horiz 1994;2:426-431.
37. Hori T et al. Effects of interleukin-1 and arachidonate on the preoptic and anterior hypothalamic neurons. Brain Res Bull 1988;20:75-82.
38. Breder CD, Dinarello CA, Saper CB. Interleukin-1 immunoreactive innervation of the human hypothalamus. Science 1988;240:321-324.
39. Kluger MJ. Fever: Role of pyrogen and cryogens. Physiological Review 1991;71:93-127.
40. Nakamori T et al. Organum vasculosum laminae terminalis (OVLT) is a brain site to produce interleukin-1 during fever. Brain Res 1993;618:155-159.
41. Hillhouse EW, Mosley K. Peripheral endotoxin induces hypothalamic immunoreactive interleukin-1 in the rat. Br J Pharmacol 1993;109:289-290.
42. Barres BA et al. A crucial role for neurotrophin-3 in oligodendrocyte development. Nature 1994;367:371-375.
43. Eide FF, Lowenstein DH, Reichardt LF. Neurotrophins and their receptors—current concepts and implications for neurologic disease. Exp Neurol 1993;121:200-214.
44. Rangel-Frausto M et al. The natural history of the systemic inflammatory response syndrome (SIRS). JAMA 1995;273:117-123.
45. Volpe BT, Hirst W. The characterization of an amnesic syndrome following hypoxic ischemic injury. Arch Neurol 1983;40:436-440.
46. Auer RN, Jensen ML, Whishaw IQ. Neurobehavioral deficit due to ischemic brain damage limited to half of the CA1 sector of the hippocampus. J Neurosci 1989;9:1641-1647.
47. Cummings JLU et al. Amnesia with hippocampal lesions after cardiopulmonary arrest. Neurology 1984;34:679-681.
48. Volpe BT, Holtzman JD, Hirst W. Further characterization of patients with amnesia after global hypoxic ischemic injury: Preserved recognition memory. Neurology 1986;36:408-411.
49. Morris RGM et al. Place navigation impaired in rats with hippocampal lesions. Nature 1982;297:681-683.
50. Scoville WB, Milner B. Loss of recent memory after bilateral hippocampal lesions. J Neurol Neurosurg Psychiatry 1957;20:11-21.
51. Therrien BA. Sex differences in the effects of hippocampal lesions on place navigation. Unpublished doctoral dissertation, The University of Michigan, Ann Arbor; 1982.
52. Waite JJ, Thal LJ. Spatial memory deficits from lesions of the cholenergic basal forebrain using ibotenic, quisqualate and AMPA. Soc Neurosci Abstracts 1992;18:1421.
53. Zola-Morgan S, Squire LR, Amaral D. Human amnesia and the medial temporal region: Enduring memory impairment following a bilateral lesion limited to field CA1 of the hippocampus. J Neurosci 1986;6:2950-2965.
54. Meyer FB. The intensive care management of cerebral ischemia. In: Andrews BT, ed. Neurosurgical intensive care. New York: McGraw Hill; 1993:329-343.
55. Sikes PJ, Segal J. Jugular bulb oxygen saturation monitoring for evaluating cerebral ischemia. Crit Care Nurs Q 1994;17:9-20.
56. Sheinberg M et al. Continuous monitoring of jugular venous oxygen saturation in head-injured patients. J Neurosurg 1992;76:212-217.
57. Hillered L et al. Neurometabolic monitoring of the ischemic human brain using microdialysis. Acta Neurochir (Wien) 1990;102:91-97.
58. Rosner M, Coley I. Cerebral perfusion pressure, intracranial pressure, and head elevation. J Neurosurg 1986;65:636-641.
59. Feldman Z et al. Effect of head elevation on intracranial pressure, cerebral perfusion pressure, and cerebral blood flow in head-injured patients. J Neurosurg 1992;76:207-211.
60. March K et al. Effect of backrest position on intracranial and cerebral perfusion pressures. J Neurosci Nurs 1990;22:375-381.
61. Durward QJ et al. Cerebral and cardiovascular responses to changes in head elevation with intracranial hypertension. J Neurosurg 1983;59:938-944.
62. Yoshida K, Marmarou A. Effects of tromethamine and hyperventilation on brain injury in the cat. J Neurosurg 1991;74:87-96.
63. Cold GE. Does acute hyperventilation provoke cerebral oligemia in comatose patients after head injury? Acta Neurochir (Wien) 1989;96:100-106.
64. Muizelaar J et al. Adverse effects of prolonged hyperventilation in patients with severe head injury. J Neurosurg 1991;75:731-739.
65. Havill JH. Prolonged hyperventilation and intracranial pressure. Crit Care Med 1984;12:72-74.
66. Young AB et al. The acute phase response of the brain-injured patient. J Neurosurg 1988;69:375-380.
67. Cunha BA, Degamin-Beltram M, Gobbo PH. Implications of fever in the critical care setting. Heart Lung 1984;13:460-465.
68. Milton AS. Thermoregulatory actions of eicosanoids in the central nervous system with particular regard to the pathogenesis of fever. Ann N Y Acad Sci 1989;559:392-410.
69. Nightingale F. Notes on nursing: What it is and what it is not. London: J.B. Lippincott; 1859.
70. Nicoll LH. Perspectives on nursing theory. 2nd ed. Philadelphia: J.B. Lippincott; 1992.
71. Chinn PL, Jacobs MK. Theory and nursing: A systematic approach. St. Louis: Mosby; 1987.
72. Stevens Barnum BJ. Nursing theory: Analysis, application, evaluation. 3rd ed. Glenview: Scott, Foresman/Little, Brown Higher Education; 1990.
73. Briones TL. Effects of music and familiar voice on ICP. Proceedings of the 5th World Congress on Intensive and Critical Care Medicine WCICCM: Kyoto, Japan; 1989.
74. Johnson SM, Omery A, Nikas D. Effects of conversation on intracranial pressure in comatose patients. Heart Lung 1989;18:56-63.
75. Bruya MA. Planned periods of rest in the intensive care unit: Nursing care activities and intracranial pressure. J Neurosurg Nurs 1981;13:184-193.

76. Rising CJ. The relationship of selected nursing activities to ICP. J Neurosci Nurs 1993;25:302-308.
77. Lehrmann E et al. Cytokines in cerebral ischemia: Expression of transforming growth factors beta-1 (TGF-(1) mRNA in the postischemic adult rat hippocampus. Exp Neurol 1995;131:114-123.
78. Locke S. Stress, adaptation, and immunity: Studies in humans. Gen Hosp Psychiatry 1982;4:49-58.
79. Graham SH, Chen J, Sharp FR, Simon RP. Limiting ischemic injury by inhibition of excitatory amino acid release. J Cereb Blood Flow Metab 1993;13:88-97.
80. Semonin-Holleran R. The use of neuromuscular blocking agents in critical care nursing practice. Crit Care Nurs Q 1993;16:37-44.
81. Caron M, Hovda D, Becker D. Changes in the treatment of head injury. Neurosurg Clin North Am 1991;2:483-491.
82. Farman C et al. The effect of hemodilution and hypercapnia on the recovery of cerebral function from experimental focal ischemia. Acta Neurochir (Wien) 1994;127-210-214.
83. Robertson CS et al. The effect of glucose administration on carbohydrate metabolism after head injury. J Neurosurg 1991;74:43-50.
84. Werner C. Cerebral perfusion and hypothermia. J Neurosurg Anesthesiol 1995;7:53-56.
85. Shiozaki T et al. Effect of mild hypothermia on uncontrollable intracranial hypertension after severe head injury. J Neurosurg 1993;79:363-368.
86. Ward J et al. Failure of prophylactic barbiturate coma in the treatment of severe head injury. J Neurosurg 1985;62:383-388.
87. Hall ED, McCall JM, Means ED. Therapeutic potential of the lazaroids (21-aminosteroids) in acute central nervous system trauma, ischemia and subarachnoid hemorrhage. Adv Pharmacol 1994;28:221-268.
88. Chan PH, Longar S, Fishman RA. Protective effects of liposome-entrapped superoxide dismutase on posttraumatic brain edema. Ann Neurol 1987;21:540-547.
89. Bokesch PM et al. Dextromethorphan inhibits ischemia-induced c-fos expression and delayed neuronal death in hippocampal neurons. Anesthesiology 1994;81:470-477.
90. Schubert P, Kreutzberg GW. Cerebral protection by adenosine. Acta Neurochir (Suppl) 1993;57:80-88.

Section 4

Management and Special Considerations

Pediatric patients and the geriatric population require special consideration because of their limited reserves and anatomic and developmental differences. Previously, management in both the adult and the pediatric patient has focused on supporting individual organs. More recent interventions aggressively target the initial resuscitation and pathophysiologic changes in volume distribution, oxygen supply and demand, and metabolism. Newer investigational therapies must move farther up the cascade to control primary events such as overwhelming activation of the inflammatory/immune response, sympathetic activation, extensive endothelial damage, and ischemia/reperfusion injury. There lies the greatest chance of reversing the vicious cycle *before* organ damage occurs.

15. The Pediatric Patient with Multiple Organ Dysfunction Syndrome
16. The Geriatric Patient with Multiple Organ Dysfunction Syndrome
17. Evaluation and Management of Oxygen Delivery and Consumption in Multiple Organ Dysfunction Syndrome
18. Multiple Organ Dysfunction Syndrome: Overview and Conclusions

CHAPTER *15*

The Pediatric Patient with Multiple Organ Dysfunction Syndrome

Patricia A. Moloney-Harmon and *Sandra J. Czerwinski*

Multiple organ dysfunction syndrome (MODS) has been studied extensively in adult populations. Until recently, the only available data concerning pediatric patients with MODS were published by Wilkinson and co-workers in 1986 and 1987.[1,2] In 1994, Proulx and colleagues[3] published study results that supported Wilkinson's data from the 1980s. The Proulx study also identified multiple risk factors associated with mortality rates in children. Because of the limited information available about infants and children with MODS, it is difficult to describe and define this syndrome for these patients and to make accurate comparisons between pediatric and adult populations. Table 15-1 provides the specific criteria that Wilkinson and co-workers established to define organ failure in children, but diagnostic criteria will vary from study to study, and no criteria for organ dysfunction has been put forth. Certain conditions that are frequently associated with the development of MODS in adult patients are also seen in children (see the box on p. 328), but no studies have been published to validate the relationship between these conditions and the development of MODS in pediatric patients. In adults and children, however, MODS is an acute and potentially reversible process that occurs in a significant number of patients admitted to the intensive care unit (ICU).

Mortality rates for children with MODS are considerably higher than those reported for critically ill children without MODS. The studies by Wilkinson and co-workers[2] and Proulx and colleagues[3] documented mortality rates of 52% to 54%, which are considerably lower than the adult mortality rates of 60% to 90%.[4-7] As with adult populations, the mortality rate in pediatric patients increases as the number of organs involved increases.[3] System dysfunction and failure can occur progressively, in sequence, or at the same time. However, pediatric patients generally develop organ failures in an overwhelming and simultaneous manner rather than progressively or sequentially.[3] The diagnosis of MODS and the maximum number of organ system failures occur very soon after admission to the pediatric ICU. Wilkinson and co-workers reported a 75% mortality rate for both medical and surgical pediatric patients when four or more organ systems were involved. Bersten and Sibbald[8] have discussed a pediatric study that showed an 88% mortality rate when four or more organ systems failed. Proulx and co-workers[3] identified that the maximum number of simultaneous organ system failures occurring during the PICU stay was an independent risk marker of death. They also identified an age of 12 months or less and the Pediatric Risk of Mortality (PRISM) score on the day of PICU admission as risk factors.[3] Respiratory failure is the most frequent organ failure seen in infants and children, followed by cardiovascular, neurologic, hematologic, and renal system involvement. No data are available on the incidence of hepatic or gastrointestinal failure, but these systems can be involved. A specific sequence of organ system failure has not been identified for children, and no specific combination of organ system failures has been found to raise mortality. Additionally, sepsis is not as strongly associated with

Table 15-1 Criteria for Failure of Specific Organ Systems

Organ system	Criteria
Cardiovascular	MAP < 40 mm Hg (infants <12 months) MAP < 50 mm Hg (children ≥12 months) HR < 50 beats/min (infants <12 months) HR < 40 beats/min (children ≥12 months) Cardiac arrest Continuous vasoactive drug infusion for hemodynamic support
Respiratory	RR > 90/min (infants <12 months) RR > 70/min (children ≥12 months) Pao_2 < 40 mm Hg (in absence of cyanotic heart disease) $Paco_2$ > 65 mm Hg Pao_2/Fio_2 < 250 mm Hg Mechanical ventilation (>24 hr if postoperative) Tracheal intubation for airway obstruction or acute respiratory failure
Neurologic	Glasgow coma scale < 5 Fixed, dilated pupils Persistent (>20 min) intracranial pressure (>20 mm Hg or requiring therapeutic intervention)
Hematologic	Hemoglobin < 5 g/dL WBC < 3000 cell/mm^3 Platelets < 20,000/mm^3 Disseminated intravascular coagulopathy (PT > 20 sec or aPTT > 60 sec in presence of positive FSP assay)
Renal	BUN >100 mg/dL Serum creatinine > 2 mg/dL Dialysis
Gastrointestinal	Blood transfusions > 20 mL/kg in 24 hr because of GI hemorrhage (endoscopic confirmation optional)
Hepatic	Total bilirubin > 5 mg/dL and SGOT or LDH more than twice normal value (without evidence of hemolysis) Hepatic encephalopathy ≥ grade II

From Wilkinson JD et al. Mortality associated with multiple organ system failure and sepsis in pediatric intensive care. J Pediatr 1987;111:325.

BUN, Blood urea nitrogen; *FSP*, fibrin split products; *HR*, heart rate; *LDH*, lactate dehydrogenase; *MAP*, mean arterial pressure; *Paco₂*, partial arterial pressure of carbon dioxide; *Pao₂*, partial arterial pressure of oxygen; *PT*, prothrombin time; *aPTT*, activated partial thromboplastin time; *RR*, respiratory rate; *SGOT*, serum glutamic-oxaloacetic transaminase; *WBC*, white blood cell.

EVENTS REPORTED TO TRIGGER MULTIPLE ORGAN SYSTEM FAILURE

Advanced age	Intraabdominal infection	Poor nutrition
Alcoholism	Liver cirrhosis	Sepsis
Atherosclerotic cardiovascular disease	Malignancy	Shock
Burns	Multiple transfusions	Splenectomy
Chronic renal failure	Neurologic trauma	Steroids
Emergency surgery (specifically abdominal)	Pancreatitis	Vascular procedure
GI bleeding	Polytrauma	Others

From Toro-Figuera L. Multiple organ system failure. In: Levin DL, Morriss FC, eds. Essentials of pediatric intensive care. St Louis: Quality Medical Publishing, Inc., 1990:186.

MODS in children as in adult populations. Wilkinson and colleagues[2] reported that more than 50% of pediatric critical care patients developed MODS in the absence of documented sepsis. Proulx[3] found that sepsis does not increase the risk of death in children.

This chapter will focus on the assessment and collaborative management of pediatric patients with MODS. Medical and nursing interventions are directed toward prevention and support of individual organ systems before failure occurs. Nurses play a key role in assessing system dysfunction, identifying abnormalities early, and minimizing complications. It is essential that nurses understand the differences in anatomy, physiology, and response to illness between children and adults, as well as the systemic consequences of nursing interventions.

PATHOPHYSIOLOGY

The pathophysiology of MODS in children is a complex process. When conditions such as sepsis or trauma disrupt the normal physiologic equilibrium, compensatory mechanisms work to regain homeostasis. However, when these mechanisms fail or become exhausted, a variety of physiologic, hemodynamic, metabolic, and inflammatory/immune dysfunctions occur.

Maldistribution of circulating blood volume

Maldistribution of circulating blood volume commonly causes the hemodynamic changes seen in the child with MODS and results in a deficit of the oxygen supply. Compensatory mechanisms attempt to restore normal circulation and use fuel stores to meet cellular oxygen demands. When the normal circulatory pattern cannot be restored quickly, the compensatory mechanisms and fuel stores are quickly exhausted. Cellular oxygen needs then go unmet (see Chapter 5).

Imbalance of oxygen supply and demand

The cellular hypoxia that results from a decreased oxygen supply damages the cell structure, which interferes with the ability of the cell to extract and use oxygen. At the same time that oxygen supply is low or underused, the initial event that triggered the MODS, together with fever, hypermetabolism, pain, and other factors greatly increases the need of the body for oxygen. The greater demand goes unmet, and further cellular hypoxia results (see Chapter 6).

Alterations in metabolism

Because the cells receive an inadequate oxygen supply, their metabolic activity becomes dysfunctional. The process that supplies energy to the cells requires oxygen. When oxygen is not present, the energy transfer is less efficient, and lactic acid is released. The buildup of lactic acid and inefficient metabolism cause generalized cell damage, unmet cellular energy needs, and cell death. Children normally have a higher metabolic rate, and conditions such as sepsis or trauma increase the rate even further. The hypermetabolic state quickly depletes the limited energy reserves of the child, and the anaerobic metabolic process cannot meet the increased energy demand. Liver failure occurs, and the hypermetabolism cannot be maintained. Cellular energy production becomes even further decreased, oxygen supply is further compromised, and cellular damage continues (see Chapter 7).

Inflammatory/immune response in children

The normal inflammatory/immune response (IIR) is a multifaceted series of events that results in phagocytic activity and the release of mediators that are directed toward destroying the invading pathogen.[9] The infant has fewer neutrophils and is less able than is the older child to replace white blood cells in the face of overwhelming infection. Complement levels are low in the infant and do not come within the normal adult range until 3 to 6 months of age, which affects chemotactic and opsonic activity in the infant. The infant is able to synthesize small amounts of immunoglobin, but most of the immunoglobulin is received through placental transfer. The lowest immunoglobin concentration occurs at approximately 4 to 5 months of age, during which time the infant is most susceptible to infections caused by viruses, *Candida* organisms, and certain bacteria. The infant and young child do have all the components to mount an immune response, but because exposure to many antigens has not occurred, a vigorous response to certain bacteria, viruses, and fungi does not occur.

When the IIR is altered, the balance between mediators is lost, and optimal protection is disrupted. Uncontrolled phagocytosis and mediator activity serve to intensify the IIR. The generalized systemic consequences that result are capillary vasodilation, increased capillary permeability, smooth muscle contraction, heightened coagulation and fibrinolytic activity, enhanced macrophage and lymphocyte function, myocardial depression, and other events.[10] (See Chapter 3.)

The inability of the child to meet cellular and metabolic needs leads to organ dysfunction, systemic disruption, and death. The generalized systemic effects elicit different reactions from individual organ systems. The remainder of this chapter focuses on the effect of systemic disruptions on the individual organ systems and the specialized nursing care needed to support the child with MODS.

RESPIRATORY SYSTEM DYSFUNCTION

Respiratory failure is generally one of the first and most common system failures seen in children.[1,10] It is classified according to both anatomic and physiologic parameters; however, the anatomic classification system is particularly useful in directing early ICU interventions (see the box below). Regardless of the cause of respiratory failure, the end result is that the metabolic oxygen needs of the tissues will not be met, and carbon dioxide excretion will be inadequate.

Anatomic and physiologic differences

Children have little respiratory reserve because of a number of anatomic and physiologic factors that are peculiar to the pediatric respiratory system.[11] Narrow airways result in high airflow resistance, and decreased cartilaginous support of the airways causes early airway closure during forced expiration. The soft compliant chest walls, more horizontal positioning of the ribs, decreased curvature of the diaphragm, and the large abdomen that pushes up on the diaphragm and restricts lung expansion will not allow generation of high intrathoracic pressures.

In addition, infants are at risk for respiratory muscle fatigue because of the immaturity and structure of respiratory skeletal muscles. These factors all

---

CAUSES OF RESPIRATORY FAILURE: ANATOMIC CLASSIFICATION

Central nervous system
Sedative overdose
Head trauma
Intracranial bleeding
Apnea of prematurity

Peripheral nervous system
Spinal cord injury
Guillain-Barré syndrome
Myasthenia gravis
Phrenic nerve paralysis

Respiratory muscles
Muscular dystrophies
Muscle wasting of cachexia
Respiratory muscle fatigue because of increased work of breathing

Chest wall and pleurae
Flail chest
Kyphoscoliosis
Pneumothorax
Hemothorax
Empyema
Chylothorax

Airways
Upper airways
  Epiglottitis
  Croup
Lower airways
  Foreign body aspiration
  Asthma
  Bronchiolitis

Parenchyma
Pneumonia
Pulmonary edema
Adult respiratory distress syndrome

Pulmonary blood flow
Pulmonary emboli
Persistent fetal circulation

From Witte M. Acute respiratory failure. In: Blumer J, ed. A practical guide to pediatric intensive care. 3rd ed. St Louis: Mosby; 1990:98.

predispose infants and children to respiratory dysfunction and failure regardless of the underlying condition.

Pathophysiologic alterations

Respiratory dysfunction in MODS is frequently manifested as adult respiratory distress syndrome (ARDS). As in adults, this syndrome results from injury to the alveolocapillary membrane and damage to the pulmonary endothelium that leads to increased pulmonary capillary permeability and leakage of fluid into the interstitium and the alveoli. The lung damage may result from direct injury such as that sustained from aspiration, inhalation of toxic gases, or pulmonary infections; or it may also be the result of indirect injury from shock, sepsis, or trauma.[12] The common denominators generally are hypotension, inflammation, and extensive tissue damage. Clinically, the child with ARDS exhibits hypoxemia that does not respond to increasing amounts of inspired oxygen, decreased pulmonary compliance, respiratory alkalosis, dyspnea, tachypnea, and the appearance of diffuse, fluffy infiltrates on chest x-ray films without evidence of cardiogenic causes.

Therapeutic management

Assessment. Successful therapeutic management of the child with ARDS depends on recognizing the basic cause and implementing effective supportive therapy. The goal of therapy is to deliver adequate oxygen to meet the metabolic needs of tissues and restore the balance of oxygen supply and demand. Close observation of the general appearance of the child is critical when assessing respiratory status. Nurses must be alert for signs of fatigue, diaphoresis, restlessness, and poor perfusion, which may indicate impending respiratory failure. Frequent nursing assessments of respiratory rate and effort, adequacy of breath sounds, and effectiveness of chest wall movements are important if the child is breathing spontaneously. Increased dyspnea, decreased respiratory rate, diminished breath sounds, altered level of consciousness, or paradoxical respirations indicate increasing respiratory dysfunction and the need for more ventilatory support.

Both invasive and noninvasive monitoring provide valuable information to the nurse caring for the child with ARDS. Cardiorespiratory monitoring is necessary, along with parameters monitored through a peripheral arterial catheter, pulse oximeter, and if indicated, a pulmonary arterial catheter. A pulmonary artery catheter will allow for evaluation of oxygen transport variables such as oxygen consumption and delivery and oxygen extraction ratio.

Ventilatory support. Rapid intervention for deteriorating respiratory status is essential to correct hypoxemia and decrease the work of breathing. Endotracheal intubation, mechanical ventilation, and the use of positive end-expiratory pressure (PEEP) will often be required to support the failing respiratory system of the child. A variety of mechanical ventilation modes can be used successfully with children. Infants are frequently ventilated using time-cycled or pressure-cycled modes that limit inspiration and cause cycling from inspiration to expiration based on a preset time or pressure. Both of these modes provide a continuous flow of gas that reduces the infant's work of breathing and energy expenditure. These modes of ventilation are not as useful in older children, since they may not provide adequate flows for children weighing more than 15 kg.

Volume-cycled ventilation is used in many critically ill children. A preset tidal volume is delivered without regard to changes that occur in the lung compliance or airway resistance of the child. High inflating pressures will be required to deliver the prescribed tidal volume in children with decreased compliance or increased airway resistance, which may lead to barotrauma. Volume-cycled ventilation can be pressure-limited to prevent the use of excessive inflating pressures that may be necessary to deliver the preset volume. This safety feature minimizes the risk of creating excessively high airway pressures and makes this mode of ventilation a good option even for small children.

Most volume ventilators that are currently used with children are equipped with options such as assist control, intermittent mandatory ventilation (IMV), synchronized IMV (SIMV), and pressure support, all of which allow the child to breathe independently between ventilator breaths. If these independent breaths are synchronized with positive pressure ventilations, the child will not have to work as hard to open the demand valve, and the risk of hypoventilation will be reduced. The combination of SIMV and pressure support will meet this requirement.

Pressure-controlled ventilation is being used more frequently in the management of pediatric patients. This mode of ventilation uses high gas flows at the beginning of inspiration; the preset inspiratory pressure are reached early in inspiration and maintained throughout the inspiratory effort. The advantage of this mode is that the sustained inspiratory pressure will keep the partially collapsed alveoli open. This occurs at lower peak airway pressures, and gas mixing is improved. Ventilator-induced lung injury is less likely to occur because both peak inspiratory pressures (PIP) and excessive alveolar volumes are reduced.[13]

All patients with acute respiratory failure require supplemental oxygen; however, the dose and duration must be carefully monitored because prolonged exposure to high levels of inspired oxygen can be toxic to lung tissue. PEEP is used routinely in ventilatory management of children and can effectively reduce the need for increasing concentrations of inspired oxygen (see the box to the right). PEEP can be particularly useful with children who have ARDS because they frequently require high concentrations of oxygen to meet their cellular needs.

There are a variety of nonconventional therapies for children with ARDS. These include high frequency ventilation, extracorporeal membrane oxygenation (ECMO), surfactant administration, nitric oxide, and liquid ventilation. These approaches attempt to address issues such as surface tension, heart-lung interaction, normalized lung function in a diseased state, and ventilation/perfusion ratio (V/Q) mismatch in ways that will reduce iatrogenic lung injury.[13] These approaches have shown promise though they still require further investigation before they become standard therapy.

Additional collaborative interventions. Management of children with respiratory failure includes continuous electrocardiogram recordings; an arterial line for continuous measurement of blood pressure; and a pulmonary artery catheter to help evaluate fluid status, measure cardiac output, and monitor pulmonary vascular pressures along with oxygen delivery and consumption. Monitoring the adequacy of ventilation is accomplished by observing chest movement and auscultating breath sounds. In addition, measurement of arterial blood gas values and oxygen saturation will help to evaluate the effectiveness of ventilatory support. Judicious fluid management, careful measurement of intake and output, and daily weighing will also be necessary. Serial chest x-ray examinations will document the progress of the

---

GUIDELINES FOR INITIATING POSITIVE-PRESSURE SUPPORT

Provision of adequate alveolar ventilation
  Select rate—physiologic norm for age
  Select tidal volume—12 to 15 mL/kg
  Select PIP—15 to 20 cm H_2O, increase as needed
  Select inspiratory time (I:E ratio)—age specific norm generally resulting in I:E ratio = 1:2
  Obstructive diseases—prolong E time, avoid prolonged I time
  Immediately assess for signs of adequate ventilation (chest excursion and breath sounds)
  Measure $Paco_2$; adjust IMV rate or tidal volume as needed to maintain $Paco_2$ between 35 and 45 mm Hg
  Decrease IMV rate to level tolerated as determined by $Paco_2$
Maintenance of adequate oxygenation
  Fio_2—1.0
  PEEP 3 cm H_2O, or higher level if needed, anticipating hemodynamic effects
  Immediately assess for signs of adequate oxygenation (color) and circulatory depression (hypotension and diminished peripheral pulses)
Measure Pao_2
  Decrease Fio_2, maintaining $Pao_2 > 70$ mm Hg
  Restrictive disease (low FRC, low compliance)—increase PEEP as needed to achieve $Pao_2 > 70$ mm Hg at $Fio_2 = 0.4$ to 0.5
  Consider direct monitoring of cardiac output if PEEP > 15 cm H_2O
  Decrease PEEP while maintaining $Pao_2 > 70$ mm Hg

From Boegner E. Modes of ventilatory support and weaning parameters in children. Clin Issues Crit Care Nurs 1990; 1:382. *E*, Expiratory; *Fio₂*, fraction of inspired oxygen; *FRC*, functional residual capacity; *I*, inspiratory; *IMV*, intermittent mandatory ventilation; *Paco₂*, partial arterial pressure of carbon dioxide; *Pao₂*, partial arterial pressure of oxygen; *PEEP*, positive end-expiratory pressure; *PIP*, peak inspiratory pressure.

disease. There is no specific drug therapy for ARDS, but generally antibiotics (chosen on the basis of Gram's stain results and culture reports) and bronchodilators are included. Paralytic agents are often used with ventilated patients and are given in conjunction with sedation.[14] Evaluation of the effectiveness of sedation is more difficult in the unconscious child, but vital sign parameters are valid indicators and are closely monitored during neuromuscular blockade. Vasoactive agents will often be necessary to support the hemodynamic status of the child.

Continuous nursing assessments of the ventilated child are critical and include observations for signs of pneumothorax or pneumomediastinum resulting from barotrauma associated with high ventilator pressures. Monitoring vital signs, color, level of consciousness, breath sounds, chest wall movements, ventilator settings, arterial blood gases, oxygen saturation, end-tidal carbon dioxide levels, and pulmonary arterial pressures is done frequently. Careful attention to peak inspiratory pressures can alert the nurse to the decreasing lung compliance and narrowing airways of the child. Meticulous pulmonary hygiene is critical, and frequent suctioning is necessary to maintain patency of the narrow endotracheal tubes required to intubate children. Hyperoxygenation is required before suctioning, and the procedure is accomplished using strict aseptic technique and caution, because the child is often immunologically and hemodynamically unstable. Elevating the head of the bed, changing position frequently, and administering chest physiotherapy are all important to ensure good pulmonary care.

Adequate rest periods are important when possible. Limb restraints are required to prevent the child from accidentally removing essential equipment, and the rationale for restraints must be explained thoroughly to parents. Attention to light and noise levels is an important nursing function, with their adverse effects being minimized without risking patient safety.

CARDIOVASCULAR SYSTEM DYSFUNCTION

The limited pediatric data available indicate that cardiovascular failure is seen clearly and relatively frequently in children with MODS.[1] It is unclear, however, if the cardiovascular changes lead to generalized organ disruption or if the cardiovascular system is compensating for organ damage that has already occurred. As in adults, the myocardium of the child can be damaged by ischemia, inflammatory mediators, and acidosis.

Anatomic and physiologic differences

Hemodynamic function is determined by cardiac output (CO) and vascular resistance. If the hemodynamic conditions change, alteration in CO or vascular resistance should occur. CO is the product of heart rate and stroke volume, and pediatric CO is greatly affected by the heart rate and body surface area of the child. Heart rates in children tend to vary over a wide range and decrease with age as shown in Table 15-2. Conversely, stroke volume is relatively fixed in infants and young children and increases with age; therefore children respond to stress and increased metabolic needs by increasing their heart rates rather than by augmenting their stroke volume.[15] To maintain optimal CO effectively and to achieve maximal cardiac index in critically ill children, the heart rate should be maintained within the high normal range for that age. Although this sustained high rate places the child at an increased risk for myocardial ischemia, it is much less of a concern in children than it is for adult patients. Children are better able to compensate for the increased myocardial oxygen consumption (MV_{O_2}) that results from the increased heart rate by increasing oxygen delivery to the myocardium (MD_{O_2}). Although it is not a common event, myocardial ischemia can occur in children of all ages during rapid heart rates. Other conditions frequently associated with myocardial ischemia include shock, thoracic trauma, head injury, asthma, and tachydysrhythmias (see the box on p. 334).

When CO is inadequate, cellular hypoxia, altered cellular metabolism, and decreased energy produc-

Table 15-2 Heart Rate Limits

Age	Low (beats/min)	High (beats/min)
0 to 24 hours	100	180
1 to 7 days	100	180
8 to 30 days	100	200
1 to 3 months	100	200
3 to 6 months	100	200
6 to 12 months	100	200
1 to 3 years	80	160
3 to 5 years	80	150
5 to 8 years	70	120
8 to 12 years	60	120
12 to 16 years	50	120

From Allen E. Basic minimal intensive care monitoring. In: Blumer J, ed. A practical guide to pediatric intensive care. 3rd ed. St Louis: Mosby; 1990:14.

> **CAUSES OF MYOCARDIAL ISCHEMIA IN CHILDHOOD**
>
> **Neonatal ischemic heart disease**
> Asphyxia neonatorum
> Increased demand
>   Persistent transitional circulation
>   Pulmonary hypertension (respiratory distress syndrome and meconium aspiration)
>
> **Congenital heart disease**
> Cyanotic heart disease
>   Total anomalous pulmonary veins
>   Transposition of great vessels
> Obstructive disease
>   Aortic or pulmonary stenosis
> Anomalous coronary arteries
>
> **Increased demand**
> Catecholamine-induced ischemia (isoproterenol treatment of asthma)
> Head injury
>
> **Vascular disease**
> Kawasaki disease
> Infantile periarteritis nodosa
> Embolism
> Atheroma (rare)
> Trauma
>
> **Trauma and head injury**

From Deshpande JK, Wetzel RC, Rogers RC. Unusual causes of myocardial ischemia, pulmonary edema, and cyanosis. In: Rogers MC, ed. Textbook of pediatric intensive care. 2nd ed. Baltimore: Williams & Wilkins; 1992:424.

tion result.[16] This state of circulatory dysfunction is clinically described as shock. It is generally caused by a reduced CO, maldistribution of circulating volume, or both, and if allowed to proceed uninterrupted, it will result in death.

Pathophysiologic alterations

The causes of shock in children are the same as in adults; however, the frequency with which they occur is different. Although shock can be classified in many ways, the categories, when based on blood flow, are low-flow shock and maldistributive shock.[17] Low-flow shock is characterized by decreased CO and may be caused by hypovolemia, cardiac failure, or blood flow obstruction. Maldistributive shock is characterized by normal or increased CO with abnormal distribution of blood flow. Neurogenic, anaphylactic, and septic shock are examples of maldistributive shock states.

Shock occurs in a wide variety of clinical settings, often without any associated illness or obvious predisposing factors. The outcome is often better for children than for adults, because the child is generally healthy before the onset of shock. Although shock occurs in children of all ages, some populations are more vulnerable to specific types of shock. Neonates, children with congenital heart disease, and oncologic and urologic patients are at greater risk for developing septic shock.[16] Organisms responsible for septic shock vary with the age of the patient. β-Hemolytic streptococci and *Haemophilus influenzae,* which are generally not associated with septic shock in adults, are seen frequently in infants and young children. Also, children with congenital heart disease are more likely to develop cardiogenic shock.

Hypovolemic low-flow shock. Hypovolemic shock is the most common cause of shock in children. It results from decreased intravascular volume generally related to water and electrolyte losses, hemorrhage, third space losses, or pathologic renal losses.[17] These losses result from a variety of insults including trauma, gastrointestinal hemorrhage, renal disease, and burns. The decreased circulating volume results in reduced venous return and preload and, therefore, decreased stroke volume and CO. Although circulating blood volume in a child is larger relative to weight than is circulating blood volume in an adult (80 ml/kg), a child can become hypovolemic with a minimal amount of fluid loss because the total circulating volume is small. The hypovolemia often results from vomiting and diarrhea because much of the total fluid volume in children is extracellular. Early symptoms usually include cool extremities, decreased peripheral perfusion, tachycardia, and decreased urine output. Cardiac output is decreased, but blood pressure is usually normal because of the efficient vasoconstrictive mechanisms in children. If volume loss is not corrected, the symptoms worsen; the child becomes hypotensive, anuric, and mentally confused, and cardiac failure results.[15]

Cardiogenic low-flow shock. Cardiogenic shock does not occur frequently in children; however, it can result from congenital heart disease, hypoxemia, acidosis, hypoglycemia, dysrhythmias, severe electrolyte imbalances, chest trauma, and drug toxicity.[17] In neonates, the usual cause of cardiogenic shock is a congenital heart defect that is characterized by outflow obstruction or systemic pulmonary shunts.[18] Tension pneumothorax, tension pneumopericardium, pericardial effusion, cardiac tamponade and massive pulmonary emboli are also causes of ventricular outflow obstruction and cardiogenic shock.[19]

Maldistributive shock. Maldistributive shock, the second most common type of shock to occur in children, is associated with an abnormal distribution of circulating volume.[18] As a result, tissues are inadequately perfused even with normal or high CO. Neurogenic shock results from massive vasodilatation related to loss of sympathetic vasomotor tone. Because of increased vascular capacity, vital organs are deprived of oxygen and nutrients. Anaphylactic shock results from a severe antigen-antibody reaction that triggers a massive release of mediators and causes vasodilatation, capillary leak, severe bronchoconstriction, and urticaria. Fortunately this is a rare occurrence in the PICU.

Sepsis is the most common cause of maldistributive shock in children. Shock may result from decreased intravascular volume, maldistribution of intravascular volume, and impaired myocardial function, all of which occur at different times during its course.[18] Critically ill children with severe burns or multiple trauma frequently develop the systemic inflammatory response syndrome (SIRS) and septic shock. Surgery, invasive devices, antibiotics, immunosuppression, hypothermia, and critical illness are all risk factors in septic shock.[19] Although the cause is usually bacterial, viral pathogens and their toxins can also cause septic shock. As in the adult, the clinical course of the child can move from the high cardiac output, hyperdynamic stage when the child looks well perfused (although tissue hypoxia may be present in some organ beds) to the uncompensated stage in which the child is cold, cyanotic, listless, anuric, and manifesting the signs and symptoms of cardiogenic shock. Adequate fluid resuscitation is vital to prevent decompensation and low CO.

Therapeutic management

The successful management of cardiovascular dysfunction is aimed at perfusing vital organs and preventing or correcting metabolic abnormalities resulting from cellular hypoperfusion. The goals of therapy are to establish and maintain the appropriate oxygen and substrate delivery to meet the metabolic needs of the child without increasing MVO_2 and to support the child until homeostasis is restored and healing begins.

Assessment. Patients in shock states warrant careful monitoring and continuous reevaluation since they undergo rapid changes. Progressive circulatory dysfunction and impaired tissue perfusion must be identified early if the child is to recover. Heart rate, blood pressure, temperature, systemic perfusion, color, level of consciousness, quality of pulses, and core temperature should be monitored continuously. An important consideration for children in shock is that blood pressure is often the last parameter to change; therefore careful consideration must be given to early changes in the systemic perfusion. Prompt identification of arrhythmias is necessary, and interventions should include correction of hypoxia, acidosis, hypocalcemia, hypokalemia, or hyperkalemia, and the use of cardioactive drugs such as atropine, isoproterenol, digoxin, adenosine, and lidocaine.[15] The use of pacemakers and cardioversion may also be necessary to increase the heart rate and maximize CO.

Both invasive and noninvasive hemodynamic monitoring are essential for assessing the child in shock. Blood pressure monitoring is accomplished using an intraarterial line if possible. This continuous display with beat-to-beat analysis of waveform and continuous display of pulse pressure is critical. This device also is valuable in the ongoing analysis of arterial blood gases. If a manual cuff is used, particular attention must be given to cuff size. The cuff should be two thirds to three fourths of the upper-arm size and should encircle the arm only once. Right atrial pressure (RAP) monitoring is an important component of optimizing preload. Pulmonary artery (PA) monitoring is necessary to evaluate left ventricular filling pressure and CO. PA catheters will also allow for mixed venous blood sampling or continuous mixed venous oxygen saturation (SvO_2) monitoring.[17]

Monitoring peripheral and core temperature is helpful in assessing peripheral perfusion, and differences in these parameters can indicate a compromised CO. Evaluation of serial arterial blood gases, electrolytes, electrocardiogram, isoenzymes, and body weight is also essential to the assessment. Sequential echocardiograms are helpful in assessing cardiac function and quantifying ventricular ejection fraction.[17] Decreased CO can often be improved by increasing preload. Children have a larger daily fluid requirement than do adults, but their total fluid requirement is smaller as illustrated in Tables 15-3 and 15-4.

Volume replacement. Volume replacement of 10 to 20 mL/kg over a 10- to 15-minute period is a priority for the child in shock. Additional replacement is based on an ongoing assessment of the vital signs, level of consciousness, systemic perfusion, urine output, and hemodynamic parameters. Urine output is measured at least hourly and should exceed 0.5 to 1.0 mL/kg/hr if renal function is normal. A urine output of less than 0.5 mL/kg/hr suggests decreased renal perfusion.[20] Accurate intake and output, including blood loss from laboratory work, is recorded to ensure close evaluation of the fluid status of the child.

Pulmonary artery catheters are often used and allow the nurse to monitor filling pressures and calculate hemodynamic indices (Table 15-5). These data allow for early detection of cardiac decompensation and pulmonary hypertension. They also provide valuable information about the volume status of the child.

Pharmacologic support. Pharmacologic support may be necessary to increase CO. Catecholamines such as dopamine, epinephrine, norepinephrine, and dobutamine are particularly effective because they work quickly, their dosage is controllable, and their half-life is short. Children receiving these agents should always be managed using invasive hemodynamic monitoring techniques. Combining inotropic drugs with vasodilators such as sodium nitroprusside will decrease afterload and increase CO without the adverse peripheral vasoconstrictor effects. A drug such as amrinone produces positive inotropic, as well as vasodilator effects. Table 15-6 lists the various vasoactive agents with the appropriate range of doses used in children. Aggressive intervention must take place to restore adequate cardiovascular

Table 15-3 Pediatric Maintenance Fluid Requirements

Body weight (kg)	Water maintenance (mL/24 hr)	Electrolyte maintenance
<10	100 mL/kg	
10 to 20	1000 mL + 50 mL for each kg	
>20	1500 mL + 20 mL for each kg above 20 kg	3 mEq of sodium + 2 mEq of potassium for each 100 mL of fluid

Recommended maintenance fluid is D5 + ¼ NS with 20 mEq of KCl/L. Do not routinely use D5W in children.

From Blumer J. Pediatric emergency guidelines. In: Blumer J, ed. A practical guide to pediatric intensive care. 3rd ed. St Louis: Mosby; 1990:inside cover.

Table 15-4 Fluid Resuscitation Requirements in Neonates and Children in Shock*

IV fluid	Amount	Rate
First D5NS	10 to 20 mL/kg	Over 5 to 10 min
Then NS or R/L	10 to 20 mL/kg†	Over 5 to 20 min
5% albumin or hetastarch	10 mL/kg for every 40 mL of crystalloid given	Over 5 to 20 min

*Physical examination: lethargic, cool extremities, mottled skin, slow capillary refill, tachycardic, and hypotensive.
†Give repeated IV boluses until vital signs improve and peripheral perfusion improves.
From Blumer J. Pediatric emergency guidelines. In: Blumer J, ed. A practical guide to pediatric intensive care. 3rd ed. St Louis: Mosby; 1990:inside cover.

Table 15-5 Normal Pressure Values for Children

Pressure	Value (mm Hg)
Central venous pressure	4 to 12
Systolic pulmonary artery pressure	20 to 30
Diastolic pulmonary artery pressure	<10
Mean pulmonary artery pressure	<20
Pulmonary capillary wedge pressure	4 to 12

Modified from Smith J, Giblin M, Koehler J. The cardiovascular system. In: Smith J, ed. Pediatric critical care. New York: J Wiley & Sons; 1983:100.

Table 15-6 Vasoactive Agents Used in Children

Agent	Site of action	Dose (μg/kg/min)	Effect
Dopamine	Dopaminergic receptors β receptors α > β receptors	0.5 to 4 4 to 10 11 to 20	Renal vasodilatation Inotropic Peripheral vasoconstriction Increased PVR Dysrhythmias
Dobutamine	β_1 and β_2 receptors	1 to 20	Inotropic Vasodilatation (β_2) Lowered PVR Weak alpha activity Tachycardic and extrasystoles
Isoproterenol	β_1 and β_2 receptors	0.05 to 2.0	Inotropic Vasodilatation Lowered PVR Increased MVo_2 Dysrhythmias
Epinephrine	β > α receptors	0.05 to 1.0	Inotropic Tachycardia Decreased renal flow Increased MVo_2 Dysrhythmias
Norepinephrine	α > β receptors	0.05 to 1.0	Profound constrictor Inotropic Increased MVo_2, SVR
Sodium nitroprusside	Vasodilator—arterial > venous	0.5 to 10	Rapid onset, short duration Increased ICP V/Q mismatch Cyanide toxicity
Nitroglycerin	Vasodilator—venous > arterial	1 to 20	Decreased PVR Increased ICP
PGE_1	Complex	0.05 to 0.2	Vasodilatation Open ductus arteriosus
Amrinone	PDE_3 inhibitor	1 to 20	Inotropic Chronotropic Vasodilatation

From Wetzel RC, Tobin JR. Shock. In: Rogers MC, ed. Textbook of pediatric intensive care. 2nd ed. Baltimore: Williams & Wilkins; 1992:600.
ICP, Intracranial pressure; *MVo₂*, myocardial oxygen consumption; *PDE₃*, phosphodiesterase inhibitor; *PVR*, pulmonary vascular resistance; *SVR*, systemic vascular resistance; *V/Q*, ventilation/perfusion.

function. If restoration of function is delayed or does not occur, additional organ dysfunction will occur, resulting in MODS.

Mechanical support. Intraaortic balloon pumping (IABP), ventricular assist devices (VADs), and extracorporeal life support (ECLS) can also play a part in managing children with cardiovascular failure.[21] The use of IABP is limited in the pediatric population. It augments diastolic and coronary blood flow by cyclic diastolic counterpulsation produced by a balloon in the descending aorta. VADs supply temporary support of ventricular function. The type most commonly used in children is the centrifugal VAD that supplies a continuous flow of blood through rotation of the centrifugal pump. A nonpulsatile flow produces a constant mean arterial pressure. ECLS is a type of cardiopulmonary bypass used to oxygenate the blood in the critically ill child.[21] Regardless of the type of therapy, the nurse caring for the child must be knowledgeable about the indications, routine care, and potential complications.

CENTRAL NERVOUS SYSTEM DYSFUNCTION
Anatomic and physiologic differences

Development of the neurologic system is rapid during the first few years of life. At birth, the infant operates at a subcortical level that consists primarily of brainstem function and spinal reflexes. Cortical development is nearly complete by 2 years of age. The brain itself grows rapidly; it is 25% of its mature adult weight at birth and reaches 75% of its mature adult weight by 2½ years. The response to injury is also different in the child compared to that in the adult. Children have a lower incidence of mass lesions in response to trauma, but a higher incidence of intracranial hypertension.

Pathophysiologic alterations

Cerebral injuries are often classified as primary or secondary. The primary injury occurs during the initial event and results in neuronal death at the time of injury. Secondary injury occurs after the primary injury and is caused by the inability of the cerebral vasculature to deliver adequate oxygen and glucose to the neurons; ischemia, hypoxia, anoxia, or metabolic derangements result.[22] Interventions must be directed at limiting secondary injury because very little can be done about the primary injury. The resulting cerebral ischemia and secondary injury cause swelling of the cerebral tissue and increased intracranial pressure (ICP). The skull of an infant does have open sutures that allow for some compensation as cerebral edema occurs. Eventually, however, if edema continues, the ICP will rise.

Therapeutic management

Assessment. Nursing management focuses on preventing secondary injury. Assessment begins with an evaluation of airway, breathing, and circulation.[23] Adequate ventilation is ensured in order to restore perfusion and oxygen delivery. Inadequate ventilation leads to increased partial arterial pressure of carbon dioxide ($PaCO_2$), which elevates the ICP. The respiratory assessment focuses on rate and rhythm and abnormal breathing patterns that may indicate changes in sensorium and ICP. The abnormal patterns can negatively affect oxygenation in the child and alter cerebral blood flow and ICP. Breath sounds are evaluated frequently to detect signs of neurogenic pulmonary edema, which is often associated with intracranial hypertension. Careful observation of the color and temperature of extremities, capillary refill, color of nailbeds and mucous membranes, pulses, blood pressure, and heart rate is valuable in assessing perfusion in the child. Changes in these parameters could indicate shock or increasing ICP.

The classic Cushing's triad, which consists of bradycardia, increasing systolic blood pressure, and widening pulse pressure, frequently indicates increasing ICP and impending herniation. This phenomenon is not often seen in infants and does not provide a reliable assessment of ICP in this group of patients.

After the airway, breathing, and circulation are evaluated, a thorough ongoing neurologic assessment is necessary using the Glasgow coma scale or other neurologic scales. These tools are used to pinpoint the level of consciousness of the patient and identify high-risk patients. The Glasgow coma scale provided in the box on p. 339 has been modified for use with children. Scores of less than 9 suggest very severe injury and are associated with high mortality. These patients will need airway support and are potential candidates for ICP monitoring and other invasive hemodynamic monitoring.[24]

Pupil size and reactivity, cranial oculovestibular reflexes, and oculocephalic reflexes need to be evaluated frequently. Cortical function can be assessed by giving the child simple directions and assessing the ability to follow them. Assessment includes observing for changes in muscle tone and posture. Observation for abnormal posturing is important. Decorticate postures are associated with cortical or hemispheric dysfunction, and decerebrate postures correlate with high pontine and midbrain lesions. Flaccidity indicates severe low brainstem dysfunction and may signal imminent death.

Seizures are often associated with severe head injuries, diffuse cerebral edema, and acute subdural hematoma and should be treated aggressively.[25,26] Seizure activity leads to increased cerebral blood

MODIFIED GLASGOW COMA SCALE FOR INFANTS

Eye opening

No response	1
Response to pain	2
Response to voice	3
Spontaneously	4

Verbal response

No response	1
Moans to pain	2
Cries to pain	3
Irritable cries	4
Coos and babbles	5

Motor response

No response	1
Abnormal extension	2
Abnormal flexion	3
Withdraws to pain	4
Withdraws to touch	5
Normal spontaneous movements	6
Maximum score	**15**

From Davis RJ et al. In: Rogers MC, ed. Textbook of pediatric intensive care. Baltimore: Williams & Wilkins; 1987:658.

flow and ICP. Immediate control can be established using diazepam or phenobarbital. Phenytoin can be given for long-term control, because posttraumatic seizures may occur for 1 to 2 years after injury.[27]

Normal ICP limits are 10 to 15 mm Hg for children and less than 10 mm Hg for infants.[28] Normal cerebral perfusion pressure is greater than 50 mm Hg. ICP can be assessed in infants by palpating the anterior fontanel. A bulging fontanel is often associated with increased ICP; however, this is a very subjective measurement. Invasive ICP monitoring techniques provide a much more objective measurement.

Current techniques for monitoring ICP include intraventricular devices, subarachnoid monitors, epidural monitors, and intraparenchymal devices.[29] Intraventricular catheters provide a very reliable measurement of ICP and allow for removal of small amounts of cerebrospinal fluid (CSF) to treat rising ICP. These devices, however, are associated with greater morbidity because of their position in the ventricle. Subarachnoid devices are simple to use and relatively noninvasive, but they are difficult to insert in infants, often significantly underestimate the ICP, and do not allow the removal of large amounts of CSF to lower the ICP.[27,29] Epidural catheters are used minimally with children and their accuracy and reliability are not well documented. Intraparenchymal devices are used more frequently and evidence supports their reliability.[30]

Control of ICP. Many methods may be used to control ICP, and expert nursing care is critical to successful management. One of the most effective means of controlling ICP is by manipulating the $Paco_2$. It is important that the $Paco_2$ be maintained between 25 and 35 mm Hg so that excessive cerebral blood flow will be prevented. Lowering the $Paco_2$ below 25 mm Hg can cause additional cerebral ischemia, and the resulting respiratory alkalosis can interfere with tissue oxygenation. Carbon dioxide levels should be continuously monitored with end-tidal carbon dioxide monitors and frequent arterial blood gas measurements.

Temperature control is very important in managing ICP and overall oxygen demand, and antipyretics and cooling blankets are frequently required to treat hyperthermia. If a blanket is used, continuous temperature monitoring and interventions to reduce shivering will be necessary. The head of the bed should be elevated and the head of the patient should be kept midline to facilitate venous drainage. Elevation may improve the compliance of the cranial vault; the optimal level of elevation may be different from patient to patient.[29] Isometric muscle contractions increase intrathoracic and intraabdominal pressures, thus decreasing cerebral venous drainage and increasing cerebral blood volume and ICP.[31] These contractions can be caused by hip and knee flexion, abnormal posturing, shivering, and pushing on the footboard. Nursing care must be directed at preventing isometric contraction by log rolling the child when turning, avoiding footboards, using high-top tennis shoes, controlling posturing with pancuronium or vecuronium, and reducing shivering with chlorpromazine (Thorazine). Rest periods should be provided between activities, and procedures should be accomplished as quickly as possible. Certain activities such as suctioning, using the bedpan, coughing, chewing, and conversations that center around the child but do not include the child have been shown to increase ICP.[32] Noxious stimuli, including loud noises, painful procedures, and nontherapeutic touch, are also associated with elevating ICP, especially during rapid eye movement (REM) sleep.[33] Purposeful touch, on the other hand, decreases ICP,[34] and families should be encouraged to talk with and touch the child as much as possible. Since suctioning causes increased ICP, it should be preceded by adequate oxygenation and limited to 10 seconds. Drugs such as lidocaine and thiopental given before suctioning may prevent an acute rise in ICP during the procedure.[29]

In general, children with a cerebral injury are fluid restricted. Two thirds of the normal requirement for maintenance is adequate for minor cerebral injuries, and one half to one third of the normal maintenance requirement is adequate for more severe injuries. This restriction is implemented upon a hemodynamically stable patient, with an adequate blood pressure, urine output, and peripheral perfusion.[29] Hypotonic fluids are avoided, with lactated Ringer's solution or half-normal saline being appropriate fluids to use.

Pharmacologic support. Diuretics are useful in reducing ICP and are usually given in conjunction with fluid restrictions. Osmotic diuretics such as mannitol, glycerol, and urea are commonly used in children to treat ICP and reduce brain bulk. Of this group mannitol is the most commonly used. Unfortunately, mannitol can draw fluid from uninjured tissue as well as damaged cells, causing fluid and electrolyte imbalances. Mannitol is given in a wide dose range from 0.25 g/kg to 2.0 g/kg.[29] Side effects of high-dose therapy are significant and include hyperosmolality, hemolysis, renal failure, and rebound intracranial hypertension. Lower doses of 0.25 g/kg are recommended and are associated with good results and fewer problems.[29] Osmolality should be maintained at normal levels (300 mOsm/L) by using judicious amounts of osmotic diuretics. If the child does become hyperosmolar, administration of hypotonic fluids to reduce the osmolality will exacerbate the cerebral edema.[29]

Loop diuretics such as furosemide and ethacrynic acid are also used in the management of ICP, but their role is less defined. These drugs reduce swelling by limiting the amount of sodium available for reabsorption into the CSF. They are often administered with other agents in order to increase the effectiveness of therapy. The recommended dose of furosemide is 0.5 to 1.0 mg/kg every 4 to 6 hours.[22]

Serum sodium and potassium levels are closely monitored in any patient receiving loop diuretics. Daily weights are also necessary.

Steroids are often used in the management of ICP, but the benefit is unclear. There is no clear evidence of their value in improving outcome, and considerable risks are associated with their use. If used, the patient is closely monitored for gastrointestinal bleeding, immunosuppression, and glucose intolerance.[29]

Another controversial therapy involves barbiturates such as pentobarbital. The purpose of this treatment, which is generally used for refractory intracranial hypertension, is to decrease cerebral metabolic rate and demand for oxygen. In addition to decreasing ICP, barbiturate coma also suppresses cardiovascular, respiratory, immunologic, and liver function. A loading dose is followed by a continuous infusion of pentobarbital to maintain a desired serum level or intracranial pressure.[29] The use of barbiturate coma eliminates the ability of the clinician to evaluate the neurologic status of the child by physical examination, and the EEG will be invalid.

HEMATOLOGIC SYSTEM DYSFUNCTION

Although hematologic failure occurs less frequently in children than in adults,[1] it is a common problem in critically ill children. Normal coagulation in children and adults is the result of an organized series of events that involves the blood vessels, platelets, plasma proteins, and the fibrinolytic system. Each component plays a vital role in the coagulation process, and a deficiency of, or damage to, any of these coagulation components can result in uncontrolled and abnormal hemostasis, blood loss, and fluid volume deficit.

Pathophysiologic alterations

Thrombocytopenia. The normal platelet count for children and adults is 150,000 to 400,000/mm^3, and thrombocytopenia is defined as a count less than 150,000/mm^3. In neonates, the normal platelet count is lower, and thrombocytopenia is defined as a count less than 100,000/mm^3.[35] Inadequate quantities of platelets or defective platelets will alter hemostasis and result in bleeding. Certain drugs that are frequently used to treat children, such as antibiotics, antihistamines, nonsteroidal antiinflammatory agents, phenothiazines, and vinca alkaloids, have been known to cause platelet dysfunction.

Even so, the most common cause of bleeding in critically ill children is not defective platelet function but inadequate quantities of platelets.[36]

Children experience a variety of bleeding disorders. Some are congenital coagulation disorders, such as hemophilia or Christmas disease, in which there is a deficiency of essential plasma proteins. More commonly, children develop acute acquired bleeding disorders generally associated with platelet defects or plasma protein dysfunction or deficiencies. Idiopathic thrombocytopenic purpura (ITP), thrombocytopenia resulting from certain diseases, autoimmune disorders, and bone marrow failure syndromes are disorders caused by platelet defects (see the box to the right). Disseminated intravascular coagulation (DIC), liver failure, and vitamin K deficiency are examples of disorders caused by plasma protein dysfunction or deficiencies.

ITP usually occurs in a healthy child after a viral infection. The physical appearance of the child is generally normal except for petechiae, ecchymosis, and hemorrhage from the nose or mouth.[30] Occasionally acute intracerebral bleeding occurs, but generally the child is not acutely ill and recovers spontaneously within several weeks. Hemolytic-uremic syndrome is a serious disorder that causes decreased platelets. It is usually characterized by acute renal failure and hemolytic anemia.[37] Children with this syndrome are hypertensive, volume overloaded, and anemic.

Bacterial and viral infections, especially in neonates, also result in low platelet counts. These infants do not hemorrhage, although they have significant thrombocytopenia. Children with bone marrow failure also have problems with platelet production and usually bleed more profusely than do other children with equivalent platelet counts.[37] Whatever the cause, treatment is aimed at correcting the underlying process and restoring normal platelet counts and functions.

Disseminated intravascular coagulation. Plasma proteins and the fibrinolytic system have similar functions in adults and children. The end-product of coagulation is a fibrin clot, and the function of the fibrinolytic system is to dissolve the clot and restore blood flow. Normally, these activities occur with precision; however, diffuse endothelial or organ destruction can lead to severe disruption of the process. DIC is characterized by uncoordinated coagulation and fibrinolysis.[38] The pathophysiology is the same for children and adults (see Chapter 4). Excessive amounts of thrombin are produced, the coagulation factors, fibrinogen, and platelets are consumed, and the fibrinolytic system is continuously activated. The result is a clinical picture of hemorrhage and microthrombosis that can lead to organ ischemia and high mortality.

DIC is not a primary disease, but results from an underlying illness or injury (see the box on p. 342). DIC is present in nearly all critically ill patients. It is often low grade and causes little clinical change because the spleen, liver, and bone marrow can compensate by increasing production of platelets and clotting factors and normalizing hemostasis. In

---

ETIOLOGY OF THROMBOCYTOPENIA

Decreased production of platelets
Bone marrow suppression (chemotherapy)
Aplastic anemia
Malignancy
Congenital amegakaryocytosis

Accelerated destruction or loss (nonimmune) of platelets
Congenital
   TORCH infections
   Giant hemangioma
Acquired
   HUS, thrombotic thrombocytopenic purpura
   Infection
   DIC
   Necrotizing enterocolitis
   Massive transfusion
   Hypersplenism

Accelerated destruction or loss (immune) of platelets
Infection
Idiopathic thrombocytopenic purpura
Neonatal passive immunization
Autoimmune disorders
Drug-induced

From Gordon JB, Bernstein ML, Rogers MC. Hematologic disorders in the pediatric intensive care unit. In: Rogers MC, ed. Textbook of pediatric intensive care. 2nd ed. Baltimore: Williams & Wilkins; 1992:1376.
DIC, Disseminated intravascular coagulation; *HUS,* hemolytic-uremic syndrome; *TORCH,* toxoplasmosis, rubella, cytomegalovirus, herpes.

> **DISORDERS ASSOCIATED WITH DISSEMINATED INTRAVASCULAR COAGULATION**
>
> Sepsis
> Shock
> Severe (penetrating) head injury
> Thermal injuries
> Snake bite
> Fresh-water drowning
> Acute promyelocytic leukemia
> Necrotizing pneumonitis
> Transfusion reactions

From Kedar A, Gross S. Disseminated intravascular coagulation. In: Blumer J, ed. A practical guide to pediatric intensive care. 3rd ed. St Louis: Mosby; 1990:518.

MODS, however, these hematologic organs often suffer damage, and they cannot adequately compensate for the disrupted coagulation. Birth depression (Apgar score <3 at 1 minute and <7 at 5 minutes) and sepsis are the most common causes of DIC in the newborn.[36] Necrotizing enterocolitis (NEC) and respiratory distress syndrome also may be associated with DIC in the neonate.

The treatment of DIC centers on identifying and treating the underlying disease process. Correction of the associated shock, acidosis, and electrolyte imbalances is critical. Laboratory findings in children are similar to those in adults. Blood component replacement therapy is controversial, but packed red blood cells, platelets, fresh frozen plasma, coagulation factors, and cryoprecipitate transfusions are often essential to treat hypovolemia and to replace clotting components. Exchange transfusions have been used in infants with limited success. Heparin infusions have been used with adults and children in an attempt to inhibit thrombin activity. This therapy is often unsuccessful and, in fact, may cause more bleeding. Antithrombin III concentrate infusions have been used in adults and neonates with some success. Other options such as low molecular weight fractions of heparin are becoming available but, in children, are still considered investigational.[36]

Liver disease. Liver disease and Vitamin K deficiency should also be considered when managing coagulopathies in children. Bleeding may be the first sign of liver disease, which is often accompanied by hepatomegaly, jaundice, and other obvious signs of liver failure. Treatment is often not necessary, but serious bleeding can occur. Vitamin K deficiency can result from inadequate nutritional status, and the onset can be rapid. Children who have illnesses that inhibit fat absorption, such as biliary atresia and cystic fibrosis, are at risk for vitamin K deficiency. Children who ingest rat poison or take certain drugs such as phenytoin, vitamin E, or aspirin are also at risk for vitamin K deficiency. Replacement therapy to restore vitamin K levels can be given orally, intramuscularly, or intravenously.

Therapeutic management

Nursing assessments are essential for early detection of hematologic dysfunction. Prolonged bleeding from venipuncture sites; oozing from wounds and catheter insertion sites; bleeding from gums and teeth; blood in gastric contents, urine, and stools; and petechiae and ecchymosis are critical nursing observations. Careful monitoring of laboratory values such as white blood count, hematocrit, platelet count, prothrombin time, and fibrin split products provides valuable information. Since thrombocytopenia is frequently present in acute DIC, the nurse must be alert for signs of bleeding and must avoid damage to the skin and mucous membranes.

Nursing measures such as meticulous skin and mouth care are essential. Accurate records of intake and output are necessary, as is continuous monitoring of vital signs. Good pulmonary hygiene is mandatory; however, caution must be used to prevent bleeding. An accurate assessment of the response of the child to blood product transfusion is necessary. Documentation of the need for blood products can help assess the progression of the hematologic failure. Nursing and medical interventions are generally aimed at supporting the child until the underlying illness is reversed.

RENAL SYSTEM DYSFUNCTION

Renal dysfunction and failure are problems seen often in critically ill children and complicate the management of these patients. However, the study by Wilkinson and co-workers documents renal failure in only 8% of the children with MSOF.[1] Even though renal failure is a significant complication in the critically ill pediatric patient, children do not die primarily from renal failure. Most cases of acute renal failure in children are potentially reversible with optimal management, such as renal replacement therapies.[39] In spite of this, the impact of renal failure in critically ill children is great. Renal failure occurs suddenly, and normal compensatory mechanisms are often unable to respond quickly enough to prevent life-threatening complications.[40] Critical illness itself adds stress to the kidneys because they work to maintain homeostasis and rid the body of by-products of tissue breakdown. Interventions for critical illness such as volume replacement, transfusions, and drug therapies place added burden on the kidneys and often have toxic side effects.[41]

Anatomic and physiologic differences

The normal urine output for a child is 1.0 mL/kg/hour. The infant has less ability to concentrate urine and, therefore, an output of 2.0 mL/kg/hour is considered normal. Also, because of the diminished ability of infants to concentrate urine urine with a low specific gravity does not indicate that the infant is adequately hydrated. Infants and young children have a larger body surface area (BSA) in relation to body weight, and maintenance fluid requirements are based on BSA. The extracellular fluid compartment of a child has a higher percentage of body water than does that of an adult. Children also have a higher amount of insensible water loss because of a higher basal metabolic rate, larger BSA, and higher metabolic rate.[42]

Pathophysiologic alterations

When acute renal failure (ARF) does occur in children, oliguric failure, which is defined as a urine output less than 0.5 mL/kg/hr, is most commonly seen. ARF can be caused by many conditions, including hypovolemia, peripheral vasodilatation and hypotension, renal vasoconstriction, nephrotoxins, or primary parenchymal renal disease (see the box below).

Causes of renal failure are usually categorized as prerenal, intrarenal, and postrenal. Prerenal and postrenal failures are reversible with rapid correction of the precipitating event. These conditions can, however, progress to intrarenal failure if not corrected, and the damage may become irreversible.

CAUSES OF ACUTE RENAL FAILURE

Prerenal disease
True volume depletion
Hemorrhage
Dehydration
Third-space sequestration

Vasodilatation
Sepsis
Antihypertensives

Edematous states
Heart failure
Hepatic disease (hepatorenal syndrome)
Hypoalbuminemia (nephrosis and protein-losing enteropathy)

Renal ischemia
High doses of vasopressor agents
Bilateral renal artery stenosis (exacerbated by ACE [angiotensin converting enzyme] inhibitors)
Nonsteroidal antiinflammatory drugs
Cyclosporin A
Renal artery thrombosis (in neonates related to umbilical artery catheter)

Intrarenal disease ("fixed" renal failure)
Postischemia: any prerenal insult, if prolonged, can result in "fixed" renal failure

Nephrotoxins
Aminoglycoside antibiotics and amphotericin B
Radiocontrast material
Chemotherapy (cisplatin and others)
Heme pigments (myoglobinuria and hemoglobinuria)

Primary renal disease
Hemolytic uremic syndrome
Glomerulonephritis (primary and secondary)
Interstitial nephritis (drug related and infectious)

Postrenal disease
Obstruction
Urethral or bladder neck
Ureterovesicle junction
Ureteropelvic junction
(Can be congenital or related to stones, blood clots, or extrinsic compression such as masses and retroperitoneal fibrosis)

From Stork J. Acute renal failure. In: Blumer J, ed. A practical guide to pediatric intensive care. 3rd ed. St Louis: Mosby; 1990:430.

The development of renal failure in the child with MODS is often attributed to acute renal tubular dysfunction, which may be caused by hypoperfusion, immune mediators, immune-complex deposition, antibiotics, or the use of vasopressors.[39] Renal function failure results in alterations in hematopoiesis, acid-base regulation, urea clearance, and electrolyte balance.[39]

Therapeutic management

The clinical picture and management of ARF are similar, regardless of the cause or the age of the patient. Patients are at risk for volume overload, hypertension, peripheral edema, skin breakdown, and infection. Electrolyte disturbances such as hyperkalemia, hyponatremia, hypernatremia, hyperphosphatemia, hypocalcemia, and hypermagnesemia are frequently seen. A severe metabolic acidosis often develops because the kidneys are unable to excrete hydrogen ions, and azotemia develops slowly as evidenced by rising blood urea nitrogen and creatinine levels.

Hypertension is commonly associated with ARF. It may be due to volume overload, especially with parenchymal renal disease. Moderate hypertension can generally be controlled by careful fluid management and efforts to decrease fluid overload. If significant hypertension persists, parenteral medication should be considered. These medications should be administered in a controlled setting with the ability to monitor mean blood pressure accurately. A rapid intravenous push of 5 mg/kg of diazoxide has a direct arterial vasodilating effect, with a peak effect in 5 minutes after administration and a duration of 4 to 12 hours. Sodium nitroprusside administered at 0.5 to 8.0 μg/kg/min has an immediate onset and acts by reducing afterload and preload and dilating arteries.[43] Hydralazine administered at 0.1 to 0.2 mg/kg may be used in moderately severe hypertension.[44]

Low-dose dopamine at 1 to 3 μg/kg/min is used to increase renal flow and improve urine output in children with ARF. Renal vasodilatation may persist with doses up to 15 μg/kg/min. Higher doses, however, are associated with renal vasoconstriction. Diuretics such as mannitol or furosemide may be used in an effort to avert ARF or improve urine output.[41]

Hyperkalemia may require emergent interventions. As a rule, a patient with a potassium level of 7.0 mEq/L or above or with symptomatic hypokalemia is treated.[45] Efforts to decrease potassium may include administration of calcium gluconate as first-line therapy for patients with ECG changes. Another therapy to decrease potassium levels is to administer sodium bicarbonate or intravenous (IV) glucose with insulin.[45] If the child continues to be hypercatabolic or has marked elevation of uremic toxins, dialysis may be indicated. Children with MODS and cardiovascular instability may not tolerate dialysis. Hemodialysis poses definite risks for the hemodynamically unstable patient because of fluid shifts. Peritoneal dialysis (PD) may not be totally effective if the child is hypotensive and has reduced splanchnic blood flow.[46] In addition, PD with large fluid volumes can create increased intraabdominal pressure, worsening hemodynamic instability, if present, and it is also associated with hypernatremia or hyponatremia. Hemofiltration through CAVH, CVVH, CAVH-D, or CVVH-D will be indicated for these children for management of fluid overload and of the metabolic abnormalities of acute renal failure. It is critical that nurses be knowledgeable about the responsibilities associated with caring for children receiving these therapies.

Anticipation is a critical component in the management of renal failure. Maintaining an adequate intravascular volume is vital. Ongoing nursing assessments focus on the state of hydration of the child to recognize dehydration or fluid overload. Dry mucous membranes, postural changes in heart rate and blood pressure, "tenting" of the skin, and a sunken fontanel may indicate dehydration. Peripheral edema, rales, liver enlargement, gallop, or hypertension may be associated with volume overload. Careful fluid management is required and includes frequent assessment and accurate documentation of intake and output, because these children are often fluid restricted or receiving fluid challenges or diuretics. Diapers are weighed to measure urine output if a catheter is not in place. All output is measured, including blood loss, gastrointestinal drainage, and stools. Daily weights are recorded using the same scale each day for accuracy. The response of the child to all interventions is documented to assess their effectiveness. Frequent monitoring of blood pressure, pulmonary capillary wedge pressures, CO, and urine specific gravity are important measures. A continuous electrocardiogram (ECG) is displayed to watch for changes associated with hyperkalemia. Serial assessment of laboratory data such as serum and urine creatinine, blood urea nitrogen, and serum and urine electrolytes is a vital nursing function.

HEPATIC DYSFUNCTION
Anatomic and physiologic differences

The normal position of the liver border varies with age and is not normally protected by the costal margin. In the newborn, the liver border may be up to 3 cm below the costal margin. The border can be up to 2 cm below the costal margin in a 1-year old, and 1 cm below the costal margin in a 4- to 5-year old. If the liver extends beyond these normal parameters, it may be a sign of early congestive heart failure, tumor, or hepatitis. However, since children sequester fluid in their livers during fluid overload, liver enlargement may not be a sign of heart failure.

Pathophysiologic alterations

The liver is assumed to play a major role in the evolution of MODS because of its diverse blood supply, multiple functions, and proximity to the gastrointestinal tract and lungs.[4] There is no consensus, however, as to whether ischemia, hypoxia, or direct cellular damage causes the MODS.[39] Hepatic failure in the child with MODS is defined as a total bilirubin level of greater than 5 mg/dL, serum glutamyl-oxaloacetic transaminase (SGOT) or lactate dehydrogenase (LDH) more than twice the normal value (without evidence of hemolysis), and hepatic encephalopathy of greater than or equal to grade II.[2] The mechanism of hepatic injury in the child with MODS has been described as a primary mechanism that occurs even when the tissues are well perfused. This mechanism is felt to be mediated by the liver macrophage (Kupffer cell).[10] A stimulus such as endotoxin activates the Kupffer cell, which then releases mediators such as prostaglandins or interleukin-1 (IL-1). These mediators injure the surrounding hepatocytes and cause cell dysfunction or death. Ischemic damage may also play a role in cellular dysfunction.

Therapeutic management

The overall goal of therapy for the child with hepatic failure is to support the child until hepatic regeneration can occur. Collaborative management of the child with hepatic dysfunction therefore revolves around preventing and treating complications such as hepatic encephalopathy, cerebral edema, gastrointestinal bleeding, infection, respiratory failure, and hepatorenal syndrome. Assessment includes monitoring for abnormal signs and symptoms associated with liver disease. Encephalopathy, jaundice, ascites, and bleeding disorders are commonly seen. Basic monitoring should include hourly observation of pulse, respirations, blood pressure, level of consciousness, urine output, and central venous pressure. Arterial blood gases should be routinely measured and a toxicology screen drawn to rule out other causes of coma.

Hepatic encephalopathy. Serial neurologic examinations are necessary to provide a clinical picture of the degree of encephalopathy, which reflects the severity of liver failure. Table 15-7 describes the stages in the development of hepatic coma. Other

Table 15-7 Stages in Development of Hepatic Coma

Stage	Mental stage	Tremor	EEG findings
I (prodrome)	Euphoria, mild confusion, slurred speech, and disorder in sleep	Slight	Normal
II	Drowsiness	Present, easily elicited	Abnormal, generalized slowing
III	Asleep or stuporous most of the time; arousable confusion is pronounced	Usually present with cooperation	Slowing delta wave
IV	Not arousable, except sometimes in pain	Usually absent	Slowing delta wave

From Halpin TJ. Acute hepatic failure. In: Blumer JL, ed. A practical guide to pediatric intensive care. 3rd ed. St Louis: Mosby; 1990:136.

conditions that can worsen the encephalopathy include excessive protein load, respiratory alkalosis, hyponatremia, hypoglycemia, infection, upper intestinal bleeding, and administration of medications that alter the level of consciousness.

Cerebral edema associated with hepatic encephalopathy is the cause of death in as many as 40% of the patients with hepatic failure.[47] The etiology is poorly understood, but both edema and encephalopathy appear to be related, because patients who develop deeper levels of encephalopathy proceed to cerebral edema if the process is not stopped. Cerebral edema associated with hepatic encephalopathy has the same clinical picture as cerebral edema associated with any other condition and is treated similarly.

Ammonia intoxication has long been suspected as one of the major problems in hepatic encephalopathy. Serial measurement of serum ammonia levels provides a guide to the effectiveness of therapy for hyperammonemia. The degree of ammonia elevation does not correlate well with the grade of encephalopathy, but changes in the ammonia level will reflect changes in the encephalopathic picture.[48]

The child with liver failure will require a decrease in dietary protein to 0.5 to 1.0 g/kg/day in an attempt to keep ammonia levels within normal limits.[49] Another therapy is to decrease ammonia production by intestinal bacteria and intestinal absorption of ammonia. This is accomplished by administering a 1 mL/kg dose of lactulose three to six times per day to maintain one to two soft stools per day and administering 125 to 500 mg of neomycin four times per day through a nasogastric tube.[49] Gastrointestinal bleeding should be treated immediately, because blood in the gastrointestinal tract will cause an increased serum ammonia as the amino acids from blood proteins are broken down.

Liver function studies. Serum transaminase levels (alanine transaminase [ALT] and aspartate transaminase [AST]) will increase to 10 to 100 times normal levels with liver dysfunction, although the degree of increase does not reflect the severity of the disease. Tracking these enzyme levels does provide important information about the progression of the liver failure. Sustained elevations may reflect a continued ability of the liver to synthesize these enzymes, with a sudden decrease indicating imminent death of the child.[47]

Although the serum enzymes reflect the integrity of the hepatic cell, hepatic function is better assessed by monitoring bilirubin, prealbumin, and coagulation. Bilirubin levels can increase to more than 20 mg/dL, and prealbumin levels can decrease to 0 mg/dL and may not respond to nutritional support. Coagulation parameters such as prothrombin and partial thromboplastin times will be increased and fibrinogen levels will be decreased because of consumption. Serial monitoring of these values will guide therapy for the bleeding patient. Profound bleeding is treated with packed red blood cell, platelet, and fresh frozen plasma replacement, and vitamin K should be administered every day. Routine correction of hepatic coagulopathy is not recommended.[49]

Hypoglycemia. Profound hypoglycemia as a result of the decrease in gluconeogenesis is common, and early identification and treatment is essential, especially in the critically ill child whose glucose stores are already low. Serum glucose should be maintained at levels greater than 130 mg/dL but below the renal threshold to avoid glycosuria.[48] Alterations in serum sodium and potassium levels also occur frequently. Large doses of potassium may be necessary to maintain a normal serum potassium level, and sodium is administered to maintain the serum sodium level at 130 mg/dL.[48]

Gastrointestinal bleeding. Gastrointestinal bleeding is a complication experienced by 70% of patients with hepatic failure and is the cause of death in 30% of these patients.[47] Bleeding is caused by stress ulcers and portal hypertension, both of which are exacerbated by the coagulopathies associated with hepatic failure. The occurrence of stress gastritis can be reduced by closely monitoring the gastric pH and maintaining it at 4.5 or greater. H_2-receptor antagonists, antacids, and gentle nasogastric suction can be used to maintain the gastric pH. Cimetidine at 30 mg/kg/day or ranitidine at 2 to 4 mg/kg/day are two commonly used H_2-receptor antagonists.[50] If gastrointestinal bleeding does occur, standard therapy is indicated. This includes nasogastric lavage and administering blood and fresh frozen plasma.

Nutritional support is paramount for the child in hepatic failure. Parenteral nutrition should be started as soon as possible, providing 50 to 60 kcal/kg/day and protein at 0.5 to 1.0 g/kg/day.[49] The addition of branched-chain amino acids to hypertonic glucose may help improve the nutritional status of the child. Aromatic amino acid-containing solutions should be avoided. Fat emulsions should be restricted to the provision of essential fatty acids only.[49]

Complications. The child with hepatic failure is at risk for infections. The three most common infections are bacteremias, urinary tract infections, and aspiration pneumonias. The use of prophylactic antibiotics is not recommended, but worsening of encephalopathy, sudden development of hepatorenal syndrome, and new onset of fever or leukocytosis may indicate infection.[47] Measures such as meticulous hand washing and aseptic care of all lines and wounds are mandatory to prevent infection. Appropriate antibiotic therapy should be initiated immediately when signs of infection are noted.

Cardiovascular, respiratory, and renal failure can all occur in the child with hepatic failure. Cardiovascular and respiratory failure will be treated in the same manner as for any child with these conditions. Renal failure related to hepatic failure may respond to the use of mannitol (0.25 g/kg) and furosemide (0.5 mg/kg).[50]

NUTRITIONAL SUPPORT
Age-related factors

Provision of adequate substrate for energy metabolism is critical for supporting the child with MODS. Critically ill children are at risk for developing malnutrition because of increased energy requirements and increased protein catabolism associated with MODS. In addition, age-related factors make nutritional depletion more likely when adequate nutritional support is not provided. Children have larger obligate energy needs and lower macronutrient stores than do adults.[51] The combination of these two factors makes the child less likely to withstand nutritional depletion when nutritional support is not provided.

Several studies have demonstrated that malnutrition does exist in critically ill children. Malnutrition and fat and protein depletions are common, especially in children under 2 years of age.[52] Also, acute malnutrition in critically ill children is associated with increased physiologic instability and increased requirements for care as evidenced by higher Physiologic Stability Index (PSI) and Therapeutic Intervention Scoring System (TISS) scores.[53]

Assessment

Nutritional needs for the child with MODS must be addressed before complications and potentially irreversible changes related to malnutrition take place. The nurse plays an important role as the child's advocate for nutritional support. Performing the initial nutritional assessment by obtaining the height, weight, and head circumference of the child, if appropriate, and obtaining a diet history as part of the data base will help identify the patient at risk for nutrition-related complications.

By obtaining daily weights the nurse can monitor weight loss in the critically ill child. An unexplained weight loss of greater than 5% of the admission weight places the child nutritionally at risk. A weight loss of greater than 10% is associated with increased morbidity, and weight loss of greater than 30% is associated with increased mortality.[54]

The assessment of the child includes noting signs of possible nutritional deficiencies such as muscle wasting or weakness, dermatitis, tetany, growth retardation, central nervous system depression, and bleeding tendencies. Mortality is increased from 3% to 33% in children with malnutrition severe enough to depress cell-mediated immunity.[54] Other clinical parameters to note are those for hair, eyes, mouth, lips, tongue, skin, and extremities. Dryness, pallor, thinness, and other abnormalities are often signs of malnutrition. An in-depth nutritional assessment will include anthropometric measurements and laboratory studies such as serum albumin, serum transferrin, serum protein, and total lymphocyte count.

Therapeutic management

Nursing interventions start with advocating early nutritional support. In critically ill patients, a short ebb phase is followed by a long flow phase in which the stress hormone response is followed by a long course of enhanced metabolic activity. Critically ill children need nutritional support to maintain lean body mass and host defense, promote growth and development, and gain time for reversal of organ failure and eradication of sepsis. Nutritional support is provided based on the nutrient needs of the child as listed in Table 15-8.

Enteral feedings are preferable because they are physiologically normal and more efficient. A variety of enteral formulas are available, including specialized pediatric formulas for infants less than 12 months of age and for children between 1 and 5

Table 15-8 Estimated Daily Nutrient Needs for Children

Age (yr)	Calories (kcal/kg)	Protein (g/kg)
0 to 0.5	115	2.2
0.5 to 1	105	2.0
1 to 3	100	1.8
4 to 6	85	1.5
7 to 10	85	1.2
Male		
11 to 14	60	1.0
15 to 18	42	0.85
Female		
11 to 14	48	1.0
15 to 18	38	0.85

Modified from Walker W, Hendricks K: Manual of pediatric nutrition. Philadelphia: WB Saunders; 1985:53.

Table 15-9 Parenteral Nutrient Doses in Critically Ill Children

Nutrient	Initial dose	Approximate maintenance dose
Protein	0.5 to 1.5 g/kg/day*	3 to 4 g/kg/day†
Dextrose	5 to 7 mg/kg/min	To obtain calorie/nitrogen ratio of 150:1 to 200:1 in low stress and 80:1 to 125:1 in high stress 70 to 90 kcal/kg/day‡
Lipid	1 g/kg/day	2 to 4 g/kg/day§

*Decrease dose for renal or hepatic insufficiency.
†Decrease dose for renal or hepatic function; desired end point is stable or increasing transferrin.
‡Caloric intake may be increased with calorimetric evidence of increased resting energy expenditure.
§Measure plasma triglycerides 4 hours after discontinuing total parenteral nutrition for evidence of clearance.
From Steinhorn DM. Nutritional strategies in organ system failure. In: Blumer JL, ed. A practical guide to pediatric intensive care. 3rd ed. St Louis, Mosby; 1990:617.

years of age. Older children can usually receive enteral formulas developed for adults. Potential complications related to enteral feedings are intolerance as evidenced by vomiting, diarrhea, abdominal distention, or gastric retention, aspiration, infection, and fluid and electrolyte imbalances.

If the child is unable to tolerate enteral feedings, then total parenteral nutrition is initiated. Table 15-9 lists appropriate doses for parenteral nutrients in the critically ill child. As noted in the table, special considerations must be taken for the child in renal or hepatic failure.

Complications related to total parenteral nutrition are infection, liver dysfunction, hyperlipidemia, metabolic problems such as hyperglycemia and electrolyte imbalances, and technical problems such as occurrence of air emboli, pneumothorax, and catheter occlusion or breakage. Close monitoring and meticulous nursing care are essential to prevent these complications.

As the critically ill child begins to tolerate enteral feedings again, total parenteral nutrition is slowly discontinued. The weaning process occurs over a 1- to 3-day period with close monitoring of serum glucose to prevent hypoglycemia.

INFECTION
Pathophysiology

MODS, medical and nursing interventions, nutritional status, and stress all lead to an increased risk for infection for the critically ill child. Anatomic and physiologic differences in the pediatric immune system also place the child at increased risk for infection.[55] Many of the conditions that trigger MODS are known to cause immunosuppression in children. Injury in the form of thermal, mechanical, or surgical trauma affects humoral immunity more in children than it does in adults.[56] Profound depression in several immune functions in children has been demonstrated after hemorrhagic shock. Depressed neutrophil motility exists at low temperatures, and the movement of immune cells and proteins in the heart-lung machine has been shown to cause cell destruction, complement activation, and other changes that lead to depressed immunity.[56]

Along with immunosuppression, overactivation of the IIR can predispose the child to secondary complications. When a child sustains a severe insult such as surgery, hypoxia, sepsis, hemorrhage, or trauma, inflammatory cells are mobilized and activated as a result of this stress, and they release inflammatory mediators. Secondary injury results from overactivation of these mediators, and the IIR becomes exaggerated and uncontrolled.[56] An unregulated IIR is involved in a number of complications, including MODS, septic shock, DIC, and ARDS.

Because environmental, anatomic, and physiologic factors place the child at risk for infection, nursing assessment for signs of infection is critical. Because of the immaturity and alterations in the immune system of infants, the child may experience an overwhelming infection without the normal systemic signs such as fever and an increased white blood cell count. The nurse should observe for other signs of infection, such as temperature instability, hyperglycemia, hemodynamic instability, and changes in the level of consciousness.

Therapeutic management

Nursing interventions begin with good hand washing before all procedures and aseptic care of all lines and wounds. Wounds and invasive line sites are inspected daily, and surveillance cultures are obtained. Skin and mucous membranes are kept as intact as possible. Frequent skin and mouth care, turning every 2 hours, and keeping the skin clean will help protect the first-line defense against infection. Antibiotics are administered as ordered, and the response of the child should be closely observed and documented.

SKIN INTEGRITY
Anatomic and physiologic differences

The integumentary system is not mature at birth; therefore, it is not a very effective barrier against physical elements or microorganisms. The skin is thinner at birth and more permeable because of smaller amounts of stratum corneum. The skin pH is more alkaline at birth, which increases susceptibility to infection, because a more acidic skin pH discourages the growth of microorganisms.[57] The infant possesses less subcutaneous fat than does the older child, so there is increased sensitivity to environmental changes.

Assessment

Nursing assessment of the skin should be conducted with adequate lighting so all areas can be viewed thoroughly. Mucous membranes, scalp, hair, and nails are included in skin assessment. Areas of dryness are noted because dry, cracked skin provides a portal of entry for bacteria. Areas where invasive lines are inserted and areas of breakdown are observed closely for signs of infection. In infants and young children, the diaper is removed and the perineal and buttock area observed for diaper rash, which can quickly lead to a severe skin breakdown.

Therapeutic management

It is critical that skin care be provided at least every 8 hours and more often, if indicated, to keep the skin clean and moist. Providing air flotation or EGGCRATE mattresses and turning the child every 2 hours will help prevent skin breakdown. Mouth care includes lubricating the mouth and cleaning the teeth every shift. Eye care in the unconscious child is provided by applying an ophthalmic ointment at least every 2 hours.

Infants and young children have larger body surface areas in proportion to their body weight and are more sensitive to environmental changes. These factors place them at risk for hypothermia, which can result in physiologic instability. Hypothermia will shift the oxyhemoglobin curve to the left, prevent the release of oxygen to the tissue, and increase oxygen consumption and glucose use in order to maintain the core temperature of the body. The child's temperature is closely monitored and measures taken to maintain a normal body temperature. Radiant warmers and hyperthermia blankets are useful for warming a child. Cooling blankets can be used for those children who are febrile and not responding to antipyretic medications. Shivering should be avoided because it increases body heat production and oxygen consumption.

PAIN MANAGEMENT
Age-related factors

Pain management is a very important part of the role of every nurse in the PICU. Pain is a complex, subjective, and elusive phenomenon.[58] The International Association for the Study of Pain describes it as "an unpleasant sensory and emotional experience with actual or potential tissue damage, as described in terms of such damage."[59] Pain is a completely subjective experience, it is defined as "what the patient says hurts" and exists "when the patient says it does."[60] Most definitions depend on the ability of the child to verbalize pain, but this is frequently not the case when dealing with infants, young children, and critically ill patients.

Many beliefs that exist about children and pain have interfered with adequate pain management. One of these beliefs is that infants and children do not feel or remember pain and therefore are unable to communicate their pain. Evidence refutes this statement, and numerous studies have documented the physiologic and behavioral responses of infants to painful stimuli.[61-63] These studies show that infants respond to stress with increased heart rate, blood pressure, and intracranial pressure. They also demonstrate simple motor responses, changes in facial expressions, and intense crying. The idea that complete nerve myelinization is necessary to experience pain is no longer supported by many clinicians. Current thinking is that the process of myelinization begins in utero, and the cortical and subcortical centers are well developed late in gestation.[64] This supports the idea that the newborn is capable of experiencing pain. There is much evidence to support the idea that infants and children do remember pain. Savedra and colleagues[65] report that children remember pain from many years earlier. Several studies have documented that children are able to describe the location and nature of their pain accurately, often using graphic words.[66,67]

Perception of pain in older children appears to be related to their level of cognitive development.[58] In theory, the preoperational child (2½ to 6 years of age) is unable to understand cause and effect relationships and will be more afraid and distressed by medical procedures than will be older children. The operational child (7 to 10 years of age), who is able to think more logically and realistically, should understand the need for procedures and exhibit less anxiety. As children get older (12 to 17 years of age), they can think more abstractly and give meaning to pain. This has been shown to increase their pain sensitivity.[68] Based on these perceptual differences, it is critical that the nurse consider the development level of the child when assessing and managing pain (Fig. 15-1).

Assessment

Assessment of pain usually involves collecting physiologic and behavioral data. The process should be ongoing and precede and follow all interventions to relieve or eliminate pain.[69] Physiologic responses indicate activation of the sympathetic nervous system, and commonly include increased heart rate, blood pressure, respiratory rate, diaphoresis, hyperventilation, pupil dilatation, and nausea and vomiting. However, nurses cannot infer or rule out pain, strictly on the basis of these parameters. Behavioral responses to pain must also be considered if a thorough assessment is desired. These responses might include crying, moaning, screaming, and facial and body expressions such as grimacing and rigidity. Behavioral observation tools have been developed that assist nurses in assessing pain. Instruments such as the Pediatric Pain Inventory,[67] Observational Scale of Behavioral Distress,[68] and CHEOPS[70] are designed for use with specific age groups to measure pain perceptions and behaviors. Other assessment tools such as the Body Outline,[71] Pain Ladder,[72] Heat Thermometer,[73] Stewart Color Scale,[74] and the McGill Pain Questionnaire[75] are age-specific and are used to describe the location, intensity, and quality of pain. Although these tools can be very valuable, their use is often impractical in the critical care environment, and they do not replace the skilled observations of the ICU nurse.

Therapeutic management

Interventions for pain are generally classified as nonpharmacologic and pharmacologic. Pharmacologic interventions must never be withheld if that is the most appropriate means to alleviate pain in a child. When administering pain medication to children, it is essential to monitor vital functions such as airway patency, ventilatory adequacy, heart rate and rhythm, and blood pressure. Pain relief must be achieved without profound respiratory or central nervous system (CNS) depression. Opiates are the most commonly used sedatives in the critical care setting, and intravenous administration is the preferred route. Morphine sulfate (0.1 to 0.2 mg/kg) has predictable analgesic and euphoric effects with an onset that is within 1 minute of administration.[76] It does cause histamine release and the potential for hypotension, tachycardia, and respiratory depression. Fentanyl (1 to 2 µg/kg) is a very potent, synthetically derived narcotic. The onset of pain relief is very rapid, the duration is short, and the side effects include respiratory and CNS depression, severe nausea and vomiting, and muscle rigidity.[60] Meperidine (1 to 2 mg/kg) is also widely used to manage pain in children. The onset and duration are similar to those of morphine sulfate, and the potential for respiratory and CNS depression also exists. Tremors, muscle twitches, and seizures sometimes occur.[60] Diazepam (0.2 to 0.5 mg/kg) is frequently used in children to achieve sedation and amnesia. Side effects include apnea, respiratory depression,

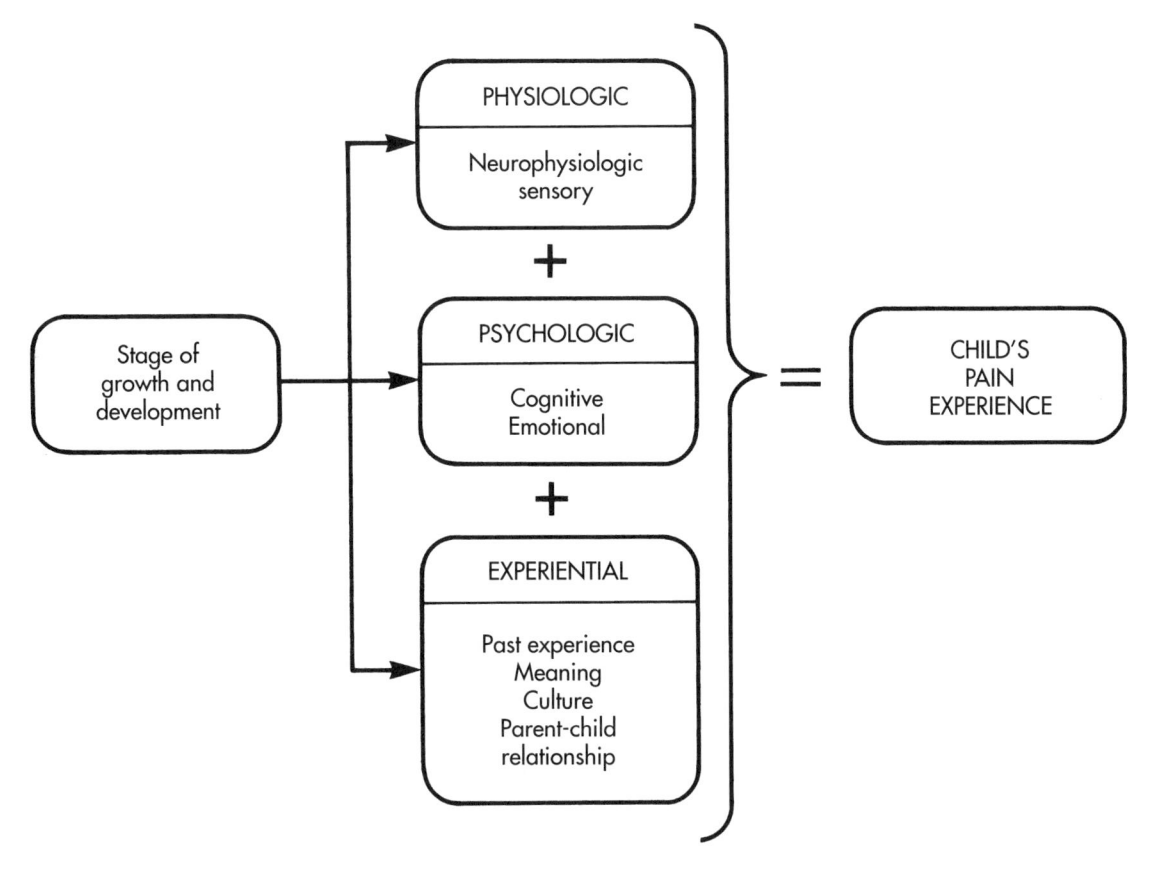

Fig. 15-1 Effect of stage of growth and development on the child's pain experience. (From Stevens B, Hunsberger M, Browne G. Pain in children: theoretical, research, and practice dilemmas. J Pediatr Nurs 1987, 2:159.)

and hypotension.[60] Other drugs, such as chloral hydrate, thiopental, midazolam, and diphenhydramine, can also play important roles in pediatric pain management. Combinations of drugs, such as fentanyl and midazolam, can be used very successfully and can reduce undesirable side effects. The response to combinations, however, may be less predictable than the response to single agents. Continuous drug infusions are also very effective and provide a more constant level of sedation instead of the uneven control provided by bolus doses.

Nurses and parents can often use nonpharmacologic techniques such as relaxation, distraction, guided imagery, and cutaneous stimulation in the critical care setting.[69] Relaxation is used to reduce the muscle tension that accompanies pain and may include simple techniques such as cuddling, holding, and rocking. Distractions are very effective with children and may include games, pop-up books, toys, songs, or stories. Guided imagery works well with children, because they can actively imagine. This technique requires that the child focus on a pleasant experience or place and then talk about the experience. Cutaneous stimulation measures are often used with children and include massage, pressure, and the use of heat and cold. Parents should be encouraged to participate in these interventions and should be taught how to perform them. Often a combination of nonpharmacologic and pharmacologic interventions will be the most effective approach to pain management in the child.

Management and Special Considerations

Minimizing the effects of the critical care environment by eliminating excess light, noise, and interruptions can also help alleviate pain. No matter what intervention is used, an ongoing assessment of the child's response is vital in order to accurately assess the effectiveness of pain management.

GROWTH AND DEVELOPMENT

A critical care unit can be a horrifying experience for the child. The child with MODS requires intensive technology and numerous, painful procedures that are completely foreign. The ability of the child to understand and develop means to cope with the experience is highly dependent on the developmental level, and nursing interventions to help the child cope must address these developmental differences.

Infants

Infants (from birth to 12 months of age) are at a stage where, according to Erikson, they are developing a sense of trust versus mistrust. They are not able to care for themselves and are totally dependent on those around them to meet their needs. Sight and sound provide stimulation, and play is important in their development. Stressors for this age group include separation from parents or primary caregivers, pain and intrusion, and immobilization. Immobilization is stressful because the infant uses motor activity as a means of exploration and also as a coping mechanism.[57]

Nursing interventions for the infant are focused upon providing a sense of trust. Infants are so acutely aware of their environment that calm, quiet, comforting surroundings are very important. Infants should be spoken to quietly, and stroking and cuddling can be used to soothe. The parents or primary caretaker need to be involved as much as possible in the child's care. Consistent caretakers help to provide a sense of security. Sudden movements are avoided, since these will startle the infant, and hands are always warmed before touching the infant. Exploration of the environment is allowed and encouraged, and mobiles should be at the bedside for the infant to look at, as well as toys for the infant to hold. Mirrors can provide hours of enjoyment because babies like to look at themselves.

Toddlers

Toddlers (1 to 3 years of age) are working at their developmental task of developing autonomy versus shame and doubt. They are assertive in expressing their will, though they are still very dependent upon their parents. They see the world from their view only. They are developing language skills quickly, though their receptive language skills are more advanced than their expressive skills. Their major stressors are separation from their parents or primary caretakers, pain and intrusion, and disruption of their rituals.[57] Ritualistic behavior provides a sense of self-control for toddlers as they develop new physical skills and abilities. Toddlers require active play as a means of furthering their social and motor development.

Toddlers need interventions that allow them to be dependent, yet be able to maintain their autonomy. Parents should be permitted to stay with their child and be encouraged to play with their child. Parents should also be encouraged to bring objects from home that will provide comfort. As the critically ill toddler becomes more stable, he or she should be allowed to play with and explore appropriate equipment such as stethoscopes, tongue blades, and syringe barrels and continue rituals. The child should be encouraged to talk about or draw pictures of the experience, if able, to have an outlet for frustration. When possible, the child should also be given choices. Explain to parents that the toddler often regresses as a means of coping when faced with stressful circumstances and that lost skills will be regained quickly.

Preschoolers

The preschooler (3 to 5 years of age) is developing a sense of initiative versus guilt. The child is acquiring more language skills, and there is a strong sense of self. The imagination is vivid and magical thinking is frequent. Major stressors for this age group are being alone, loss of self-control, pain and intrusion, and fear of mutilation.[57]

Effective nursing interventions for the preschooler include good explanations of equipment and procedures. Procedures should be explained immediately before they take place, and the nurse can help the child cooperate by explaining what is expected of him or her. Realistic limits on behavior should be set, and the child needs to be reassured that the procedure is necessary and is not a punishment. The child should be encouraged to ask questions and discuss feelings, using the ability to fantasize constructively. When possible, the child should participate in care. Like the toddler, the preschooler is comforted by favorite items from home.

School-age children

The school-age child (6 to 12 years of age) is developing a sense of industry verus inferiority. The child has well-developed language skills and is capable of verbalizing concerns and responding to reason and compromise. The child has a strong need to accomplish and will feel inferior if unable to achieve. The school-age child has an incomplete understanding of death. Major stressors for the school-age child include separation from parents and peer group, loss of self-control, loss of privacy, fear of the unknown, pain and intrusion, fear of disfigurement, and fear of death.[57]

The school-age child requires concrete answers to questions and can usually understand pathophysiology and treatment. Procedures are explained well beforehand, and, if possible, the child should be offered choices. The child should be encouraged to discuss his or her understanding of the event, which can help the child retain a sense of worth. Parents should be encouraged to visit, though the child may not want them present during procedures. Communication from siblings and schoolmates should also be suggested. At all times, the child's sense of modesty should be respected.

Adolescents

The adolescent (12 to 19 years of age) is seeking identity versus role confusion. Adolescence is characterized by rapid growth and emotional lability related to hormonal changes. The adolescent's cognitive level is comparable to that of an adult, yet adolescents have not had the adult life experiences that bring their thinking to a more mature level. They are usually able to and want to make their own decisions. Their peer group is very significant, because they are attempting to establish their own sense of belonging and self-esteem. Major stressors for adolescents include separation from their peers, loss of group status and acceptance, dependency, loss of self-control, and permanent disability and death.[57]

The autonomy of the adolescent needs to be respected at all times. Choices and control should be permitted as much as possible. Adolescents should be encouraged to maintain contact with their peers and family, although parents may need assistance in understanding their child's wish to be independent of them. Adolescents should be prepared for procedures as far in advance as possible to allow for questions and corrections of any misconceptions. Nurses should help the adolescent verbalize fears. Privacy must be maintained, and flexibility with hospital routines should be provided when possible.

FAMILY SUPPORT

Having a child with MODS in the critical care unit is an extremely stressful experience for the family. The child is critically ill with a dramatically changed appearance, and the family must cope with this frightening situation in a world of strangers. Nurses play a critical role in helping family members cope with this crisis. If the parents or primary caretakers are unable to cope with the hospitalization, then their ability to support and comfort their child will be disrupted.[77]

Parental needs

Miles and Carter[78] assessed parental needs and identified stressors in the pediatric critical care unit. Stressors identified were the environment, the appearance of the child, procedures, communication with staff, staff behavior, and changes in the parental role. Eberly and co-workers[79] studied parents of children in the pediatric ICU and found that the areas of highest stress were parental role, communication, and response to their child's behavior and appearance. Philichi[77] identified other parental needs in the pediatric critical care unit including the need to be with the child, to receive accurate and truthful information, to have a place to sleep and rest near the unit, to participate in the child's care, and to feel assured that the child's care and treatment are appropriate. Kirschbaum[80] found that parents had a need for information and for hope.

Therapeutic management

Based on these and many other research findings, there are many nursing interventions that can help the parents of a child with MODS in the critical care unit. Parents must be allowed to visit and stay with their child on a continuous, 24-hours-a-day basis. Questions should be answered honestly and accurately. The child's primary nurse should be with the parents when the physician talks to them to explain any issues that they may not understand. Nurses can guide parents to where they can sleep, bathe, and eat, and they should facilitate these activities as much as possible. Nurses can assist parents in touching and talking to their critically ill child. Encouragement to bathe and massage their child, read a story, and bring familiar items from home helps the parents feel that they are still maintaining their parental role. Sibling visitation should be an option especially if the parents request it. This requires careful preparation of the sibling by both the nurse and the parents.

A study conducted by Curley[81] validates the importance of nursing interventions in reducing parental stress. Parents were assigned randomly to two groups. One was a control group that received routine nursing contact. The treatment group received nursing intervention designed to allow the parents to participate in the care of their child to the extent that the parents wished and that the child's condition permitted. The parents in the intervention group reported significantly lower stress scores than the control group for four of the seven dimensions that have been reported as stressful for parents. An important finding in this study was that the nursing intervention was effective in reducing stress and that time, alone, did not account for stress reduction. This finding was further validated when the study was replicated and similar results were obtained.[82]

Parental grief

Mortality rates are high for children with MODS, so nurses will often be supporting parents whose child has died. At this time, care shifts entirely to the family, and support from the nursing staff must continue. It is important to assure parents that all possible measures were taken to save their child and that their child did not suffer. Further conversation can be guided by the parent's need for information. The presence of the nurse while the parents begin to experience the tremendous loss is helpful. Parents will often not remember the exact words that were said, but they will remember that someone cared enough to be with them during their grief. Parents should be allowed to spend as much time as they need to say goodbye to their child, and expressions of grief such as crying or screaming should not be discouraged.

It is helpful to the parents if the nurse who cared for the child makes contact with them shortly after the child's death. Usually the child with MODS was a patient in the critical care unit for a number of days or weeks, and the primary nurse has developed a relationship with the parents. Talking to the nurse gives the parents the opportunity to ask questions and express feelings that may have developed since the child's death. Many parents need continued reassurance and support as they experience the various stages of grief, and the nurse can play a key role in providing that support. Also, if appropriate, the nurse can recommend grief support groups for the parents.

CONCLUSION

MODS is the result of a variety of conditions in the critically ill child. In the child with MODS, the normal equilibrium between organ systems and protective responses does not exist. Disruption of organ function occurs, and the body attempts to compensate and regain equilibrium. Compensation and intervention will benefit certain organs but harm others, and when compensation and regulatory mechanisms fail, organ dysfunction occurs. The pathophysiology of MODS in the child is not tremendously different from the pathophysiology in adults. Anatomic and physiologic differences in each child, however, will affect his or her response to organ dysfunction and to treatment. No single therapy is based on treating MODS as a primary entity; therefore nursing and medical interventions focus on maximizing oxygen delivery, providing nutritional support, and supporting individual organ systems. The interventions must be based on reversing the primary entity, minimizing infection and inflammation, and preventing cellular damage.[10]

Although overall mortality rates are high, children have a better chance for survival than do adults. Expert nursing management is essential to maximize the potential for a positive outcome. More research on MODS in children is necessary, especially in the area of nursing interventions and their effect on patient outcomes.

REFERENCES

1. Wilkinson JD et al. Outcomes of pediatric patients with organ system failure. Crit Care Med 1986;14:271-274.
2. Wilkinson JD et al. Mortality associated with multiple organ system failure and sepsis in pediatric intensive care. J Pediatr 1987;111:324-328.

3. Proulx F et al. Timing and predictors of death in pediatric patients with multiple organ system failure. Crit Care Med 1994;22:1025-1030.
4. Cerra FB, Bihari D. Multiple organ failure: Critical care, state of the art. Soc Crit Care Med 1989;3:1-397.
5. Barton R, Cerra F. The hypermetabolism-multiple organ failure syndrome. Chest 1989;96:1151-1155.
6. Knaus WA, Wagner DP. Multiple systems organ failure: Epidemiology and prognosis. Crit Care Clin 1989;5:218-222.
7. Tran DD et al. Age, chronic disease, sepsis, organ system failure and mortality in a medical intensive care unit. Crit Care Med 1990;18:471-475.
8. Bersten A, Sibbald WJ. Circulatory disturbances in multiple system failure. Crit Care Clin 1989;5:229-235.
9. Graham P, Brass NJ. Multiple organ dysfunction: Pathophysiology and therapeutic modalities. Crit Care Nurs Q 1994;16:8-15.
10. Toro-Figuera LO. Multiple organ system failure. In: Levin DL, Morriss FC, eds. Essentials of pediatric intensive care. St. Louis: Quality Medical Publishing; 1990:186-193.
11. Witte M. Acute respiratory failure. In: Blumer J, ed. A practical guide to pediatric intensive care. 3rd ed. St. Louis: Mosby, 1990:95-103.
12. Eigen H. Adult respiratory distress syndrome. In: Blumer J, ed. A practical guide to pediatric intensive care. 3rd ed. St. Louis: Mosby, 1990:348-352.
13. Ring RC, Stidham GL. Novel therapies for acute respiratory failure. Pediatr Clin North Am 1994;41:1325-1363.
14. Tobias JD, Rasmussen GE. Pain management and sedation in the pediatric intensive care unit. Pediatr Clin North Am 1994;41:1269-1292.
15. Wetzel R, Rogers MC. Dysrhythmias and their management. In: Rogers M, ed. Textbook of pediatric intensive care. 2nd ed. Baltimore: Williams & Wilkins, 1992:532-562.
16. Blumer J. Shock. In: Blumer J, ed. A practical guide to pediatric intensive care. 3rd ed. St. Louis: Mosby, 1990:71-81.
17. Curley MAQ. Shock. In: Curley MAQ, Smith JB, Moloney-Harmon PA, eds. Critical care nursing of infants and children. Philadelphia: WB Saunders, 1996.
18. Rimar J. Recognizing shock syndromes in infants and children. MCN 1988;13:32-37.
19. Perkin R, Levin D. Shock. In: Levin DL, Morriss FC, eds. Essentials of pediatric intensive care. St. Louis: Quality Medical Publishing, 1990:78-97.
20. Schleien C et al. Postoperative management of the cardiac surgical patient. In: Rogers MC, ed. Textbook of pediatric intensive care. 2nd ed. Baltimore: Williams and Wilkins, 1992:467-531.
21. Philichi L. Multiple system organ failure in the pediatric population. Crit Care Nurs Q 1994;16:96-105.
22. Rekate H. Increased intracranial pressure. In: Blumer J, ed. A practical guide to pediatric intensive care. 3rd ed. St Louis: Mosby, 1990:239-246.
23. Aumick JE. Head trauma guidelines for care. RN 1991;54:27-31.
24. Hahn SE et al. Theories of brain resuscitation. In: Rogers MC, ed. Textbook of pediatric intensive care. 2nd ed. Baltimore: Williams & Wilkins, 1992:698-732.
25. Hahn YS et al. Factors influencing posttraumatic seizures in children. Neurosurgery 1988;22:864.
26. Moloney-Harmon PA. Pediatric issues in multisystem trauma. Crit Care Nurs Clin North Am 1989;1:85-94.
27. Luchka S. Working with ICP monitors. RN 1991;54:34-37.
28. Shapiro K, Giller CA. Increased intracranial pressure. In: Levin DL, Morriss FC, eds. Essentials of pediatric intensive care. St. Louis: Quality Medical Publishing, 1990:49-53.
29. Dean JM, Rogers MC, Traystman RJ. Pathophysiology and clinical management of the intracranial vault. In: Rogers MC, ed. Textbook of pediatric intensive care. 2nd ed. Baltimore: Williams and Wilkins, 1992:639-666.
30. Filloux F, Dean JM, Kirsch JR. Monitoring the central nervous system. In: Rogers MC, ed. Textbook of pediatric intensive care. 2nd ed. Baltimore: Williams and Wilkins, 1992:667-697.
31. Andrus C. Intracranial pressure: Dynamics and nursing management. J Neurosci Nurs 1991;23:85-91.
32. McQuillan K. Intracranial pressure monitoring: Technical imperatives. AACN Clin Issues Crit Care Nurs 1991;2:623-636.
33. Jastremski CA. Traumatic brain injury. Crit Care Nurs Clin North Am 1994;5:473-481.
34. Walleck CA. The effect of purposeful touch on intracranial pressure. 1983 National Teaching Institute, unpublished data.
35. Gordon JB et al. Hematologic disorders in the pediatric intensive care unit. In: Rogers MC, ed. Textbook of pediatric intensive care. Baltimore: Williams and Wilkins, 1987:1181-1222.
36. Gordon JB, Bernstein ML, Rogers MC. Hematologic disorders in the pediatric intensive care unit. In: Rogers MC, ed. Textbook of pediatric intensive care. 2nd ed. Baltimore: Williams & Wilkins, 1992:1357-1402.
37. Roloff J. Disseminated intravascular coagulation and other acquired bleeding disorders. In Levin DL, Morriss FC, eds. Essentials of pediatric intensive care. St. Louis: Quality Medical Publishing, 1990:151-174.
38. Kedar A, Gross S. Disseminated intravascular coagulation. In: Blumer J, ed. A practical guide to pediatric intensive care. 3rd ed. St. Louis: Mosby, 1990:517-519.
39. Nadkarni VM. Multiple organ system failure. In Holbrook PR, ed. Textbook of pediatric critical care. Philadelphia: WB Saunders, 1994:155-161.
40. Maxwell LG, Colombani PM, Fivush BA. Renal, endocrine, and metabolic failure. In: Rogers MC, ed. Textbook of pediatric intensive care. 2nd ed. Baltimore: Williams and Wilkins, 1992:1182-1234.
41. Stork J. Acute renal failure. In: Blumer J, ed. A practical guide to pediatric intensive care. 3rd ed. St. Louis: Mosby, 1990:429-437.
42. Moloney-Harmon PA, Rosenthal CH. Nursing care modifications for the child in the adult ICU. In: Stillwell S, ed. Critical care nursing reference. St. Louis: Mosby, 1992:588-670.
43. Seikaly MG. Hypertensive crisis. In: Levin DL and Morriss FC, eds. Essentials of pediatric intensive care. St. Louis: Quality Medical Publishing, 1990:410-417.
44. Ruley EJ. Hypertension. In: Holbrook PR, ed. Textbook of pediatric critical care. Philadelphia: WB Saunders, 1994:602-612.
45. Paschall JA, Melvin T. Fluid and electrolyte therapy. In: Holbrook PR, ed. Textbook of pediatric critical care. Philadelphia: WB Saunders, 1994:653-702.
46. Ongkingco JRC, Bock GH. Diagnosis and management of acute renal failure in the critical care unit. In: Holbrook PR,

ed. Textbook of pediatric critical care. Philadelphia: WB Saunders, 1994:585-601.
47. Rogers EL, Perman JA. Gastrointestinal and hepatic failure. In: Rogers MC, ed. Textbook of pediatric intensive care. 2nd ed. Baltimore: Williams & Wilkins, 1992:1132-1160.
48. Halpin TJ. Acute hepatic failure. In: Blumer J, ed. A practical guide to pediatric intensive care. 3rd ed. St. Louis: Mosby, 1990:135-139.
49. Belknap WM. Acute hepatic failure. In: Levin DL, Morriss FC, eds. Essentials of pediatric intensive care. St. Louis: Quality Medical Publishing, 1990:137-143.
50. Mohan P, Kerzner B. Hepatic failure. In Holbrook PR, ed. Textbook of pediatric critical care. Philadelphia: WB Saunders, 1994:621-637.
51. Gaedeke Norris MK, Steinhorn DM. Nutritional management during critical illness in infants and children. AACN Clin Issues Crit Care Nurs 1994;5:485-492.
52. Pollack M et al. Malnutrition in critically ill infants and children. JPEN 1982;6:20-24.
53. Pollack M, Ruttimann U, Wiley J. Nutritional depletions in critically ill children: Associations with physiologic instaility and increased quantity of care. JPEN 1985;9:309.
54. Pollack M. Nutritional failure and support in pediatric intensive care. In: Shoemaker WC et al, eds. Textbook of critical care. 2nd ed. Philadelphia: WB Saunders, 1989:1125-1128.
55. Rosenthal CH. Immunosuppression in pediatric critical care patients. Crit Care Nurs Clin North Am 1989;1:775-784.
56. Hauser GJ, Holbrook PR. Immune dysfunction in the critically ill infant and child. Crit Care Clin 1988;4:711-729.
57. Foster RL. Nursing strategies: Altered skin integrity. In: Foster RL, Hunsberger M, Anderson J, eds. Family centered nursing care of children. Philadelphia: WB Saunders, 1989:1612-1637.
58. Stevens B, Hunsberger M, Browne G. Pain in children: Theoretical, research, and practice dilemmas. J Pediatr Nurs 1987;2:154-164.
59. Beyer JE, Aradine CR. Content validity of an instrument to measure young children's perception of the intensity of their pain. J Pediatr Nurs 1986;1:386-395.
60. Yaster M et al. Pain, sedation and postoperative anesthetic management in the pediatric intensive care unit. In: Rogers MC, ed. Textbook of pediatric intensive care. 2nd ed. Baltimore: Williams and Wilkins, 1992:1518-1568.
61. Beyer JE, Wells N. The assessment of pain in children. Pediatr Clin North Am 1989;36:837-854.
62. McGrath PJ, Craig KD. Developmental and psychological factors in children's pain. Pediatr Clin North Am 1989; 36:823-836.
63. Anand KJ, Carr DB. The neuroanatomy, neurophysiologic and neurochemistry of pain, stress, and analgesia in newborns and children. Pediatr Clin North Am 1989;36:795-822.
64. Anand KJ, Hickey PR. Pain and its effects in the human neonate and fetus. New Engl J Med 1987;317:1321-1329.
65. Savedra M et al. Description of the pain experience: A study of school-age children. Issues Compr Pediatr Nurs 1981;5:373-380.
66. Lollar DJ, Smits SJ, Patterson DL. Assessment of pediatric pain: An empirical perspective. J Pediatr Psychol 1982;7: 267-277.
67. Jay SM et al. Behavioral management of children's distress during painful medical procedures. Behav Res Ther 1985;5:513-520.
68. Ross DM, Ross SA. Childhood pain: The school-aged child's viewpoint. Pain 1983;20:179-191.
69. Savedra M, Eland J, Tesler M. Pain management. In: Craft MJ, Denehy JA, eds. Nursing interventions for infants and children. Philadelphia: WB Saunders, 1990:304-325.
70. McGrath PJ, Unruh AM. Pain in children and adolescents. Amsterdam: Elsevier, 1987:1-351.
71. Margolis RB, Tait RC, Krause SJ. A rating system for use with patients with pain drawings. Pain 1986;24:57-65.
72. Jeans ME, Johnston CC. Pain in children: Assessment and management. In: Lipton S, Miles J, eds. Persistent pain: Modern methods of treatment. Vol 5. London: Grune & Stratton, 1985:111-127.
73. Molsberry D. Young children's subjective qualifications of pain following surgery [master's thesis]. Iowa City, Iowa: University of Iowa, 1979.
74. Stewart ML. Measurement of clinical pain. In: Jacox AV, ed. Pain: A source book for nurses and other health professionals. Boston: Little, Brown, 1977:107-138.
75. Melzak R. The McGill pain questionnaire: Major properties and scoring methods. Pain 1975;1:277-299.
76. Marx C. Sedation and analgesia. In: Blumer J, ed. A practical guide to pediatric intensive care. St. Louis: Mosby, 1990:92-308.
77. Philichi LM. Supporting the parents when the child requires intensive care. Focus Crit Care 1988;15:34-37.
78. Miles MS, Carter MC. Assessing parental stress in the intensive care unit. MCN 1983;8:354-359.
79. Eberly TW, Miles MS, Carter MC. Parental stress after the unexpected admission of a child to the intensive care unit. Crit Care Q 1986;8:57-65.
80. Kirschbaum MS. Needs of parents of critically ill children. Dimens Crit Care Nurs 1990;9:344-352.
81. Curley MAQ. Effects on the nursing mutual participation model of care on parental stress in the pediatric intensive care unit. Heart Lung 1988;17:683-688.
82. Curley MAQ, Wallace J. Effects of the nursing mutual participation model of care on parental stress in the PICU: A replication. J Pediatr Nurs 1992;7:377-385.

CHAPTER *16*

The Geriatric Patient with Multiple Organ Dysfunction Syndrome

Carol A. Rauen and *Christine A. Stamatos*

"Old age is a tyrant which forbids the pleasures of youth on pain of death."
   Cato (Roman Stoic philosopher), 45 BC
"We have elevated the desire for health, youth and longevity to the position of a religion."
   Stephen S. Wise (American rabbi), 1940

Many researchers have found advanced age to be a contributing factor to the development of multiple organ dysfunction syndrome (MODS).[1-6] The elderly suffer a higher rate of MODS than do other segments of society. Sepsis and sepsis-related syndromes are a major precursor in the development of MODS and the most common cause of death in intensive care units in the United States.[7] The Centers for Disease Control and Prevention ranks septicemia as the thirteenth leading cause of death in this country and the tenth leading cause of death in the elderly.[8] The incidence of sepsis increased 139% between 1977 and 1987 in the general population, yet it rose 162% in patients over the age of 65.[9] Rates of organ dysfunction and resulting mortality are also elevated in the elderly. Kass and co-workers[10] studied organ failure in the elderly and found single organ failure mortality rates to be 30% to 70% and the mortality rates for two organ failure to be 80% to 100% in the group over 85 years of age. The statistics in the general adult population are mortality rates of 10% to 40% for single organ failure and 41% to 67% for two organ failure.[11,12]

The two major reasons for the differences in incidence and outcome between critically ill young and critically ill older adults is the increased occurrence of preexisting illnesses in the elderly and the lack of physiologic reserve caused by the aging process.[6,13-15] The degenerative process and the presence of chronic illnesses make it difficult for the aging body to combat and compensate during times of stress resulting from anemia, hypovolemia, hypervolemia, sepsis, hypoperfusion states, surgery, or trauma. Tran and colleagues[16] studied the relationship between age, preexisting chronic disease, sepsis, organ system failure, and mortality in a medical ICU patient population and found age, chronic disease, and number of failing organs to be major determinants of mortality. Interestingly, the occurrence of sepsis alone was not found to be statistically significant in the Tran study. Knaus and Wagner[5] identified age as a major risk factor for the development of MODS.

Demographics and changing statistics

The elderly are the fastest growing portion of the American population today. Individuals over the age of 65 represent 13% (35 million) of the U.S. population and account for 33% of health care spending.[17] The U.S. Senate Special Committee on Aging[18] estimates that the group over 85 years of age will triple in number between 1980 and 2030 and the group over 100 years of age will expand from 61,000 individuals in 1985 to 100,000 by 2050. The significant increase in the elderly population results from the aging, as a critical mass, of the segment of society known as the "baby boomers" (those born between 1946 and 1964).[19] This large group of aging individuals, combined with medical advances, lower birth rates, and increased life expectancy has expanded the population of the elderly.[20] The geriatric patient population has unique health care needs and these needs will be witnessed more and more as the number of elderly individuals continues to grow.

The changing demographics noted above are being felt in critical care units across the country. People in the group over-65 years of age are hospitalized three times more frequently than are younger adults, have higher complication rates, have longer lengths of stay both in critical care units and in the hospital, and have higher mortality rates.[18,21-24] The aged body responds differently to stress states because of the physiologic changes that occur with time. The traditional protocols for caring for the critically ill will not always meet the needs of the elderly and, in fact, may sometimes be harmful. The health care team needs to become knowledgeable about geriatric assessment, the biology of aging, and treatment options for this patient group. The inclusion of a chapter on the elderly in the special considerations and management section in the second edition of this book demonstrates the importance and uniqueness of this patient population.

This chapter will outline the immune response of the elderly and the physiologic changes that occur over time. The current criteria used in the diagnosis of MODS will be challenged and new criteria will be offered integrating aging physiology. Treatment options for caring for the elderly suffering from MODS will be reviewed and possible changes in current practice will be suggested.

MODS in the elderly

To identify MODS in the elderly, the clinician must be familiar with both the physiology of aging and the pathology of organ dysfunction. The degenerative process makes the identification of MODS difficult in this high-risk population. Many of the changes that occur over time mask, inhibit, or prevent the "normal" physiologic response to hypoperfused states. Most of the research on organ dysfunction or failure has not specifically involved the elderly population, therefore the physiologic influence of advanced age has not been directly considered. Lack of physiologic reserve is the classic description of the biology of aging and the natural degenerative process. In fact, many of the normal physiologic and structural changes associated with aging are dangerously similar to the criteria used to describe early organ failure reported in the MODS literature. Compelling evidence suggests that the criteria used for identifying patients with sepsis or MODS patients may require modification.[25] New definitions for organ failure should be established and scientifically evaluated to enhance prompt identification of elderly patients particularly at risk for the development of MODS. Cerra[26] established a four-phase theory of organ failure. Figure 16-1 outlines how the process is hindered by the physiology of aging.[1] Only through early identification and initiation of appropriate treatment strategies will the overwhelming morbidity and mortality associated with multiple organ dysfunction in the elderly be reduced.

Organ dysfunction criteria in the elderly

MODS has been extensively studied over the last 25 years in both clinical and laboratory settings. Much knowledge has been gained and many new therapies and treatments have been developed for predicting, preventing, and treating this syndrome. One very active area of clinical research has been identifying the physiologic criteria for diagnosing organ dysfunction and failure. Despite these efforts, the 1992 consensus conference between the American College of Chest Physicians (ACCP) and the Society of Critical Care Medicine (SCCM)[9] was unable to delineate specific criteria for organ dysfunction. In fact, their report stated that "specific descriptions of this continuous process are not currently available" and that "MODS is subject to modulation by numerous factors at varying time periods, both interventional and host-related."[9]

Researchers, however, have found commonalities among groups of patients who suffer from MODS. They have identified physiologic criteria that are common for single and multiple organ dysfunction. These physiologic criteria are very useful in clinical research and in comparing populations of patients. Listed in Table 16-1 is a summary of criteria from Deitch,[28] Fry,[20] and Knaus and Wagner.[5]

Knaus and Wagner[5] identified the severity of the patient's underlying disease to be the strongest predictor of MODS, followed by sepsis, respiratory infection, and the age of the patient. Fry[20] found the sequence of specific organ dysfunction to be most likely determined by the physiologic reserve of each system (a factor of chronologic age or chronic disease). In subsequent retrospective and prospective studies comparing survivors with nonsurvivors, age was found to be a clinically and statistically significant factor.[16,28-32]

The Geriatric Patient with Multiple Organ Dysfunction Syndrome 359

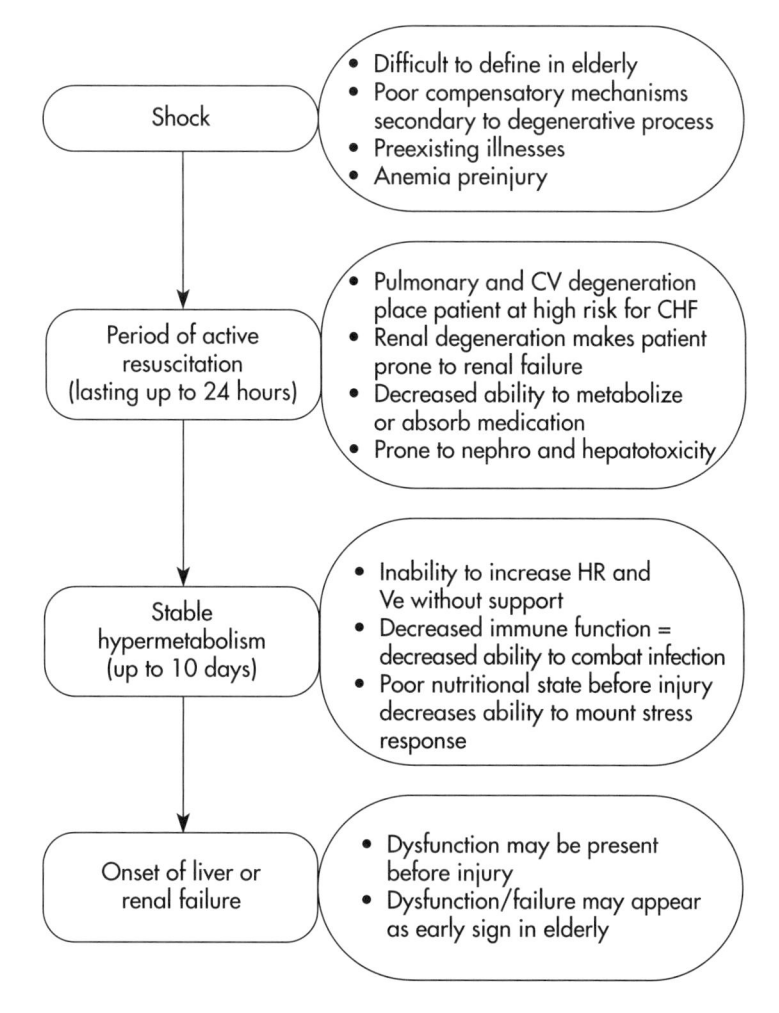

Fig. 16-1 The effect of the degenerative process on organ dysfunction. *CV,* Cardiovascular; *CHF,* congestive heart failure; *HR,* heart rate; *Ve,* minute ventilation. (Rauen C. Too old to live. Too young to die. Multiple organ dysfunction syndrome in the elderly. Crit Care Nurs Clin North Am 1994;6:535-542.)

The criteria for organ dysfunction listed in Table 16-1 and the physiologic criteria identified by the ACCP/SCCM consensus conference for systemic inflammatory response syndrome (SIRS) (Table 16-2) reflect the consequences of physiologic stress on individual organ systems. The natural process of aging slowly and methodically stresses the functional capabilities of cells and organs. The criteria listed in Table 16-1 unfortunately are not reflective of organ dysfunction frequently demonstrated in the critically ill elderly population. Based on existing mortality statistics associated with MODS or SIRS, these criteria would imply a nearly 100% mortality rate for all critically ill elderly patients. Iberti and co-workers[5] tested the criteria on a sample group of the elderly and concluded that standards for identifying septic patients may require modification when caring for the elderly. A new and more specific set of criteria needs to be established in order to clearly identify those older patients truly threatened by MODS.

When diagnosing organ dysfunction or failure in the acutely ill geriatric person, it is imperative that

Table 16-1 Organ Dysfunction Criteria

Pulmonary
Respiratory rate ≤5 breaths/min or ≥49 breaths/min*
Pao_2 >50 mm Hg*
Serum pH ≤7.24 with a $Paco_2$ of ≤49 torr*
$AaDo_2$ >350 mm Hg, $AaDo_2 = Fio_2 - Paco_2 - Pao_2$; normal = 713*
Five or more consecutive days on the ventilator to treat hypoxemia†
Hypoxia requiring assistive ventilation for at least 3-5 days (early)‡
Progressive ARDS requiring PEEP >10 cm H_2O and Fio_2 >.50 (late)‡

Cardiovascular
Heart rate <54 beats/min*
MAP ≤49 mm Hg (systolic blood pressure <60 mm Hg)*
Ventricular tachycardia or ventricular fibrillation*
Decreased ejection fraction or capillary-leak syndrome (early)‡
Hypodynamic response refractory to inotropic support (late)‡

Renal
Urine output ≤479 ml/24 hours or ≤159 ml/8 hours*
BUN ≥100 mg/dL*
Creatinine ≥3.5 mg/dL*
Creatinine >2.0 mg/dL†
Preexisting renal disease†
Doubling of the admission serum creatinine level†
Oliguria ≤479 ml/24 hours or creatinine >3 mg/dL (early)‡
Requires dialysis (late)‡

Hepatic
Bilirubin >6 mg %*
Prothrombin time >4 seconds over control*
Bilirubin >2.0 mg/dL†
Serum glutamic-oxaloacetic transaminase and lactate dehydrogenase >2 times normal†
Serum bilirubin ≥2-3 mg/dL or liver function tests ≥2 times normal (early)‡
Clinical jaundice with bilirubin ≥8-10 mg/dL (late)‡
Blood albumin ≤3.0 g/dL*

Gastrointestinal
Ileus with intolerance to enteral feeding >5 days (early)‡
Stress ulcers requiring transfusion†, (late)‡
Acalculus cholecystitis (late)‡
GI bleeding requiring 2 U of blood therapy within 24 hours for presumed stress bleeding or endoscopic examination to confirm gastric ulcerations†

Hematologic
WBC ≤1,000/mm^3*
Platelet ≤20,000/mm^3*
Hematocrit ≤20%*
PT and PTT >25% or platelets <50-80,000/mm^3 (early)‡
Disseminated intravascular coagulation (late)‡

Neurologic
Glasgow Coma Score ≤6 (in absence of sedation)*
Confusion—mild disorientation (early)‡
Progressive coma (late)‡

---

*From Knaus W, Wagner D. Multiple systems organ failure: Epidemiology and prognosis. Crit Care Clin 1989; 5:223.
†From Fry D. Multiple system organ failure. St. Louis: Mosby, 1992.
‡From Deitch E. Overview of multiple organ failure. In Prough D, Trystman R, eds. Critical care state of the art. Society of Critical Care Medicine 1993;14:134.

Table 16-2 Systemic Inflammatory Response Syndrome (SIRS)—Definition

Temperature >38° C or <36° C
Heart rate >90 beats/min
Respiratory rate >20 breaths/min or $PaCO_2$ <32 mm Hg
White blood cell count >12,000/mm^3 or <4000/mm^3 or >10% immature (bands)

From Bone RC et al. Definitions for sepsis and organ failure and guidelines for the use of innovative therapies in sepsis. Chest 1992;101:1644-1655.

clinicians be familiar with the physiology of aging. Entire texts have been written on the biology of the aging process, and therefore, this section will only analyze the specific criteria for organ dysfunction or failure listed in Table 16-1 with respect to geriatric physiology. Through this discussion new criteria to define organ dysfunction in the elderly will be suggested.

PHYSIOLOGY OF AGING
Theory of aging

Since the beginning of time, man has been attempting to identify the secret of the aging process. Prior to documented history, East Indian legend told of a fountain of youth. It was the quest for this fountain that brought Ponce de Leon to discover Florida in the 1500s. Through this knowledge man hoped to control his own mortality. Through the work of many researchers and philosophers several theories of aging have emerged over the years: the cellular/mechanical theory, the systems theory, and the immune theory. These theories revolve around one primary question: Does aging cause physiologic changes or do physiologic changes cause aging? The cellular/mechanical theory examines aging as a process of the system falling apart as a result of genetic alterations leading to self-destruction. The systems theory is aimed at defining the failure to maintain homeostasis in response to acute stress as a function of changes in the neuroendocrine or immune systems. The immune theory also examines the possibility that the system slowly destroys itself through the development of autoantibodies. There is general agreement that no single cause of aging exists. Scientific efforts should be aimed at identifying and controlling factors that can be manipulated in order to enhance quality and quantity of life.

Always progressive and often silent, aging is associated with increased vulnerability and decreased viability. Although these changes may not affect normal daily activities, aging is recognized as the progressive deterioration of the physiologic processes necessary for the maintenance of homeostasis in response to acute stressors. There is extreme variability among the aged in terms of the rate at which evidence of senescent changes begin to appear, particularly in response to physiologic insult.

Response to insult

Neuroendocrine response in the elderly. Multiple organ dysfunction syndrome is associated with a dysregulation of both the neuroendocrine and the inflammatory/immune response. Aging is also associated with dysregulation of the neuroendocrine and immune systems. Therefore it becomes imperative that a differentiation be made between the normal regulatory changes associated with aging and the development of multiple organ dysfunction often associated with critical illness in the elderly.

The neuroendocrine response to acute stress involves a number of complex, integrated, and highly coordinated events and is characteristically blunted in older individuals.[33-36] Age-related changes in the neuroendocrine response may be caused by decreased hormone secretion or by alterations in the response to hormones effected by a variety of receptor and effector alterations associated with aging. In 1990, Bursztyn[33] measured serum concentrations of various hormones associated with the stress response (epinephrine, norepinephrine, insulin, cortisol, and vasopressin) in nonstressed healthy young individuals (22 to 34 years of age) and older individuals (66 to 74 years of age). Interestingly, norepinephrine and cortisol levels were found to be higher in older subjects and insulin, vasopressin, and epinephrine levels to be the same in the two groups. Such findings suggest that mechanisms other than hormone secretion or concentration are responsible for the decline in the stress response.

The sympathetic nervous system (SNS) is activated by injury, illness, or acute shock. Various chemoreceptors and baroreceptors are responsible for triggering SNS activation. Significant evidence indicates that there is a reduction in sensitivity to these receptors with advanced age.* For example,

---
*References 15, 23, 24, 34, 35, 37-39.

decreased baroreceptor sensitivity is attributed to a diminution of arterial distensibility in response to changes in arterial pressure, which decreases the amount of "stretch" perceived by the baroreceptors. Chemoreceptors are less responsive to hypercapnic and hypoxic conditions over time, resulting in decreased stimulation of these receptors.[38,39] In addition, efferent pathways from the brain may be less effective with advanced age because of changes in neuronal impulse transmission.[34,40] Together, these changes result in an overall reduction in sympathetic outflow (Fig. 16-2).

Metabolic stress response in the elderly. The physiology of aging is associated with a failure to mobilize the appropriate metabolic resources needed to respond to acute stress. Although recent research reveals that older persons are capable of mounting a substantial response to acute stress, the pattern of this response is quite different from that of their younger counterparts.[41-44] For example, older persons are able to mount a substantial hypermetabolic response to acute illness or injury, equal to that of younger persons.[42,44] Unfortunately, these efforts may be at a significant cost to the entire sys-

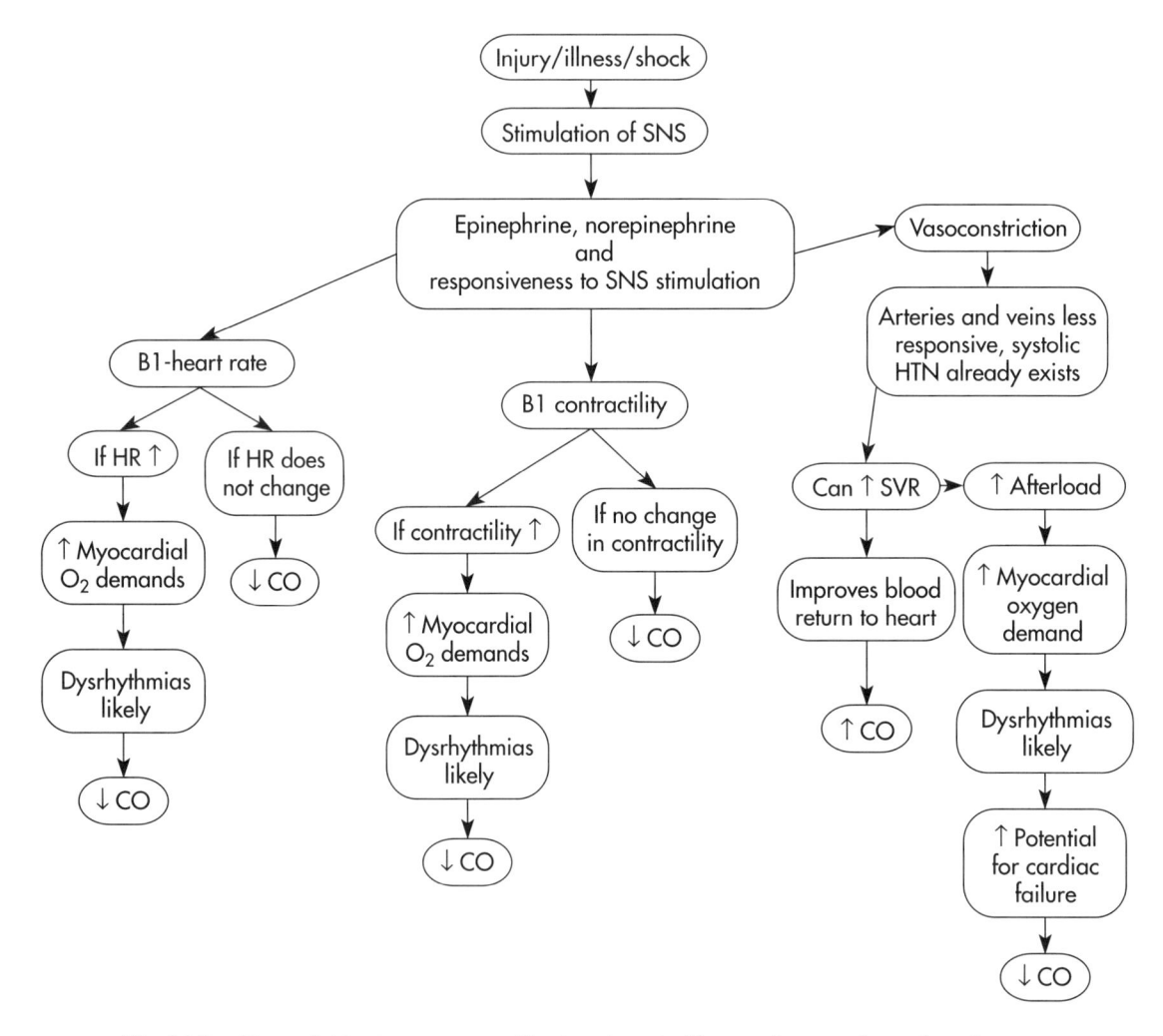

Fig. 16-2 The geriatric stress response. Treatment: control loss or decrease demands, volume resuscitate based on cardiovascular parameters, administer blood products for blood loss, inotropes, vasodilators, early mechanical ventilation. *CO,* Cardiac output; *HR,* heart rate; *HTN,* hypertension; *SNS,* sympathetic nervous system.

tem. In one study of younger versus older trauma victims, sustained hypermetabolism for more than 3 days was associated with a 20% mortality in the younger group and a 100% mortality in the elderly group.[44]

The ability to increase oxygen and substrate delivery during periods of acute stress is directly related to the amount of active muscle (metabolic) tissue. There is a significant reduction in muscle mass and a progressive increase in adipose tissue over a person's lifespan. As a result, the ability to increase oxygen consumption in order to meet the increased metabolic demands imposed by critical illness may be significantly blunted. The decreased response to catecholamines also contributes to the altered ability to rally appropriate metabolic resources.

Fuel utilization patterns during acute stress are considerably different in the elderly.[41,43-45] Older patients are slower to mobilize fat stores and tend to oxidize more carbohydrates to meet energy requirements. There is a characteristic persistent hyperglycemic response, earlier lipid intolerance, and sluggish protein synthesis. A pronounced insulin resistance influences the utilization and disposal of glucose. Several researchers have attempted to determine whether this insulin resistance also affects the anabolic properties of insulin on protein synthesis. Aging does not bring about a significant deterioration in the response to anabolic signals of insulin.[45,46] Unfortunately, there is a substantial reduction in growth hormone levels with advancing age that is largely responsible for the loss of muscle mass and sluggish protein synthesis during periods of acute stress.[34,47] Existing research provides strong evidence that age-dependent metabolic dysfunctions may limit the capacity of the aged to generate the metabolic fuels necessary to deal with internal and external environmental challenges.

The inflammatory/immune response in the elderly. It is generally accepted that immune competence declines with advancing age. Evidence suggests that aging affects immune competence, and also that immune competence affects the aging process. To what extent the two mechanisms are distinctly responsible for the overall loss in immune function remains controversial. Through careful orchestration of events, the body works to prevent infection. Age-related changes in the immune response are associated with all levels of defense (Table 16-3). Changes in the immune system result from extrinsic factors such as environmental exposure, medications, preexisting pathology, and malnutrition. Intrinsic factors such as failure of the external defense mechanisms, involution of the thymus gland, alterations in lymphocyte proliferation and differentiation, alterations in macrophage activity, and increased formation of autoantibodies also account for the relative lack of immunocompetence demonstrated in older individuals.[13,47-50]

Physical barriers, such as skin and mucous membranes, provide the first line of defense against infection. However, a number of age-related changes influence the reliability of these barriers against foreign invasion (Table 16-4). For example, collagen, fat, and water content of skin is decreased leaving

Table 16-3 Immune Dysfunction or Alterations Associated with Advanced Age

Immune function	Status in elderly
Neutrophil counts	Decreased
Phagocytic activity	Decreased
Lymphocyte counts	Decreased
Monocyte and basophil counts	Decreased
Chemotaxis	Decreased
Phagocytosis	Decreased
Interleukin-1 (IL-1) levels	Unchanged/decreased
Interleukin-2 (IL-2) levels	Decreased
Antibody production (due to changes in T cells)	Decreased
Autoantibody production	Increased
IL-2 receptors on T cells	Decreased
Natural killer cell activity	Decreased
Macrophage-T cell interaction	Decreased
Antigen processing and presentation	Increased/unchanged
Helper T (CD4+) cell proliferation/cytokine production	Decreased
Supressor T (CD8+) cell activity	Decreased
CD4+:CD8+ ratio (not much data available)	Unchanged
Cytotoxic T cell activity	Decreased
MHC class II expression	Decreased
PGF$_2$ production by macrophages	Increased
Lymphocyte traffic out of lymph nodes	Decreased
Cell-mediated immunity	Decreased
Humoral immunity	Decreased/unchanged
Febrile response	Decreased

Table 16-4 External Defense Mechanisms in the Critically Ill Elderly Patient

Barrier	Normal disruption with age
Intact epithelium	Dry, thin skin; decreased elasticity
	Decreased sensitivity to heat and cold
	Decreased subcutaneous fat of face and limbs
	Decreased number of blood vessels and water content of skin
	Delayed epithelialization and contraction of wounds
	Abnormal proliferation of GI epithelium
Acidic pH	Frequent utilization of H_2 blockers results in increased gastric pH
	Decreased basal HCl production by parietal cells
	Decreased urinary acidification
	Decreased saliva production
Resident flora	Bacterial overgrowth because of changes in pH
	Decreased mucus production favors bacterial growth and increased adherence
Mechanical removal	Loss of elastic tissue surrounding alveoli
	Weakened respiratory muscles
	Weakened cough and sneezing reflex
	Diminished saliva production
	Decreased mucociliary function
	Slowed esophageal and gastric emptying
	Decreased peristalsis
	Urinary retention because of prostatic hypertrophy
	Pelvic floor relaxation in women, inefficient bladder emptying
Ciliary activity	Decreased throughout (both size and function of cilia)
Mucus production	Decreased production throughout
Bactericidal secretions	Decreased numbers of sweat glands and decreased perspiration production
	Decreased saliva and tear production

the skin thin and fragile. Mucus production throughout the body is reduced, resulting in the loss of effective barriers against injury and invasion. The ability to regulate pH closely is significantly reduced with age; the maintenance of an acid pH is important for the prevention of bacterial overgrowth within the respiratory, gastrointestinal, and genitourinary systems.[35,51-54]

The most striking senescent changes in the immune system are seen in the T lymphocytes and in cell-mediated immunity (CMI). As the thymus involutes over time (Fig. 16-3), T cell maturation and differentiation are impaired, resulting in alterations in subpopulations of T cells (helper and cytotoxic) and inefficient CMI.[13,35,50,55] As a person ages, the T cells produce less Interleukin 2 (IL-2) and are also less sensitive to its stimulatory effects. Therefore, the elderly population has less effective CMI and an increase in susceptibility especially to fungal, viral, and mycobacterial infections. Subtle changes are noted in antigen-presenting cells such as macrophages, monocytes, and Kupffer cells (Table 16-3).

Numerous experiments have demonstrated a restoration of CMI through strategies to improve thymic activity with hormone (hypophysial, growth, and thyroid hormones) injections and thymus grafts.[50] Although these results are promising, more research is needed before manipulation of thymic activity in clinical practice can be advocated.

Although humoral immunity (HI) is relatively well preserved with age, it is indirectly influenced by the decline in CMI. Optimal antibody responses require normal helper T-cell activity. Therefore, a decline in helper T-cell activity decreases the production of antibodies in response to foreign antigens. Increased autoantibody production may also be responsible for some of the normal physiologic changes associated with aging.

Decreased growth hormone levels reduce production of IL-1, IL-2, and tumor necrosis factor factors common to all critically ill patients, the elderly have the influences of advanced age, probable malnutrition (present in 65% of acutely ill geriatric patients), and the likelihood of two or more preexisting medical conditions (in 25% to 65% of elderly trauma victims).* These combined factors work synergistically to significantly alter the inflammatory/immune response, the incidence of sepsis and MODS, and the clinical presentation associated with these syndromes.

Critically ill geriatric patients may develop a syndrome of multiple organ dysfunction that can remain clinically occult until the organ failure is irreversible.[57] The presentation of infection in the elderly is often associated with a delay in recognition of impending organ failure 20% to 50% of the time.[13,58] The dampened inflammatory response manifests as less severe fever, reduced leukocytosis, and fewer signs and symptoms associated with bacteremia, sepsis, and SIRS.[13,58] Many of the criteria listed in Tables 16-1 and 16-2 parallel the expected changes that occur over time in the body. This does not mean that all elderly people have organ failure, but that they are experiencing diminished reserves. In order to diagnose organ dysfunction as a result of sepsis or critical illness in the elderly, the clinician must first be aware of the changes that may be attributed to the normal aging process.

Fever and leukocytosis, the most common early signs of infection, are likely to be absent from the geriatric patient. In fact, hypothermia and normal-to-low white cell counts may be present.[59,60] Individuals over the age of 65 have an increased risk of both hypothermia and hyperthermia because of their decreased basal metabolic rate, changes in the autonomic and neuroendocrine centers of the hypothalamus, decreased amount of body fat, and diminished intake of both calories and fluid.[60] Because of changes in thermoregulation, the elderly maintain a lower basal temperature and show less elevation when harboring an infection or a stress state. Fever, the classic warning sign of infection, is not a reliable indicator in this age group.

Symptoms such as pain, redness, and swelling may also, dangerously, be absent owing to the delayed inflammatory response, changes in peripheral

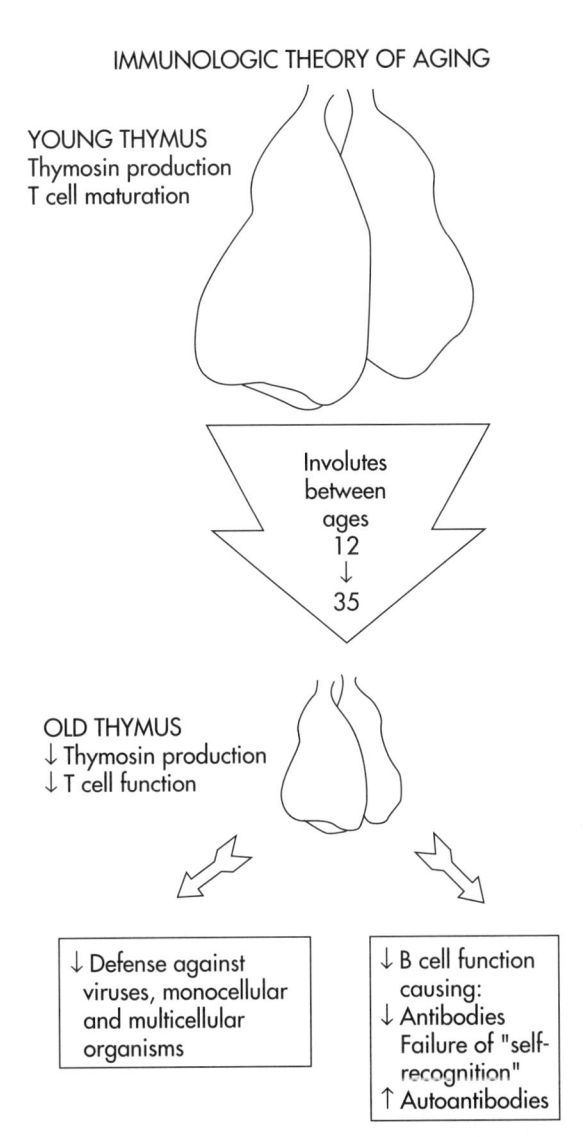

Fig. 16-3 The geriatric immune response to illness: thymus involution. (From Timiras P. Physiological basis of geriatrics. New York: MacMillan 1988:55.)

(TNF). These changes are actually thought to improve overall immune function and potentially result in a diminished systemic inflammatory response.[49,50]

Blunted response and clinical presentation

A multitude of factors increases the risk of infection or sepsis in the elderly. In addition to the risk

---

*References 5, 6, 13, 15, 56.

vasculature, and diminished peripheral pain receptors. Tachycardia, tachypnea, hypotension, and increased cardiac index will probably not be the early signs of a systemic inflammatory response because of the preexisting prevalence of hypertension and decreased cardiopulmonary function in this particular population. However, acidosis, hypoglycemia, or hyperglycemia may be likely to provide early evidence of impending SIRS.*

Acute-phase protein production in response to infection may be a fairly reliable indicator of the presence and severity of infection and the response to antimicrobial therapy.[53] In a prospective study of 114 patients (62 to 92 years of age) admitted to a geriatric unit at a large teaching hospital, various acute-phase proteins were measured at regular intervals to evaluate their predictive capacity in determining severity of infection. C reactive protein (CRP) (normal levels, 0 to 20 mg/L) was greatly increased in most elderly patients with significant infection, whereas a number of patients with minor infections had normal values (1 to 109 mg/L in mild infection; 72 to 159 mg/L in SIRS).[53] Therefore, CRP levels may be monitored clinically as a means of distinguishing severe infection from other grades of infection.[53]

EFFECTS OF AGING ON ORGAN STRUCTURE AND FUNCTION

As discussed, early recognition of MODS in critically ill elderly victims is difficult to determine, and compelling evidence suggests that the criteria used for identifying patients with septis or MODS may require modification.[25] This section is a discussion of the normal physiologic changes associated with each organ. Attempts to redefine criteria based on the current state of the art have been made (Table 16-5). These criteria or any other new definitions for organ failure in the elderly should be scientifically evaluated in order to apply them clinically to the prompt identification of elderly patients particularly at risk for the development of MODS.

The aging respiratory system: effects on oxygenation and ventilation

The criteria for pulmonary dysfunction listed in Table 16-1 are not sufficient when evaluating the respiratory status of an elderly individual. The changes that occur in the pulmonary system over time affect the ability of the elderly individual to combat critical illness and increase the incidence of complications (Table 16-6). Mortality from pneumococcal pneumonia is approximately four times greater in the elderly than in young adults.[61] In a study involving over 2000 elderly patients admitted to intensive care units for respiratory problems, pneumonia was the most frequent diagnosis (in 31% of the patients) with a mortality rate of 24%.[62]

The occurrence of respiratory failure increases with age because of the changes in respiratory mechanics, drive, and muscle strength.[63] Chelluri and colleagues[64] studied critically ill patients 85 years of age and over and found that 82% required intubation and ventilatory assistance and 39% of those patients did not survive. Gee and co-workers reported a 69% rate of mortality from adult respiratory distress syndrome (ARDS) in elderly patients as compared to a 12% rate for patients under 60 years of age.[65]

The anatomic and physiologic changes that occur in the geriatric group require different assessment strategies and treatment plans in managing both oxygenation and ventilation.[66] The anatomic changes affect pulmonary compliance and gas diffusion in the alveolar capillary bed. There is a decrease in alveolar surface area and total parenchyma. The decreased compliance from collagen deposition and decreased surfactant production over time cause higher residual lung volumes and air trapping in small airways.[67] When auscultating breath sounds of the elderly, there will be decreased air exchange in the bases of the lung fields because of this air trapping and decreased lung expansion.[71] Standard pulmonary function test results are altered in the aged, for example the forced expiratory volume (FEV_1) drops a minimum of 20 ml per year after 25 years of age, and a 20% change in closing volume occurs between 20 and 80 years of age.[68]

The combination of these changes over time creates changes in gas exchange with an increase in alveolar-arterial oxygen difference ($A\text{-}aO_2$),[53] increase in ventilation-to-perfusion (V/Q) mismatch (approximately 4 mm Hg per decade), and progressive reduction in arterial oxygen tension PaO_2 (PaO_2 of 70 mm Hg by 80 years of age).[35,63] "Normal" arterial blood gas (ABG) results are rarely seen in people over the age of 65. There is a decrease in ar-

---

*References 7, 13, 25, 36, 57.

Table 16-5 Recommended Organ System Failure Criteria in the Elderly*

Pulmonary

Ten or more consecutive days on the ventilator
Respiratory rate <10 breaths/min or >40 breaths/min
Serum pH ≤7.24 with a $Paco_2$ ≤49 torr
Pao_2 <60 mm Hg with a Sao_2 <88%
Hypoxia requiring assistive ventilator for at least 5 to 7 days (early)
Progressive ARDS requiring PEEP >5 cm H_2O and Fio_2 >.70 (early)

Cardiovascular

Mean arterial pressure <60 mm Hg or <20% below baseline
Dysrhythmias—atrial/ventricular ectopy, tachycardia/bradycardia, or fibrillation
Decreased ejection fraction 10% below baseline levels
Demonstration of decreased end organ perfusion—decreased level of consciousness, decreased urine output, hemodynamic instability

Hematologic/immune

Normal to low-grade temperature
C reactive protein levels >100 mg/L
WBC <1,000/mm^3
Platelets <50,000-80,000/mm^3; PT and PTT >25% (early)
Platelet <30,000/mm^3 (with change in function)
Hematocrit <20% below baseline
GI bleeding (with or without requirements for blood transfusions)
Disseminated intravascular coagulation (late)

Renal

BUN ≥100 mg/dL
Serum creatinine level 1.5 to 2 times admission level
Urine output <0.5 ml/kg/hr for 8 hr or more
Creatinine clearance of 5-50 ml/min (early) or <5 ml/min (late); (for a younger population, creatinine clearance is 15-80 ml/min for prerenal failure and <5 ml/min for ARF)
Preexisting renal disease (or age >75 yrs)
Requiring dialysis

Hepatic

Bilirubin >2.8 mg/dL (increased because of normal elevation with age)
Prothrombin time >4 seconds above control values
Serum glutamic-oxaloacetic transaminase >2 times normal levels
Lactate dehydrogenase >2 times normal levels (normal level for ages 65 and over is 2.7-7.3 mg/dL)
Alkaline phosphatase >2 times normal levels (normal level for ages 65 and over is 0.7-6.6 mg/dL)
Clinical jaundice

Gastrointestinal/metabolic

Ileus with intolerance to enteral feedings >3 days (early) (in younger population: >5 days)
Abdominal distention (qualified by >20% increase above admission level)
Evidence of stress ulcers with or without transfusion requirements (early)
Acalculus cholecystitis (late)
Negative nitrogen balance >5 days

Neurologic

Mild confusion, disorientation, or lethargy (early)
Progressive coma

*Developed by the authors as suggestions based on a review of the literature. The criteria have not been studied for validity or reliability in predicting outcome.

Table 16-6 Age-Related Changes in Pulmonary Structure and Function after Age 30*

Structure

4% decrease per decade in alveolar surface area after 30 years of age
Stiffened trachea
Diminished actual lung weight
Weakened respiratory muscles
Structural changes to chest (kyphosis, shortened thorax, increased wall stiffness, increased anteroposterior diameter)

Function

Blunted cough and laryngeal reflexes
Decreased vital capacity, forced expiratory volume in one minute, lung recoil pressure, diffusing capacity, and arterial O_2 tension (PaO_2)
Increased closing volume, functional residual capacity, and residual volume
Progressive reduction of PaO_2
Increased alveolar-arterial oxygen gradient (A-aO_2)
Increased ventilation-perfusion (V/Q) mismatch by approximately 4 mm Hg per decade
Drop in 2,3-diphosphoglycerate levels
50% reduction in response to hypercapnia and hypoxia

*References 35, 53, 66-69.

terial oxygen tension but little change in carbon dioxide tension.[68] Changes in the pH from pulmonary causes are rare because alterations in arterial carbon dioxide tension ($PaCO_2$) are minimal in normal aging; therefore, abnormalities in these values (pH and $PaCO_2$) are usually related to pulmonary pathology or metabolic alterations rather than to the degenerative process. The decrease in 2,3-diphosphoglycerate with age will also affect saturation and oxygen release because of the shift to the left in the oxyhemoglobin disassociation curve.[53] The elderly may demonstrate a slower clinical response to oxygen administration secondary to this shift to the left.[70]

The central and peripheral chemoreceptors undergo changes with time.[35] Because the elderly display as much as a 50% delayed response to hypoxia and hypercapnia,[38,72] changes in respiratory rate will not occur as quickly, if at all, when there are changes in the blood chemistry. Changes in breathing patterns may also affect respiratory rate and compensation. Breathing patterns like Cheyne-strokes respirations (periodical breathing and apnea) are common in individuals over 65 years of age.[63]

Both Fry[11] and Deitch[28] identified the length of time that a patient was on the ventilator as an indication of respiratory dysfunction. The structural and endurance alterations in the elderly pulmonary system lead to longer periods on the ventilator. The aged must expend more energy to accomplish the same respiratory effect as do individuals under 65 years of age.[73] This is due to chest wall structural changes, osteoporotic changes, and weakening of the respiratory muscles.[82] The high potential for and the incidence of pneumonia in the elderly also increase the period of ventilatory support required. Enright and co-workers[74] studied the maximal inspiratory and expiratory pressures and found age to be a negative predictor of successful weaning.

Deitch[28] identified the need for high levels of positive end expiratory pressure (PEEP) to combat hypoxia as an indicator of ARDS. Levels greater than 10 cm H_2O are not usually necessary when treating the elderly.[63] Because of their increased closing volume, older persons have increased intrinsic PEEP (PEEP$_i$). The lack of cardiovascular reserves in the elderly makes it very difficult to increase positive pressure without a concomitant decrease in cardiac output and oxygen delivery (DO_2). Maintaining a PaO_2 of 60 mm Hg and SaO_2 ≥88% should be adequate when managing hypoxia in the geriatric patient.[63]

Pulmonary status cannot be assessed in isolation from other organ systems, especially in the elderly population. The challenge for the critical care practitioner is to differentiate between "normal degeneration" and true dysfunction. Preexisting conditions such as cardiovascular disease, renal failure, and malnutrition will greatly affect the functional ability of the respiratory system. The criteria for evaluating pulmonary dysfunction in this age group must reflect longer ventilator times, decreased gas exchange, and lack of functional reserve (Table 16-5).

The aging liver: effects on homeostasis and clinical management

The liver appears to be severely affected by aging[35,53]; however, specific changes in the aging liver remain fairly controversial. Liver weight decreases

18% to 24% between 20 and 80 years of age.[51] Although the weight of the liver may decrease, the overall size of the liver tends to increase with age. With a reduction in the number of hepatocytes, the surviving cells become larger but not necessarily more functional.[35,51,53] There is a reduction in the amount of endoplasmic reticulum necessary for synthesis of organic substances. Liver blood flow also decreases over time by as much as 60% by 65 years of age.[53]

As a result of these structural changes there is a slight reduction in the rate of protein synthesis and carbohydrate metabolism. One of the most significant clinical changes is an overall reduction in the capacity of the liver to metabolize drugs. This is thought to result from changes in hepatic blood flow, as well as reduced activity of hepatic enzymes. Older persons clearly require more time for drug clearance.[75,76] The extent of these changes is not altogether clear because of the heterogenous nature of the elderly population. There is no significant difference in elimination patterns and protein synthesis.[33] For example, prothrombin and partial thromboplastin times, and various liver enzyme studies are relatively unchanged in the elderly.[64] Indications of metabolic function that progressively change with age are levels of triglycerides, total protein and albumin (decrease as much as 50%), lactate dehydrogenase (LDH), alkaline phosphatase (increase 2.5 times the normal level), and bilirubin (increase 1.5 times the normal level) (Table 16-7).[64,65,77,78] These changes should be considered when examining the existing criteria for liver failure. Perhaps the threshold for dysfunction should be adjusted because of a lack of hepatic reserve (Table 16-5).

The aging gastrointestinal tract: effects on nutrition and infection

Table 16-1 outlines criteria for gastrointestinal (GI) dysfunction in MODS but many of these changes are already present in the elderly because of the degenerative process. The gut plays a prominent role in maintaining immune competence and contributing to the development of sepsis in critically ill patients, with many of the organisms that cause sepsis existing within its walls (see Chapter 10). The GI tract is a vital component of the immune system, with half of all immune cells in the body living within its confines.[79] The vast quantity of gut-associated lymphoid tissue (GALT) located in the GI tract is responsible for sampling foreign antigenic material within the intestinal lumen and mounting cell-mediated and humoral immune responses as needed.[79,80]

The older gut goes through a number of changes that challenge the integrity of this immunologic organ (Table 16-8). There is both a qualitative and a quantitative decline in T- and B-cell activity within GALT, contributing to the diminution of cell-mediated and humoral immunity noted in the elderly.[52]

Table 16-7 Significant Differences in Laboratory Data in the Elderly*

Value	Normal range	Elderly range
WBC count (per mm^3)	4800-10,800	3700-4600
Hb (g/dL)	M, 14-18; F, 12-16	M, 13.6-13.9; F, 11.4-16.6
HCT (%)	M, 42-52; F, 37-47	M, 38.8-41.6; F, 32.8-49.0
Fasting glucose (mg/dL)	70-125	60-136
Serum CO$_2$ (mEq/L)	24-30	23-31
Total protein (g/dL)	6.0-8.5	5.3-5.9
Albumin (g/dL)	3.0-5.5	2.7-2.9
Triglycerides (mg/dL)	10-190	191-327
PO$_4$ (mg/dL)	2.5-4.6	2.2-2.4
Total bilirubin (mg/dL)	0-1.2	1.4-2.0
Alkaline phosphatase (units/L)	30-115	129-169
AST (units/L)	1-41	53-85

*Results reported in a study of 15 persons 65 to 80 years of age. Only results significantly different from normal ranges are recorded here.
AST, Aspartate aminotransferase; *Hb,* hemoglobin; *HCT,* hematocrit; *PO$_4$,* phosphate; *WBC,* white blood cell.
Modified from Coodley EL: Laboratory tests in the elderly: What is abnormal? Postgrad Med 1989;85:336-337.

Reductions in peristalsis, gastric acid secretion, and mucus production throughout the gut contribute to bacterial overgrowth, injury, and finally entry of bacteria or their products into the systemic circulation (Table 16-8).[51,53,79,80]

Maintenance of mucosal integrity is dependent upon normal epithelial cell production and mucociliary activity. As splanchnic blood flow to the mucosal villi falls, the senescent GI tract becomes threatened by a reduction in the size and quantity of cilia necessary for normal gut motility and absorption. As a result of these changes, nutrient absorption through the GI tract is significantly impaired, contributing to the fragile mucosa associated with the normal aging process. Mucosal integrity is further challenged by alterations in epithelial cell production (hyperproliferation and abnormal production) and turnover (25% reduction) with advancing age.[53,81] Improper diet, medications, and alcohol ingestion may also contribute to the disruption of mucosal integrity observed in the elderly.[35,75]

The prevalence of digestive disorders in the elderly must also be considered when attempting to define organ failure in the aged. A 50% incidence of chronic or acute gastritis is reported in this population.[33,49] As a result of the normal changes in mucosal integrity, older persons are much more likely to develop acute GI bleeding during critical illness.[51] Because of underlying medical problems and the lack of adequate physiologic reserve, the elderly also have a higher morbidity and mortality rate associated with GI bleeding.[49,64] Another common complaint among the elderly is constipation. Large-bowel motility is frequently decreased because of changes in innervation and muscle strength; however, this is highly related to diet, exercise, and pathology.[33,51] During acute illness, constipation can contribute to bacterial colonization, intolerance to tube feedings, abdominal distention, pain, or bowel obstruction.

Specific criteria for the evaluation of GI failure should therefore be slightly modified in order to incorporate the chronic changes in the GI tract (Table 16-5). For example, the combined impact of these changes and the stress imposed by gut starvation result in an exacerbation of intestinal atrophy, decreased gastric motility, and reduced transit time through the small bowel, resulting in malabsorption and intolerance of feedings, ileus formation, and breakdown of the protective mucosal barrier. In addition, there is a reduced capacity to regulate blood flow to the GI tract adequately in response to hypoperfusion, further reducing motility and the protective capacity of the mucosal wall. As a result, stress ulcer formation should be considered early evidence of GI failure with or without the need for

Table 16-8 Changes in Gut Integrity and Function with Age

Function	Alteration
Gastric acid	Decreased gastric acid production under basal conditions leading to bacterial overgrowth and aspiration pneumonia
	Increased gastric acid production with illness leading to mucosal wall disruption
Peristalsis	Dysphagia
	Decreased esophageal motility
	Decreased gastric emptying
	Decreased motility throughout small intestine
	Decreased muscle mass in large intestine leading to potential for aspiration, small or large bowel obstruction, or constipation
Microflora	Changes in acid-base balance leading to a potential for bacterial overgrowth and translocation
Desquamation	Hyperproliferation of epithelial cells and abnormal development or up to a 25% reduction in proliferation contributing to fragility of mucosal barrier
Mucus	Decreased mucosal cell activity leading to reduced mucus content and increased likelihood of breakdown
Bile	Remains fairly stable with adequate nutrient intake

transfusions. The presence of decreased bowel sounds, abdominal distention, and pain should be carefully monitored in order to diagnose the presence of ileus and GI bleeding. Daily measurements of abdominal girth and microscopic evidence of blood in the upper and lower GI tracts should be noted in all critically ill older patients.

The aging pancreas: effects on endocrine and exocrine function

Uncertainty exists regarding the extent of exocrine and endocrine dysfunctions in the aging pancreas. There appears to be a loss of secretory cells and an increase in fatty tissue. A decrease in glucose tolerance with advanced age that appears to be multifactorial in nature rather than a consequence of aging alone is well documented. In fact, insulin levels may actually be elevated in some elderly patients, with increasing evidence of insulin resistance being noted, similar to that seen with the hypermetabolic stress response.[34,36,43] The following factors contribute to decreased glucose tolerance with age: (1) loss of hepatic sensitivity to reduce gluconeogenesis and glycogenolysis, (2) increased glucagon levels, and (3) changes in diet and exercise.

The pancreas is also responsible for producing digestive enzymes (amylase, lipase, and trypsin) and bicarbonate. Amylase and bicarbonate levels remain relatively unchanged over time, while lipase and trypsin levels are reduced dramatically with age. Lipase is responsible for lipid metabolism, which has been shown to be altered with advancing age.[42,44] Trypsin is necessary for protein metabolism, and the effects of these changes have not yet been determined. In general the age-related changes in pancreatic function do not seriously compromise overall pancreatic function because of a large functional reserve.[53]

The aging cardiovascular system: effects on transport and perfusion

The cardiovascular system undergoes many changes over the lifetime of an individual (Table 16-9). The degree to which these changes are realized by the individual is directly related to the workload required to meet the needs of the body. There is a substantial loss of cardiac reserve by 65 years of age.[35,53,66,82] This lack of reserve may not affect the day-to-day functioning of the individual. However, when placed in a physiologically stressful situation

Table 16-9 Changes in Cardiovascular Structure and Function after 30 Years of Age[35,53,67]

Structure
Hypertrophied heart muscle
Increased fibrous tissue and calcium deposits on valves
Increased diameter of aorta
Increased heart wall rigidity
Loss of elasticity in large arteries

Function
Decreased resting cardiac output and cardiac index
Increased systolic blood pressure
Decreased vasomotor tone
Increased myocardial irritability
Decreased adrenergic modulation of cardiovascular function
Decreased responsiveness to beta-adrenergic stimulation
Decline in myocardial catecholamine concentration
Decreased resting left ventricular performance
Slowed myocardial contraction rate
Drop in maximal coronary artery flow
Increased peripheral vascular resistance

such as hypoperfusion states (sepsis, dysrhythmias, hypovolemia, or volume overload), the lack of reserve is evidenced by cardiac dysfunction.

By 70 years of age there is a significant drop in the resting heart rate. There is actual cell loss in the sinoatrial (SA) and atrioventricular (AV) nodes, the bundle of His, and bundle branches beginning in the second decade of life.[53] The sinus rate is also decreased because of blockade of both sympathetic and parasympathetic stimulation.[83] In addition to the physiologic changes affecting heart rate, the elderly may have pharmacologically induced effects on cardiac function as well. There is an increased likelihood that the elderly might be taking oral cardiac drugs such as beta-blockers, calcium channel blockers, or cardiac-glycosides that will slow their resting heart rate for therapeutic reasons. The use of these drugs will certainly delay the cardiac response to stress and sepsis in the elderly.

Arterial blood pressure increases with age secondary to increased peripheral vascular resistance over time, cardiac muscle hypertrophy, and atrial stiffening.[83] These factors, as well as aortic outflow impedance from valvular changes, contribute to an increase in systolic pressure.[35,66] Elevation of diastolic pressure occurs as a result of the progressive atherosclerosis associated with the normal aging process. Fluid and electrolyte changes naturally occurring in the elderly also contribute to higher resting blood pressures. For example, sodium excretion is diminished secondary to a decline in the glomerular filtration rate, which will elevate intravascular volume.[32] It is, therefore, essential to have a baseline blood pressure (BP) value on older critically ill patients. This information will be useful when interpreting the cardiac assessment of a geriatric patient. What appears normotensive may actually be a hypotensive state for that patient.

The third criterion in Table 16-1 is an increased incidence of ventricular tachycardia or V-fibrillation. The elderly heart is prone to both atrial and ventricular dysrhythmias because of changes in the electrical conduction system.[82] Changes in the SA node and decreased activity of the AV node make it more difficult to suppress ectopic foci. As a result the heart muscle is more irritable and less responsive to impulses from the SNS. Therefore, the elderly are more likely to develop reentry-type dysrhythmias.[82,66] Kane and co-workers[84] found an increased incidence of premature ventricular contractions with age. This occurred in 10% of ECG-monitored and 30% to 40% of Holter-monitored geriatric patients. Ischemia-related ectopy also increases with age because of the increased incidence of coronary artery disease (CAD) in this group.

A decreased ejection fraction (EF) is commonly seen in victims of MODS. This decrease has been attributed to many factors including myocardial depressant factor, tissue hypoxia, dysrhythmias, decreased preload, and anaerobic metabolism.[85,86] EF is decreased as a function of the normal aging process as well. Between the ages of 20 and 80 there is an estimated 42% decrease in stroke volume.[53] Additionally, typical changes in heart rate and rhythm will affect the percentage of blood volume ejected with each beat. Decreased coronary perfusion secondary to CAD will also impede cardiac output and EF. Changes in heart muscle structure and function can also affect ejection capacity. There is a nearly 50% reduction in cardiac output by age 65. This can be attributed to the 30% increase in muscle mass and collagen deposition, as well as failure within the excitation-contraction coupling process, changes in oxidative metabolism, and decreased competence of myocardial valves.[53,57,82,83]

The last criterion identified in Table 16-1 is a hypodynamic response that is refractory to inotropic support. Adrenergic modulation of the cardiovascular system decreases with age.[34,36,83] The degenerative process affects the number and function of receptor sites and responsiveness to circulating neurotransmitters and hormones that are usually stimulated to induce cardiac compensation. As a result, the response to beta-adrenergic stimulation diminishes, as does the systemic response to endogenous and exogenous catecholamines.[83] The changes in the pulmonary and renal systems over time affect the acid-base balance of the body, which also affects the physiologic response to inotropic therapy.

If organ assessment were based solely on the criteria in Table 16-1, most individuals over 65 years of age would qualify for cardiac dysfunction. However, when assessing the cardiac status of the elderly, the ability to compensate during stress and specific symptoms associated with cardiac dysfunction must be examined. Criteria for cardiovascular failure in the elderly must be individualized and based on such factors as prestress cardiac function and evidence of adequate end-organ perfusion, such as level of consciousness, urine output, and hemodynamic stability (Table 16-5).

An essential component for evaluating cardiac dysfunction in the elderly is obtaining a detailed cardiac history and determining whether observed cardiovascular (CV) assessment findings are primarily related to the degenerative process or to MODS. The general criteria for establishing CV dysfunction are the same as those listed in Table 16-1 with modifications for the biology of aging (Table 16-5). The elderly who are acutely ill are more likely to demonstrate a decreased or increased heart rate and elevated blood pressure. The EF in this group will be lower, accompanied by a decreased stroke volume and cardiac output. These parameters will be further decreased if the patient has had myocardial infarction. The decreased or delayed response to inotropic support will be an early, rather than a late, sign of failure. The critically ill elderly are also at a higher risk for ventricular and atrial ectopy than are their younger counterparts.

The aging renal system: effects on fluid and electrolyte balance

Normal changes in the structure and function of the senescent kidneys primarily affect functional reserve rather than baseline values (Table 16-10). Under basal conditions, fluid and electrolyte balance and acid-base status remain relatively "normal." However, aging significantly impairs the ability of the older person to adapt to stressors such as dehydration, hypotension, ischemia, acidosis, exposure to multiple nephrotoxic agents, and other clinical situations associated with critical illness.

The most significant structural change affecting renal function is the reduction in kidney size (400 gm at 40 years of age reduced to 250 gm by 80 years of age), principally within the cortex of the kidney, which dramatically affects glomerular structure and function.[54] Glomerular filtration rates (GFRs) decrease by as much as 50% by age 60 because of the reduction in the size, number, and function of the nephrons, as well as chronic changes in renal blood flow (649 ml/min in the fourth decade reduced to an average of 289 ml/min in the ninth decade).[54] A number of factors are responsible for the decrease in renal blood flow such as decreased cardiac output, atherosclerosis, and changes in the amount of and responsiveness to renin. Together, these conditions lead to a reduction in creatinine clearance (CrCl) and slightly elevated levels of blood urea nitrogen (BUN) and serum creatinine (Cr).

In many ways normal renal function in the elderly resembles chronic renal failure specifically because of the noted reduction in diluting and concentrating ability when the older kidney is stressed. One of the most specific and consistent changes associated with advanced age is the loss of the ability to regulate and maintain normal volume status. In addition to a decrease in renal blood flow, several other factors contribute to the inability to regulate fluid volume.[34-36,87] For example, although antidiuretic hormone (ADH) levels may be normal or even slightly elevated, responsiveness to ADH by the renal tubules is extremely variable in the elderly. At the same time, circulating levels of aldosterone may be decreased by as much as 60% to 70%, con-

Table 16-10 Alterations in Renal Function Associated with the Aging Process*

Function	Alteration
Regulation of water balance	Ineffective thirst mechanism Dilution or concentration of urine slower secondary to decreased responsiveness to ADH, decreased GFR, decreased production of renin, or decreased number and function of nephrons
Electrolyte balance	Decreased reabsorption of PO_4^- Decreased maximal ability to excrete glucose Limited ability to handle K loads Impaired conservation of Na secondary to decreased aldosterone and response to ADH Total body K^+ and Mg^{++} levels down related to common use of diuretics that affect K^+ and Mg^{++} levels
Acid-base balance	Inability to excrete acid load maximally Metabolic alkalosis associated with aggressive diuretic therapy
Excretion of end product	Creatinine clearance reduced, BUN increased secondary to decreased GFR, decreased number and function of nephrons Serum creatinine unchanged related to decreased muscle mass Slower clearance of various drugs
Regulation of RBC production	Anemia secondary to decreased erythropoietin production

*Not all patients will present with each criterion.
ADH, Antidiuretic hormone; *BUN,* Blood urea nitrogen; *GFR,* Glomerular filtration rate; K^+, Potassium; Mg^{++}, Magnesium; *Na,* Sodium; PO_4^-, Phosphate; *RBC,* Red blood cell.

tributing to an increased susceptibility to dehydration and impaired fluid conservation capabilities.[36] One of the primary mechanisms for maintaining adequate hydration is the sensation of thirst transmitted to the cerebral cortex through stimulation of osmoreceptors. As with other receptors, osmoreceptors become less sensitive over time, which leads to an increased tolerance of osmoreceptors to higher serum osmolarities and a decreased sensation of thirst.

The efficiency of acid-base homeostasis is also decreased in the elderly. Elimination of acid loads is markedly prolonged in older persons when compared with younger subjects. Minor decreases in serum bicarbonate levels and delayed renal elimination of bicarbonate contribute to the inefficiency of this system.[59] The ability of the respiratory system to compensate for metabolic acid-base abnormalities is also diminished with age.

Criteria to determine failure of the renal system should be based on the lack of reserve and the assumption that most older persons have some element of preexisting renal disease or dysfunction. Because of the preexisting compromise in renal blood flow and the sensitivity of the elderly to physiologic alterations such as dehydration, hypotension, sepsis, and exposure to various nephrotoxic substances, acute renal failure is more likely to occur early in the course of critical illness for the geriatric patient. The use of urine output as a determinant of renal failure should also be specifically individualized in the elderly compared with existing criteria established for organ system failure.

CrCl studies may be fairly reliable as an indicator of renal function in the elderly because there is a characteristic decline in CrCl associated with an age-related decrease in renal function.[54] The Baltimore Longitudinal Study on Aging demonstrated a decline in CrCl in normal subjects followed over a 10-year period.[88] Mean CrCl values fell from 140 ml/min/1.73m^2 at 25 to 34 years of age to 97 ml/min/1.73m^2 in octogenarians.[88] However, there is some evidence that not all persons will experience a decline in CrCl. Therefore, it is postulated that this decline is not part of the "normal" aging process, but instead, is due to chronic pathologic changes commonly noted in the elderly: undetected glomerulonephritis, immunologic insults, drugs or other toxic exposures, vascular occlusions, and urinary tract infections.

Serum Cr levels have not been shown to be significantly different over time. This is probably due to a reduction in Cr production reflecting the decrease in muscle mass that occurs with aging. As a result, serum Cr levels alone should not be used as a primary criterion for determining renal failure in the elderly. It may be more reliable to measure the change in serum Cr during acute illness, such as a doubling of the admission Cr level (Table 16-5).[53,54,87-89]

Although BUN levels must be examined in the context of hydration status, protein intake, and renal blood flow they may reflect actual changes in renal function with age better than do serum Cr values. It is unlikely that protein intake is the leading cause for the elevation in BUN levels in normal, healthy, well-hydrated older subjects. Consequently, it is believed that changes in BUN levels may directly reflect the reduction in renal blood flow associated with aging.[53,54,87-89] Therefore, in the older critically ill patient BUN values should be utilized more specifically in order to determine whether renal failure is present.

Older persons are more likely to develop acute renal failure (ARF) early in the course of critical illness because of chronic renal insufficiency. Therefore, the requirement for dialysis may need to be considered an earlier criterion of organ system dysfunction or failure (Table 16-5) than that determined by Dietch[28] in the younger patient population group (Table 16-1).

The aging neurologic system: effects on regulation and behavior

It is very difficult to assess and identify the causes of neurologic dysfunction in the critically ill patient. Pathology of any organ system can cause some degree of neurologic malfunction. For example, decreased cardiac output, impaired gas exchange, and electrolyte imbalances can all potentially cause a change in level of consciousness, confusion, and coma. Conversely, neurologic dysfunction can also affect regulatory function in numerous organ systems. However, there are some biologic changes that occur over time that also affect neurologic function and capability.

The central and peripheral nervous systems are affected by the aging process. The actual weight of the brain decreases over time and there is a decline in nerve and cerebral functions.[53] The elderly have a reduction in the number of neurons and synapses resulting in a decrease of conduction speed and an increase in the time required for processing information.[53] Biochemical alterations affect behavioral and regulatory systems.[57] Cerebral perfusion also decreases over time. In individuals 70 years of age, cerebral perfusion may be as low as 40 ml/min/100 g,[53] which is a 50% drop from the perfusion rate in young adults. This may be of great significance in the hypoperfusion states that occur in patients suffering from MODS. The elderly may demonstrate a decreased level of consciousness related to these changes.

There are a multitude of reasons for the geriatric patient to become confused. The problem could be as simple as difficulty with sensory input. Hearing and visual deficits are common in this age group.[67] These changes may affect the ability of the patient to understand the unusual surroundings of the intensive care unit. The sleep pattern changes that occur over time place the elderly at even higher risk for sleep deprivation than younger critically ill patients.[90] Or the confusion could be caused by complex factors such as changes in metabolism, or fluid and electrolyte disturbances. Level of consciousness could also be affected by prescription or over-the-counter medications the individual may be taking. Fein and Niederman[61] found that the most common presenting complaint of geriatric patients suffering from infection was lethargy or confusion.

The criteria for identifying neurologic dysfunction in the elderly are similar to those established for younger adults (Tables 16-1 and 16-5). The challenge when performing a neurologic assessment on a geriatric patient is to determine whether the findings are a result of normal aging, are metabolic in nature, or are a result of MODS.

THERAPEUTIC MANAGEMENT
Treatment considerations

The management of the geriatric patient suffering from MODS is more difficult than that of the adult patient. As stated throughout this chapter, the elderly population is unique because of the physiologic changes that occur over time, causing a decrease in functional reserve and an inability to compensate during periods of stress. The goal in caring for these patients is to incorporate the biology of aging into every assessment interpretation and treatment decision.

The conservative decision to delay treatment for fear of complications is a very dangerous one. A conservative approach has been shown to have a very high mortality rate.[22,57,91] Pellicane and colleagues[22] found that preventable complications contributed to mortality in 62% of their geriatric patients with documented MODS. They discovered that the majority of these complications occurred because the elderly had not been monitored aggressively. Scalea and co-workers[57] improved survival from 7% to 53% in injured elderly patients by early invasive monitoring and treatment, and they state: "Evaluation of multiply injured geriatric patients may be misleading as those seemingly stable may have dangerously low CO. Untreated, this hypoperfusion state will proceed to cardiogenic shock and may produce multiple organ failure (MOF) if treated late. Emergent invasive monitoring identifies occult shock early, limits hypoperfusion, and will help prevent MOF and improve survival." Santora and co-workers[91] strongly recommend the use of early invasive monitoring to calculate oxygen transport variables, which allows for more precise and adequate planning of treatment. The ethical decision to treat or not to treat is one that should be made very early in the course of the illness and evaluated on a regular basis. If the decision to treat is made, it should be done as aggressively as possible, given the information available at the time.

Specific considerations must be addressed when aggressively treating the elderly patient suffering from actual or impending MODS. Preinjury laboratory values should be acquired from the patient's private physician if possible. Blood chemistry assays can help identify the functional level of various organs. A thermodilution pulmonary artery catheter is very helpful when determining the ability of the cardiopulmonary system to withstand and respond to volume resuscitation, inotropic support, and the cardiovascular stress imposed by critical illness and hyperdynamic states. Knowledge of prescription and nonprescription medication is essential. All drug doses should be considered carefully and levels evaluated frequently.

Most adult critical care practitioners deliver care to individuals 18 years of age and older. Because the elderly are different, it is necessary to have two bodies of knowledge for "normal" physiology: one for the 18 to 65 years of age group and another for those over 65 years of age. Unfortunately, as a group, the elderly are very heterogenous. The degenerative process occurs at different rates based on variations in life style, genetic makeup, social support systems, and chronic illnesses. To meet the challenge of caring for this patient population, the practitioner must be familiar with the physiology of aging, have a complete and detailed physical and psychosocial history of the patient, perform a comprehensive physical and laboratory assessment, be knowledgeable of critical care principles and treatment options available for MODS, and apply all of this information to create an individual plan of care for each patient.

Improved outcomes can only be realized through knowledge of the geriatric response to injury or shock and the employment of management strategies that will reduce the incidence of pulmonary, cardiac, and septic complications. The elderly frequently display shock in a precipitous fashion, masking the early warning signs and providing very little time for intervention between the first manifestation of distress and blatant shock.

The use of early invasive monitoring to assess cardiovascular function and intravascular volume status should be instituted as soon as possible. Resuscitation should otherwise be similar to the management of any patient that presents with shock. Blood loss should be replaced with blood products as soon as possible to maintain intravascular volume and oxygen-carrying capacity.[23,37,57] It may be necessary to utilize low-dose dopaminergic agents in an effort to improve perfusion of the kidneys and splanchnic bed during acute low-flow states. It is also important to remember that urine output may not reflect perfusion states because of chronic changes in renal function associated with advanced age.

Once the aging process has been taken into consideration, the basic theory of caring for the elderly MODS patient is similar in principle to that of all critically ill adult patients. Recognizing risk factors (preexisting conditions, medications, age), early recognition of organ failure, and prevention of infection and hypoperfusion are undoubtedly the most important treatment goals. Because of the lack of physiologic reserve in the critically ill elderly patient, prevention of MODS is paramount. Prompt recognition of the early warning signs associated with activation of the inflammatory/immune response is essential. Once activated, the cascade of MODS is treated with source control, oxygen supply and demand balance, nutritional support, and individual organ support as outlined in Chapters 17 and 18 of this book. This section will review principles of therapy that are unique to the geriatric population.

Prevention. The most critical element of treatment for all patients at risk for sepsis, SIRS, or MODS is prevention. Regardless of the age of the patient, the basic course of prevention remains the same. A thorough history and physical assessment, rapid resuscitation, surgery if necessary, prompt stabilization of fractures, aggressive monitoring, early nutritional support, and management of all infectious processes are essential. However, it is vital that in addition to these, the clinician must consider the other unique characteristics of aging when caring for the elderly. Most important is the delayed presentation of symptoms of infection and even sepsis frequently observed in the elderly. The typical presentations of tachycardia, increased minute ventilation, increased white blood cell count, and fever are all delayed and may possibly be absent in the septic elderly patient. A change in mental status or general malaise may be the first and possibly the only clinical symptom of infection until the patient develops frank septic shock.[61] These subtle signs should be methodically investigated and specific infection or SIRS should be ruled out. Remember, however, that MODS is not always associated with sepsis but rather with a systemic inflammatory response gone awry.

The elderly must be carefully protected against infection because of their chronic immunosuppressed state. They have a decreased CMI and altered humoral immunity, and are also on a variety of medications (steroids, nonsteroidal antiinflammatory drugs) for chronic illnesses that may impair the normal immune response to injury, illness, or acute infection. The box on p. 377 outlines some of the preventive measures that can be taken with this vulnerable patient group.

Successful prevention of MODS in the aged population requires a collaborative, multidisciplinary plan of care. Aggressive invasive monitoring is usually required. The need to identify the physical reserve status (true physiologic age) of the patient usually outweighs the risks associated with invasive monitoring. Once instituted, the need for continued maintenance of any line, tube, or drain should be discussed daily. Frequent turning, aggressive pul-

> **CLINICAL TREATMENT PERSPECTIVE FOR ELDERLY SEPTIC PATIENTS**
>
> 1. Skin and urinary tract colonization is a greater problem the elderly than in younger patients. Thus, the need for commonly used devices such as indwelling urinary catheters must be carefully considered, and the importance of regular skin care must be emphasized in the elderly.
> 2. The elderly, due in part to changes in immune competence, face a different spectrum of pathogens than younger patients. Therefore, the elderly must have limited exposure to fungal, viral, and mycobacterial pathogens that might be unrecognized as problems in younger patients.
> 3. The elderly do not show typical signs of infection. Common "atypical" presentations of infection include change in mental status, weakness, malaise, anorexia, repeated falls, normothermia or hypothermia, failure to thrive, and alteration in hemostasis. Typical presenting findings including fever, chills, tachypnea, tachycardia, and leukocytosis are frequently absent in elderly patients with significant infection.
> 4. The key to blunting the effects of sepsis in the elderly in rapid diagnosis with immediate resuscitation. Elimination of infection source is also critical. Effective early resuscitation may coincide with institution of broad-spectrum antibiotic coverage until appropriate cultures are available to narrow the antibiotic spectrum.
> 5. Proper systemic care, particularly nutrition, may be essential in the elderly as these patients frequently present with preexisting deficits coinciding with infection problems.
> 6. Although a variety of mediators and blockers for the sepsis syndrome are receiving current attention, recent studies suggest that appropriate application of these agents in the elderly may be compromised by failure to recognize appropriate signs indicating the need for intervention because of altered response to infection.

From Stengel J, Dries D. Sepsis in the elderly. Crit Care Nurs Clin North Am 1994;6:426.

monary toilet, and early ambulation are essential to decrease the risk of pneumonia and other complications of immobility. Prevention is the key, attention must be paid to each organ system, and support must be provided.

Source identification and control. Early identification and control of infection are important goals when treating all patients with MODS. In some situations the source is not easily identified. Although cultures, hemodynamic monitoring, radiographic tests, and detailed physical assessment are very useful, sometimes the source cannot be identified without surgical intervention. Once a cause is identified every measure should be undertaken to eradicate it. This is usually accomplished by specific antibiotic administration, surgical débridement, and removal or drainage of abscesses resulting from infectious sources. The elderly should be placed on antibiotics, based on clinical features, and the coverage should be specific for a particular organism as soon as one is identified.[92,93] The patient with a positive culture should be treated with specific antibiotics even if there is a strong potential for organ toxicity. These organs must be monitored carefully and supported to the fullest extent. If surgery is indicated it should not be delayed. The primary goals are to remove the source, restore hemostasis, and prevent further mediator release and damage. Unfortunately there are times when a source is never identified. In these instances organ support is often the only option.

The decrease in functional reserve not only contributes to the development of MODS in the elderly but also influences their response to treatments. For example, the potential for nephrotoxicity with antibiotic administration is increased in the aged. Fluid resuscitation must be carefully monitored to ensure appropriate replacement without complications of hypovolemia or hypervolemia. Drug doses may need to be modified for renal or hepatic dysfunction. Aggressive treatments must be ordered with knowledge of aging physiology and must be individualized for each specific patient.

Oxygen supply and demand balance. As stated earlier, the goal of treatment is to return the patient to homeostasis. In the patient with MODS this is predominantly accomplished by optimizing oxygen supply, repaying any oxygen debt that may have accumulated, and decreasing oxygen demands. Optimizing oxygen supply is achieved, as outlined in Chapter 17, by volume resuscitation, inotropic and vasopressor administration, and achieving an optimal hemoglobin level and arterial saturation. Shoemaker and colleagues[94] demonstrated improved survival rates when supranormal values for cardiac index, oxygen delivery, and oxygen consumption were achieved (in adults). The same therapies should be initiated in geriatric patients (Fig. 16-4), but unfortunately the aged do not respond as quickly or as well to treatment. The decreased functional ability of the cardiac and pulmonary systems in the elderly specifically affects many treatment modalities. In fact, some treatments can actually cause more harm than good if not ordered and administered with geriatric physiology in mind. Last, the actual goal of therapy must be modified. The definitions of optimal cardiac output and oxygen saturation are different when evaluating the elderly.

Therapies that are usually effective in optimizing cardiac output are fluid resuscitation and inotropic or vasoactive drug infusions. These therapies should certainly be instituted when caring for elderly patients, but the physical response of the patients can be varied, because of the normal changes in the cardiovascular system with age. The cardiac output of a healthy 80-year-old may be as much as 50% below the "normal" output for a younger adult.[65] Therefore, it is not likely that volume resuscitation or pharmacologic agents will achieve a "normal" result for cardiac output (4 to 6 L/min). Chronic disorders that affect pulmonary, cardiac, or renal function may affect the response to fluid administration as well. The elderly who have a chronic increase in

$$DaO_2 = CO \times Hgb \times SaO_2 \times 1.34 \times 10$$

- HR × SV
  - Optimize 90-110 beats/min
- 10-12 gm/dL
- Support early with ventilator
  Maintain SaO_2 > 88%

Preload
- Give volume
  Goal: optimize WP (15-20 mmHg, highly individualized)
- Monitor cardiac function during fluid replacement

Afterload
- Maintain SVR > 800
  MAP > 80
  Use vasopressors after volume adequately replaced
- Maintain SVR < 1500 through afterload reducing agents after volume is adequately replaced

Contractility
- Early inotropic support
  Optimize CO >5 L/min
  Monitor for tolerance
  —Failure to respond
  —Dysrhythmias
  —ECG changes
  —End organ dysfunction

Monitoring for Evidence of Adequate Tissue Perfusion
- Mental status
- Skin color, temperature, moisture, quality pulses
- Liver and renal function
- Acid base balance
- Hemoglobin and hematocrit

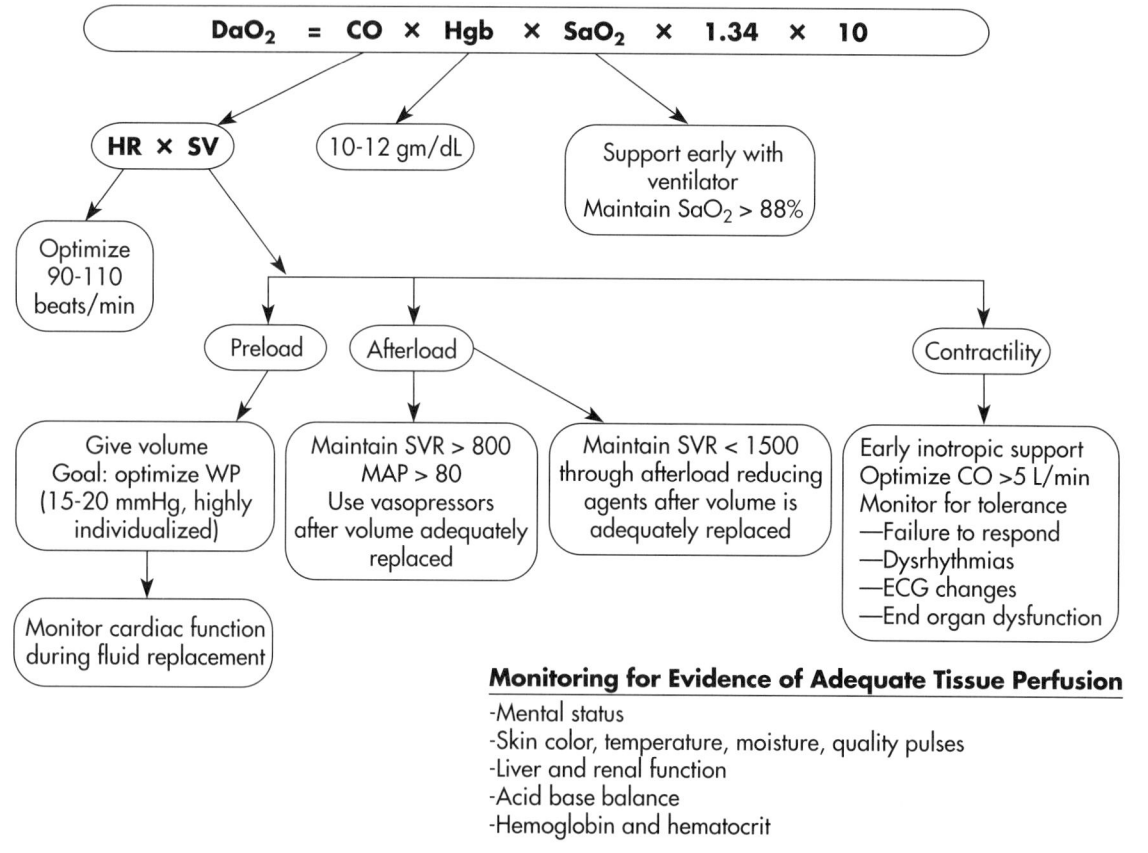

Fig. 16-4 Therapeutic goals for critically ill elderly cardiopulmonary support.[6,7,57,94,97] *CO*, Cardiac output; *ECG*, electrocardiogram; *MAP*, mean arterial pressure; *SVR*, systemic vascular resistance; *WP*, wedge pressure.

preload or afterload may respond with worsening shock when fluid is administered (Fig. 16-4). The use of invasive monitoring is essential to determine the best treatment option and evaluate the effectiveness of therapies.

The response to drug administration may be varied in the elderly as well, because of changes in the levels of circulating catecholamines and the receptor response. As outlined in the physiology section, the elderly will probably need higher doses of vasoconstrictors to achieve a therapeutic response. An increase in afterload could cause increased work and oxygen demands on the heart resulting in decreased cardiac output, ST segment changes, dysrhythmias, and eventually, cardiac decompensation. The physical assessment findings of improved mentation, urine output, and warm skin may be better indicators of improved cardiac output than the thermodilution number obtained.

Tissue perfusion can be impaired in the elderly for a variety of reasons. In addition to optimizing cardiac output, another way to improve oxygenation and tissue perfusion is to administer oxygen or blood (hemoglobin), recognizing again that the geriatric patient has lower than "normal" values of both of these indices. In this era of conservative blood administration for reasons related to infection and cost , it must be remembered that hemoglobin is essential to oxygen delivery. Therefore, age should always be a consideration in the decision of whether to administer blood in order to optimize tissue perfusion.

One mechanism to improve the oxygen supply and demand balance is to decrease demand. This is very important in the elderly critically ill patient population. Because of the decreased functional reserve in this group, they are, by nature, out of balance. Every effort should be made to decrease any demands on all of the systems. For example ventilator support is frequently necessary to decrease demands on the respiratory system (work of breathing) and deliver adequate amounts of oxygen. Because of the weakness and degeneration that has occurred over time in the pulmonary structures of the elderly patient, the addition of positive pressure ventilation is sometimes a welcome break from the increased expenditure of energy necessary for normal ventilation. As a result, geriatric patients frequently require a longer time on the ventilator and a more structured weaning program. The elderly benefit from work and rest periods throughout the day and rest at night. The use of pressure support modes and muscle training are helpful. Attempts to wean the elderly using the same parameters as for younger patients may be unsuccessful; therefore, parameters should be individually determined based on preexisting pulmonary function. There is sometimes a hesitancy to initiate ventilator support in geriatric patients for fear of making them ventilator dependent. Nevertheless, if the decision is made to aggressively treat the elderly suffering from MODS, the only way to optimize oxygen delivery may be through ventilator management.

Patients should be kept as free of pain as possible. This may require asking them directly if they have pain and extensive education regarding pain management strategies. Anxiety should be treated because of its effects on cardiac and pulmonary work. Something as simple as allowing the patients to wear their glasses or a hearing aid may relieve anxiety. Sedatives should be utilized, if needed, to decrease oxygen demands and make the patient more comfortable. High or low temperature swings will also increase demands and should be prevented, along with preventing hypovolemic or hypervolemic states and wide swings in blood pressure. Although decreasing the oxygen demands is a goal when caring for all critically ill patients, it is of even greater importance with the elderly because of their diminished reserve prior to illnesses.

Nutritional support in the elderly critically ill. Early feeding with enteral and parenteral nutritional support is necessary for this fragile critically ill population. Unfortunately, there are a variety of barriers and challenges that prevent the adequate and appropriate delivery of nutritional support to the critically ill elderly patient.[44,56,95] The overall goal of nutritional support is to minimize depletion of active muscle tissue in order to optimize oxygen consumption and prevent wasting of vital muscle tissue such as pulmonary and skeletal mass in order to promote optimal recovery and minimize functional losses. Specific support should be guided by two major principles. First, the older person has minimal reserves to call upon in times of acute stress starvation. Therefore, nutritional support should begin as soon as acute shock has resolved (within 24 to 48 hours). In fact some researchers are examining the possibility of providing nutritional support as early as 8 to 12 hours after surgery or traumatic injury with good results.[80] The second principle focuses on maintaining integrity of the GI system. This will minimize the hypermetabolic response to acute illness and optimize immune function.

Bowel rest, frequently associated with critical illness and the delivery of total parenteral nutrition, exacerbates mucosal atrophy and could contribute to the development of bacterial translocation and endotoxemia.[79,80,96] These pathophysiologic complications potentiate the hypermetabolic stress response and act as a stimulus for the development of sepsis and multiple organ dysfunction. Myocardial depressant factor may also be released as the mucosal wall breaks down, leading to further organ system failure.[79,80] Thus, whenever possible, enteral support should be considered as a first choice for the delivery of energy substrates.

The integrity of the GI system is totally dependent upon direct exposure to nutrients through the GI tract. If full alimentation is not possible, small amounts of enteral nutrition should be provided to the gut beyond the ligament of Treitz in order to maintain mucosal integrity (10 to 20 ml/hr has been recommended,[96,97] although there is very little scientific research to support a specific infusion rate). Another very important consideration is the enteral delivery of glutamine, a conditionally essential amino acid. Glutamine plays a very important role in the immunologic structure of the GI tract, providing a fuel source for lymphocytes and macrophages. Unfortunately, glutamine is currently not stable in parenteral solutions and, therefore, can only be delivered through enteral alimentation. Without this amino acid the mucosal surface atrophies and CMI is further compromised.* Additionally, there are a number of disease-specific formulas that can be employed in order to minimize further organ system dysfunction.[97]

Full nutritional support through enteral nutrition alone may not be achievable. Every effort should be taken, however, to utilize mixed delivery techniques for the older critically ill patient in order to protect the gut, while at the same time providing adequate nutritional support. As GI function returns, parenteral support should be slowly titrated down and enteral provisions gradually increased until the desired nutritional goal is achieved.[44,56,80,96] Of course, there are certain conditions such as small- or large-bowel obstruction that completely preclude the implementation of any enteral support, in which case total parenteral nutrition should be provided without hesitation.

Specific nutrient requirements depend upon the level of stress, the presence and type of organ dysfunction, and the goals of nutritional support (based on preexisting nutritional status and the phase of the acute stress response). Although there are a variety of strategies to estimate actual energy requirements, the most common method of determining energy requirements is the use of the Harris-Benedict equation as a measure of basal energy expenditure multiplied by a stress factor or activity factor such as those developed by Long and co-workers.[98] Once initiated, specific substrate delivery will need to be adjusted on a daily basis depending on the level of patient tolerance.[99]

Recommendations for nutrient delivery are based on knowledge of altered patterns of substrate utilization during critical illness in the elderly.[42,44,56] It is best to start with a higher percentage of carbohydrates than is utilized in younger acutely ill patients. In order to achieve the desired goal, exogenous administration of insulin will most likely be necessary. Fats should be administered on a 12- to 24-hour basis in order to improve uptake and minimize lipid intolerance. Protein replacement will depend on renal function, but should ideally start with 2.0 gm/kg/day and be titrated to the desired effect or protein tolerance.[45,46,95] A positive nitrogen balance is the ultimate goal; however, depending on the particular phase of stress it may be possible only to minimize losses or maintain an even nitrogen balance.

Individual organ support. Individual organ support is an important component of prevention and of maintaining the oxygen supply and demand balance. The lack of reserve in most organ systems in the elderly may require initiation of therapy or support earlier in the course of treatment than with younger patients. The amount of support necessary to maintain function and combat failure may also be greater in the elderly. As noted above, the elderly may need ventilator support earlier and require it for longer periods of time. Geriatric patients may have a greater need for dialysis as well. If active resuscitation and support is the treatment choice, therapies should be initiated as soon as their use can be beneficial. Many studies have demonstrated that the

---

*References 56, 79, 80, 96, 97.

mortality and morbidity of elderly critically ill patients can be improved when they are managed aggressively.[16,22,64,100] However, before initiating individual organ support, the clinician must verify that the dysfunction of the organ is acute and not from the aging process alone.

The goals of management for the victims of MODS are similar regardless of the age of the patients. Prevention, source identification and control, maintaining oxygen supply and demand balance, nutritional support, and individual organ support are the cornerstones of therapy. It is increasingly difficult to achieve these goals when caring for the elderly population. The barriers of diminished physiologic reserve, preexisting conditions, and decreased responses to treatments are difficult to overcome. Successful treatments are those that apply the physiology of aging to all assessment and treatment decisions, differentiate dysfunction from degeneration, and initiate therapies early with meticulous follow up and monitoring to prevent complications.

Ethical considerations

Buehler states: "Caring for critically ill people contains elements not only of scientific and intellectual challenge, but also challenges to one's moral values, ethical reasoning, and belief systems, not to mention one's most deeply felt emotions."[101] These challenges are increased when delivering care to elderly victims of MODS. Caring for people with this disorder is labor intensive and a financial burden to family, institution, and society. Despite intense research and investigation, only minimal improvements in outcomes have resulted over the last 20 years. The questions facing the critical care team, patient, and family are the most difficult questions in health care. When is treatment futile? When is death a better option?

Although difficult, these questions must be answered. A multidisciplinary approach is essential to determine what treatments most benefit the elderly patient.[102] Informed consent on the part of the patient and family is vital.[103] Ideally, a preillness discussion with the primary care provider will have been held and legal documentation of the patient's wishes in the form of a durable power of attorney for health care decisions will have been executed. Decisions must be made utilizing a physical, psychologic, and financial cost-benefit analysis. The relationship between critical care, elderly patients, and their quality of life requires more vigorous scientific and ethical investigation.[104]

CONCLUSION

Caring for patients suffering from MODS offers the greatest challenge in the critical care setting. Elderly patients bring a unique set of problems and considerations for the health care team. This patient population is growing at an astonishing rate and occupies an increasingly higher percentage of beds in acute care units. Successful treatment and improved outcomes will be realized when the physiology of aging is incorporated into all treatment decisions. Prevention, early identification, and aggressive treatment are the key to patient survival. Because of the decreased functional reserve characteristic of the aged, mortality rates increase once the organs cross the fine line from dysfunction to failure. Although these patients have many obstacles to recovery, outcomes can be positive if they are treated with aggressive, state of the art supportive care.[100,105]

"To be happy we must be true to nature and carry our age along with us"
William Hazlitt (English critic and author), 1830

REFERENCES

1. Bone R et al. Definitions for sepsis and organ failure and guidelines for the use of innovative therapies in sepsis. Chest 1992;101:1648-1655.
2. Darling G et al. Multiple organ failure in critically ill patients. Can J Surg 1988;31:172.
3. Hotter A. The pathophysiology of multi-system organ failure in the trauma patient. AACN Clin Issues Crit Care Nurs 1990;1:465-471.
4. Demling R et al. Multiple organ dysfunction in the surgical patient: Pathophysiology, prevention, and treatment. Curr Probl Surg 1993;30:345-424.
5. Knaus WA, Wagner DP. Multiple systems organ failure: Epidemiology and prognosis. Crit Care Clin 1989;5:221-232.
6. Morris J, Mackenzie E, Edelstein S. The effect of preexisting conditions on mortality in trauma patients. JAMA 1990; 263:1942-1946.
7. Panlilio A, Culver D, Gaynes R. Methicillin resistant Staphylococcus aureus in U.S. hospital 1975-1991. Infection Control and Hospital Epidemiology 1992;13:10.
8. NCHS. Public health focus: Surveillance, prevention, and control of nosocomial infection. MMW 1990;41:42.
9. Centers for Disease Control and Prevention. Surveillance Report 3rd quarter. 1994;5.
10. Kass J, Castriotta R, Malakoff F. Intensive care unit outcome in the very elderly. Crit Care Med 1992;20:1666-1671.
11. Fry D. Multiple system organ failure. Surg Clin North Am 1990; 68:541-547.

12. Knaus W et al. Prognosis in acute organ system failure. Ann Surg 1985;202:685.
13. Stengle J, Dries D. Sepsis in the elderly. Crit Care Nurs Clin North Am 1994;6:421-427.
14. Reilly E, Yucha C. Multiple organ failure syndrome. Crit Care Nurse 1994;14:25-31.
15. Smith DP, Enderson BL, Maull KI. Trauma in the elderly: Determinants of outcome. South Med J 1990;83:171-177.
16. Tran D et al. Age, chronic disease, sepsis, organ system failure and the mortality in medical intensive care unit. Crit Care Med 1990;18:474-479.
17. Beck M. The gray nineties. Newsweek 1993; Oct. 4, 65-66.
18. U.S. Senate Special Committee on Aging. Aging of America: Trends and projections 1991 edition. U.S. Federal Printing Office, 1991.
19. American Medical Association Council on Scientific Affairs. Societal effects and other factors affecting health care for the elderly. Arch Intern Med 1990;150:1184-1189.
20. Castillo P, Pausada L. Emergency services use by elderly individuals. Clin Geriatr Med 1993; 9:491-497.
21. Graves E. Centers for Disease Control and Prevention, 1992 summary: National hospital discharge survey. Advance Date 1994;249.
22. Pellican J, Byrne K, DeMaria E. Preventable complications and death from multiple organ failure among geriatric trauma victims. J Trauma 1992;3:440-444.
23. Levy D, Hanlon D, Townsed R. Geriatric trauma. Clin Geriatr Med 1993;9:601-620.
24. Zietlow S et al. Multisystem geriatric trauma. J Trauma 1994;37:985-988.
25. Iberti R et al. Are the criteria used to determine sepsis applicable for patients >75 years of age? Crit Care Med 1993;S130.
26. Cerra F. The multiple organ failure syndrome. Hosp Prac 1990; August 15:169-176.
27. Finelli F et al. A case study for major trauma in geriatric patients. J Trauma 1989;29:541-548.
28. Deitch E. Overview of multiple organ failure. In: Critical care state of the art. Society of Critical Care Medicine, 1993; 14:131-168.
29. Johnson C et al. Trauma in the elderly: An analysis of outcomes based on age. Am Surg 1994;6:899-902.
30. McCoy G, Johnstone R, Duthe R. Injury to the elderly in road traffic accidents. J Trauma 1989;29:494-497.
31. Osler T et al. Trauma in the elderly. Am J Surg 1988;156:537-543.
32. Ross N et al. High cost of trauma care in the elderly. South Med J 1989;82:857-859.
33. Bursztyn M et al. Effect of aging on vasopressin, catecholamines, and alpha2-adrenergic receptors. J Am Geriatr Soc 1990;38:628-632.
34. Gregerman R. Mechanisms of age-related alterations of hormone secretion and action. An overview of 30 years of progress. Exp Gerontol.1986;21:345-365.
35. Timiras P. Physiological basis of geriatrics. New York: MacMillan Publishing Company; 1988.
36. Waters JM, Wilmore DW. Physiology of aging: The response to injury. In: Meakins JL, McClaran JC, eds. Surgical care of the elderly. St. Louis: Mosby; 1988.
37. Schwab CW, Kauder DR. Trauma in the geriatric patient. Arch Surg 1992;127:701-706.
38. Kronenberg RS, Drager CW. Attenuation of the ventilatory and heart rate response to hypoxia and hypercapnia with aging in normal man. J Clin Invest 1973;52:1812-1819.
39. Levitsky MG. Effects of aging on the respiratory system. Physiology 1984;27:102-107.
40. Collins KJ et al. Functional changes in autonomic nervous responses with aging. Age Ageing 1980;9:17-24.
41. Desai D, March R, Watters JM. Hyperglycemia after trauma increases with age. J Trauma 1989;29:719-723.
42. Jeevanandam M, Young DH, Schiller WR. Energy cost of fat-fuel mobilization in geriatric trauma. Metabolism 1990; 39:144-149.
43. Odio MR, Brodish A. Effects of age on metabolic responses to acute and chronic stress. Am J Physiol 1988;254:E617-E624.
44. Stamatos CA, Fontaine D, Frankenfield D. A comparative analysis of the metabolic response to trauma in the elderly (abstract). Heart Lung 1992;21:294.
45. Jeevanandam M et al. Effect of major trauma on plasma free amino acid concentrations in geriatric patients. Am J Clin Nutr 1990;51:1040-1045.
46. Young V. Amino acids and proteins in relation to the nutrition of elderly people. Age Ageing 1990;19:S10-24.
47. Rudman D. Growth hormone, body composition, and aging. J Am Geriatr Soc 1985;33:800-809.
48. Busby J, Caranasos G. Immune function, autoimmunity, and selective immunoprophylaxis in the aged. Med Clin North Am 1985;69:465-474.
49. Ismail N, Hakim RM, Helderman JH. Renal replacement therapies in the elderly: Part II. Renal transplantation. Am J Kidney Dis 1994;23:1-15.
50. Lesourd BM, Meaume S. Cell mediated immunity changes in ageing, relative importance of cell subpopulation switches and of nutritional factors. Immunol Lett 1994;40:235-242.
51. Isaacs KL. Severe gastrointestinal bleeding. Clin Geriatr Med 1994;10:1-17.
52. Kawanishi H. Recent progress in senescence-associated gut mucosal immunity. Dig Dis 1993;11:157-72.
53. Kenney R. Physiology of aging: A synopsis. 2nd ed. Chicago: Mosby, 1989.
54. Lindeman RD. Renal physiology and pathophysiology of aging. Contrib Nephrol 1993;105:1-12.
55. Rose NR. Thymus function, ageing and autoimmunity. Immunol Lett 1994;40:225-230.
56. Opper F, Burakoff R. Nutritional support of the elderly patient in an intensive care unit. Clin Geriatr Med 1994;10:31-49.
57. Scalea TM et al. Geriatric blunt multiple trauma: Improved survival with early invasive monitoring. J Trauma 1990;30:129-136.
58. Finkelstein MS et al. Pneumococcal bacteremia in adults: Age-dependent differences in presentation and in outcome. J Am Geriatr Soc 1983;31:19-27.
59. Watters JM, Bessey PQ. Critical care for the elderly patient. Surg Clin North Am 1994;74:187-197.
60. Brody G. Hyperthermia and hypothermia in the elderly. Clin Geriatr Med 1994;10:213-229.
61. Fein A, Niederman M. Severe pneumonia in the elderly. Clin Geriatr Med 1994;10:121-143.
62. Heuser M, Case L, Ettinger W. Mortality in intensive care patients with respiratory disease: Is age important? Arch Intern Med 1992;152:1683.

63. Krieger B. Respiratory failure in the elderly. Clin Geriatr Med 1994;10:103-119.
64. Chelluri L, Pinsky M, Grenvik A. Outcome of intensive care of the "oldest-old" critically ill patients. Crit Care Med 1992;20:757-761.
65. Gee M et al. Physiology of aging related to outcome in the adult respiratory distress syndrome. J Appl Physiol 1990;69:822-829.
66. Miller C. Nursing care of older adults. Glenview, Illinois: Foresman and Company 1990.
67. Pathy M, Finucane P. Geriatric medicine. New York: Springer-Verlag, 1989.
68. Brandstetter R, Kazemi H. Aging and the respiratory system. Med Clin North Am 1983;67:419-431.
69. Krumpe P et al. The aging respiratory system. Clin Geriatr Med 1985;1:143-175.
70. Matteson MA, McConnell ES. Gerontological nursing. Philadelphia: W.B. Saunders, 1988.
71. Kidd P, Murakami R. Common pathologic conditions in elderly persons: Nursing assessment and intervention. J Emerg Nurs 1987;13:27-32.
72. Sparrow D, Weiss S. Pulmonary system. In Rowe J, Besdine R, eds. Geriatric medicine. Boston: Little, Brown, 1988:266-275.
73. Rauen C. Too old to live. Too young to die. MODS in the elderly. Crit Care Nurs Clin North Am 1994;6:535-542.
74. Enright P et al. Respiratory muscle strength in the elderly. Am J Resp Crit Care Med 1994;149:430-438.
75. Nielson. C. Pharmacologic considerations in critical care of the elderly. Clin Geriatr Med 1994;10:71-89.
76. Walker MK. Pharmacology and drug therapy in critically ill elderly patients. AACN Clin Issues Crit Care Nurs 1992; 3:137-148.
77. Kelso T. Laboratory values in the elderly: Are they different? Emerg Med Clin North Am 1990; 8:241-254.
78. Coodley EL. Laboratory tests in the elderly: What is abnormal? Postgrad Med 1989;85:333-338.
79. Lord LM, Sax HC. The role of the gut in critical illness. AACN Clin Issues Crit Care Nurs 1994;5:450-458.
80. Phillips MC, Olson LR. The immunologic role of the gastrointestinal tract. Crit Care Nurs Clin North Am 1993;5:107-120.
81. Atillasoy E, Holt PR. Gastrointestinal proliferation and aging. J Gerontol 1993;48:B43-49.
82. Harris R. Cardiovascular diseases in the elderly. Med Clin North Am 1983;67:379-394.
83. Schneider E, Rowe J. Handbook of the biology of aging. 3rd ed. New York: Academic Press, 1990.
84. Kane RL, Ouslander JG, Abrass IB. Essentials of clinical geriatrics. 3rd ed. New York: McGraw-Hill, 1994.
85. Gates DM. In Huddleston VB, ed. Multisystem organ failure: Pathophysiology and clinical implications. St. Louis: Mosby, 1992:178-203.
86. Cunnion RE, Parrillo JE. Myocardial dysfunction in sepsis. Crit Care Clin 1989;5:99-118.
87. Tinetti ME. Effects of stress on renal function in the elderly. J Am Geriatr Soc 1983;31:174-180.
88. Rowe JW et al. The effect of age on creatinine clearance in men: A cross-sectional and longitudinal study. J Am Geriatr Soc 1976;31:155-163.
89. Sica D. Renal disease, electrolyte abnormalities, and acid-base imbalance in the elderly. Clin Geriatr Med 1994: 10:197-211.
90. Fontaine D. Measurement of nocturnal sleep patterns in trauma. Heart Lung 1989;18:402-409.
91. Santora TA, Schinco MA, Trooshin SZ. Management of trauma in the elderly patient. Surg Clin North Am 1994;74:163-185.
92. Bender B. Sepsis. Clin Geriatr Med 1992;24:365-368.
93. Fontanarosa P, Kaeberlein F, Gerson L. Difficulty in predicting bacteremia in elderly emergency patients. Ann Emerg Med 1992;21:842-848.
94. Shoemaker WC et al. Hemodynamic and oxygen transport monitoring to titrate therapy in septic shock. New Horiz 1993;1:145-159.
95. Rolandelli RH, Ullrich JR. Nutritional support in the frail elderly surgical patient. Surg Clin North Am 1994;74:79-91.
96. Kaminski MV, Blumeyer TJ. Metabolic and nutritional support of the intensive care patient. Ascending the learning curve. Crit Care Clin 1993;9:363-366.
97. Zaloga G, Ackerman MH. A review of disease-specific formulas. AACN Clin Issues Crit Care Nurs 1994;5:421-435.
98. Long CL et al. Metabolic response to injury and illness: Estimation of energy and protein needs from indirect calorimetry and nitrogen balance. J Parenter Enter Nutr 1979;3:452-456.
99. Stamatos C, Reed E. Nutritional needs of trauma patients: Challenges, barriers, and solutions. Crit Care Nurs Clin North Am 1994;3:501-514.
100. Broos P et al. Multiple trauma in elderly patients. Factors influencing outcome: Importance of aggressive care. Injury 1993;24:365-368.
101. Buehler D. Informed consent and the elderly: An ethical challenge for critical care nursing. Crit Care Nurs Clin North Am 1990;2:461-471.
102. Field B, Devich L, Carlson R. Impact of a comprehensive supportive care team on management of hopelessly ill patients with multiple organ failure. Chest 1989;96:353-356.
103. Jillings C. Shock: Psychosocial needs of the patient and family. Crit Care Nurs Clin North Am 1990;2:325-330.
104. Adelman RA, Berger JT, Macina LO. Critical care for the geriatric patient. Clin Geriatric Med 1994;10:19-29.
105. Van Aalst JA et al. Severely injured geriatric patents return to independent living: A study of factors influencing function and independence. J Trauma 1991;31:1098-1102.

CHAPTER *17*

Evaluation and Management of Oxygen Delivery and Consumption in Multiple Organ Dysfunction Syndrome

Kathryn T. Von Rueden and C. Michael Dunham

Cellular hypoxia has been implicated as a progenitor and protractor of the systemic inflammatory response syndrome (SIRS) and multiple organ dysfunction syndrome (MODS). Hypoxia, oxygen debt accumulation, and the resulting cellular dysfunction are due to inadequate systemic oxygen delivery or impairment of cellular oxygen uptake. In addition, normal compensatory responses that limit hypoxic injury may be defective in the presence of inflammatory mediators associated with SIRS and MODS. These mediators also contribute to cardiopulmonary and microvascular dysfunction, thereby reducing oxygen availability and creating cellular hypoxia. Thus, a vicious cycle is perpetuated in critically ill patients with SIRS or MODS. The pathophysiologic mechanisms of hypoxia in relation to SIRS and MODS are described in Chapter 6.

Because cellular hypoxia can incite SIRS and MODS, it is intuitive that oxygen debt should be rapidly reversed and systemic oxygen delivery and consumption maintained. However, the aggression with which these tenets are embraced is controversial. Intensive efforts to observe and describe oxygen dynamics in the critically ill have been undertaken in the past decade. Documentation exists that seriously injured patients and patients with sepsis and adult respiratory distress syndrome (ARDS) usually have enhanced systemic oxygen delivery (Da_{O_2}) and consumption (V_{O_2}).[1-3] Other investigators report that postoperative[4] and injured[5] patients developing ARDS have an antecedent decrease of Da_{O_2} and V_{O_2} and that failure to therapeutically enhance V_{O_2} is associated with a poor outcome.[6,7]

The relationship between Da_{O_2} and V_{O_2} in the critically ill is debated, with some investigators claiming that there is a clear biphasic relationship,[7,8] while others refute this premise on the basis that the pathologic relationship is a mathematical artifact.[2,9-11] Poor outcomes in patients with blunted Da_{O_2} has prompted advocacy for early, therapeutically induced supranormal Da_{O_2}.[12-15] Recent clinical trials suggest that achievement of supranormal Da_{O_2} is beneficial in mitigating MODS.[16-18] However, others conclude that increasing Da_{O_2} does not improve outcome[1,19] and that the level of critical Da_{O_2} is relatively low.[2]

Indicators of oxygen debt, such as elevated serum lactate, may identify critically ill patients who could potentially benefit from Da_{O_2} enhancement. However, some researchers argue that persistent acidosis is only a predictor of a poor outcome.[6,7] Still others claim that global measures of oxygen debt, such as lactate levels, should be replaced with more discriminate measures that reflect regional perfusion deficits.[20,21]

This chapter will review the clinical evaluation of Da_{O_2}, V_{O_2} and oxygen debt and explore these controversial issues. Practical strategies are suggested for managing oxygen delivery and consumption dynamics in the patient with SIRS or MODS.

CLINICAL EVALUATION OF OXYGEN DELIVERY, OXYGEN CONSUMPTION, AND OXYGEN DEBT
Oxygen delivery

Normal cell function, and therefore tissue and organ function, is in large part dependent on the delivery of sufficient oxygen and other substrates to meet the metabolic requirements. Delivery of oxygen to cells is normally influenced by arterial oxygen content and blood flow to the tissue beds (cardiac output and microcirculatory responses). DaO_2 is the product of arterial oxygen content (CaO_2) and cardiac output. Critically ill individuals at risk for or with MODS may require serial monitoring of DaO_2 including the components of cardiac output and CaO_2. Table 17-1 summarizes the clinical parameters utilized to assess oxygen delivery.

Determinants of cardiac output. Cardiac output is a function of heart rate and stroke volume (SV), which is determined by cardiac preload, afterload, and contractility. An impairment in cardiac output requires analysis of these variables to direct appropriate interventional strategies.

Preload. Preload is the resting myofibril (sarcomere) length at ventricular end-diastole that is principally influenced by ventricular end-diastolic volume (VEDV). Preload is primarily affected by circulating blood volume, intravascular distribution of blood volume, and atrial contraction. Within the limits of the Frank-Starling law, adequate VEDV causes lengthening of the myofibrils to enhance the force of contraction, thereby increasing stroke volume and cardiac output. Although the relationship of ventricular end-diastolic pressure and volume is not linear,[22] cardiac pressures are commonly measured at the bedside to assess both right and left ventricular end-diastolic volume. Pressures frequently measured include pulmonary artery occlusion pres-

Table 17-1 Oxygen Delivery Variables

Parameter	Formula	Normal values
CO	Heart rate × Stroke volume	4-8 L/min
CI	$\dfrac{CO}{Body\ surface\ area}$	2.5-4 L/min/m²
SVI	$\dfrac{CI}{Heart\ rate}$	33-47 mL/beat/m²
RAP	Direct measurement	0-8 mm Hg
PAOP	Direct measurement	8-12 mm Hg
RVEDVI	$\dfrac{Stroke\ volume\ index}{RV\ ejection\ fraction}$	60-100 mL/m²
SVRI	$\dfrac{(MAP - RAP)}{CI} \times 80$	1360-2200 dynes/sec/cm⁻⁵
PVRI	$\dfrac{(MPAP - PAOP)}{CI} \times 80$	<425 dynes/sec/cm⁻⁵
LVSWI	SVI (MAP − PaOP) × 0.0136	40-70 gm-m/m²/beat
RVSWI	SVI (PAP − RAP) × 0.0136	5-10 gm-m/m²/beat
CaO_2	(Hb × 1.37 × SaO_2) + (0.003 × PaO_2)	20 mL O_2/dL
CvO_2	(Hb × 1.37 × SvO_2) + (0.003 × PvO_2)	15 mL O_2/dL
DaO_2I	CI × CaO_2 × 10	500-600 mL O_2/min/m²
DvO_2I	CI × CvO_2 × 10	375-450 mL O_2/min/m²

CaO_2, Arterial oxygen content; *CI*, cardiac index; *CO*, cardiac output; *CvO_2*, venous oxygen content; *DaO_2I*, arterial oxygen delivery index; *DvO_2I*, venous oxygen delivery index; *Hb*, hemoglobin; *LVSWI*, left ventricular stroke work index; *MAP*, mean arterial pressure; *MPAP*, mean pulmonary artery pressure; *PAOP*, pulmonary artery occlusion pressure; *PVRI*, pulmonary vascular resistance index; *RAP*, right atrial pressure; *RVEDVI*, right ventricular end-diastolic volume index; *RVSWI*, right ventricular stroke work index; *SVI*, stroke volume index; *SVRI*, systemic vascular resistance index.

sure (PAOP) and pulmonary artery diastolic pressure (PADP) as indicators of left ventricular end-diastolic pressure, and right atrial pressure (RAP) and central venous pressure (CVP) for right ventricular end-diastolic pressure. Recently, measurement of right ventricular end-diastolic volume via ejection fraction has become a practical method to evaluate VEDV and, therefore, preload.[23]

Afterload. Afterload, the impedance to ejection of blood from the ventricle, is inversely related to SV and cardiac output. Elevation of afterload reduces stroke volume unless a substantial increase in ventricular end-diastolic pressure or contractility is generated to overcome ventricular outflow impedance. Conversely, arterial vasodilatation can reduce excessive vascular resistance (impedance) and enhance ventricular ejection, thus improving SV and cardiac output. Systemic vascular resistance (SVR) is the clinical measurement that reflects left ventricular afterload. Before intervening to normalize an elevated SVR, preload and contractility must be scrutinized. A reduction in preload or contractility elicits a compensatory arterial vasoconstriction and produces an increase in SVR. If this is the cause of the increased SVR, the interventions should focus on improving preload or contractility rather than on lowering the SVR. Right ventricular afterload, important because of its impact on not only right ventricular function but also left ventricular preload and compliance,[22] is assessed by calculating pulmonary vascular resistance (PVR).

Contractility. Myocardial contractility is the intrinsic rate and force of myofibril shortening at a constant preload and afterload. Contractility is influenced predominantly by the status of beta-1 sympathetic receptors, electrolyte and acid-base balance, the presence of circulating mediators, and myocardial oxygen supply and consumption balance. Although myocardial contractility cannot be measured directly, an alteration in contractility is assumed when a change in cardiac output is apparently unrelated to preload and afterload. Indirectly, stroke work index reflects the efficiency of cardiac work because it incorporates two of the determinants of work, the mass to be moved (the SV) and the resistance to flow (mean arterial pressure).

Determinants of oxygen content. Arterial oxygen content is determined by the amount of oxygen dissolved in plasma (PaO_2), the oxygen carrying capacity (hemoglobin level), and the oxygen saturation of hemoglobin (SaO_2). Hemoglobin and SaO_2 are the most significant contributors to CaO_2 because only a very small percentage of oxygen is actually dissolved in the plasma (Table 17-1). Although sufficient oxygen-carrying capacity is necessary to ensure adequate oxygen transport, excessive elevation of hematocrit increases blood viscosity and reduces microcirculatory blood flow and oxygen transport.[24,25]

Assessment of the adequacy of CaO_2 includes monitoring PaO_2 and SaO_2 and their primary determining factors, namely, intrapulmonary shunting (Qs/Qt) and inspired oxygen (FiO_2). Oxygenation of pulmonary capillary blood is affected by a multitude of factors that are commonly deranged in MODS or SIRS and that cause hypoxemia and suboptimal SaO_2. These include alveolar ventilation and oxygenation; blood volume and flow in the pulmonary vasculature; transit time of hemoglobin past ventilated alveoli; and diffusion distance between ventilated alveoli and pulmonary capillaries.

Mechanical ventilation, commonly employed in critically ill patients with MODS or SIRS to improve ventilation and oxygenation, can have deleterious effects on cardiac output, thereby affecting oxygen transport. Assessment of the impact of ventilatory support on venous return, pulmonary vascular resistance and right ventricular afterload, and left ventricular preload and compliance is important to achieve optimal arterial oxygenation without sacrificing cardiac output and reducing oxygen transport.[26]

The oxyhemoglobin dissociation curve depicts the normal, reversible affinity of oxygen and hemoglobin and the relationship of PaO_2 to SaO_2. Alterations in the affinity of hemoglobin for oxygen are reflected in a shift of the curve to the left or to the right. Increased affinity, a shift to the left, enhances the binding of oxygen to hemoglobin and inhibits the release of oxygen to the cells. Reduced 2,3-diphosphoglycerate (2,3-DPG) levels (e.g., by infusion of banked blood that is depleted of 2,3-DPG during storage), hypothermia, and alkalosis are associated with a shift to the left and increased oxygen-hemoglobin affinity and decreased release of oxygen at the tissue level. A shift to the right, as seen in febrile and acidotic states, reduces the binding affinity of oxygen to hemoglobin; however, the decreased affinity facilitates hemoglobin release of oxygen to the tissues. Thus, a shift to the right enhances release of oxygen to cells and improves oxygen supply to the tissues, whereas, a shift to the left increases oxygen-hemoglobin affinity and can cause cellular hypoxia in the critically ill.[27] The oxyhe-

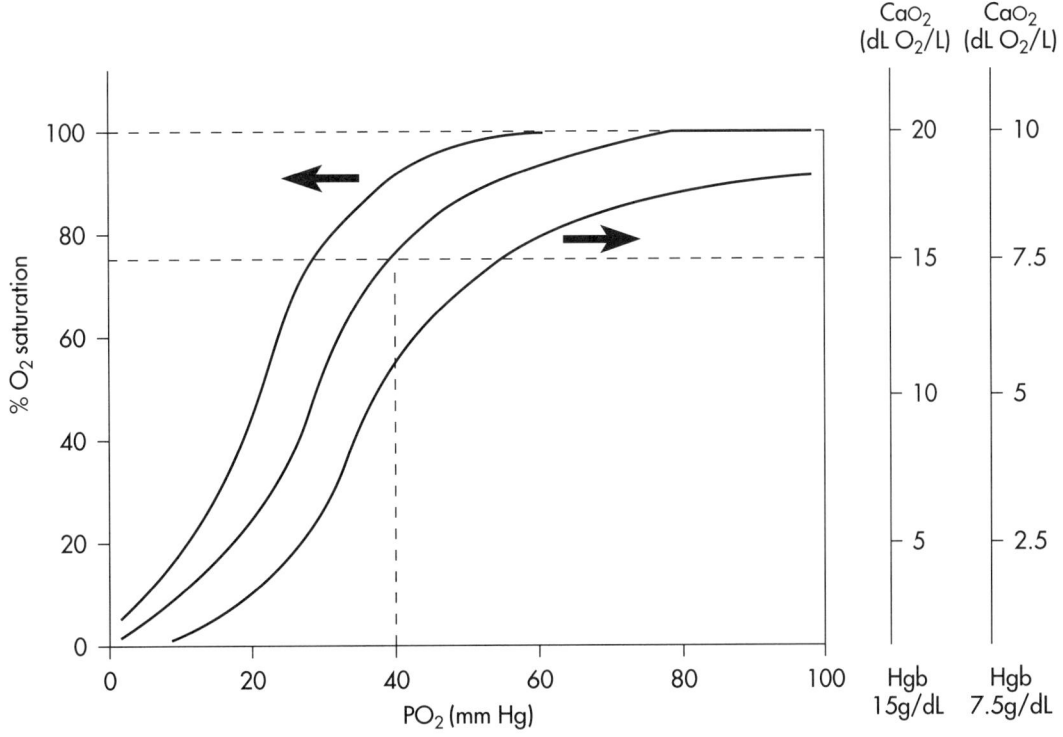

Fig. 17-1 The relationship of oxygen saturation and partial pressure on the oxyhemoglobin dissociation curve. The effect of So_2, Po_2, shifts to the left (<-) or right (->) and hemoglobin are depicted to estimate the significance of alteration of these variables on oxygen content (right axis). (Modified from Snyder JV, Pinsky MR, eds. Oxygen transport in the critically ill. Chicago: Mosby, 1989:4.)

moglobin dissociation curve and the effect of reduced hemoglobin on Cao_2 in relation to the curve is shown in Figure 17-1.

Oxygen consumption

Tissue and cellular oxygen consumption is influenced by the availability of microcirculatory oxygen and cellular extraction of oxygen from systemic capillaries to meet cellular oxygen requirements (demand). In normal conditions of oxygen transport and demand, the cells utilize approximately 25% of the available oxygen (Dao_2). Oxygen extraction is evaluated by the arterial and venous oxygen content difference (Ca-vo_2) and the oxygen extraction ratio (OER) (Table 17-2). Typically, oxygen extraction is inversely related to cardiac output and oxygen transport. For example, as the supply of oxygen to the cells exceeds their requirements, a smaller percentage of oxygen is extracted from the blood and is reflected by a smaller OER or a narrower Ca-vo_2.

Mixed venous Po_2 and So_2 are principal components of venous oxygen content (Cvo_2), and OER is, in part, a derivation of these values. Pvo_2 and Svo_2 may be indicators of oxygen extraction as the values usually decrease with increased cellular utilization of oxygen from arterial blood or rise in states of reduced tissue oxygen extraction. However, Pvo_2 and Svo_2 need to be assessed with respect to cardiac output, Cao_2, and oxygen consumption to elucidate their meaning fully. Regional alterations in oxygen transport and uptake in underperfused tissue beds, as in SIRS, shock, or MODS are often not reflected by changes in global values such as mixed Pvo_2 and Svo_2.[28]

Vo_2 is the clinical measure of global cellular oxygen utilization. Normal cell and organ function require adequate oxygen availability and uptake to fuel efficient aerobic metabolism. Pathologic reduction in oxygen consumption (decompensated SIRS or MODS) may be caused by altered micro-

Table 17-2 Oxygen Utilization Variables

Parameter	Formula	Normal values
Svo_2	Direct measurement	60%-80%
Pvo_2	Direct measurement	35-45 mm Hg
O_2 extraction	$Cao_2 - Cvo_2$	3-5 mL O_2/dL
OER	$\dfrac{Cao_2 - Cvo_2}{Cao_2}$	22%-30%
Vo_2I	$(Cao_2 - Cvo_2) \times CI \times 10$	120-170 mL/min/m^2
pHa	Direct measurement	7.35-7.45
pHi	Direct measurement	7.32-7.37
BE/BD	Direct measurement	-2-$+2$
Lactate	Direct measurement	0.5-2.2 mmol/L

BE/BD, Base excess/base deficit; *pHa*, arterial pH; *pHi*, gastric mucosal pH; *OER*, oxygen extraction ratio; *Vo₂I*, oxygen consumption index; for all other abbreviations see Table 17-1.

circulatory oxygen delivery or the inability of cells to extract oxygen, for example, in cytotoxicity or cell death. Vo_2 can be calculated using oxygen delivery and extraction parameters (Table 17-2) in the inverse Fick formula or measured from inspired and expired oxygen concentration and flow analysis. Controversy exists regarding the accuracy of the Dao_2 and Vo_2 relationship when Vo_2 is calculated by the Fick method because cardiac index, hemoglobin, and Sao_2 are factors common to both formulas, and the relationship may be a reflection of mathematical coupling. Verification of Vo_2 measurement by gas analysis may be appropriate when the Dao_2-Vo_2 relationship is in question. This issue is explored later in this chapter.

Global and regional oxygen debt

Pathophysiology. Cellular oxygen deficit occurs (1) when oxygen requirements are greater than oxygen delivery and extraction or (2) where there is a defect in cellular oxygen uptake and utilization. In either case, the actual Vo_2 is less than the required Vo_2 (Fig. 17-2). Insufficient oxygen availability or extraction mandates reliance on less efficient anaerobic metabolism to support cell function. Aerobic metabolism and normal oxidation of glucose result in the net synthesis of 36 molecules of adenosine triphosphate (ATP) via glycolysis and the Krebs cycle as a fundamental energy source for cell function. Without sufficient oxygen, cells rely on anaerobic metabolism and produce only two molecules of ATP because pyruvate is converted to lactic acid that does not enter the Krebs cycle in the mitochondria. Lactic acid accumulates and causes a metabolic acidosis.[29] Oxygen debt can be "paid back" with restitution of oxygen delivery, extraction, and consumption; however, severe and prolonged oxygen deficit causes irreversible oxygen debt and cell death (Fig. 17-2).

Clinical evaluation of oxygen debt. Clinical evaluation of oxygen debt accumulation may be based on measurement of Vo_2 and indicators of metabolic acidosis. A decreased Vo_2 or even unchanging Vo_2 in the presence of metabolic acidosis, may be evidence that a critically ill patient has or is accumulating an oxygen debt. Currently, arterial pH (pHa), gastric mucosal pH (pHi), base deficit (BD), and serum lactate are readily available clinical parameters to aid evaluation of the presence and magnitude of oxygen debt.

Arterial pH. Arterial pH (pHa) is affected by pulmonary CO_2 elimination and renal acid-base buffering systems. Consideration of the arterial Pco_2, bicarbonate, and the rapidity of the decrease in pH is required in the analysis of pHa and oxygen debt. An acute reduction in bicarbonate and pHa, not fully explained by a relative or absolute hypercarbia, is an indication to suspect a perfusion deficit and oxygen debt accumulation. Survivors of septic shock have been shown to have significantly higher pHa in both the initial and final phases of shock (pHa of 7.38 and 7.42 respectively) than do nonsurvivors (initial and final pHa of 7.32 and 7.31 respec-

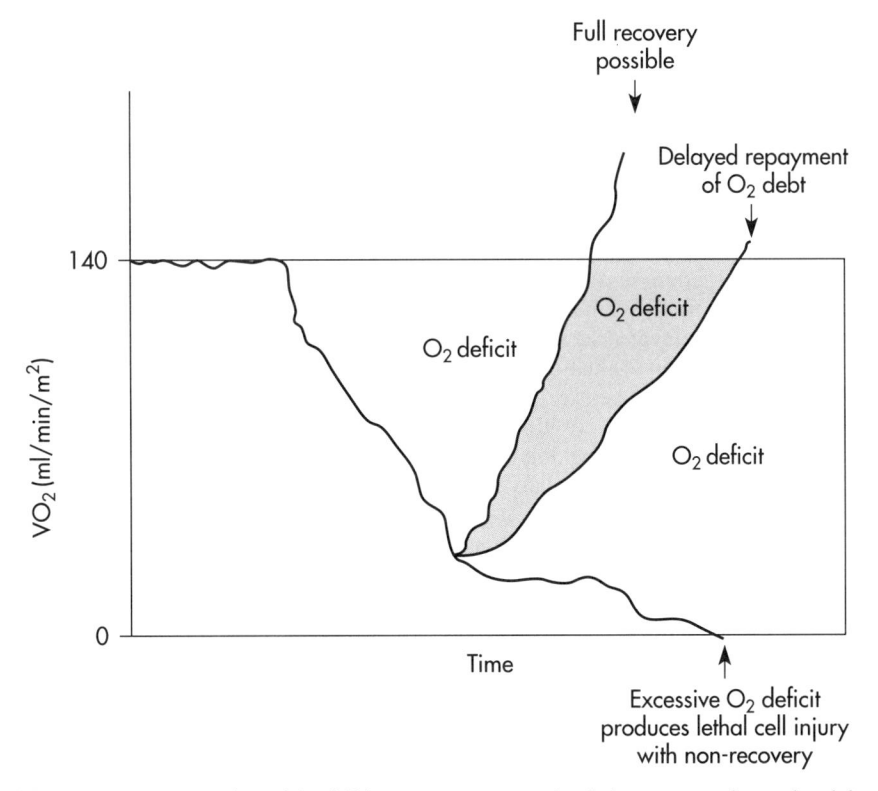

Fig. 17-2 The representation of the fall in oxygen consumption below oxygen demand and the accumulation of oxygen debt that ensues following loss of cellular perfusion. Restitution of perfusion can reverse oxygen deficit accrual if interventions are adequate and initiated before irreversible cell injury occurs. (From Siegel JH. Trauma: Emergency surgery and critical care. New York: Churchill Livingstone, 1992:205.)

tively).[30] Patients with documented SIRS and sepsis who developed MODS also had arterial and venous acidemia within the first 24 hours of the onset of sepsis.[20] Similarly, a relative acidosis was present (pHa of 7.35) in patients who developed MODS or died compared with a mean pHa of 7.44 in those who did not develop MODS or those who survived.[31]

Base deficit. Hemorrhagic shock and the associated oxygen debt are acknowledged triggers of SIRS and MODS. BD, obtained from routine blood gas analysis, has been shown to be of use in evaluating oxygen debt and predicting MODS and mortality in hemorrhagic shock. Normalization of BD and resolution of metabolic acidosis can be indicators of adequate resuscitation and resolution of oxygen debt.[32-35] BD reflecting metabolic acidosis is related to oxygen debt, mortality, and MODS when associated with hemorrhage.[32,33] A BD in the range of -18.8 to -19.7 mmol/L is associated with high morbidity and mortality (LD_{50}) in clinical[32] and animal investigations.[33]

Serum lactate. Accumulation of lactate to serum levels above normal (>2.2 mmol/L) may be classified as hyperlactatemia or lactic acidosis. Hyperlactatemia is related to factors that increase pyruvate concentration such as catecholamine administration, alkalosis, or hypermetabolic states; however, acidosis is not present.[36] Lactic acidosis (increased lactate and pHa <7.35) results from the sequence of tissue hypoperfusion, cellular hypoxia, decreased pyruvate oxidation, and increased lactate production. Lactic acidosis is associated with oxygen debt,[37] acute myocardial infarction,[38] severe traumatic injury,[32,34,37] and sepsis.[28,30,31,38]

Dunham and colleagues[37] identified several inflammatory markers, including an elevated admission serum lactate, which were associated with development of MODS in blunt trauma patients (mean Injury Severity Score of 41; admission lactate of 4.8 mmol/L). Nonsurvival in septic shock has also been associated with persistently elevated lactate levels of >2.0 mmol/L.[30,31] However, an evaluation of predictors of MODS and death in septic patients showed that although lactate levels were higher in septic patients who developed MODS and in those who died, the differences were not statistically significant.[20]

Persistent hyperlactatemia in septic patients may also, in part, be due to delayed skeletal muscle uptake and reduced hepatic clearance of lactate.[20,36,38] Conversely, lactate levels may be normal in the early stages of anaerobic metabolism and oxygen debt accumulation until the production of lactate exceeds tissue uptake.[36]

Gastric mucosal pH. Recent attention has been directed toward the evaluation of tissue hypoxia in the splanchnic bed. Splanchnic vasoconstriction, which increases flow to vital organs, but causes hypoperfusion, hypoxia, and acidosis of the gut mucosa,[39] is an early compensatory response to shock. Measurement of gastric mucosal pH (pHi) via tonometry utilizes a nasogastric tube with a saline-filled silicone balloon. After 30 or more minutes of equilibration time, the saline is aspirated, Pco_2 analyzed, and pHi calculated. This parameter has been studied in several critically ill populations as a monitor of therapeutic interventions and a predictor of MODS and death. A pHi of <7.32 has been associated with nonsurvival in critically ill patients, the majority (16 out of 22 patients) diagnosed with sepsis or ARDS.[40] A study of septic patients showed a strong correlation of low pHi (<7.15), measured within 24 hours of the onset of sepsis, with MODS and death.[20] Severely injured trauma patients with a pHi of <7.32 at 24 hours after injury had a higher incidence of MODS and mortality. A threshold value of 7.10 for pHi was noted, that is, all patients with a pHi ≤7.10 developed MODS.[41]

RELATIONSHIP OF OXYGEN DELIVERY, OXYGEN CONSUMPTION, AND OXYGEN DEBT
Delivery-dependent and delivery-independent oxygen consumption

The relationship of oxygen delivery and consumption may be depicted as a biphasic curve (Fig. 17-3). The slope of the curve represents delivery-dependent oxygen consumption, both in normal and high oxygen demand states, when oxygen delivery is not sufficient to permit adequate oxygen consumption. When oxygen delivery increases and additional oxygen is available to meet the metabolic requirements, oxygen consumption increases. Beyond a level of critical oxygen delivery, oxygen demand is met and the consumption of oxygen plateaus (delivery-independent oxygen consumption). Levels of critical Dao_2 and Vo_2 in high-demand states are greater than the baseline values in normal oxygen demand states, that is, delivery must be higher to meet the increased demand, or consumption becomes dependent. The plateauing of Vo_2 and normalization of metabolic indicators of oxygen debt (e.g., pH and lactate) are, typically, evidence that cellular oxygen requirements have been met and that oxygen debt is not accruing.[36]

Compensated SIRS state

Several compensatory mechanisms are initiated to assure adequate oxygen availability to cells in high oxygen demand states (Fig. 17-4). A compensated SIRS state is present when cardiac output increases, secondary to the normal stress response and inflammatory mediator and hormone release, to augment oxygen delivery to the tissues. The additional metabolic requirements for oxygen mandate the increase in oxygen delivery to prevent oxygen debt accumulation. In this state, oxygen consumption reaches a plateau and indicators of oxygen debt are normal. An early and sustained compensatory increase in cardiac output and Dao_2 is associated with higher Vo_2 in survivors of septic shock compared with Vo_2 in nonsurvivors.[42,43]

When oxygen delivery is inadequate to meet metabolic requirements, oxygen consumption and cell function may be maintained by increased cellular extraction of oxygen from the blood. This is manifested by a widened Ca-vo_2, greater OER, and lower Svo_2, and is associated with a rise in Vo_2 to a

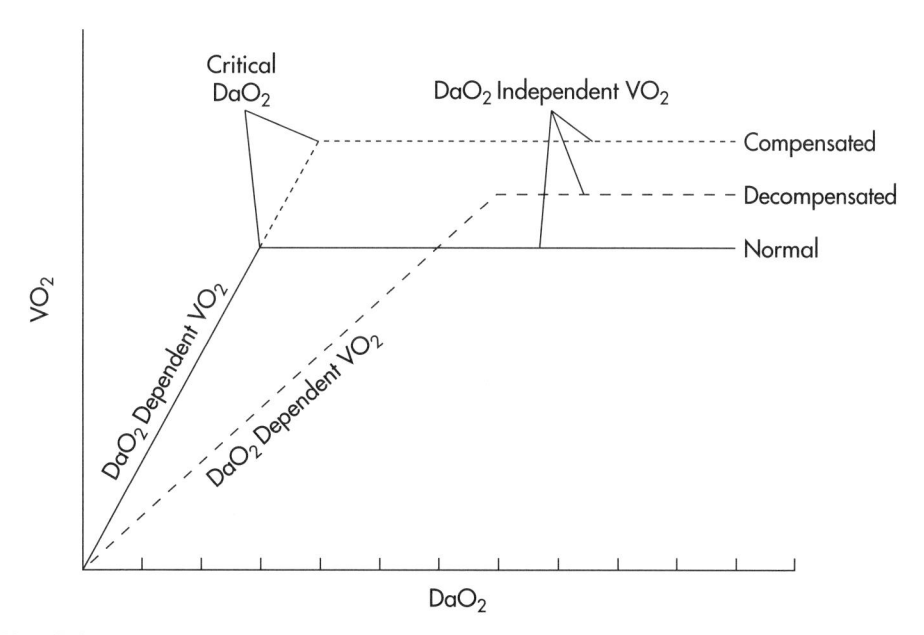

Fig. 17-3 The biphasic relationship of oxygen delivery (DaO_2) and consumption (VO_2) showing the dependence of oxygen consumption on oxygen delivery up to a critical level of oxygen delivery where VO_2 becomes independent of DaO_2. Three conditions are depicted: (1) Normal, increase in DaO_2 is associated with a rise in VO_2 when oxygen demand is normal (solid line); (2) compensated SIRS/MODS, where oxygen demand is high and the increase in VO_2 is commensurate with increased DaO_2 (dotted line); and (3) decompensated SIRS/MODS, where VO_2 is impaired despite an increased DaO_2 (dashed line).

plateau and a lack of global oxygen debt. In septic shock, the inability to maintain the critical level of oxygen transport is associated with a higher, but inadequate, oxygen extraction ratio, lower VO_2, and death.[42,43]

Uncompensated SIRS state

In an uncompensated SIRS or MODS state, oxygen demand is not met by increases in cardiac output, oxygen delivery, and oxygen extraction and a cellular oxygen deficit is created (Fig. 17-4). Additional compensatory mechanisms are stimulated to preserve vital organ function. Arterial vasoconstriction and closure of precapillary sphincters in, for example, the splanchnic bed, shunt blood from "nonessential" organs and enhance preferential perfusion of vital organs such as the heart, lungs, and brain. Hypoxia and oxygen debt may develop in the underperfused tissue beds and are clinically evident initially by regional acidosis and subsequently by organ dysfunction. SvO_2 or systemic pH and lactate may not reflect regional hypoperfusion (covert tissue hypoxia) and oxygen debt accumulation because provincial flow into and out of these tissue beds is significantly reduced, particularly in the early stages of shock. Therefore, the metabolic byproducts of anaerobic metabolism in these regions contribute minimally to global indicators of hypoxia and are insufficient to alter these parameters of oxygen debt.[36,39] Therapeutic measures that enhance cardiac output and oxygen delivery and/or increase oxygen extraction can convert the patient from an uncompensated to a compensated SIRS state.

Decompensated SIRS state

A decompensated SIRS or MODS state is one in which there is a failure in oxygen extraction, and it manifests with a low oxygen consumption relative to the level of oxygen delivery and oxygen debt ac-

392 *Management and Special Considerations*

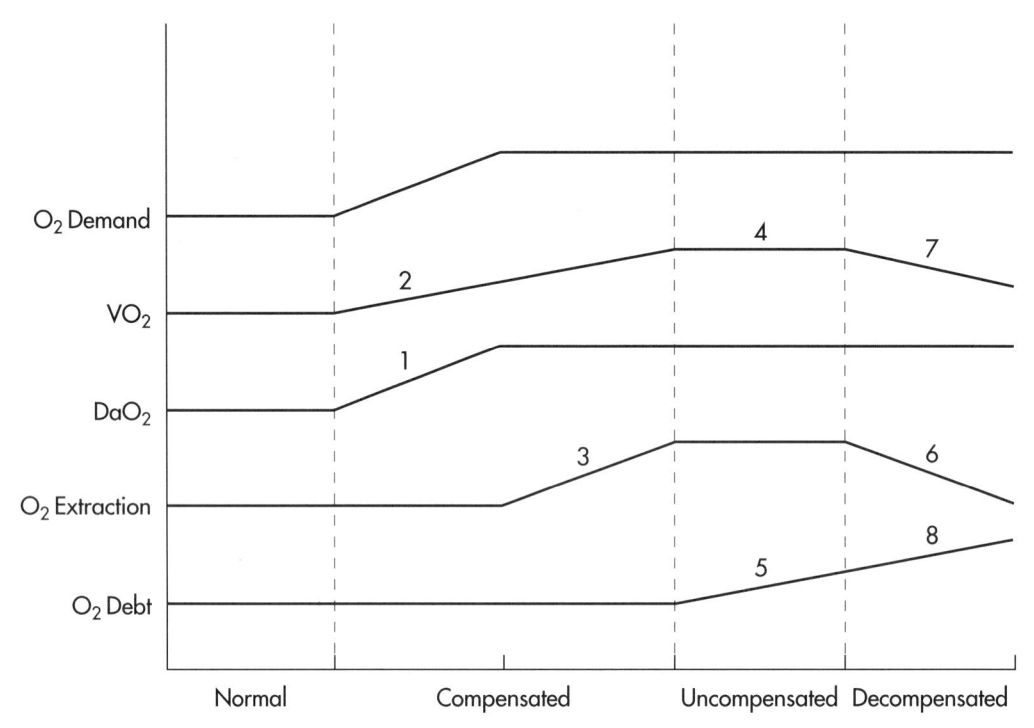

Fig. 17-4 The conceptual oxidative response to rising oxygen demand associated with SIRS/MODS. Compensated state: increased oxygen demand is compensated by cardiac output and oxygen delivery (DaO_2) *(1)* with a rise in oxygen consumption *(2)*. Failure of DaO_2 to meet oxygen demand elicits an increase in oxygen extraction *(3)*, further increasing VO_2 *(4)*. Uncompensated SIRS/MODS: patient self-generated DaO_2 and oxygen extraction are insufficient to meet oxygen demand, VO_2 plateaus and oxygen debt accumulates *(5)*. Decompensated SIRS/MODS: impairment of oxygen extraction *(6)* relative to the level of cardiac output and DaO_2 and despite resuscitation, manifested by a fall in VO_2 *(7)* and continued oxygen debt accumulation *(8)*.

cumulation (Fig. 17-4). Evidence exists that in ARDS and sepsis, VO_2 may not change or significantly increase in response to increases in DaO_2, despite the presence of a hypermetabolic state.[31,44-47] Also, some investigators have reported unchanged or lower oxygen extraction associated with sepsis compared with nonseptic states, when DaO_2 is increased.[48,49] Defective cellular oxygen extraction secondary to inflammatory mediator activity, capillary occlusion by neutrophil or platelet aggregation, and maldistribution of blood flow, hinders an increase in oxygen consumption even in the presence of enhanced DaO_2.[7,50,51] This decompensated state of SIRS or MODS is clinically evidenced by no change or by a persistently low VO_2, and oxygen extraction associated with regional or global oxygen debt accumulation and cell death, despite deliberate interventions that increase DaO_2 (Figs. 17-3 and 17-4).

MANAGEMENT TARGETS RELATED TO OXYGEN DELIVERY AND CONSUMPTION
Cardiopulmonary targets

A number of clinical investigations have shown that early achievement of supranormal cardiopulmonary values decreases organ failure and mortality.[13,18,52,53] Establishment of therapeutic physiologic goals is directed toward maximizing cardiac output, DO_2, and VO_2, and thereby preventing or eliminating oxygen debt accumulation and organ hypoxia. Most frequently quoted therapeutic goals are in reference to critically ill trauma patients and high risk surgical patients. These treatment objectives include a cardiac index ≥4.5 L/min/m^2, Do$_2$I ≥600 mL/min/m^2, and Vo$_2$I ≥170 mL/min/m^2.[53] Despite aggressive interventions, investigators report that high risk surgical and trauma patients who fail to achieve these supranormal values, especially within the first 24 hours postinjury and 48 hours after major surgery, have significantly higher mortality, higher rate of organ failure, increased number of ventilator days, and increased length of stay in the ICU.[6,13,18,53] Therapeutic cardiopulmonary goals for septic patients have been estimated at slightly higher values than those used for surgical or trauma patients. Investigators recommend increasing cardiac index >5.5-6.0 L/min/m^2, Do$_2$I >1000 mL/min/m^2, and Vo$_2$I >190 mL/min/m^2.[43,52]

Some controversy exists regarding the effect of supranormal cardiopulmonary values on outcome and also regarding the relationship of Do$_2$ to Vo$_2$. The concept of a critical oxygen delivery level in septic and MODS patients has been challenged because of the failure of supranormal Do$_2$ to consistently increase Vo$_2$ and improve outcome. Several investigators have not been able to demonstrate an increase in Vo$_2$ associated with achievement of supranormal Do$_2$ in critically ill patients, primarily those with sepsis or ARDS.[17,54] Yu and co-workers described patients with sepsis, ARDS, or hypovolemic shock, who, when treated to achieve a Do$_2$I of > 600 mL/min/m^2, had the same mortality as those who were not managed to reach supranormal values. Interestingly, survivors of both groups had elevated Do$_2$, whether achieved as response to therapy or as a self-generated compensatory response.[14]

One group of investigators suggests that interventions to increase Do$_2$ to supranormal values, with the aim of increasing Vo$_2$, may be inappropriate because elevation of Do$_2$ was not associated with an increase in Vo$_2$ in patients with ARDS or sepsis.[2,46,47] Also, the level of critical oxygen delivery in septic and nonseptic patients, with or without ARDS, was not different and was lower than previously reported levels.[2,3] However, to some degree, all patients did exhibit the biphasic relationship of Do$_2$ and Vo$_2$ depicted in Figure 17-3.[2,3,43]

Mathematical coupling

The conflicting evidence in the literature regarding the impact of achieving supranormal levels of Do$_2$ and Vo$_2$ on the outcome of the illness and the relationship between the two values may be the result of Vo$_2$ measurement techniques and mathematical coupling of Do$_2$ and Vo$_2$ calculations. The most common type of mathemetical coupling occurs when a measured value (such as CO, hemoglobin, or Sao$_2$) is used to determine a calculated value (such as Do$_2$ or Vo$_2$). If two calculated values have a common measured component, a change in the measured value guarantees a change in both calculated values and may produce an artificial relationship between the two calculated values.[55] The measured values of cardiac output, hemoglobin, Pao$_2$, and Sao$_2$ are common to the calculation of both Do$_2$ and Vo$_2$. Use of these shared variables may result in mathematical coupling of Do$_2$ and Vo$_2$ and is a potential source of error when analyzing the relationship between Do$_2$ and Vo$_2$.[55-57]

Measurement of Vo$_2$ using analysis of respiratory gases (spirometry) via indirect calorimetry is independent of calculations based on thermodilution cardiac output, hemoglobin, Pao$_2$, and Sao$_2$ and avoids the errors related to mathematical coupling. Smithies and associates[56] describe good reproducibility of spirometric measurement of Vo$_2$ in mechanically ventilated critically ill patients (with Fio$_2$ of 0.23-0.60). Smithies[56] also found a close relationship between spirometric measurement of Vo$_2$ and Vo$_2$ calculated using thermodilution cardiac output, although spirometric values were significantly higher than calculated Vo$_2$ values. A recent study examined the relationship of spirometric Vo$_2$ and/or calculated Vo$_2$ to Do$_2$ in hemodynamically stable patients with ARDS.[57] Deliberate elevation of Do$_2$ with dobutamine infusion produced a significant increase from the baseline level in the calculated Vo$_2$, consistent with reports of oxygen delivery-dependent oxygen consumption. However, there was no change in Vo$_2$ and no dependence of Vo$_2$ on Do$_2$ when Vo$_2$ was measured by respiratory gas analysis. The authors conclude that previously demonstrated dependent relationships of calculated Vo$_2$ on Do$_2$ are due to mathematical coupling.[57] These findings support other reports of a lack of oxygen supply-dependency in patients with ARDS and sepsis in whom increases in Do$_2$ did not produce an increase in Vo$_2$ when Vo$_2$ was measured by indirect calorimetry.[45-47]

Regional perfusion targets

Gastric mucosal pH. Recent emphasis has been placed on utilization of measures of regional perfusion such as gastric mucosal pH (pHi) and hepatic venous oxygen saturation (ShvO$_2$) to direct therapy toward increasing oxygen delivery in critically ill patients. Because persistently low pHi caused by gut hypoperfusion is associated with development of MODS and a higher mortality,[20,39-41] elevation of Do$_2$ to correct gut hypoperfusion, guided by normalization of pHi, appears to be a rational therapeutic approach and may avoid the controversy surrounding management based on the relationship of Do$_2$ to Vo$_2$. In a large prospective randomized trial,[58] the use of gastric tonometers was evaluated in critically ill patients. The control group was managed conventionally and the practitioners were blinded to the pHi. Interventions for the protocol group were designed to increase oxygen transport to achieve and maintain a pHi >7.35. Therapy guided by pHi improved survival in the protocol patients whose pHi was normal on admission to the critical care unit. Interestingly, there was no difference in survival between the patients in either group who were admitted with a low pHi (<7.35) despite treatment which raised pHi to >7.35 in the protocol patients.[58]

In a separate study, septic patients receiving volume and dobutamine infusions to increase Do$_2$I to >600 mL/min/m^2 did not increase their pHi until the Do$_2$I was increased to 825 mL/min/m^2 with additional volume infusion. The survivors had significantly higher pHi after volume infusion than did the nonsurvivors. Neither group of patients had a significant change in Vo$_2$.[59] In a similar investigation, dobutamine was administered to septic patients with a pHi <7.32. Do$_2$ and pHi both increased as the dobutamine infusion was increased from 5 to 10 μg/kg/min. Vo$_2$ remained unchanged in response to therapy and enhanced Do$_2$, even in those patients with elevated serum lactate levels.[60]

Hepatic venous saturation. Measurement of systemic venous oxygen saturation has been shown to have limited value in determining tissue hypoxia in patients with maldistribution of volume and underperfusion of various organ beds that is thought to occur in sepsis, ARDS, or MODS. However, use of a regional splanchnic bed monitor of Svo$_2$ may be more valuable than measurement of systemic Svo$_2$ in detecting covert tissue hypoxia and in evaluating the need for and effectiveness of interventions that enhance oxygen delivery. Mean hepatic venous saturation (ShvO$_2$) has been reported to be 15% lower than Svo$_2$ in septic shock patients, despite a normal Svo$_2$ in these patients.[21] In an attempt to increase Do$_2$ via use of alpha-mimetic agents, epinephrine or norepinephrine administration decreased ShvO$_2$ of these patients while having little or no effect on Svo$_2$. The widened difference between ShvO$_2$ and Svo$_2$ suggests reduced perfusion to the liver despite an increased DaO$_2$. Conversely, administration of beta-2 and dopaminergic agents to these patients did not change the difference between ShvO$_2$ and Svo$_2$, suggesting maintenance or enhancement of hepatic perfusion in septic shock.[21] A similar comparison of ShvO$_2$ and Svo$_2$ in cardiac surgery, respiratory failure, and septic patients showed no consistent gradient between these variables. For example, when the Svo$_2$ was >65%, the ShvO$_2$ range was 31% to 71%,[61] evidence that global Svo$_2$ response to changes in DaO$_2$ may not be a reliable indication of adequate management of oxygen transport and uptake at the organ level.

THERAPEUTIC INTERVENTIONS

Therapeutic interventions to support oxygen transport and consumption in sepsis, ARDS, and MODS are aimed toward preserving organ function and preventing or reducing oxygen debt accumulation. Interventions are specifically related to maintaining adequate Do$_2$ and improving cellular oxygen consumption. These include increasing cardiac output by optimizing preload, afterload, and contractility; maintaining hemoglobin at a level sufficient to provide adequate oxygen-carrying capacity; achieving optimal ventilation and oxygenation; and maintaining an internal therapeutic environment conducive to cellular oxygen uptake and reducing excessive metabolic demands (e.g., euthermia and acid-base balance). Although controversy exists regarding therapeutic goals and the efficacy of supranormal Do$_2$ and Vo$_2$ values, clinicians and investigators are in agreement that maintenance of sufficient oxygen transport and uptake is necessary to preserve organ function.

Interventions to increase cardiac output

Fluid administration. A mainstay of therapy to enhance cardiac output is administration of fluids (crystalloids or colloids) to assure that intravascular volume and, thus, preload is optimized. The oxygen flux test (deliberately increasing cardiac output and DaO$_2$, then evaluating Vo$_2$ for a commensurate response) may be useful in establishing the presence of an oxygen debt and the requirement for increasing DaO_2.[29] However, several previously mentioned investigators[31,44-47] report no change in VO_2 after increasing DaO_2, and use of additional parameters such as lactate or pHi may provide more specific evidence of covert tissue hypoxia. Meier-Hellman and colleagues[59] administered hydroxyethylstarch to septic shock patients with a pHi <7.35 who were hemodynamically stable with previous volume and dobutamine infusion (mean DaO_2 of 717 mL/min/m^2). The additional volume infusion further increased the DaO_2 of the patients and increased their pHi, but did not elicit a change in VO_2.

Consideration and monitoring of the effect of hemodilution on DaO_2 is required because the reduced oxygen-carrying capacity that is associated with asanguinous volume infusion may not be offset by the increase in cardiac output.[62] Another consideration related to volume infusion concerns the increased vascular permeability that occurs with SIRS or MODS and its influence on the effective duration of intravascular volume administration. Although crystalloids are known to have a shorter intravascular half-life than do colloids,[63] leakage of colloids into the interstitial space through widened endothelial junctions may enhance plasma flux from the vascular to the interstitial space and potentially contribute to intravascular volume depletion and exacerbate interstitial edema.[64] Consensus has not been reached regarding the most appropriate type of fluid for intravascular volume resuscitation and maintenance in patients with SIRS or MODS.

Inotropic agents. Inotropic support of cardiac output is another conventional means to optimize DaO_2. Dobutamine is the most frequently described positive inotrope in the research literature related to increasing cardiac output and DaO_2. Gutierrez and co-workers[60] showed improvement in DaO_2 and a rise in pHi, but no change in VO_2 (negative O_2 flux test) in a group of patients with sepsis and pHi <7.32 after short-term infusion of dobutamine. Patients with elevated serum lactate levels had a reduction in lactate concentration, whereas those with normal lactate levels showed no change despite the increase in their pHi. The authors concluded that inotropic support with dobutamine effectively increases DaO_2 and reduces regional hypoperfusion and that systemic indicators of oxygen uptake may not reliably evaluate the efficacy of inotropic therapy to increase DaO_2, improve perfusion, or reveal covert hypoxia.

Epinephrine infusion has been investigated as an inotrope in septic shock patients. One such study increased the infusion rate incrementally by 3 μg/min, after intravascular volume resuscitation, to restore systolic blood pressure and attempt to increase DaO_2 to more than 600 mL/min/m^2. Epinephrine infusion up to 18 μg/min increased heart rate and mean arterial pressure in a linear fashion. Cardiac index, stroke index, DaO_2, and VO_2 also increased significantly; however, the mean values decreased at infusion rates greater than 12 μg/min, possibly because of the increase in SVRI (1079 dyne/sec/m^2 increased to 1448 dyne/sec/m^2), which although not a statistically significant change, may have some clinical importance.[65]

Vasoactive agents. Other pharmacologic agents that affect peripheral vascular tone and afterload have been studied in the critically ill. The utility of prostacyclin (PGI_2) has been compared to that of dobutamine in patients with sepsis and normal lactate concentrations.[66] Both drugs increased cardiac output, DaO_2, and, to a lesser degree, VO_2 but did not affect oxygen extraction. PGI_2, however, was not as well tolerated as dobutamine because it caused a profound reduction in blood pressure and PaO_2 because of its vasodilatory effects on the arterial and pulmonary vasculatures. The investigators caution that the relationship of DaO_2 and VO_2 may have been affected by several factors including mathematical coupling and drug-induced increases of VO_2 associated with both agents.

Epinephrine and norepinephrine have been compared with dobutamine and dopamine in the manipulation of cardiac output and blood pressure in septic patients. One group of investigators reported that both epinephrine and norepinephrine, when titrated to attain the same arterial blood pressure as achieved with dobutamine, produced a reduction in splanchnic perfusion that was determined by a significant decrease in $ShvO_2$. The authors concluded that use of these catecholamines may be counterproductive in septic shock patients because of the redistribution of perfusion away from the splanchnic bed.[21] Conversely, Ruokonen and colleagues[61] suggest that infusion of norepinephrine and high-dose dopamine (mean dose of 21 μg/kg/min) does not compromise splanchnic perfusion as demonstrated by an increase in the mean ShvO$_2$ in a group of cardiac surgery, septic, and respiratory failure patients. Analysis of data for the separate diagnoses was not presented, although the authors stated that the gradient between SvO$_2$ and ShvO$_2$ was not consistent or related to the diagnosis.[61]

Increasing evidence supports the use of norepinephrine to correct hemodynamic abnormalities in hyperdynamic septic shock. A comparison was made of norepinephrine (0.5-5.0 μg/kg/min) and dopamine (up to 25 μg/kg/min) in septic shock patients utilizing supranormal therapeutic endpoints for cardiac index, DaO$_2$ and VO$_2$, and normalization of SRVI and blood pressure. Norepinephrine infusion improved SVRI, blood pressure, urine output, and VO$_2$ in 93% of the patients, including those who did not respond to dopamine, whereas only 31% of the patients showed improved hemodynamics and urine output with dopamine infusion.[67] Similarly, Redl-Wenzl and co-workers[68] reported significantly increased SVRI, blood pressure, and creatinine clearance associated with norepinephrine in a group of patients with severe septic shock who did not respond to high-dose (>20 μg/kg/min) dopamine, dobutamine, or fluid therapy.[68] Norepinephrine did not significantly change cardiac index, DaO$_2$, or VO$_2$ in the patients in this study. Norepinephrine has also shown efficacy in increasing mean arterial blood pressure and improving right ventricular function, determined by right ventricular EDVI and ejection fraction, of patients with hyperdynamic septic shock.[69]

In a review of the literature related to correcting the hemodynamic alterations of septic shock, Vincent[70] makes the following practical recommendations for enhancing DaO$_2$ to reverse maldistribution of blood flow and to restore and maintain organ perfusion: (1) repletion of intravascular volume is essential prior to pharmacologic interventions; (2) a combination of vasoactive and inotropic therapy is indicated in most patients; and (3) therapy should be guided and evaluated not only by systemic blood pressure, but also by serial and multiple assessment parameters including DaO$_2$, VO$_2$, lactate, and indicators of the metabolic function of organs.[70]

Interventions to increase arterial oxygen content

Patients with MODS or SIRS typically require interventions to enhance arterial oxygen content in addition to therapies directed toward improving cardiac output. Maintenance of oxygen-carrying capacity, alveolar ventilation and perfusion, and pulmonary gas exchange is a necessary tenet of management to support oxygen delivery.

Red blood cell administration. Oxygen-carrying capacity, determined primarily by hemoglobin concentration, has a significant impact on DaO$_2$. A sufficient quantity of hemoglobin is required for adequate delivery of oxygen; however, elevation of hemoglobin and hematocrit increases blood viscosity, which can reduce cardiac output, blood flow, and perfusion, particularly in the microvasculature.[24] Recommended values for maintenance of sufficient oxygen-carrying capacity balanced with cardiac output are 10 to 12 g/dL of hemoglobin and a hematocrit in the 30% to 35% range.[24,25] Although blood transfusion is an important means to enhance DaO$_2$, evidence exists that it may not significantly improve VO$_2$[71] or regional perfusion,[24,72] perhaps because of the temporary increase in the affinity of oxygen and hemoglobin caused by infusion of stored packed red blood cells that may be cold and depleted of 2,3-DPG.

Mechanical ventilation. Acute lung injury or ARDS, and subsequently impaired oxygenation and ventilation, may be primary in nature and precede MODS or result from secondary injury related to SIRS and the failure of other organ systems in patients with MODS.[73] Regardless of the etiology of respiratory failure, therapeutic interventions are required to assure adequate oxygenation of the blood and to a lesser, but nonetheless essential, degree, removal of carbon dioxide.

The primary objectives of mechanical ventilation in ARDS are to attain the "best" PaO$_2$ without incurring additional lung injury or impairing cardiovascular function and to eliminate excess carbon dioxide from the blood to prevent an acute onset of intracellular acidosis. Current literature supports the use of pressure-controlled ventilation as opposed to volume-controlled ventilation.[74-76] Pressure-controlled ventilation employs decelerating inspiratory flow and limits cycling pressure. Compared to volume-controlled ventilation, pressure-controlled ventilation maintains mean and peak airway pressures at lower levels; therefore, stress to the alveoli and airways is reduced.[75] Further injury to the lung endothelium and epithelium from high pressures may thereby be retarded. Additionally, use of permissive hypercapnea ($PaCO_2$ >45 mm Hg), especially in conjunction with pressure control ventilation has shown improved outcomes in patients with ARDS by reducing peak airway pressure through the use of smaller tidal volumes.[74,76]

Therapeutic positioning. Patient positioning is a necessary adjunct to mechanical ventilation to limit the degree of pulmonary dysfunction in critically ill patients. Lateral turning and prone positioning redistribute ventilation and perfusion, as well as reduce atelectasis and facilitate drainage of secretions from previously dependent portions of the lungs.[77] Clinical and animal studies of the prone position in acute pulmonary failure show improved oxygenation (PaO_2)[78,79] and reduced intrapulmonary shunting through improved ventilation and perfusion matching.[79,80] Continuous lateral turning in a 120-degree arc (kinetic therapy) has been shown to improve intrapulmonary shunting and arterial oxygenation, and to reduce peak airway pressures in blunt trauma patients with ARDS.[81] The patients on kinetic therapy beds in this study had a lower mortality than the conventionally positioned patients, although this was not significant. Meta-analysis of prospective kinetic therapy research indicates that early institution of kinetic therapy (within 72 hours of admission to the ICU) reduced the number of pneumonias, ventilator days, and days spent in the ICU. However, no measurable effect on the incidence or development of ARDS was demonstrated.[82] To date, no research has been identified that directly explores the effect of prone positioning or kinetic therapy on morbidity or mortality in ARDS.

Investigational therapies. Recent investigational management strategies for ARDS include use of nitric oxide and extracorporeal carbon dioxide removal ($ECCO_2R$). $ECCO_2R$ permits use of near apneic ventilation with tracheal insufflation of oxygen, allowing lung rest and healing because airway pressures are maintained at a very low level to prevent alveolar collapse.[83] Although $ECCO_2R$ appears to be potentially more efficacious than extracorporeal membrane oxygenation (ECMO) in ARDS, further investigation and refinement of technology is indicated.

Evidence exists that nitric oxide has a role in immune system modulation, sepsis, and ARDS; however, additional clinical investigations are required before it can be widely advocated and employed.

Inhaled nitric oxide may be an important advance in the treatment of ARDS because it causes bronchodilatation and selective dilatation of the pulmonary vasculature, improving alveolar ventilation and perfusion, and thus, PaO_2.[84] A comparison of nitric oxide and PGI_2 showed that although both improved cardiac output and reduced pulmonary artery pressure and resistance, nitric oxide inhalation improved intrapulmonary shunting and oxygenation with no change in mean arterial blood pressure, whereas PGI_2 increased the intrapulmonary shunt, severely reduced PaO_2, and lowered mean arterial blood pressure.[85] Until research is available to clarify the indications, appropriate administration, and short- and long-term effects, the precise clinical role of nitric oxide will remain unclear.

PRACTICAL CONSIDERATIONS AND CONCLUSIONS

Until a "magic bullet" is discovered for the treatment of sepsis, ARDS, or MODS, supportive therapy will remain the hallmark of care for these patients. A logical approach to assessment of oxygen transport and uptake and to the management and evaluation of the response to therapy related to oxygen transport is paramount. Early identification of SIRS and those patients at risk for developing SIRS and MODS guides the need for increasingly invasive assessment. Close surveillance for subtle changes in clinical indicators of oxygen debt, organ dysfunction (see the box on p. 398, upper left), or the SIRS criteria[86] at the onset of MODS provides initial clues that a patient may require a higher level of monitoring technology. Likewise, clinical conditions associated with an increased risk for the development of MODS (see the box on p. 398, lower left), particularly when there is evidence of an uncompensated state (see the box on p. 398, upper right), are an indication for more invasive monitoring, and the use of technologies such as a gastric tonometer, $ShvO_2$ monitor, or pulmonary artery catheter should be considered. Table 17-3 summarizes the clinical scenarios and oxidative responses associated with SIRS and MODS. It is critical that interventions to increase DaO_2 are directed by known, specific derangements in cardiac output and oxygen content. Objective evaluation of the response of the patient to these interventions is likewise a fundamental aspect of care for the patient with SIRS or MODS.

> **CLINICAL CRITERIA FOR MULTIPLE ORGAN DYSFUNCTION SYNDROME**
>
> Two or more of the following:
> Adult respiratory distress syndrome
> Renal insufficiency
> Hypoalbuminemia
> Hyperglycemia
> Metabolic acidosis
> Hyperbilirubinemia

> **RISK FACTORS FOR MULTIPLE ORGAN DYSFUNCTION SYNDROME**
>
> Hemorrhagic shock
> Septic shock
> Major burns
> Infection with SIRS
> Severe injury
> Coma
> Emergency surgery
> Pancreatitis
> Comorbidities with the above factors:
>   Age
>   Preexisting or chronic conditions

> **COMMON MANIFESTATIONS OF THE UNCOMPENSATED SIRS STATE: INDICATIONS FOR MONITORING OXYGEN DELIVERY AND CONSUMPTION**
>
> 1. Patients who are at risk for MODS (see the box to the lower left)
> 2. Patients who are at the onset of MODS
> 3. Patients who have progression of MODS and display the following conditions:
>   Hypotension
>   Elevated serum lactate
>   Persistent acidemia
>   Regional hypoperfusion
>   Decreased venous oxygen saturation
>   Tachydysrhythmias
>   Persistent oliguria
>   Increased serum creatinine
>   Decreased creatinine clearance

The use of advanced monitoring technology and multiple sources of assessment data are necessary to evaluate oxygen delivery, consumption and debt, and to guide interventions, particularly in the critically ill patients at high risk for developing SIRS and MODS and those in uncompensated and decompensated states. However, several considerations are important to assure appropriate use of resources regardless of the strategies and technology employed. Although much of the recent literature addressing the issue of appropriate use of advanced technologies is directed toward the "use and abuse of pulmonary artery catheters,"[87] the tenets are applicable to all monitoring devices. These are as follows: understanding the data provided and their limitations; obtaining data at appropriate frequencies; recognizing the mechanical and physiologic influences on the validity of the data; accurately obtaining the data; and incorporating data from multiple sources, not only from the particular technology.[88-91] Use of advanced monitoring technology is not appropriate unless the data is fully integrated into assessment and management of the patient. As Thomas Iberti[92] so eloquently stated: "Insertion of a pulmonary artery catheter is not a therapeutic maneuver." Integration of the data requires comprehension of the data, a prerequisite that, unfortunately, is often deficient.[92,93]

Appropriate utilization of data thereby guides initiation of interventions to reverse or prevent oxygen debt and tissue hypoxia and includes monitoring the response to therapy. Diligent evaluation and conscientious maintenance of oxygen transport and uptake are cornerstones in the care of all patients with MODS. Whether or not cellular hypoxia is the cause or effect of SIRS or MODS, prevention and treatment of oxygen deficiency is essential to preserve organ function and impact patient outcome.

Table 17-3 Clinical Scenarios: Interventions and Expected Response

Scenario	Dao$_2$	O$_2$E	Vo$_2$	O$_2$ debt	Intervention	Expected response to therapy
Compensated SIRS No organ dysfunction, acidosis, etc.	↑	0/↑	↑	0	None	N/A
Uncompensated SIRS Organ dysfunction and/or metabolic signs of hypoxia	↑/0	↑/0	0	↑	↑ Dao$_2$	↑ Dao$_2$ and Vo$_2$, ↑ or no change in O$_2$E, O$_2$ debt parameters WNL
Decompensated SIRS/MODS Organ dysfunction, metabolic signs of hypoxia	0/↑/↓	↓	↓	↑	↑ Dao$_2$ and seek cause of cellular dysfunction; correct metabolic abnormalities, e.g. hypothermia, hypophosphatemia	*Desired:* ↑ Dao$_2$, Vo$_2$, and O$_2$E; O$_2$ debt parameters WNL *Probable:* No ↑ in O$_2$E or Vo$_2$, and persistent O$_2$ debt, despite Dao$_2$ increase
SIRS abatement	↑/0	↑/0	↑/0	0	Stop any inotrope	Normal Dao$_2$, O$_2$E, Vo$_2$, and O$_2$ debt parameters

↑, Increase; ↓, decrease; *0*, no change; *Dao$_2$*, arterial oxygen delivery; *N/A*, not applicable; *O$_2$E*, oxygen extraction; *Vo$_2$*, oxygen consumption; *O$_2$ debt*, oxygen debt; *WNL*, within normal limits.

REFERENCES

1. Steltzer H et al. The relationship between oxygen delivery and uptake in the critically ill: Is there a critical or optimal therapeutic value? A meta-analysis. Anaesthesia 1994;49:229-236.
2. Ronco JJ et al. Identification of the critical oxygen delivery for anaerobic metabolism in critically ill septic and nonseptic humans. JAMA 1994;270:1724-1730.
3. Ronco JJ et al. No differences in hemodynamics, ventricular function, and oxygen delivery in septic and nonseptic patients with adult respiratory distress syndrome. Crit Care Med 1994;22:777-782.
4. Shoemaker WC, Appel PL, Bishop MH. Temporal patterns of blood volume, hemodynamics, and oxygen transport in pathogenesis and therapy of postoperative adult respiratory distress syndrome. New Horiz 1993;1:522-537.
5. Meade P et al. Temporal patterns of hemodynamics, oxygen transport, cytokine activity, and complement activity in the development of adult respiratory distress syndrome after severe injury. J Trauma 1994;36:651-657.
6. Moore FA et al. Incommensurate oxygen consumption in response to maximal oxygen availability predicts postinjury multiple organ failure. J Trauma 1992;33:58-67.
7. Hayes MA et al. Response of critically ill patients to treatment aimed at achieving supranormal oxygen delivery and consumption. Relationship to outcome. Chest 1993;103:886-895.
8. Schumacker PT, Cain SM. The concept of critical oxygen delivery. Intensive Care Med 1987; 13:223-229.
9. Krachman SL et al. Effect of dobutamine on oxygen transport and consumption in the adult respiratory distress syndrome. Intensive Care Med 1994;20:130-137.
10. Annat G et al. Oxygen delivery and uptake in the adult respiratory distress syndrome. Lack of relationship when measured independently in patients with normal blood lactate concentrations. Am Rev Respir Dis 1986;133:999-1001.
11. Marik PE, Mohedin M. The contrasting effect of dopamine and norepinephrine on systemic and splanchnic oxygen utilization in hyperdynamic sepsis. JAMA 1994;272:1354-1357.
12. Spec-Mann A et al. Oxygen delivery-consumption relationship in adult respiratory distress syndrome patients: The effect of sepsis. J Crit Care 1993;21:43-50.
13. Bishop MH et al. Relationship between supranormal circulatory values, time delays, and outcome in severely traumatized patients. Crit Care Med 1993;21:56-63.

14. Yu M et al. Effect of maximizing oxygen delivery on morbidity and mortality rates in critically ill patients: A prospective, randomized, controlled study. Crit Care Med 1993; 21:830-838.
15. Grootendorst AF. Hemodynamic aspects of multiple organ failure. Intensive Care Med 1990;2:S165-S167.
16. Shoemaker WC, Appel PL, Kram HB. Role of oxygen debt in the development of organ failure, sepsis, and death in high-risk surgical patients. Chest 1992;102:208-215.
17. Boyd O, Grounds RM, Bennett ED. A randomized clinical trial of the effect of deliberate perioperative increase of oxygen delivery on mortality in high risk surgical patients. JAMA 1993;270:2699-2707.
18. Flemming A et al. Prospective trial of supranormal values as goals of resuscitation in severe trauma. Arch Surg 1992;127:1175-1181.
19. Russell JA, Phang PT. The oxygen delivery/consumption controversy. Approaches to management of the critically ill. Am J Respir Crit Care Med 1994;149:533-537.
20. Marik PE. Gastric mucosal pH. A better predictor of multiorgan dysfunction syndrome and death than oxygen derived variables in patients with sepsis. Chest 1993;104:225-229.
21. Meir-Hellmann A et al. The relationship between mixed venous and hepatic venous O_2 saturation in patients with septic shock. Adv Exp Med Biol 1994;345:701-707.
22. Headley JM, Von Rueden KT. The right ventricle: Significant anatomy, physiology, and interventricular considerations. J Cardiovasc Nurs 1991;6:1-11.
23. Santora TA, Schinco MA, Trooskin SZ. Are volumetric hemodynamic parameters better predictors of "recruitable" myocardial function in septic hearts? (abstract) Crit Care Med 1995;23(suppl):A133.
24. Marini CP et al. Effect of hematocrit on regional oxygen delivery and extraction in an ARDS model (abstract). Crit Care Med 1995;32(suppl):A140.
25. Dhainaut JF et al. Practical aspects of oxygen transport: Conclusions and recommendations of the Roundtable Conference. Intensive Care Med 1990;16(Suppl 2):S179-S180.
26. Pinsky MR. Heart-lung interactions during positive-pressure ventilation. New Horiz 1994;2:443-456.
27. Dauberschmidt R et al. Increased oxygen affinity contributes to tissue hypoxia in critically ill patients with low oxygen delivery. Adv Exp Med Biol 1994;345:781-788.
28. Astiz ME et al. Relationship of oxygen delivery and mixed venous oxygenation to lactic acidosis in patients with sepsis and acute myocardial infarction. Crit Care Med 1988; 16:655-658.
29. Epstein CD, Henning RJ. Oxygen transport variables in the identification and treatment of tissue hypoxia. Heart Lung 1993;22:328-343.
30. Bakker J et al. Blood lactate levels are superior to oxygen-derived variables in predicting outcome in human septic shock. Chest 1991;99:956-962.
31. Groeneveld ABJ et al. Relation of arterial blood lactate to oxygen delivery and hemodynamic variables in human shock states. Circ Shock 1987;22:35-53.
32. Siegel JH et al. Early predictors of injury severity and death in blunt multiple trauma. Arch Surg 1990;125:498-508.
33. Dunham CM et al. Oxygen debt and metabolic acidemia as quantitative predictors of mortality and the severity of the ischemic insult in hemorrhagic shock. Crit Care Med 1991;19:231-243.
34. Dunham CM et al. The rapid infusion system: A superior method for the resuscitation of trauma patients. Resuscitation 1991;21:207-227.
35. Davis JW et al. Base deficit as a guide to volume resuscitation. J Trauma 1988;28:1464-1467.
36. Mizock BA. Lactic acidosis in critical illness. Crit Care Med 1992;20:80-93.
37. Dunham CM et al. Inflammatory markers: Superior predictors of adverse outcome in blunt trauma patients? Crit Care Med 1994;22:667-672.
38. Astiz ME et al. Oxygen delivery and consumption in patients with hyperdynamic septic shock. Crit Care Med 1987;15:26-28.
39. Mythen MG. The role of gut mucosal hypoperfusion in the pathogenesis of post-operative organ dysfunction. Intensive Care Med 1994;20:203-209.
40. Gutierrez G et al. Comparison of gastric intramucosal pH with measures of oxygen transport and consumption in critically ill patients. Crit Care Med 1992;20:451-457.
41. Chang MC et al. Gastric tonometry supplements information provided by systemic indicators of oxygen transport. J Trauma 1994;37:1-7.
42. Shoemaker WC et al. Temporal hemodynamic and oxygen transport patterns in medical patients. Chest 1993;104:1529-1536.
43. Shoemaker WC et al. Sequence of physiologic patterns in septic shock. Crit Care Med 1993;21:1876-1889.
44. Vallet B et al. Prognostic value of the dobutamine test in patients with sepsis syndrome and normal lactate values: A prospective, multicenter study. Crit Care Med 1993; 21:1868-1875.
45. Mira JP et al. Lack of oxygen supply dependency in patients with severe sepsis. Chest 1994;106:1524-1531.
46. Ronco JJ et al. Oxygen consumption is independent of changes in oxygen delivery in severe adult respiratory distress syndrome. Am Rev Respir Dis 1991;143:1267-1273.
47. Ronco JJ et al. Oxygen consumption is independent of increases in oxygen delivery by dobutamine in septic patients who have normal or increased plasma lactate. Am Rev Respir Dis 1993;147:25-31.
48. Silance PG, Simon C, Vincent JL. The relation between cardiac index and oxygen extraction in acutely ill patients. Chest 1994;105:1190-1197.
49. Zhang H, Vincent JL. Oxygen extraction is altered by endotoxin during tamponade-induced stagnant hypoxia in the dog. Circ Shock 1993;40:168-176.
50. Siegel JH, Vary TC. Sepsis, abnormal metabolic control, and the multiple organ failure syndrome. In Siegel JH, ed. Trauma: Emergency surgery and critical care. New York: Churchill Livingston, 1987:411-501.
51. Siegel JH et al. Physiologic and metabolic correlations in human sepsis. J Surg 1979;86:163-193.
52. Tuchschmidt J et al. Elevation of cardiac output and oxygen delivery improves outcome in septic shock. Chest 1992; 102:216-220.
53. Shoemaker WC, Kram HB, Appel PL. Therapy of shock based on pathophysiology, monitoring and outcome prediction. Crit Care Med 1990;18:S19-S25.
54. Hayes MA et al. Elevation of oxygen delivery in the treatment of critically ill patients. N Engl J Med 1994;330:1717-1722.

55. Archie JP. Mathematical coupling of data. Ann Surg 1981;193:296-303.
56. Smithies MN et al. Comparison of oxygen consumption measurement: Indirect calorimetry versus the reversed Fick method. Crit Care Med 1991;19:1401-1406.
57. Phang PT et al. Mathematical coupling explains dependence of oxygen consumption on oxygen delivery in ARDS. Am J Respir Crit Care Med 1994;150:318-323.
58. Gutierrez G et al. Gastric intramucosal pH as a therapeutic index of tissue oxygenation in critically ill patients. Lancet 1992;339:195-199.
59. Meier-Hellman A et al. The relevance of measuring O_2 supply and O_2 consumption for assessing regional tissue oxygenation. Adv Exp Med Biol 1994;345:741-746.
60. Gutierrez G et al. Effect of dobutamine on oxygen consumption and gastric mucosal pH in septic patients. Am J Respir Crit Care Med 1994;150:324-329.
61. Ruokonen E, Takala J, Uusaro A. Effect of vasoactive treatment on the relationship between mixed venous and regional oxygen saturation. Crit Care Med 1991;19:1365-1369.
62. Beards SC et al. Comparison of hemodynamic and oxygen transport responses to modified fluid gelatin and hetastarch in critically ill patients: A prosective, randomized trial. Crit Care Med 1994;22:600-605.
63. Golster M, Berg S, Lisander B. Blood volume and colloid osmotic pressure in crystalloid and colloid infusion. Crit Care Med 1995;23 (supp):A88.
64. Kaminski MV, Haase TL. Albumin and colloid osmotic pressure implications for fluid resuscitation (abstract). Crit Care Clin 1992;8:311-321.
65. Moran JL et al. Epinephrine as an inotropic agent in septic shock: A dose-profile analysis. Crit Care Med 1993;21:70-77.
66. DeBacker D et al. Relationship between oxygen uptake and delivery in septic patients: Effects of prostacyclin versus dobutamine. Crit Care Med 1993;21:1658-1664.
67. Martin C et al. Norepinephrine or dopamine for the treatment of hyperdynamic septic shock? Chest 1993;103:1826-1831.
68. Redl-Wenzl EM et al. The effects of norepinephrine on hemodynamics and renal function in severe septic shock states. Intens Care Med 1993;19:151-154.
69. Martin C et al. Effects of norepinephrine on right ventricular function in septic shock patients. Intens Care Med 1994;20:444-447.
70. Vincent JL. Inotropic agents. New Horiz 1993;1:137-144.
71. Lorente JA et al. Effects of blood transfusion on oxygen transport variables in severe sepsis. Crit Care Med 1993;21:1312-1318.
72. Silverman HJ, Tuma P. Gastric tonometry in patients with sepsis: Effects of dobutamine infusions and packed red blood cell transfusions. Chest 1992;102:184-188.
73. Demling RH. Adult respiratory distress syndrome: Current concepts. New Horiz 1993;1:388-401.
74. Marini JJ. New options for the ventilatory management of acute lung injury. New Horiz 1993;1:489-503.
75. Armstrong BW, MacIntyre NR. Pressure-controlled, inverse ratio ventilation that avoids air trapping in the adult respiratory distress syndrome. Crit Care Med 1995;23:279-285.
76. Hickling KG et al. Low mortality rate in adult respiratory distress syndrome using low-volume, pressure-limited ventilation with permissive hypercapnea: A prospective study. Crit Care Med 1994;22:1568-1583.
77. Doering LV. The effect of positioning on hemodynamics and gas exchange in the critically ill: A review. Am J Crit Care 1993;2:208-216.
78. Pappert D et al. Influence of positioning on ventilation-perfusion relationships in severe adult respiratory distress syndrome. Chest 1994;106:1511-1516.
79. Gattinoni L et al. Body position changes redistribute lung computed-tomographic density in patients with acute respiratory failure. Anesthesia 1991;74:15-23.
80. Lamm WJE, Graham MM, Albert RK. Mechanism by which the prone position improves oxygenation in acute lung injury. Am J Respir Crit Care Med 1994;150:184-193.
81. Pape HC et al. The effect of kinetic positioning on lung function and pulmonary haemodynamics in posttraumatic ARDS: A clinical study. Injury 1994;25:51-57.
82. Choi SC, Nelson LD. Kinetic therapy in critically ill patients: Combined results based on meta-analysis. J Crit Care 1992;7:57-62.
83. Reynolds HN, Habashi N, Borg U. New directions and applications for extracorporeal cardiopulmonary support. Adv Trauma Crit Care 1994;9:99-133.
84. Cioffi WG, Ogura H. Inhaled nitric oxide in acute lung disease. New Horiz 1995;3:73-85.
85. Rossaint R et al. Inhaled nitric oxide for the adult respiratory distress syndrome. N Engl J Med 1993;328:399-405.
86. ACCP/SCCM Consensus Conference Committee. American College of Chest Physicians/Society of Critical Care Medicine Consensus Conference: Definitions for sepsis and organ failure and guidelines for the use of innovative therapies in sepsis. Crit Care Med 1992;20:864-874.
87. Shoemaker WC. Use and abuse of balloon tipped pulmonary artery catheter: Are patients getting their money's worth? Crit Care Med 1990;18:1294-1295.
88. Tuman KJ, Carroll GC, Ivankovich AD. Pitfalls in interpretation of pulmonary catheter data. J Cardiothorac Anesth 1989;3:625-637.
89. Sibbald WJ et al. New technologies, critical care, and economic realities. Crit Care Med 1993;21:1777-1779.
90. Naylor CD et al. Pulmonary artery catheterization: Can there be an integrated strategy for guideline development and research promotion? JAMA 1993;269:2407-2411.
91. American Society of Anesthesiologists Task Force. Practice guidelines for pulmonary artery catheterization. Anesthesiology 1993;78:380-394.
92. Iberti TJ et al. A multicenter study of physicians' knowledge of the pulmonary artery catheter. JAMA 1990;264:2928-2932.
93. Iberti TJ et al. Assessment of critical care nurses' knowledge of the pulmonary artery catheter. Crit Care Med 1994;22:1674-1678.

CHAPTER *18*

Multiple Organ Dysfunction Syndrome: Overview and Conclusions

Virginia Huddleston Secor

Through the years following its initial description, the multiple organ dysfunction syndrome (MODS) has become known as the final common pathway to death in the twentieth century Intensive Care Unit (ICU) and is now considered the leading cause of death in the surgical ICU.[1,2] Although questions remain concerning the development and progression of MODS,[3] major conceptual advances have occurred over the past 20 years (see the box on p. 403).[4-6] The fundamental role of the inflammatory response in the development and progression of organ dysfunction and failure is now recognized through the use of terms such as the systemic inflammatory response syndrome (SIRS).[7-12]

As emphasized throughout this text, many investigators believe the common thread running through the different patient populations who progress to MODS is the dysregulation of the inflammatory/immune response (IIR).[7,13-20] Control is lost in the systems initially designed to protect and defend the patient. Exaggerated and overwhelming inflammation ensues leading to maldistribution of circulating volume, imbalance of oxygen supply and demand, and alterations in metabolism (Fig. 18-1).

SUMMARY OF PATHOPHYSIOLOGY
Primary events and pathophysiologic changes

Predisposing factors and primary events triggering mediator release are presented in Chapter 1. The mechanisms of infection, inflammation, and ischemia along with preexisting factors such as chronic disease, age, and nutritional status are common physiologic insults and conditions associated with the development of MODS.[1,4,21-25] Primary events such as neuroendocrine activation, triggering of the IIR, endothelial damage and ischemia/reperfusion injury occurring with insult or following resuscitation trigger the elaboration of numerous mediators.[6,26] Neuroendocrine activation and the IIR protect the host, limit the extent of injury, and promote rapid healing of involved tissue when under tight control; however, if control is lost, the pathophysiologic changes develop and progress to the clinical presentation common in sepsis, SIRS, and MODS (Fig. 18-2).

Chapter 2 presents a brief overview of the IIR, with a special emphasis on the immunosuppressant roles of trauma, stress, hemorrhage, blood transfusions, general anesthesia, and malnutrition. Key assessment findings including the role of both natural host defenses and laboratory values are also discussed. An increasing amount of evidence points to ineffective macrophage-T cell interaction as one source of this immunosuppression.[27-29] Liberation of glucocorticoids, decreased antibody production, alterations in cytokine production, and increased T-cell suppressor activity are also implicated in the immunosuppression seen in critically ill patients that places them at added risk for septic complications.[27,28,30,31]

Chapter 3 presents an in depth explanation of both the physiologic role and pathophysiologic effects of the mediators playing a significant role in the pathophysiology of sepsis, SIRS, and MODS.[25,32,33] Tumor necrosis factor (TNF), interleukin-1 (IL-1), toxic oxygen metabolites (TOMs),

> **CONCEPTUAL ADVANCES IN THE STUDY OF MODS**
>
> Pathophysiologic events are set into motion immediately postinsult.
> Reperfusion of ischemic tissue can trigger an inflammatory response and may cause additional tissue injury.*
> Although organ function may not appear impaired clinically, damage to the ultrastructure may already be occurring.†
> Insults are synergistic, with the first insult priming the inflammatory cells and tissues such that a second hit could produce an exaggerated response.†
> Organs interact in their physiologic and pathophysiologic states. Failure of one organ potentiates failure in another.‡
> Inflammatory "septic" state can occur in the absence of infection.§
> Treatment of the primary event or removal of the initial inflammatory stimuli may not halt the process.
> "The host is not an innocent bystander or victim whose tissues are being ravaged by invading bacteria but instead is an active participant in this destructive process."§

*From Welbourn et al. Pathophysiology of ischaemia reperfusion injury: Central role of the neutrophil. Br J Surg 1991;78:651-655.
†From Schlag G, Redl H. Introduction. In: Schlag G, Redl H, eds. Pathophysiology of shock, sepsis, and organ failure. Berlin: Springer-Verlag; 1993:1-3.
‡From Matuschak GM. Organ interactions in critical illness: Paradigms and mechanisms. New Horiz 1994;2:413-414.
§From Deitch EA. Multiple organ failure: Pathophysiology and potential future therapy. Ann Surg 1992;216:117-134.

arachidonic acid (AA) metabolites, and proteases are dominant mediators. Consequently, their presence implicates the neutrophil (source of TOMs, AA, and proteases) and the macrophage (source of TNF and IL-1) as principal elements in the pathogenesis of SIRS and MODS.[34,35] The endothelium and the products that it generates constitutively and during injury (nitric oxide, endothelin, adhesion molecules, tissue factor) have also been implicated in the pathogenesis of the secondary complications common in critical illness.[36-40]

In Chapter 4, Bell comprehensively examines the role of DIC in MODS progression showing endothelial damage and microvascular thrombi as key factors in the development and progression of ischemic organ damage and dysfunction.[26,39-41] Removal of the underlying pathology in DIC remains the definitive therapy.

The cyclical, autoactivating nature of the IIR and endothelial damage constitutes the major danger in MODS and contributes to the self-propagation of the major pathophysiologic changes. Robins extensively describes maldistribution of volume at the systemic, organ, and local levels in Chapter 5. The pathophysiology and role of ischemia/reperfusion injury are also addressed. Robins emphasizes that despite a hyperdynamic circulation and increased cardiac output, perfusion may be submaximal in some tissue beds. Patchy areas of low flow or ischemia may exist in an organ even when the overall flow in the organ is normal or increased.[20,42-44] The elegant balance of oxygen supply and demand and autoregulatory capacities is often lost, thus setting the stage for organ dysfunction and failure. Increased capillary permeability, vasodilatation, selective vasoconstriction, and vascular obstruction all contribute to the maldistribution of volume. Without volume delivery, no oxygen and nutrient delivery occurs, which exacerbates the balance between oxygen supply and demand.

In Chapter 6, Kearney emphasizes the role of ischemia, oxygen debt, and anaerobic metabolism in the pathophysiology of MODS. Perfusion abnormalities, pathology at the microcirculatory level, and defects in oxygen extraction and utilization are examined in the discussion of the oxygen supply and demand imbalance common in sepsis and MODS.[44-47] In addition to the decreased oxygen supply, the oxygen demand is also elevated secondary to hyperthermia, shivering, increased work of breathing in ARDS, and, very profoundly, by the hypermetabolism.[48,49]

The nutritional and metabolic status of the patient, both before and after admission, greatly influence the pathophysiology and survival rates of MODS. Kimbrell presents the hypermetabolic state as a primary pathophysiologic mechanism in MODS.[50-52] In Chapter 7, inappropriate substrate

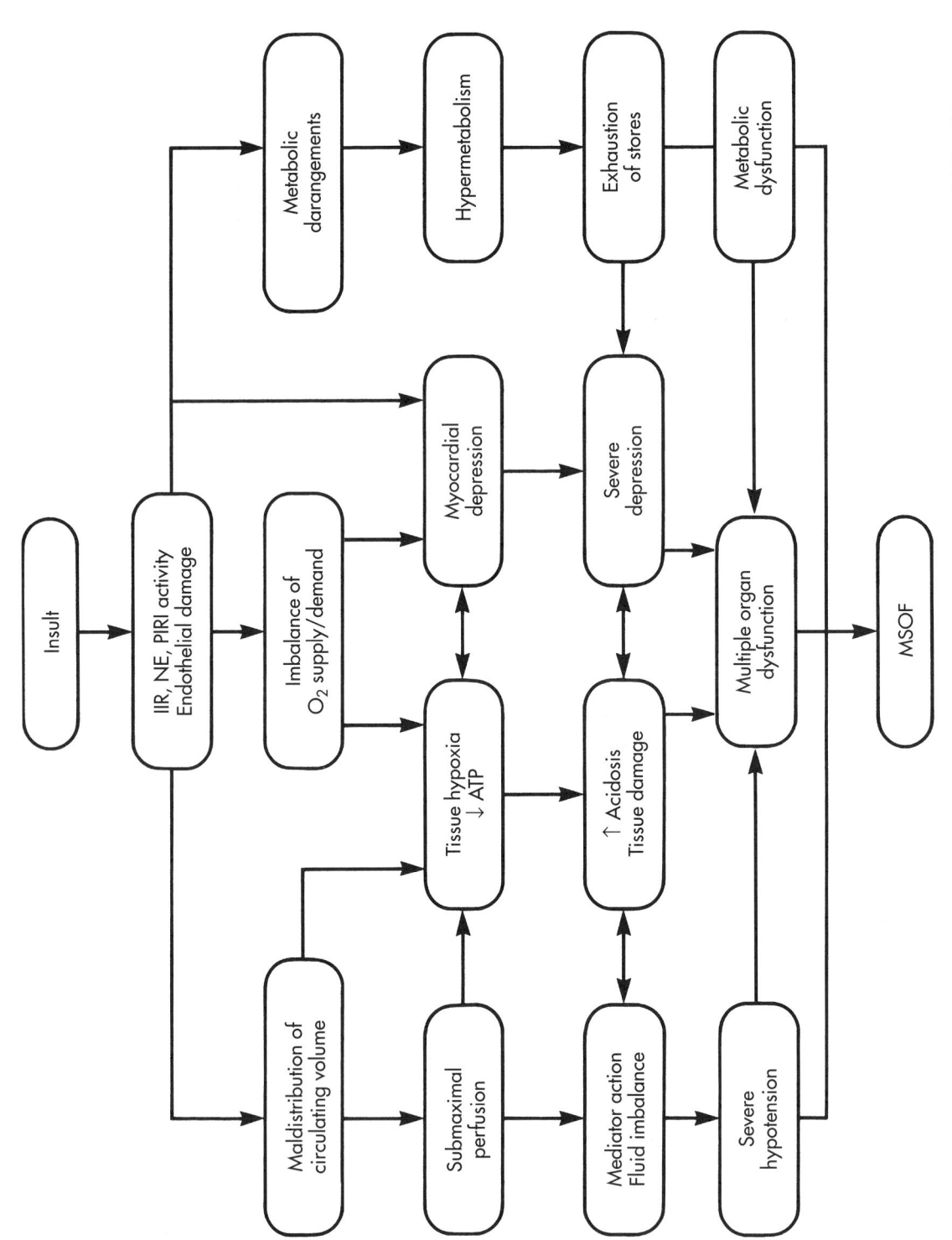

Fig. 18-1 Pathophysiologic cascade mechanism of MODS. *ATP*, Adenosine triphosphate; *IIR*, inflammatory/immune response; *MSOF*, multisystem organ failure; *NE*, neuroendocrine activation; *PIRI*, postischemic reperfusion injury.

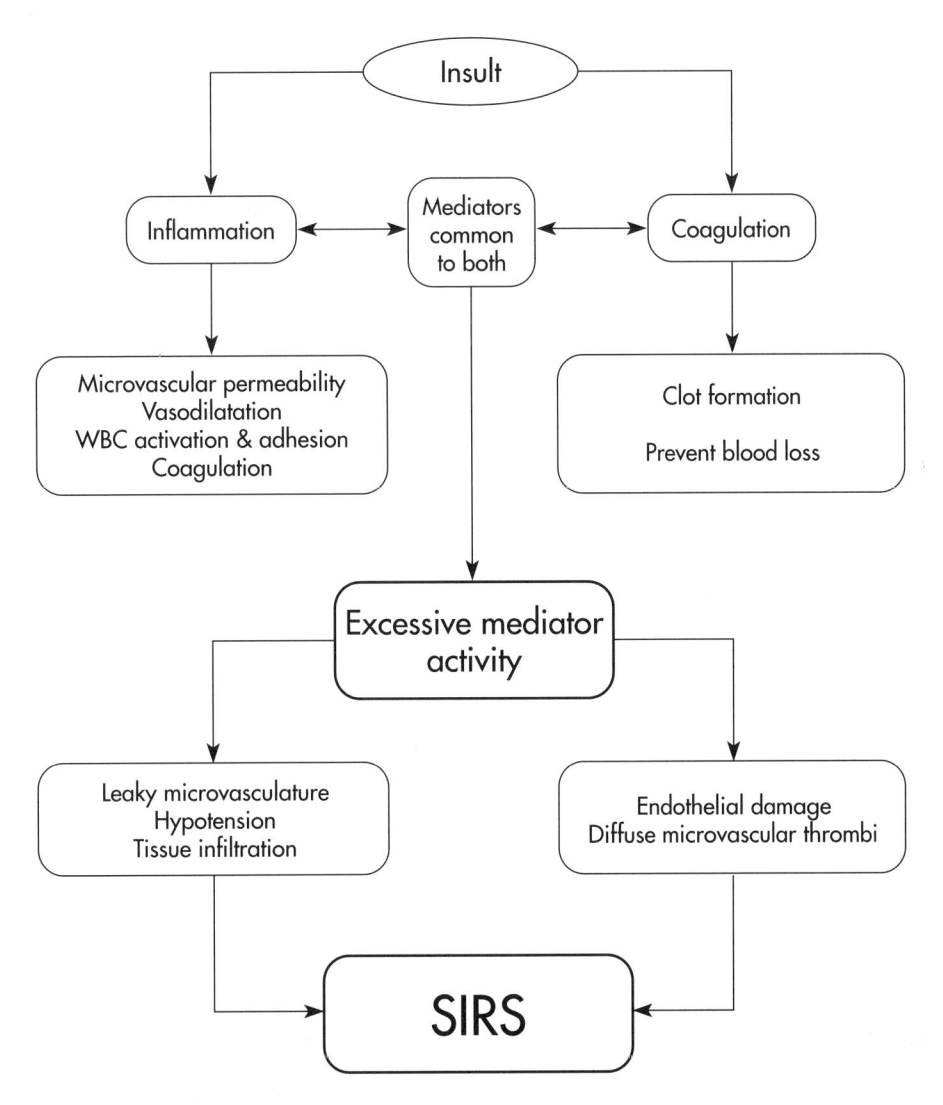

Fig. 18-2 Interactive cascades of inflammation and coagulation. *SIRS,* Systemic inflammatory response syndrome; *WBC,* white blood cell. (From Secor VH. The inflammatory/immune response in critical illness: role of the systemic inflammatory response syndrome. Crit Care Nurs Clin North Am 1994;6:255.)

metabolism of carbohydrates, proteins, and lipids are addressed. As gluconeogenesis increases, muscle mass is severely depleted, and visceral protein stores fall prey to the metabolic machine. Immunocompetence is affected, along with diaphragmatic muscle strength, mobility, and organ system integrity.

Liver dysfunction compounds the immune dysfunction and metabolic abnormalities. In Chapter 9 Lohrmann presents evidence implicating liver involvement as a major determinant of MODS development and progression.[50,53,54] While controversy exists concerning the exact etiology and pathogenesis of the liver dysfunction (ischemic versus cell-to-cell interaction), the failure does occur much earlier than previously thought.[55,56] Cerra[50] and others believe that the severity of MODS parallels the severity of the liver dysfunction; therefore, when the liver can no longer meet the metabolic demands of the body, the patient dies.

Role of the individual organ

The systemic pathophysiologic derangements (Chapters 5 through 7) set the stage for malfunction in each individual organ. Not all organs have equal susceptibility to injury, nor does each failure impact patient survival with the same magnitude. Dysfunction of any particular organ depends on (1) sensitivity of the organ's vascular bed to mediators and hypoperfusion, (2) regional degree of inflammation, that is, the proximity of a given organ to the primary site of trauma, infection, inflammation, or ischemia, and (3) responsiveness to therapeutic regimen; for example, what may help one organ may harm another.

The pulmonary system is commonly the first organ system to display signs of dysfunction. This may be related to its increased susceptibility to damage or the fact that it receives the entire cardiac output and thus is exposed to the multitude of mediators circulating during sepsis and SIRS. In Chapter 8, Morris discusses the adult respiratory distress syndrome (ARDS) and presents the updated definitions and diagnostic criteria put forth at the American-European Consensus Conference on ARDS held in 1992.[57] Acute lung injury represents a major insult to the body, and the inability of the lungs to adequately oxygenate the cardiac output from the right heart potentiates hypoxemia that is often refractory to therapy. Ventilation-perfusion mismatching and intrapulmonary shunting are responsible for the hypoxemia. While ARDS can occur in isolation, it is more frequently associated with sepsis and MODS, both as a cause and as a secondary complication.

Although each organ may have varying degrees of damage related to numerous factors, MODS is *not* a series of isolated failures. Although each of the organs may be a victim or a target of the syndrome, each organ has the potential to impact the process and contribute to failure of other organs, thus perpetuating the self-propagating nature of MODS (Fig. 18-3). Although the gut is very sensitive to hypoxia and often suffers ischemic damage and mucosal atrophy, it is also the source of other complications. As O'Neill points out in the discussion on gastrointestinal involvement (Chapter 10), the gut is a ready source of bacterial contamination. Although not consistently demonstrated, bacteria, yeast, endotoxin, or other bacterial products and inflammatory stimuli may translocate across the injured gut barrier into the lymphatics or portal circulation.[58-61] If the hepatic Kupffer cells do not clear this foreign debris adequately or are overly activated by the debris, systemic infection or inflammation could result. The patient may also develop nosocomial pneumonia by aspirating gastric contents or contaminated oropharyngeal secretions.[62,63]

The pancreas is also more commonly identified as a trigger of the process rather than as a victim of the syndrome. Sensing provides an in depth overview of the etiology and pathophysiologic derangements seen in acute pancreatitis (Chapter 11). The chief problem related to pancreatitis is the massive necrosis and liberation of inflammatory mediators.[64] Major derangements in pulmonary and cardiovascular function are common.

Gates, in the discussion on myocardial involvement (Chapter 12), eloquently lays out the role of myocardial depression in sepsis, integrated with a background of normal myocardial physiology. Gates dispels the commonly held assumption that most patients experience both the hyperdynamic and hypodynamic state during the evolution of septic shock, citing evidence to show that only 10% of septic nonsurvivors experience a true hypodynamic presentation. Most patients die from refractory hypotension and low systemic vascular resistance (SVR) or move into MODS.[42] The presence of a falling cardiac output is more likely to be related to inadequate fluid resuscitation, the most common mistake in managing patients in septic shock and MODS. Along with Robins, Gates discusses several hypotheses related to myocardial depression, including maldistribution of flow within the myocardium itself, direct mediator activity (myocardial depressant factor, TNF), and myocardial edema. It is of primary importance to note that myocardial depression is present early, even in the face of a high cardiac output and that a high cardiac output does not guarantee sufficient oxygen delivery to all tissues because the preexisting maldistribution of volume precludes adequate flow to all regions.[20,42]

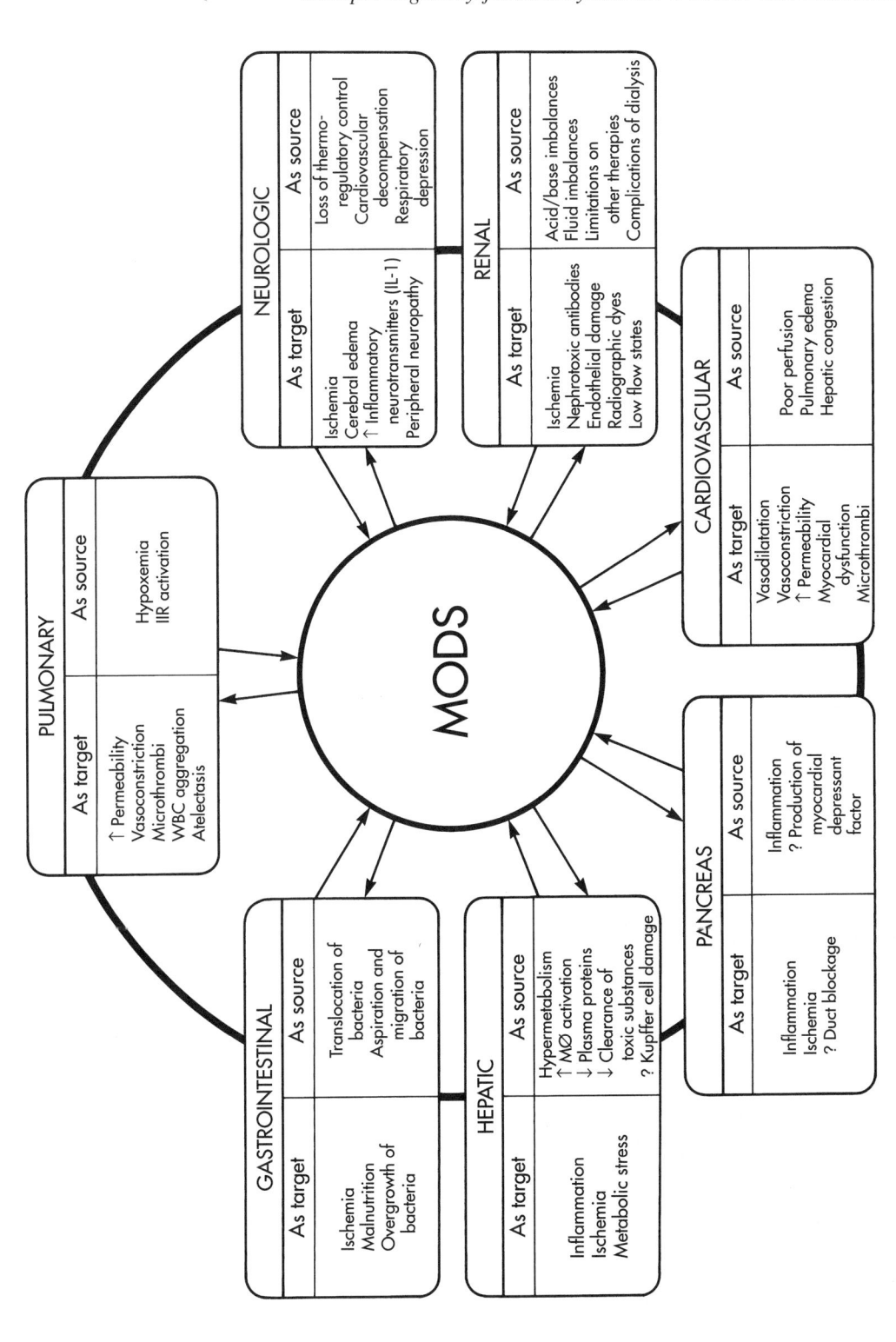

Multiple Organ Dysfunction Syndrome: Overview and Conclusions   407

Fig. 18-3 The circle of MODS. Each organ may be a target of damage in the process or a contributor to MODS progression. As the number of failing organs increases, other organs are affected and mortality approaches 100 percent. *IIR*, Inflammatory/immune response; *IL-1*, interleukin-1; *MØ*, macrophage.

While isolated renal failure was a common finding in casualties of war and trauma patients in the 1950s and 1960s, improvement in fluid resuscitation techniques and aggressive monitoring have greatly reduced the incidence of prerenal failure. Today, renal failure is more commonly associated with ischemic acute tubular necrosis (ATN) and nephrotoxic factors such as antibiotic treatment. In Chapter 13, Toto reviews pertinent renal anatomy and physiology, and then examines the classification and differential diagnosis of acute renal failure, with an emphasis on the updated clinical course and management of acute tubular necrosis. The systemic hemodynamic changes and mediators common in SIRS and MODS greatly impact the renal vasculature and flow dynamics, thus setting the stage for ischemic ATN.[65]

In relation to other organs, little is known concerning the nervous system and MODS. Briones (Chapter 14) points out that shock and sepsis frequently induce ischemic brain injury. Autoregulatory mechanisms fail and the blood-brain barrier becomes more permeable to toxic substances. As in other organs, reperfusion may actually exacerbate the damage because petechial and subarachnoid hemorrhage and transudation of colloid occur secondary to increased capillary permeability and restoration of flow. Studies also identify peripheral neuropathies in MODS.[66]

ASSESSMENT

The presentation of sepsis and SIRS represents a dynamic continuum in which the patient may recover or die from the multiple organ dysfunction. Table 18-1 outlines the clinical findings of the hyperdynamic presentation along with their etiologies. No consensus has been reached concerning the definition of criteria to routinely identify and study MODS. The older criteria such as those of Knaus and Wagner[67] focused on failure of the organs rather than on dysfunction. Moore and colleagues[23] have developed a set of criteria at their institution to identify organ dysfunction (Table 18-2). Although these criteria are continuously being updated and refined, they represent an attempt to view this syndrome not as an all-or-none phenomenon, but as a dynamic process with a wide range of clinical presentations.

Special consideration must be taken with the pediatric and elderly populations because of their anatomic and physiologic differences, as well as their more limited reserves in responding to an insult. Moloney-Harmon and Czerwinski discuss specific assessment findings and management strategies for the pediatric population in Chapter 15. While the pathophysiology follows a similar cascade of events as that seen in the adult population, the anatomic and physiologic differences in infants and young children require specialized assessment skills and alterations in therapy.

In Chapter 16, Rauen and Stamatos comprehensively delineate the unique challenges involved in the elderly patient with MODS, most interestingly that many of the criteria used to define organ dysfunction in the general population are actually baseline values in many healthy elderly individuals. The presence of chronic disease also compounds the ability of the elderly to respond to and withstand a major physiologic insult. Therefore, these authors propose new criteria specifically for the elderly based on a thorough review of the literature concerning the structural and functional changes associated with the aging process. As with Moore's criteria, these criteria await testing for validity and reliability; however, they represent a major step forward in the early identification and management of this special population.

OVERVIEW OF THERAPEUTIC MANAGEMENT
Goals

The management of MODS remains difficult and, in many areas, controversial. It requires a multidisciplinary approach including nursing, medicine, respiratory therapy, nutritional support, physical therapy, occupational therapy, social services, and rehabilitation. Collaborative management concentrates on four major goals*:

1. Prevention, early identification, and control of infectious or inflammatory stimuli
2. Restoration of oxygen supply and demand balance
3. Provision of nutritional support and metabolic requirements
4. Individual organ support

Prevention

Once triggered, the systemic IIR continues with minimal exogenous stimuli. Even aggressive treat-

---

*References 2, 4, 21, 56, 68.

Table 18-1 Hyperdynamic Clinical Presentation and Etiology

Clinical presentation	Etiology
Increased cardiac output	Fluid resuscitation in vasodilated patient → increased circulating volume Vasodilatation → decreased SVR Sympathetic nervous system activation → increased venous return Increased heart rate Ventricular dilatation and low afterload → increased stroke volume
Decreased systemic vascular resistance	Mediator activity → vasodilatation Increased oxygen needs in the periphery Decreased responsiveness to catecholamines
Hypotension	Vasodilatation secondary to mediators Relative volume deficit Cardiac dysfunction Volume losses as fluid leaks into extravascular spaces
Tachycardia	SNS activation Fever Compensatory mechanism for hypotension Increased metabolic rate
Metabolic acidosis	Anaerobic metabolism Rhabdomyolysis and cell death Impaired renal function
Respiratory alkalosis → respiratory acidosis	Hyperventilation (early) Compensation for metabolic acidosis (early) Respiratory acidosis in latter stages secondary to poor gas exchange and ARDS Respiratory depression secondary to CNS depression
Decreased level of consciousness	Direct action of mediators Decreased cerebral blood flow Decreased cerebral perfusion pressure Loss of cerebral autoregulation Reperfusion injury Fever Acid-base abnormalities
Decreased urine output	Relative volume deficit Selective renal vasoconstriction Poor perfusion pressures Acute renal failure
Fever → hypothermia	Increased metabolic rate Direct action of mediators on hypothalamus May be low in late stages secondary to thermoregulatory failure of hypothalamus, decreased metabolic activity → decreased heat production

Leukocytosis → leukopenia	Immune response
	Stress response
	May be decreased in latter stages secondary to
	    consumption of WBCs
	    sequestration in lungs and other organs
	    bone marrow exhaustion

Increased lactate	Anaerobic metabolism Hepatocellular dysfunction → decreased lactate clearance

Continued.

Table 18-1 Hyperdynamic Clinical Presentation and Etiology—cont'd

Clinical presentation	Etiology
Hyperglycemia→ hypoglycemia	Increased gluconeogenesis Catecholamine release (SNS activation) Insulin resistance Glucocorticoid release May be hypoglycemic in late stages secondary to liver failure or inadequate substrate metabolism
Hypoxemia accompanied by shortness of breath, decreased respiratory depth, and crackles	Pulmonary endothelial damage and microthrombi Increased atelectasis and secretions ARDS and high permeability pulmonary edema CHF and cardiogenic pulmonary edema V/Q mismatching and intrapulmonary shunting Pneumonia and supra-infections
$S\bar{v}o_2$ > 80% (early)	Decreased oxygen extraction/utilization secondary to microvascular pathology and obstruction

$S\bar{v}o_2$ < 60% (This value is often abnormally high and difficult to interpret in septic and hyperdynamic states and should be used with caution.)	Falls in late stages secondary to
	  low CO
	  low Sao_2
	  low Hgb

Decreased platelets and clotting factors	Accelerated clotting Increased consumption DIC
Increased fibrin degradation products (FDPs)	Accelerated fibrinolysis DIC

From Secor VH: Complications of critical illness and injury: Sepsis, DIC, and multiple organ dysfunction [monograph]. Atlanta, copyright 1994 Virginia Huddleston Secor, p 23-26.
ARDS, Adult respiratory distress syndrome; *CHF,* congestive heart failure; *CNS,* central nervous system; *CO,* cardiac output; *DIC,* disseminated intravascular coagulation; *FDP,* fibrin degradation product; *Hgb,* hemoglobin; *Sao₂,* arterial oxygen saturation; *SNS,* sympathetic nervous system; *Sv̄o₂,* mixed venous oxygen saturation; *SVR,* systemic vascular resistance; *V/Q,* ventilation-perfusion; *WBC,* white blood cell.

ment of the initial insult may not halt the vicious cycle of inflammation once it becomes malignant. Therefore, the ultimate and most effective weapon against MODS is prevention. Iatrogenic complications are a common source of infectious or inflammatory stimuli.[69] Early interventions must focus on infection control, early identification of complications, and prompt, aggressive resuscitation and ongoing therapy. Often referred to as "front-loading" therapy, complications are prevented or minimized by early intervention, rather than being treated only when compromise and decompensation occur.

All treatable injuries should be managed upon admission. Removal of all necrotic tissue, early débridement of burn eschar, and prompt stabilization of fractures minimize further soft tissue damage, inflammation, and infection.[2,4,56] A secure airway and frequent oral care are crucial in reducing aspiration and nosocomial pneumonia. Meticulous line, site, and catheter care and observation, along with aggressive wound and skin care minimize iatrogenic complications. Hand washing remains a key factor in preventing nosocomial colonization and infection.[70] Antibiotic therapy is based on the initial Gram stain results and the clinical status of the patient and is altered according to patient response and culture reports.[71] The use of empiric antibiotics and empiric laparotomy remains controversial. Although corticosteroids are potent antiinflammatory agents, their routine use is not ad-

Table 18-2 Postinjury MOF Score*

Organs	Grade 1	Grade 2	Grade 3
Pulmonary dysfunction	ARDS score >5†	ARDS score >9	ARDS score >13
Renal dysfunction	Creatinine >1.8 mg/dL	Creatinine >2.5 mg/dL	Creatinine >5 mg/dL
Hepatic dysfunction‡	Bilirubin >2.0 mg/dL	Bilirubin >4.0 mg/dL	Bilirubin >8.0 mg/dL
Cardiac dysfunction§	Minimal inotropes	Moderate inotropes	High inotropes

*MOF score = A + B + C + D, not due to chronic disease.
†ARDS score, see below.
‡Not due to biliary obstruction or resolving hematoma.
§Cardiac index <3.0 L/min/M² requiring inotropic support: minimal dose = dopamine or dobutamine <5 µg/kg/min; moderate dose = dopamine or dobutamine 5-15 µg/kg/min; high dose = dopamine or dobutamine >15 µg/kg/min.

Postinjury ARDS Score*

Variables	Grade 1	Grade 2	Grade 3	Grade 4
Pulmonary/radiographic	Diffuse, mild interstitial marking/opacities	Diffuse, marked interstitial/mild air-space opacities	Diffuse, moderate air-space consolidation	Diffuse, severe air-space consolidation
PaO_2/FiO_2 (mm Hg)	175-250	125-174	80-124	<80
Minute ventilation (L/min)	11-13	14-16	17-20	>20
PEEP (cm H_2O)	6-9	10-13	14-17	>17
Static compliance	40-50	30-39	17-20	<20

*ARDS SCORE = A + B + C + D + E when PCWP ≤ 18 mm Hg or when there is no clinical reason to suspect hydrostatic pulmonary edema.
PCWP, Pulmonary capillary wedge pressure; PEEP, positive end-expiratory pressure.

vocated in sepsis, SIRS, and MODS.[72] Because they are associated with significant side-effects, particularly immunosuppression, corticosteroids actually predispose the patient to greater complications.[73-75]

Restoration of oxygen supply and demand balance

A major focus of both monitoring and intervention involves restoration of the oxygen supply and demand balance.[76] While arterial blood gases (ABGs) provide crucial patient information, they only assess the amount of oxygen brought into the blood stream, not the amount actually delivered to the tissues. An arterial saturation (SaO_2) of 99% matters little if the cardiac output is so low that the oxygenated blood cannot be delivered to the tissues. Likewise, assessing oxygen delivery without considering the amount of oxygen that tissues actually consume leads to misinterpretation of assessment findings and clinical condition. Oxygen transport formulas such as oxygen delivery (DO_2) and oxygen consumption (VO_2) provide the clinician with much more valid information concerning oxygen delivery and tissue oxygenation. All parameters of oxygenation must be assessed, including the variables that define those parameters. Cardiac output, hemoglobin concentration, and arterial saturation are principal variables in both DO_2 and VO_2 formulas; therefore, aggressive efforts are aimed at optimizing cardiac output, hemoglobin level, and arterial saturation in MODS.

Information and data concerning oxygen delivery and consumption continue to expand rapidly. Therefore, in this second edition, an entire chapter is devoted to a discussion of the evaluation and management of oxygen delivery and consumption. In Chapter 17, Von Rueden and Dunham extensively examine the wealth of literature in this controversial area. The relationship of oxygen delivery, consumption, and debt to the SIRS state is presented along with management considerations. The use of supranormal values is addressed in depth. Although the use of global measures of oxygen debt such as arterial pH, base deficit, and lactate levels is common, Von Rueden and Dunham emphasize the need for more specific indicators of regional oxygen transport and uptake at the organ level.

Decrease oxygen demand

Because oxygen demand is greater than supply, any condition such as fever, pain, shivering, tachycardia, or an increased work of breathing that increases oxygen demand places a severe strain on an already compromised balance.[77] Interventions that decrease the demand are as vital as those aimed at increasing the supply. While fever shifts the oxyhemoglobin dissociation curve to the right and also enhances immune system function, excessive body temperatures need to be reduced and controlled.[78]

Optimizing sedation in critically ill patients is crucial in increasing patient comfort and decreasing oxygen demand.[79] Procedural pain and distress are a common source of anxiety and increased oxygen demand in many patients.[80] Pain medication and antianxiety medication not only increase patient comfort, but also decrease restlessness, tachycardia, and work of breathing, thus "freeing up" additional oxygen for use by the major organ beds. Analgesics also enhance toleration of invasive procedures and interventions such as turning, suctioning, dressing changes, and line insertions; therefore, desaturation is minimized.

Provision of nutritional support

Nutritional support must be provided early. For each day that this is delayed, hypermetabolism and muscle catabolism continue unabated.[49] In the future, antioxidants and other nutritional supplements may be used to alter the host inflammatory response and its sequelae.[81,82] In Chapter 7, Kimbrell discusses the advantages and complications of total parenteral nutrition and enteral feedings, along with nutritional assessment and investigational therapies. Goals of nutritional support include the following*:

1. To support organ structure and function
2. To prevent substrate-limited metabolism
3. To support metabolic pathways
4. To maintain nitrogen equilibrium

Increasing evidence points to enteral feedings as being superior to total parenteral nutrition in terms of both the number of resulting complications and the maintenance of gut barrier function.[50,52,59,83] Advantages of early enteral feedings include (1) enhancement of enteral immune function, (2) prevention of GI atrophy and maintenance of mucosal integrity, thus aiding in the prevention of bacterial translocation, (3) decrease in bile sludging to minimize cholestasis and cholecystitis, (4) decrease in incidence of stress ulceration, and (5) support of hepatic function.

Individual organ support

The fourth major goal of therapy is support of individual organs; however, the treatment of the patient must focus on the entire disease process and on removing the stimulus of the IIR. Supportive care treats manifestations and does not remove the source of the problem. Monitoring must include parameters such as oxygen delivery and consumption that measure the effects of therapy on more than one system. The box on p. 413 summarizes the general therapeutic goals and interventions for MODS.

INVESTIGATIONAL THERAPIES

The National Heart, Lung, and Blood Institute of the National Institutes of Health recently reported the work of the Task Force on Research in Cardiopulmonary Dysfunction in Critical Care Medicine. This task force was designated to "assess the current state of knowledge in cardiopulmonary dysfunction in adults in the critical care environment and recommend future research approaches that would lead to improved understanding of the pathophysiology of critical illness, better management of critically ill patients, and improved health care."[85] In their report they identified areas in both basic science and clinical research that needed to be addressed. Their recommendations highlight the importance of MODS pathophysiology and management through their emphasis on tissue injury and repair, intrinsic tissue defense mechanisms, and determinants of tissue oxygenation. They specifically highlighted organ-organ interaction and MODS.[85] The impact of MODS cannot be underestimated. It is a major source of morbidity and mortality, personal pain and loss, increased expenditures, and utilization of resources. As the population ages, it will only become a greater problem. Research into the pathogenesis and management of the syndrome must continue.

Investigational therapies for MODS are extremely broad in scope. All therapy from tube feed-

---

*References 50, 52, 59, 83, 84.

GENERAL THERAPEUTIC GOALS AND INTERVENTIONS FOR MODS

Prevention and early identification of inflammatory stimuli

Obtain thorough history and physical to prevent overlooking injuries or other significant information
Use rapid resuscitation to decrease shock and ischemic time
Perform surgical débridement or drainage of necrotic tissue or abscesses
Stabilize fractures early to prevent further tissue damage and promote early ambulation
Replace lines inserted in the field within 12 to 24 hours
Secure airway to prevent aspiration and enhance oxygen delivery
Perform frequent oral care to minimize oropharyngeal contamination and risk of silent aspiration
Perform meticulous line, site, and catheter care and observation and documentation
Maintain closed systems: capped ports, fewer stopcocks, inline suctioning, manual ventilator breaths for hyperoxygenation or hyperventilation
Perform meticulous wound care
Recognize changes promptly: cultures, WBC counts, fever, and radiographic changes
Administer intravenous antibiotics based on Gram's stain, patient condition, culture reports, and patient response
Remove potential contaminants such as cut flowers or standing water
Ensure proper terminal cleaning of bedside and other reusable equipment
Ensure early, aggressive supportive therapy: nutrition, intravenous fluids, mobilization, and pulmonary toilet
Wash hands before and after patient contact

Restoration of oxygen supply and demand

Optimize cardiac output
    Pulmonary artery catheterization
    Fluid resuscitation
    Inotropic therapy
    Vasoactive therapy
    Control severe acidosis
Optimize hemoglobin level
    Maintain level at 10 to 12 g/dL
    Monitor CBC
Optimize Sao_2
    Ventilatory support
    Prevent nosocomial pneumonia
        Sterile technique with suctioning
        Frequent oral care
        Consider sucralfate for stress bleeding prophylaxis
        Monitor for aspiration of gastric contents, tube feedings, and oral secretions
Change position frequently and encourage early mobility

Nutritional support

Provide early tube feedings if possible
Provide total parenteral nutrition as necessary to meet metabolic needs

Individual organ support as indicated

Provide mechanical ventilation
Provide hemodialysis/continuous arteriovenous hemofiltration
Administer inotropic and vasoactive agents
Use therapeutic beds

CBC, Complete blood count; *WBC*, white blood count.

ings to cutting-edge immunotherapy has the potential to impact the MODS process. Numerous organ-specific therapies are discussed in Section III. Other investigational therapies such as antimediator therapies are more "syndrome-specific." These new therapies focus on the triggers and mediators of the IIR, including endotoxin, cytokines, and the cells of the IIR, rather than targeting any particular organ. Even gene therapy is now seen as a potential resource for the future.[86] Steadily making its way from the basic science laboratory to the clinical arena, immunotherapy focuses on inhibiting or controlling the IIR and minimizing mediator activity and damage.[87-95]

Antimediator therapy can be designed along two courses: (1) neutralizing the mediator in the circulation or (2) blocking interaction between the mediator and its cell-surface receptors and, thus, preventing the mediator from sending its message to a particular target.[87] Monoclonal antibodies (mAbs), along with other pharmacologic agents, have been studied in both forms of therapy.

Monoclonal antibodies

One of the major breakthroughs to move from the bench to the bedside is the clinical application of mAb techniques.[96] Monoclonal antibodies against endotoxin, endotoxin receptors, TNF, and TNF receptors have been developed. In the case of actual *mediators* such as endotoxin and TNF, the mAb should bind to the mediator and neutralize the ability of the mediator to impair host tissues. In the case of mAbs against specific *mediator receptors,* the mAb competes with the mediator at the target cell by binding the receptor and blocking it so that the mediator itself cannot bind and cause damage. Because white blood cell–endothelial cell interaction and adhesion can cause significant endothelial damage secondary to free radical and protease activity, mAbs to adhesion molecules on white blood cells are also being examined. If the adhesion molecule is bound with mAbs, the white blood cell should not be able to adhere to the endothelial wall and injure it.[97-99]

Development. Each B cell is dedicated to binding only with a specific antigenic determinant. The binding of antigen with surface immunoglobulin on a B cell stimulates that particular B cell to proliferate (clonal selection) and ultimately differentiate into antibody-producing plasma cells and memory cells. Many foreign agents are complex and contain many antigenic determinants, each capable of stimulating a different B cell clone; therefore, a heterogeneous mixture of antibodies (polyclonal antibodies) is produced as different B cells bind with different determinants (Fig. 18-4).

In 1975 Köhler and Milstein[100] developed the mAb technique that produced homogeneous, specific antibodies. Before this discovery, production of therapeutic antibodies required volunteers to be injected with an antigen. A response then occurred in which antibodies with several different specificities (idiotypes) were formed. The blood was then drawn from the volunteer, and serum containing the different antibodies was collected. Because the response was variable, reproducibility from one collection to the next was difficult to achieve. Conversely, mAbs are specific for one antigenic determinant, and therefore, their specificity and affinity are more potent, and toxic interactions are minimized.[101,102]

Clinical trials. In the past 5 years, several mAbs have gone through various stages of clinical trials. Although two antiendotoxin antibodies (known as HA-1A and E5) initially showed much promise,[103-106] several concerns were raised regarding their efficacy and therapeutic potential.[107] A subsequent study of HA-1A was terminated because of higher mortality in the study group at interim analysis;[108] however, in a recent multicenter clinical trial, Bone and the E5 Sepsis Study Group[109] once again demonstrated clinical promise for the antiendotoxin mAb E5. The E5 group did not show a significant decrease in overall mortality; however, a significantly greater percentage of patients with gram-negative sepsis experienced resolution of major organ failure after they received E5, compared with those patients who received placebo (p = .005).[109] Further study is needed to clarify the role of E5 in sepsis, SIRS, and MODS. Other antiendotoxin therapies are under investigation.[110,111]

Although sepsis from gram-negative bacteria and endotoxemia are major etiologic factors in the development of MODS, they are not the only factors. Overwhelming inflammation without a septic source is documented in 25% to 50% of cases.[1] Anti-TNF or anti-TNF receptor mAbs may be more helpful in these patients when ischemia and other conditions have triggered the systemic inflammatory response and TNF release.[112-120]

Anti-TNF mAbs are presently in clinical trial. In earlier animal studies, anti-TNF mAbs were shown to attenuate many of the signs and symptoms associated with sepsis and organ failure[112,113,121]; however, in a recent clinical trial, anti-TNF mAbs did not decrease mortality except in a small subset of patients identified retrospectively to have had high entry-level plasma TNF levels.[122] The potential for mAbs in clinical therapy is promising, but future research is necessary to define their therapeutic role.

Receptor antagonists

Receptor antagonists also block the effects of select mediators. IL-1 acting in isolation or in concert with TNF inflicts cellular and tissue injury.[11,34] By binding and blocking the IL-1 receptor on the target site, the IL-1 receptor antagonist inhibits IL-1–induced activity.[123,124] Wakabayashi and co-workers[123] documented a significant reduction in the severity of *Escherichia coli*–induced sepsis in laboratory animals given recombinant IL-1 receptor an-

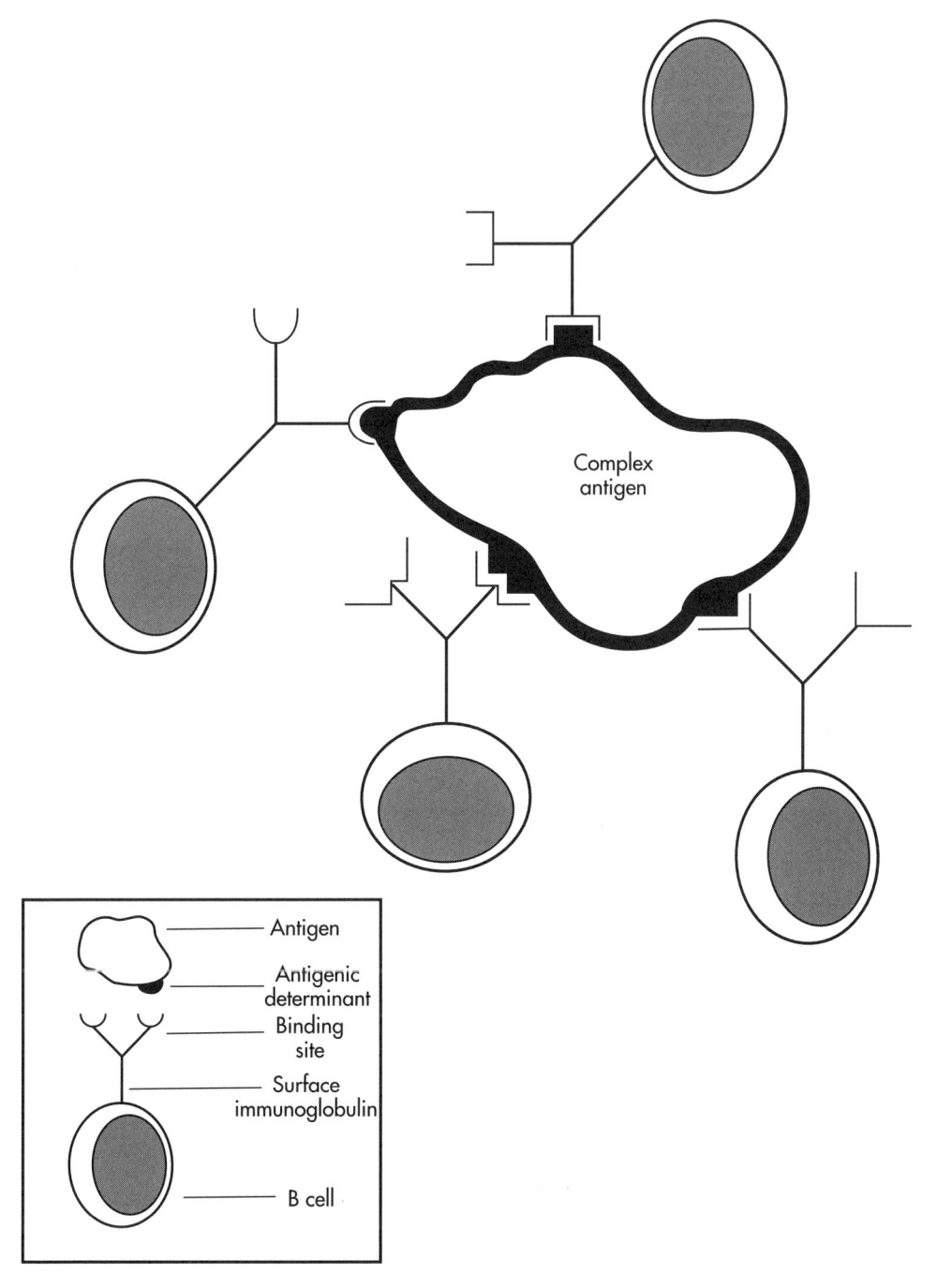

Multiple Organ Dysfunction Syndrome: Overview and Conclusions **415**

Fig. 18-4 Polyclonal stimulation and antibody production. As surface immunoglobulins on specific B cells bind with their predefined antigen, the B cell is stimulated to proliferate. Because complex antigens have numerous antigenic determinants, more than one B cell clone is activated. Several different antibody clones are produced, yielding serum with polyclonal antibodies.

tagonist. A recent prospective, randomized, double-blind clinical trial of this drug in SIRS has been completed.[125] Although the overall mortality rate was not significantly reduced in the group receiving IL-1 receptor antagonist, a retrospective analysis suggested that the drug may reduce mortality in a subset of patients with worsening disease.[125]

Antioxidant therapy

Another large area of interest and research concentrates on TOM production and damage during WBC activation and reperfusion injury.[126-130] In the body, several mechanisms generate free radicals (oxidants) after insult and injury. These include increased xanthine oxidase activity seen with reperfusion injury and histamine release; activated neutrophils undergoing respiratory burst activity; and increased arachidonic acid metabolism (see Chapters 3 and 5). The release of intracellular iron from injured cells also increases production of the more toxic oxidant, hydroxyl radical.

Free radicals incite lipid peroxidation of cell membranes and cell damage, causing local and systemic tissue inflammation and organ dysfunction. Whether lipid peroxidation incites cell and tissue damage and increased capillary permeability or the tissue damage induces increased lipid peroxidation remains controversial. Lipid peroxidation also generates arachidonic acid, leading to increased production of eicosanoids (prostaglandins, thromboxanes, and leukotrienes). Antioxidants, including free radical scavengers,[131] xanthine oxidase inhibitors, and iron-chelating agents are under investigation (see the box below).

N-acetylcysteine. N-acetylcysteine is a free radical scavenger and also boosts the natural antioxidant defenses (glutathione system) of the body.[127] Clinical improvement has occurred following administration of N-acetylcysteine in both animal models and human studies of ARDS.[128,132,133]

Ibuprofen. Ibuprofen and allopurinol both attenuate inflammatory changes seen after an insult, although the exact physiologic mechanism is not completely defined.[134-136] Proposed antiinflammatory effects of ibuprofen include cyclooxygenase inhibition leading to decreased production of prostaglandins and thromboxane; stabilization of neutrophils leading to decreased production of free radicals and other TOMs; and decreased lipid peroxidation leading to membrane stability.[134-136] Other research by Demling and LaLonde and others highlights the iron-chelating activity of ibuprofen as an important antiinflammatory mechanism. Because continued hydroxyl radical generation re-

---

FUTURE TRENDS IN THE MODULATION OF SIRS

Anticytokine therapy[11,87-94]
Anti-TNF monoclonal antibodies[112,113-119,122]
Soluble TNF receptors[120]
Anti–IL-6 therapy[154]
IL-1ra[11,124,125]
IL-10[148]
Pentoxifylline[137-142]

Antiendotoxin therapy[110,111]
Antiendotoxin monoclonal antibodies[101-109]
Peptides and lipoproteins that bind endotoxin
Lipid A derivatives

Antioxidant therapy[126-130]
Allopurinol[135,136]
Superoxide dismutase[131]
Catalase
Iron chelators[135,136]
N-acetylcysteine[132,133]
Mannitol[6]

Miscellaneous antiinflammatory therapy[88-90]
Ibuprofen[132-134]
Adhesion molecule blockade[97-99,151]
Protease inhibitors[149,153]
Complement inhibitors[144]
Arachidonic acid inhibitors[145,147]

Modulators of coagulation
Antithrombin III
Aprotinin[146]
Protein C
Heparin
Anti-clotting factor monoclonal antibodies
Nitric oxide
Hirudin

quires iron, iron-chelating agents such as ibuprofen and deferoxamine inhibit production of free radicals and may decrease cell and tissue injury caused by free radical-induced lipid peroxidation of cell membranes (Fig. 18-5).[134]

Pentoxifylline

Pentoxifylline, a methylxanthine used to decrease blood viscosity in chronic vascular disease, has shown promise in the treatment of tissue perfusion and oxygenation in sepsis and MODS.[137-140] Noel and colleagues[141] reported that pentoxifylline decreased the sequestration of neutrophils, inhibited TNF activity, and decreased severe morbidity in animals given intravenous endotoxin. Waxman and associates[142] reported improved tissue oxygenation and oxygen consumption with pentoxifylline administration after experimental hemorrhage. Improved microcirculatory blood flow and a possible decrease in neutrophil adherence to the endothelium are hypothesized mechanisms of action.

Other therapies

In addition to the therapeutic agents listed above, other investigational therapies are being developed and put through trial in either animal or human studies.[143-154] Many have antioxidant and other antiinflammatory effects. Modulators of coagulation are also being examined. A summary of investigational agents and their category of action are listed in the box on p. 416.

Summary of investigational therapies

Routine therapy has made little impact on the mortality statistics of sepsis, SIRS, and MODS over the last 20 years. As clinical investigation progresses, only a few of these investigational therapies will actually prove feasible and effective for use in the general patient population. The others will be dismissed, and new therapies will surface. Many therapies may appear inadequate only because they were implemented too late in the course of the disease. Timing may be just as crucial as the therapy itself. It is unlikely that any single therapy will halt the entire inflammatory cascade because of its intricacy and the presence of redundant pathways; therefore "cocktails" containing several antimediator agents are likely to be investigated.

Investigations are difficult to conduct in the MODS patient because of the complexity of the

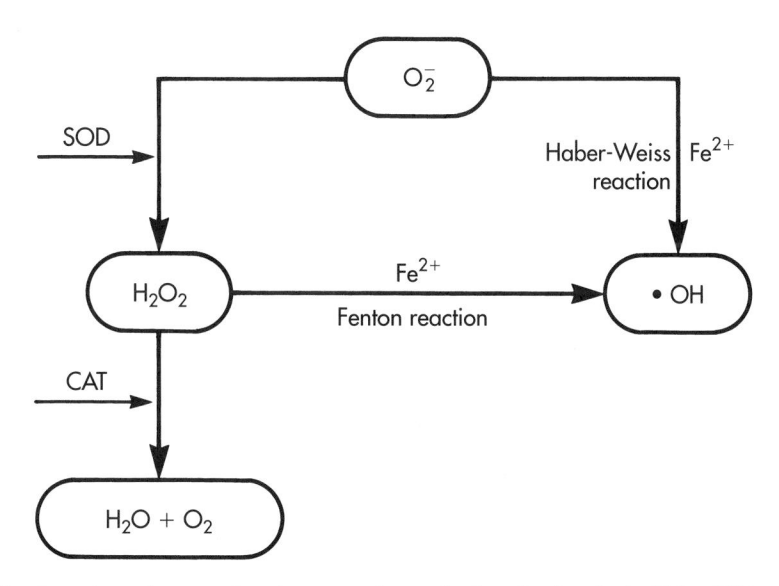

Fig. 18-5 Iron-dependent reactions in oxygen-free radical production. In the Haber-Weiss and Fenton reactions, iron is required for the production of hydroxyl radicals; therefore iron-chelating agents inhibit the reactions and thus hydroxyl radical production. Because the hydroxyl radical is more toxic than the other radicals, inhibiting its formation may attenuate free radical injury. *CAT,* Catalase; *SOD,* superoxide dismutase.

syndrome and the number of confounding variables involved.[155] The patient most likely to benefit from the therapy is difficult to define.[156] Although initial studies involving laboratory animals under controlled conditions are necessary to control confounding variables and protect the patient from unforeseen complications, caution must be taken in extrapolating all animal findings to the human response.

One major drawback in immunotherapy is the potential to actually inhibit not only the uncontrolled aspect of the IIR response but also the protective aspect.[157] Corticosteroid therapy is a perfect example: by blocking specific mediator function and activity, protective host mechanisms are impaired, predisposing the patient to overwhelming microbial invasion. Knowledge of the IIR is vital not only for understanding the pathophysiology of clinical conditions but also for ensuring safe and effective delivery of pharmacologic agents and for accurate assessment of the patient's response to therapy.

ETHICAL AND PSYCHOSOCIAL CONSIDERATIONS

With a mortality approaching 100% in some patient populations with MODS, numerous ethical dilemmas surface in the ICU. As controls over availability of resources tighten and critical care costs skyrocket, care decisions regarding limiting or withdrawing treatment are being made at an earlier time point. Costs approaching $200,000 have been quoted for a 21-day stay in the ICU. Rehabilitation costs for the survivor may approach $300,000 during the year after discharge from the unit. What role does the cost/benefit ratio play in our decisions? When is enough, enough? Or too much?[156,158] It is hoped that these decisions will continue to be made by compassionate health care professionals in conjunction with patient and family wishes and not by legislative bodies.[159] Unfortunately, many end-stage patients are comatose and cannot verbalize their desires. The weight of the decision often falls on distraught and anxious family members, who also have emotional and psychologic needs.[160] The stress on the family is great, particularly in an acute illness, where there was no warning or emotional preparation. Every attempt should be made to develop family-focused care, particularly during the acute phase when it may actually be the most difficult to do.[161]

The development of a Comprehensive Supportive Care Team for hopelessly ill patients with multiple organ failure has been reported.[162] The multidisciplinary team consisted of a clinical nurse specialist, staff physician, chaplain, social worker, respiratory therapist, and the patient's bedside nurse. The team assumed patient responsibility in accordance with patient or family wishes for those patients deemed hopelessly ill by the organ failure criteria of Knaus.[67] Patient and family preferences regarding heroic measures, physical comfort, psychosocial comfort, and family support were incorporated into decision-making. Although mortality did not decrease (100% as expected), the length of ICU stay and the number of therapeutic interventions decreased significantly. The high technologic maintenance of hopelessly ill patients presents a psychologic burden to family and staff, a financial burden to family and the health care industry, and a gross intrusion into the patient's privacy and death. Moving patients out of the ICU greatly increases patient-family interaction and enhances patient dignity and privacy.

CONCLUSION

Assessment and treatment of this complex syndrome focuses primarily on minimizing infectious or inflammatory stimuli, maintaining adequate preload and circulating volume, enhancing oxygen delivery and consumption, minimizing oxygen demand, and meeting metabolic requirements. Individual organ support and other standard critical care regimens are used to maintain the patient during this state; although, they often do not treat the underlying problem. Unfortunately, many therapies treat one problem, only to initiate a new one. Standard prophylaxis of stress bleeding with antacids and H_2-receptor antagonists protects against gastric ulceration, but may predispose the patient to overgrowth of bacteria in the stomach. Total parenteral nutrition increases the risk of infection, gut atrophy, and fatty liver. Positive end-expiratory pressure (PEEP) decreases venous return and cardiac output, affecting renal function and renin secretion. Benefits and risks of routine therapies and investigational interventions must be carefully weighed for each patient.

Attention is now being diverted from the classic cardiopulmonary etiologies to more novel sources of complications, such as the role of the gut and the wound in MODS. Are they the ultimate culprit in

MODS or, at the very least, a major contributor to continual inflammation?[56,58,59,163] Until newer therapies are readily available that can control the inflammatory process without increasing the risk of infection, efforts must be focused on prevention and early identification.

As Deitch[3] states in his text on the syndrome: "Although many facets of multiple organ failure remain shrouded in mystery, confusion, or controversy, progress is being made. Testable hypotheses on the cause and pathophysiologic features of organ failure have been generated and a consensus has been reached on multiple aspects of the care of these patients." Although the morbidity and mortality of MODS remain high, major breakthroughs in our understanding of the physiologic response to insult, resuscitative techniques, and the role of the IIR in MODS promise a brighter future for the critically ill patient at risk for the development of MODS. The future will not only test our ability to intervene aggressively but also our willingness to appropriately limit or withdraw that intervention when the condition and wishes of the patient warrant such action.

REFERENCES

1. DeCamp MM, Demling RH. Posttraumatic multisystem organ failure. JAMA 1988;260:530-534.
2. Demling RH, Lalonde C, Ikegami K. Physiologic support of the septic patient. Surg Clin North Am 1994;74:637-658.
3. Deitch EA, ed. Multiple organ failure. New York: Thieme Medical Publishers, 1990.
4. Deitch EA. Multiple organ failure. Adv Surg 1993;26:333-356.
5. Goris RJA. Shock, sepsis, and multiple organ failure: The result of whole-body inflammation. In: Schlag G, Redl H, eds. Pathophysiology of shock, sepsis, and organ failure. Berlin: Springer-Verlag, 1993:7-24.
6. Welbourn et al. Pathophysiology of ischaemia reperfusion injury: Central role of the neutrophil. Br J Surg 1991;78:651-655.
7. American College of Chest Physicians/Society of Critical Care Medicine Consensus Conference Committee. Definitions for sepsis and organ failure and guidelines for the use of innovative therapies in sepsis. Crit Care Med 1992;20:864-874.
8. Bone RC. Toward an epidemiology and natural history of SIRS (systemic inflammatory response syndrome). JAMA 1992;268:3452-3455.
9. Beal AL, Cerra FB. Multiple organ failure syndrome in the 1990s: Systemic inflammatory response and organ dysfunction. JAMA 1994;271:226-233.
10. Rangel-Frausto M et al. The natural history of the systemic inflammatory response syndrome (SIRS). JAMA 1995;273:117-123.
11. Dinarello CA, Gelfand JA, Wolff SM. Anticytokine strategies in the treatment of the systemic inflammatory response syndrome. JAMA 1993;269:1829-1835.
12. Ackerman MH. The systemic inflammatory response, sepsis, and multiple organ dysfunction: New definitions for an old problem. Crit Care Nurs Clin North Am 1994;6:243-250.
13. Anderson BO, Harken AH. Multiple organ failure: Inflammatory priming and activation sequences promote autologous tissue injury. J Trauma 1990;30:S44-S49.
14. Border JR. Hypothesis: Sepsis, multiple systems organ failure, and the macrophage [editorial]. Arch Surg 1988;123:285-286.
15. Goris RJ. Multiple organ failure: Generalized autodestructive inflammation. Arch Surg 1985;120:1109-1115.
16. Goris RJ et al. Multiple organ failure and sepsis without bacteria. Arch Surg 1986;121:897-901.
17. Goris RJ. Multiple organ failure: Whole body inflammation? Schweizer Med Wochenschr 1989;119:347-353.
18. Nuytinck HKS et al. Whole-body inflammation in trauma patients. Arch Surg 1988;123:1519-1524.
19. Pinsky MR. Multiple systems organ failure: Malignant intravascular inflammation. Crit Care Clin 1989;5:195-198.
20. Pinsky MR, Matuschak GM. Multiple systems organ failure: Failure of host defense homeostasis. Crit Care Clin 1989;5:199-220.
21. Demling R et al. Multiple organ dysfunction in the surgical patient: Pathophysiology, prevention, and treatment. Curr Probl Surg 1993;30:348-414.
22. Secor VH. The inflammatory/immune response in critical illness: Role of the systemic inflammatory response syndrome. Crit Care Nurs Clin North Am 1994;6:251-264.
23. Moore FA, Moore EE. Evolving concepts in the pathogenesis of postinjury multiple organ failure. Surg Clin North Am 1995;75:257-277.
24. Waydas C et al. Inflammatory mediators, infection, sepsis, and multiple organ failure after severe trauma. Arch Surg 1992;127:460-467.
25. Abraham E, ed. Sepsis: Cellular and physiologic mechanisms. New Horiz 1993;1:1-159.
26. Müller-Berghaus G. Pathophysiologic and biochemical events in disseminated intravascular coagulation: Dysregulation of procoagulant and anticoagulant pathways. Semin Thromb Hemost 1989;15:58-87.
27. Faist E et al. Mediators and the trauma induced cascade of immunologic defects. Prog Clin Biol Res: Second Vienna Shock Forum 1989;308:495-506.
28. Ertel W et al. Immunoprotective effect of a calcium channel blocker on macrophage antigen presentation function, major histocompatability class II antigen expression, and interleukin-1 synthesis after hemorrhage. Surgery 1990;108:154-160.
29. Ayala A et al. Differential effects of hemorrhage on Kupffer cells: Decreased antigen presentation despite increased inflammatory cytokine (IL-1, IL-6, and TNF) release. Cytokine 1992;4:66-75.
30. Chaudry IH, Ayala A. Mechanisms of increased susceptibility to infection following hemorrhage. Am J Surg 1993;165:59S-67S.
31. Waymack JP et al. Effect of blood transfusion and anesthesia on resistance to bacterial peritonitis. J Surg Res 1987;42:528-535.

32. Secor VH. Mediators of coagulation and inflammation: Relationship and clinical significance. Crit Care Nurs Clin North Am 1993;5:411-433.
33. Bone RC. The pathogenesis of sepsis. Ann Intern Med 1991;115:457-469.
34. Beutler B. Endotoxin, tumor necrosis factor, and related mediators: New approaches to shock. New Horiz 1993;1:3-12.
35. Ghosh S et al. Endotoxin-induced organ injury. Crit Care Med 1993;21(suppl):S19-S24.
36. Talbott GA et al. Leukocyte-endothelial interactions and organ injury: The role of adhesion molecules. New Horiz 1994;2:545-554.
37. Albina JE, Reichner JS. Nitric oxide in inflammation and immunity. New Horiz 1995;3:46-64.
38. Vallance P, Moncada S. Role of endogenous nitric oxide in septic shock. New Horiz 1993;1:77-86.
39. Schiffrin EL. The endothelium and control of blood vessel function in health and disease. Clind Invest Med 1994;17:602-620.
40. Morrissey JH, Drake TA. Procoagulant response of the endothelium and monocytes. In: Schlag G, Redl H, eds. Pathophysiology of shock, sepsis, and organ failure. Berlin: Springer-Verlag, 1993:564-574.
41. ten Cate H et al. Disseminated intravascular coagulation: Pathophysiology, diagnosis, and treatment. New Horiz 1993;1:312-323.
42. Parrillo JE. Pathogenetic mechanisms of septic shock. N Engl J Med 1993;328:1471-1477.
43. Bersten A, Sibbald WJ. Circulatory disturbances in multiple organ failure. Crit Care Clin 1989;5:233-254.
44. Crouser ED, Dorinsky PM. Gastrointestinal tract dysfunction in critical illness: Pathophysiology and interaction with acute lung injury in adult respiratory distress syndrome/multiple organ dysfunction syndrome. New Horiz 1994;2:476-487.
45. Cain SM, Curtis SE. Experimental models of pathologic oxygen supply dependency. Crit Care Med 1991;19:603-612.
46. Gutierrez G. Cellular energy metabolism during hypoxia. Crit Care Med 1991;19:619-626.
47. Moore FA et al. Incommensurate oxygen consumption in response to maximal oxygen availability predicts postinjury multiple organ failure. J Trauma 1992;33:58-67.
48. Buran MJ. Oxygen consumption. In: Snyder JV, Pinsky MR, eds. Oxygen transport in the critically ill. Chicago: Mosby, 1987:16-21.
49. McClave SA, Snider HL. Understanding the metabolic response to critical illness: Factors that cause patients to deviate from the expected pattern of hypermetabolism. New Horiz 1994;2:139-146.
50. Cerra FB. Hypermetabolism, organ failure, and metabolic support. Surgery 1987;101:1-14.
51. Baue AE. Nutrition and metabolism in sepsis and multisystem organ failure. Surg Clin North Am 1991;71:549-565.
52. Clevenger FW. Nutritional support in the patient with the systemic inflammatory response syndrome. Am J Surg 1993;165(suppl 2A):68S-74S.
53. Lekander BJ, Cerra FB. The syndrome of multiple organ failure. Crit Care Nurs Clin North Am 1990;2:331-342.
54. Matuschak GM. Liver-lung interactions in critical illness. New Horiz 1994;2:488-504.
55. Wang P, Hauptman JG, Chaudry IH. Hepatocellular dysfunction occurs early after hemorrhage and persists despite fluid resuscitation. J Surg Res 1990;48:466-470.
56. Baue AE. Multiple organ failure: Patient care and prevention. St. Louis: Mosby, 1990.
57. Bernard GR, Artigas A, Brigham KL. The American-European Consensus Conference on adult respiratory distress syndrome: Definitions, mechanisms, relevant outcomes and clinical trial coordination. Am J Resp Crit Care Med 1994;149:818-824.
58. Deitch EA. The role of intestinal barrier failure and bacterial translocation in the development of systemic infection and multiple organ failure. Arch Surg 1990;125:403-404.
59. Deitch EA. Gut failure: Its role in the multiple organ failure syndrome. In: Deitch E, ed. Multiple organ failure: Pathophysiology and basic concepts of therapy. New York: Thieme Medical Publishers, 1990:40-59.
60. Ryan CM et al. Increased gut permeability early after burns correlates with the extent of burn injury. Crit Care Med 1992;20:1508-1512.
61. Zhi-Yong S, Dong YL, Wang XH. Bacterial translocation and multiple system organ failure in bowel ischemia and reperfusion. J Trauma 1992;32:148-153.
62. Driks MR et al. Nosocomial pneumonia in intubated patients given sucralfate as compared with antacids or histamine type 2 blockers. N Engl J Med 1987;317:1376-1382.
63. Meijer K, van Saene HK, Hill JC. Infection control in patients undergoing mechanical ventilation: traditional approach versus a new development—selective decontamination of the digestive tract. Heart Lung 1990;19:11-20.
64. Marshall JB. Acute pancreatitis: A review with an emphasis on new developments. Arch Intern Med 1993;153:1185-1198.
65. Wardle EN. Acute renal failure and multiorgan failure. Nephrol Dial Transplant 1994;9:104-107.
66. Safar P, Bircher NG. Cardiopulmonary cerebral resuscitation. 3rd ed. London: WB Saunders, 1988:229-278.
67. Knaus WA, Wagner DP. Multiple systems organ failure: Epidemiology and prognosis. Crit Care Clin 1989;5:221-232.
68. Fry DE, ed. Multiple system organ failure. St. Louis: Mosby, 1992.
69. Giraud T et al. Iatrogenic complications in adult intensive care units: A prospective two-center study. Crit Care Med 1993;21:40-51.
70. Doebbeling BN et al. Comparative efficacy of alternative hand-washing agents in reducing nosocomial infections in intensive care units. N Engl J Med 1992;327:88-93.
71. Beam TR Jr. Anti-infective drugs in the prevention and treatment of sepsis syndrome. Crit Care Nurs Clin North Am 1994;6:275-293.
72. Nicholson DP. Review of corticosteroid treatment in sepsis and septic shock: Pro or con. Crit Care Clin 1989;5:151-155.
73. Bernard GR et al. High-dose corticosteroids in patients with the adult respiratory distress syndrome. N Engl J Med 1987;317:1565-1570.
74. Veterans Administration Systemic Sepsis Cooperative Study Group. Effect of high-dose glucocorticoid therapy on mortality in patients with clinical signs of systemic sepsis. N Engl J Med 1987;317:659-665.

75. Bone RC et al. A controlled clinical trial of high-dose methylprednisolone in the treatment of severe sepsis and septic shock. N Engl J Med 1987;317:653-658.
76. Fiddian-Green RG et al. Goals for resuscitation of shock. Crit Care Med 1993;21(suppl):S25-S31.
77. Manthous CA et al. The effect of mechanical ventilation on oxygen consumption in critically ill patients. Am J Resp Crit Care Med 1995;151:210-214.
78. Manthous CA et al. Effect of cooling on oxygen consumption in febrile critically ill patients. Am J Resp Crit Care Med 1995;151:10-14.
79. Bizek KS. Optimizing sedation in critically ill, mechanically ventilated patients. Crit Care Nurs Clin North Am 1995;7:315-325.
80. Porter LA. Procedural distress in critical care settings. Crit Care Nurs Clin North Am 1995;7:307-314.
81. Grimble RF. Nutritional antioxidants and the modulation of inflammation: Theory and practice. New Horiz 1994;2:175-185.
82. Lowry SF, Thompson WA I. Nutrient modification of inflammatory mediator production. New Horiz 1994;2:164-174.
83. Alexander JW. Immunoenhancement via enteral nutrition. Arch Surg 1993;128:1242-1245.
84. Ackerman MH, Evans NJ, Ecklund MM. Systemic inflammatory response syndrome, sepsis, and nutritional support. Crit Care Nurs Clin North Am 1994;6:321-340.
85. Lenfant C. Task force on research in cardiopulmonary dysfunction in critical care medicine. Am J Resp Crit Care Med 1995;151:243-248.
86. Brigham KL, Stecenko AA. Gene therapy in acute critical illness. New Horiz 1995;3:321-329.
87. Christman JW, Holden EP, Blackwell TS. Strategies for blocking the systemic effects of cytokines in the sepsis syndrome. Crit Care Med 1995;23:955-963.
88. Giroir BP. Mediators of septic shock: New approaches for interrupting the endogenous inflammatory cascade. Crit Care Med 1993;21:780-789.
89. Hazinski MF. Mediator-specific therapies for the systemic inflammatory response syndrome, sepsis, severe sepsis, and septic shock: Present and future approaches. Crit Care Nurs Clin North Am 1994;6:309-319.
90. St John RC, Dorinsky PM. Immunologic therapy for ARDS, septic shock, and multiple organ failure. Chest 1993;103:932-943.
91. Shapiro L, Gelfand JA. Cytokines and sepsis: Pathophysiology and therapy. New Horiz 1993;1:13-22.
92. Lowry SF. Anticytokine therapies in sepsis. New Horiz 1993;1:120-126.
93. Molloy RG, Mannick JA, Rodrick ML. Cytokines, sepsis, and immunomodulation. Br J Surg 1993;80:289-297.
94. Klein DM, Witek-Janusek L. Advances in immunotherapy of sepsis. Dimens Crit Care Nurs 1992;11:75-89.
95. Natanson C et al. Selected treatment strategies for septic shock based on proposed mechanisms of pathogenesis [NIH conference]. Ann Intern Med 1994;120:771-783.
96. Dunn DL. Monoclonal antibodies for diagnosis and treatment. Arch Surg 1993;128:1274-1280.
97. Tuomanen EI et al. Reduction of inflammation, tissue damage, and mortality in bacterial meningitis in rabbits treated with monoclonal antibodies against adhesion-promoting receptors of leukocytes. J Exp Med 1989;170:959-968.
98. Mileski WJ et al. Inhibition of CD18-dependent neutrophil adherence reduces organ injury after hemorrhagic shock in primates. Surgery 1990;108:206-212.
99. Ward PA, Mulligan MS. Strategies for in vivo blocking of adhesion molecules. Agents Actions 1993;Suppl #43:173-186.
100. Köhler G, Milstein C. Continuous cultures of fused cells secreting antibody of predefined specificity. Nature 1975;256:495-497.
101. Fisher CF et al. Initial evaluation of human monoclonal anti-lipid A antibody (HA-lA) in patients with sepsis syndrome. Crit Care Med 1990;18:1311-1315.
102. Teng NNH et al. Protection against Gram-negative bacteremia and endotoxemia with human monoclonal IgM antibodies. Proc Natl Acad Sci 1985;82:1790-1794.
103. Ziegler EJ et al. Treatment of gram-negative bacteremia and septic shock with HA-1A human monoclonal antibody against endotoxin. N Engl J Med 1991;324:429-436.
104. Greenman RL et al. A controlled clinical trial of E5 murine monoclonal IgM antibody to endotoxin in the treatment of gram-negative sepsis. The XOMA Sepsis Study Group. JAMA 1991;266:1097-1102.
105. Gorelik KJ et al. Multicenter trial of antiendotoxin antibody E5 in the treatment of gram-negative sepsis [abstract]. Crit Care Med 1990;18:S253.
106. MacIntyre NR et al. E5 antibody improves outcome from multi-organ failure in survivors of gram-negative sepsis [abstract]. Crit Care Med 1991;19(4 suppl):S14.
107. Fink MP. Adoptive immunotherapy of gram-negative sepsis: Use of monoclonal antibodies to lipopolysaccharide. Crit Care Med 1993;21(2 suppl):S32-S39.
108. Luce JM. Introduction of new technology into critical care practice: A history of HA-1A human monoclonal antibody against endotoxin. Crit Care Med 1993;21:1233-1241.
109. Bone RC et al. A second large controlled clinical study of E5, a monoclonal antibody to endotoxin: Results of a prospective, multicenter, randomized, controlled trial. Crit Care Med 1995;23:994-1006.
110. Lynn WA, Golenbock DT. Lipopolysaccharide antagonists. Immunol Today 1992;13:271-276.
111. Zanetti G, Glauser M, Baumgartner J. Anti-endotoxin antibodies and other inhibitors of endotoxin. New Horiz 1993;1:110-119.
112. Tracey KJ et al. Anticachectin/TNF monoclonal antibodies prevent shock during lethal bacteraemia. Nature 1987;330:662-665.
113. Hinshaw LB et al. Survival of primates in LD100 septic shock following therapy with antibody to tumor necrosis factor (TNF alpha). Circ Shock 1990;30:279-292.
114. Shalaby MR et al. Binding and regulation of cellular functions by monoclonal antibodies against human tumor necrosis factor receptors. J Exp Med 1990;172:1517-1520.
115. Espevik T et al. Characterization of binding and biological effects of monoclonal antibodies against a human tumor necrosis factor receptor. J Exp Med 1990;171:415-426.
116. Exley AR et al. Monoclonal antibody to TNF in severe septic shock. Lancet 1990;335:1275-1277.

117. Stellin G et al. Hypoxia stimulates release of tumor necrosis factor from human macrophages [abstract]. Crit Care Med 1991;19(4 suppl):S57.
118. Wherry JC, Pennington JE, Wenzel RP. Tumor necrosis factor and the therapeutic potential of anti-tumor necrosis factor antibodies. Crit Care Med 1993;21:S436-S440.
119. Bodmer M, Fournel MA, Hinshaw LB. Preclinical review of anti-tumor necrosis factor monoclonal antibodies. Crit Care Med 1993;21:S441-S446.
120. Mohler KM et al. Soluble tumor necrosis factor (TNF) receptors are effective therapeutic agents in lethal endotoxemia and function simultaneously as both TNF carriers and TNF antagonists. J Immunol 1993;151:1548-1561.
121. Beutler B, Milsarek IW, Cerami AC. Passive immunization against cachectin/tumor necrosis factor protects mice from lethal effect of endotoxin. Science 1985;229:869-871.
122. Fisher CJ Jr et al. Influence of an anti-tumor necrosis factor monoclonal antibody on cytokine levels in patients with sepsis. The CB0006 Sepsis Syndrome Study Group [see comments]. Crit Care Med 1993;21:318-327.
123. Wakabayashi G et al. A specific receptor antagonist for interleukin-1 prevents Escherichia coli-induced shock in rabbits. FASEB J 1991;5:338-343.
124. Ohlsson K et al. Interleukin-1 receptor antagonist reduces mortality from endotoxin shock. Nature 1990;348:550-552.
125. Fisher CJ et al. Recombinant human interleukin 1 receptor antagonist in the treatment of patients with sepsis syndrome: Results from a randomized double-blind, placebo-controlled trial. JAMA 1994;271:1836-1843.
126. Eugui EM et al. Some antioxidants inhibit, in a co-ordinate fashion, the production of tumor necrosis factor-alpha, IL-beta, and IL-6 by human peripheral blood mononuclear cells. Intl Immunol 1994;6:409-422.
127. Goode HF, Webster NR. Free radicals and antioxidants in sepsis. Crit Care Med 1993;21:1770-1776.
128. Christman BW, Bernard GR. Antilipid mediator and antioxidant therapy in adult respiratory distress syndrome. New Horiz 1993;1:623-630.
129. Schiller HJ, Reilly PM, Bulkley GB. Antioxidant therapy. Crit Care Med 1993;21(suppl):S92-S102.
130. Tanswell AK, Freeman BA. Antioxidant therapy in critical care medicine. New Horiz 1995;3:330-341.
131. Marzi I et al. Value of superoxide dismutase for prevention of multiple organ failure after multiple trauma. J Trauma 1993;35:110-120.
132. Bernard GR. N-acetylcysteine in experimental and clinical acute lung injury. Am J Med 1991;91(suppl 3C):54-59.
133. Suter PM et al. N-acetylcysteine enhances recovery from acute lung injury in man: A randomized, double-blind, placebo-controlled clinical study. Chest 1994;105:190-194.
134. Kennedy TP et al. Ibuprofen prevents oxidant lung injury and in vitro lipid peroxidation by chelating iron. J Clin Invest 1990;86:1565-1573.
135. Demling RH, LaLonde C. Identification and modification of the pulmonary and systemic inflammatory and biochemical changes caused by a skin burn. J Trauma 1990;30(suppl 12):S57-S62.
136. Demling RH, LaLonde C. Early postburn lipid peroxidation: Effect of ibuprofen and allopurinol. Surgery 1990;107:85-93.
137. Schade UF. Pentoxifylline increases survival in murine endotoxin shock and decreases formation of tumor necrosis factor. Circ Shock 1990;31:171-181.
138. Haas F et al. Pentoxifylline improves pulmonary gas exchange. Chest 1990;97:621-627.
139. Refsum SE et al. Pentoxifylline modulates cytokine responses in a sepsis model. Prog Clin Biol Res 1994;388:323-333.
140. Zhang H et al. Pentoxifylline improves the tissue oxygen extraction capabilities during endotoxic shock. Shock 1994;2:90-97.
141. Noel P et al. Pentoxifylline inhibits lipopolysaccharide-induced tumor necrosis factor and mortality. Life Science 1990;47:1023-1029.
142. Waxman K et al. Pentoxifylline in resuscitation of experimental hemorrhagic shock. Crit Care Med 1991;19:728-731.
143. Cobb JP, Cunnion RE, Danner RL. Nitric oxide as a target for therapy in septic shock [editorial]. Crit Care Med 1993;21:1261-1263.
144. Bone RC. Inhibitors of complement and neutrophils: A critical evaluation of their role in the treatement of sepsis. Crit Care Med 1992;20:891-898.
145. Bone RC. Phospholipids and their inhibitors: A critical evaluation of their role in the treatment of sepsis. Crit Care Med 1992;20:884-890.
146. Cumming AD, Nimmo GR. Hemodynamic, renal, and hormonal actions of aprotinin in an ovine model of septic shock. Crit Care Med 1992;20:1134-1139.
147. Fink MP et al. A novel leukotriene B4-receptor antagonist in endotoxin shock: A prospective, controlled trial in a porcine model. Crit Care Med 1993;21:1825-1837.
148. Howard M et al. Interleukin 10 protects mice from lethal endotoxemia. J Exp Med 1993;177:1205-1208.
149. Jochum M et al. The role of phagocyte proteinases and proteinase inhibitors in multiple organ failure. Am J Respir Crit Care Med 1994;150(6 Pt 2):S123-30.
150. Muizalaar JP et al. Improving the outcome of severe head injury with the oxygen radical scavenger polyethylene glycol-conjugated superoxide dismutase: A phase II trial. J Neurosurg 1993;78:375-382.
151. Mulligan MS et al. Protective effects of oligosaccharides in P-selectin-dependent lung injury. Nature 1993;364:149-150.
152. Sekido N et al. Prevention of lung reperfusion injury in rabbits by a monoclonal antibody against interleukin-8. Nature 1993;365:654-657.
153. Tani T et al. Treatment of septic shock with a protease inhibitor in a canine model: A prospective, randomized, controlled trial. Crit Care Med 1993;21:925-930.
154. Vanderpoll T et al. Elimination of interleukin-6 attenuates coagulation activation in experimental endotoxemia in chimpanzees. J Exp Med 1994;179:1253-1259.
155. Solomkin JS. Very large-scale, randomized, clinical trials in sepsis and septic shock [editorial]. Crit Care Med 1994;22:1-2.
156. Sibbald WJ et al. New technologies, critical care, and economic realities. Crit Care Med 1993;21:1777-1780.
157. Bromberg JS, Chavin KD, Kunkel SL. Anti-tumor necrosis factor antibodies suppress cell mediated immunity in vivo. J Immunol 1992;148:3412-3417.

158. Atkinson S et al. Identification of futility in intensive care. Lancet 1994;344(8931):1203-1206.
159. Rushton CH. Creating an ethical practice environment: A focus on advocacy. Crit Care Nurs Clin North Am 1995; 7:387-397.
160. Jillings CR. Shock: Psychosocial needs of the patient and family. Crit Care Nurs Clin North Am 1990;2:325-330.
161. Titler MG, Bombei C, Schutte DL. Developing family-focused care. Crit Care Nurs Clin North Am 1995;7:375-386.
162. Field BE, Devich LE, Carlson RW. Impact of a comprehensive supportive care team on management of hopelessly ill patients with multiple organ failure. Chest 1989;96:353-356.
163. Baxter CR. Future prospectives in trauma and burn care. J Trauma 1990;30(Suppl 12):S208-S209.

APPENDICES

A. Inflammatory Mediators
B. Abbreviations
C. Glossary

Appendix A

Inflammatory Mediators

Plasma Enzyme Cascades

Component	Function	Source	Stimulated by	Action
Complement	Activation and enhancement of IIR Induction of inflammation via anaphylatoxin (C3a, C5a) formation Mediator between tissue injury and cellular activation	Circulating pool—complex series of proteins and proteases produced by macrophages and endothelial cells of liver and gut	Classic pathway: Ag-Ab complex (IgG and IgM only) Alternate pathway: tissue trauma cell debris kinins endotoxin plasmin	Opsonization Cellular activation: Stimulate PMN chemotaxis, phagocytosis, and aggregation Stimulate PMN oxidative metabolism and release of mediators Stimulate degranulation of mast cells and basophils leading to histamine and serotonin release Direct target cell lysis Vasodilatation ↑ Microvascular permeability Activation of kinin cascade ↑ Arachidonic acid metabolism ? Induction of TF expression by PMN and MØ Smooth muscle contraction Induce MØ release of TNF/IL-1 Enhancement of Ab neutralization of virus
Coagulation	Prevention of hemorrhage and isolation of injury site	Circulating pool—complex series of proteins produced by liver, endothelium, MØ, and megakaryocytes	Intrinsic pathway: endothelial damage and collagen exposure leading to activation of Hageman factor (factor XII) Extrinsic pathway: tissue trauma and long bone fracture leading to release of tissue factor	Fibrin formation and deposition

Fibrinolysis	Promotion of clot breakdown Working in concert with other natural anticoagulants to prevent intravascular thrombosis	Circulating pool—proteins produced by liver	Activation of plasminogen to plasmin by: t-PA thrombin activated Hageman factor kallikrein lysosomal enzymes	Clot degradation
Kallikrein/kinin (bradykinin)	Enhancement of IIR activity Enhancement of fibrinolytic cascade Possible role in renal blood flow and blood pressure regulation	Circulating pool—protein precursors produced in liver	Hageman factor Tissue trauma Complement WBCs and their mediators	Potent vasodilatation ↑ Microvascular permeability PMN chemotaxis, respiratory burst, and mediator release Smooth muscle contraction Pain

Cellular Components

Component	Function	Origin or location	Stimulated/attracted by	Action

Lymphocytes	Participation in inflammatory/immune response
	Regulation of IIR
		Bone marrow/thymus
		Lymphatic tissue
		Circulating pool
			APCs with antigen + MHC
			IL-1 and IL-2
			Cancerous cells
			Foreign donor tissue
			Intracellular infections
			Virus-infected cells
				T cell:
				  Helper (CD4+ cell) activity via mediator release:
				    enhance B cell proliferation and antibody production
				    enhance MØ activity
				    enhance further T cell activity
				  Suppressor activity-regulator
				  Cytotoxic activity (CD8+ cell) against cancer cells, virus-infected cells, and intracellular infections
				B cell:
				  Antibody production
				  Memory response
				  Antigen presentation

Mast cells and basophils	Participation in inflammatory/immune response	Bone marrow
		Mast cell—body tissues, primarily those near external environment
		Basophil—circulating pool
			Direct injury
			Endotoxin
			Complement
			Bradykinin
				Induction of inflammation via mediator release:
				  histamine
				  proteases
				  eicosanoids
				  heparin
				  chemotactic factors

Monocyte/macrophage family	Participation in inflammatory/immune response
	Link between nonspecific and specific responses
	Wound microdébridement
		Bone marrow
		Circulating pool
		Lymphatic tissue
		Marginal pool
		Peripheral tissue
			Endotoxin
			Complement
			Cytokines
			Monocyte chemotactants: complement fragments
			PMN fragments
			bacterial fragments
			cytokines
			Ag-Ab complexes
			Certain viruses
				Phagocytosis
				Antigen processing and presentation
				Mediator release:
				  IL-1
				  TNF
				  proteases
				  eicosanoids
				  colony stimulating factors
				  TOMs
				  interferon
				  PAF
				  plasminogen activator
				  complement proteins
				  coagulation factors

Neutrophil	Participation in inflammatory/immune response
	Mediation of acute inflammation
		Bone marrow
		Marginal pool
		Circulating pool
			Complement
			Kinins
			Cytokines: TNF, IL-1
			PAF
			Endotoxin
			Cell debris
			Clotting factors
			Eicosanoids
			Proteases
			Fibrin fragments
			Collagen fragments
				Phagocytosis
				Mediator release:
				  TOMs
				  proteases
				  PAF
				  eicosanoids
				  interleukins
				  TF

Platelets	Coagulation
	Participation in inflammatory/immune response
		Bone marrow
		Spleen
		Circulating pool
			Vessel wall components
			Exposed collagen
			Thrombin
			Fibrin
			PAF
			Immune complexes
			Epinephrine
				Aggregation and plug formation
				Mediator release:
				  eicosanoids, particularly thromboxane
				  serotonin
				  chemotactants
				  PAF
				  histamine
				↑ PMN aggregation
				Fibrinogen binding site

Cytokines and Other Intercellular Mediators

Mediator	Function	Source	Release stimulated by	Action
Arachidonic acid metabolites (eicosanoids)	Participation in inflammatory/immune response Physiologic homeostasis	Cell membrane phospholipids (made by all cells except RBCs)	Catecholamines, tissue injury, hypoxia, ischemia, endotoxin, neurogenic and hormonal stimulation, collagen, thrombi, bradykinin, Ag-Ab complexes, TOM, TNF ↓ cell membrane disruption ↓ phospholipid availability ↙ ↘ arachidonic acid ↙ ↘ lipoxygenase cyclooxygenase pathway pathway ↓ ↓ leukotrienes prostaglandins and thromboxane	Biologic targets: Vasomotor tone Microvascular permeability Platelet aggregation Macrophage-T cell interaction Temperature regulation Cellular activation and mediator release Bronchial smooth muscle tone GI motility, secretion, blood flow
PGI$_2$ (prostacyclin)	Major vascular AA metabolite Participation in IIR and coagulation	Endothelium most active producer Platelets		Vasodilatation ↓ Platelet aggregation
Thromboxane		Macrophages		Vasoconstriction ↑ Platelet aggregation
PGE$_2$	Feedback inhibition of macrophage response	Macrophages		↓ MØ-T cell interaction Induction of T-cell suppressor activity
Leukotrienes	Participation in inflammatory/immune response	Lipoxygenase pathway of arachidonic acid metabolism		↑ Microvascular permeability Pulmonary vasoconstriction Smooth muscle contraction Activation of IIR cells PMN chemotaxis

Inflammatory Mediators **433**

Hageman factor	Activation of coagulation and kinin systems
	Link between coagulation and IIR
		Circulating pool
		Produced by the liver
			Endotoxin
			Contact with damaged tissue:
			  Collagen
			  Cartilage
			  Basement membrane
			Contact with Ag-Ab complexes
			Kallikrein
			Contact with negatively charged particles
				Conversion of prekallikrein to kallikrein
				Initiation of intrinsic coagulation cascade

Histamine	Induction of inflammation	Mast cells Basophils Platelets Gastric mucosa Skin	Binding of complement, antigen, and endotoxin to cells Direct cell trauma Neurogenic stimulation	Vasodilatation ↑ Microvascular permeability Smooth muscle contraction Gastric acid secretion
Interferon-γ (IFN-γ)	Participation in inflammatory/immune response Enhance host defense, particularly T-helper activity Antiviral effects	T cells (CD4+ and CD8+) Virus-infected cells NK cells Fibroblasts Macrophages	IL-2 Viral infections Ag recognition by TCR Microorganisms Endotoxin	Antiviral properties Induces MHC class II expression on APC ↑ T cell, B cell, MØ, and NK activity and mediator activity ↑ PMN-endothelium adhesion Fever Triggers acute phase response
Interleukin-1 (IL-1)	Participation in inflammatory/immune response Synergistic activity with TNF Psycho/neuroendocrine/immune link	Monocytes/macrophages NK cells Fibroblasts Perturbed endothelium Other APCs	Phagocytosis of foreign debris T cell cytokines or TNF acting on MØ Hemorrhage Thrombin	Links IIR with neuroendocrine system, such as fever induction Leukocytosis ↑ T cell, B cell, NK cell, MØ, PMN activity and proliferation ↑ Antibody production Stimulates production of acute-phase reactants Stimulates hematopoiesis ↑ PMN/endothelium adhesion Stimulates release of IL-2 from T cell ↑ Amino acid flux and muscle proteolysis Stimulates endothelium to express mediators and procoagulant activity ↑Fibroblast activity and wound healing

Cytokines and Other Intercellular Mediators—cont'd

Mediator	Function	Source	Release stimulated by	Action
Interleukin-2 (IL-2)	Participation in inflammatory/immune response	T cells NK cells	Interleukin-1 MØ-T cell interaction	↑ T cell proliferation and mediator release (powerful T cell growth factor) ↑ T cell receptors for IL-2 ↑ B cell proliferation Further activation of MØ and NK cell
Interleukin-6 (IL-6)	Participation in inflammatory/immune response Acute phase response Messenger in neuro-endocrine-immune axis	Macrophages and other APCs Helper T cells Cells throughout the body: brain, pituitary, adrenal glands, ovaries, testes, immune system	Injury Cytokines: TNF, IL-1	Acute phase response Lymphocyte differentiation Stimulation of CRH-HPA-cortisol release Fever
Nitric oxide (NO)	Exertion of vasoregulatory control Messenger between and within cells	Endothelial cells Brain tissue Smooth muscle Hepatic tissue Macrophages Platelets Others	Calcium Alteration in blood flow Inflammatory/immune response	Vasodilatation ↓ Platelet aggregation ↓ PMN adhesion/plugging Stimulates AA metabolism Messenger molecule in CNS, gut, kidney
Platelet activating factor (PAF)	Participation in inflammatory/immune response and coagulation	Platelets Mast cells Basophils Monocytes/macrophages PMNs Endothelium	Anything stimulating source cells Decreased coronary artery flow Hypotension Renal dysfunction	Platelet shape change leading to platelet aggregation Serotonin release PMN chemotaxis PMN activation leading to respiratory burst and degranulation ↑ Microvascular permeability Smooth muscle contraction Vasodilatation and vasoconstriction Bronchoconstriction Myocardial depression
Proteases (elastase, collagenase)	Participation in inflammatory/immune response Remodeling of tissue	PMNs Macrophages Mast cells	PMN, macrophage, and mast cell activation secondary to tissue trauma, ischemia, necrosis, microorganisms, and other foreign matter	Degradation of tissue for wound healing and remodeling Degradation of vasculature and parenchyma leading to damage and fibrosis

Serotonin	Vasoactive amine Neurotransmitter	Intestinal tissue Central nervous system Platelets	Activated platelets Neurogenic stimulation	Vasodilatation and vasoconstriction Inhibition of pain pathways
Toxic oxygen metabolites (Oxygen-derived free radicals, reactive oxygen species) (TOM)	Killing of microorganisms	PMN and MØ oxidative metabolism (respiratory burst) By-product of reperfusion AA metabolism Xanthine oxidase systems	Perfusion deficit Inflammatory cellular activity Reperfusion ↑ Fio$_2$	Endothelial damage Lipid peroxidation of cell membranes leading to loss of membrane fluidity, secretory function, and ionic gradients ↑ Microvascular permeability Altered cell receptor function Denaturation of proteins, including antiproteases
Transforming growth factor-β (TGF-β)	Down-regulation of IIR and hematopoietic function	T cells Macrophages Platelets	Inflammatory stimuli	↑ Connective tissue growth ↑ Collagen formation ↓ Hematopoiesis ↓ Immune function ? Role in angiogenesis
Tumor necrosis factor/ cachectin (TNF)	Participation in inflammatory/ immune response	Primarily macrophages T cells NK cells	Endotoxin Microorganisms Ischemic tissue Tissue debris	Induction of fever Trigger release of other cytokines Enhancement of MØ, PMN, and eosinophil function ↑ hepatocyte resistance to infection, particularly parasitic ↑ WBC-endothelium adhesion Lipoprotein lipase suppression leading to ↓ fat uptake Anorexia/wasting Stimulation of ↑ collagenase production Endothelial damage ↑ procoagulant activity of endothelium ↓ vascular responsiveness to catecholamines Fibrosis Trigger generation of adhesion molecules

AA, Arachidonic acid; *Ab*, antibody; *Ag*, antigen; *APC*, antigen-presenting cell; *APR*, acute phase response; *CRH*, corticotropin releasing hormone; *CNS*, central nervous system; *GI*, gastrointestinal; *HPA*, hypothalamic-pituitary-adrenal; *IIR*, inflammatory/immune response; *IL*, interleukin; *MHC*, major histocompatibility complex; *MØ*, macrophage; *NK*, natural killer; *NO*, nitric oxide; *PG*, prostaglandin; *PMN*, polymorphonuclear granulocyte (neutrophil); *RBC*, red blood cell; *TCR*, T cell receptor; *TF*, tissue factor; *TNF*, tumor necrosis factor; *TOM*, toxic oxygen metabolite; *t-PA*, tissue plasminogen activator; *WBC*, white blood cell.

Appendix B

Abbreviations

AA	arachidonic acid
Ab	antibody
ABG	arterial blood gas
ADH	antidiuretic hormone
Ag	antigen
APC	antigen-presenting cell
APR	acute phase response
ARDS	adult respiratory distress syndrome
ARF	acute renal failure
AT III	antithrombin III
ATN	acute tubular necrosis
ATP	adenosine triphosphate
BUN	blood urea nitrogen
C3a, C5a	complement split products
CaO_2	arterial oxygen content
CAVH	continuous arteriovenous hemofiltration
CBC	complete blood count
CBF	cerebral blood flow
CI	cardiac index
$CMRO_2$	cerebral metabolic rate of oxygen
CO	cardiac output
CO_2	carbon dioxide
CPP	cerebral perfusion pressure
CRRT	continuous renal replacement therapy
CSF	cerebrospinal fluid
CSF	colony stimulating factor
CvO_2	mixed venous oxygen content
CVP	central venous pressure
DIC	disseminated intravascular coagulation
DO_2	oxygen delivery
EAA	excitatory amino acids
EDRF	endothelial-derived relaxant factor
EDV	end-diastolic volume
EF	ejection fraction
ESV	end-systolic volume
FDP	fibrin/fibrinogen degradation product
FiO_2	fraction of inspired oxygen
GALT	gut-associated lymphoid tissue
GFR	glomerular filtration rate
GI	gastrointestinal
HLA	human leukocyte antigen
HMWK	high molecular weight kininogen
HR	heart rate
ICP	intracranial pressure
IIR	inflammatory/immune response
IL-1, IL-2	interleukin-1(-2)
ITP	idiopathic thrombocytopenic purpura
LDH	lactate dehydrogenase
LT	leukotriene
LV	left ventricle
LVAD	left ventricle assist device
LVEF	left ventricular ejection fraction
LVSWI	left ventricular stroke work index
MØ	macrophage
mAb	monoclonal antibody
MAP	mean arterial pressure
MDF	myocardial depressant factor
MDO_2	myocardial oxygen delivery
µg	microgram
MHC	major histocompatibility complex
MODS	multiple organ dysfunction syndrome
MSOF	multisystem organ failure
MVO_2	myocardial oxygen consumption
NK	natural killer
NO	nitric oxide
ODFR	oxygen-derived free radical
PA	pulmonary artery
PAD	pulmonary artery diastolic
PAF	platelet activating factor
PAP	pulmonary artery pressure
PCWP	pulmonary capillary wedge pressure
PEEP	positive end-expiratory pressure
PF-3	platelet factor-3
PG	prostaglandin
PMN	polymorphonuclear granulocyte
PVR	pulmonary vascular resistance
RES	reticuloendothelial system
RV	right ventricle

RVAD	right ventricular assist device
RVEF	right ventricular ejection fraction
RVSWI	right ventricular stroke work index
SaO_2	arterial oxygen saturation
SDD	selective decontamination of digestive tract
SNS	sympathetic nervous system
SOD	superoxide dismutase
SV	stroke volume
SvO_2	mixed venous oxygen saturation
SVR	systemic vascular resistance
SWI	stroke work index
TBI	traumatic brain injury
TF	tissue factor
TGF	transforming growth factor
TNF	tumor necrosis factor
TOM	toxic oxygen metabolites
t-PA	tissue plasminogen activator
TX	thromboxane
VO_2	oxygen consumption
V/Q	ventilation/perfusion ratio
WBC	white blood cell

Appendix C

Glossary*

agonist A substance that promotes normal biologic activity of a given system usually through binding to a receptor on the cell surface.

anaphylatoxin Active complement peptides (C3a, C5a) that cause mast cell degranulation (release of mediators such as histamine) and smooth muscle contraction.

antagonist A substance that opposes the activity of a given system.

arachidonic acid A fatty acid derived from the phospholipids of most cell membranes. Its metabolism produces three distinct groups of mediators, collectively known as eicosanoids.

autocatalytic A reaction or series of reactions whose by-products continue to stimulate (catalyze) the reaction so that a continuous cycle is established.

cascade A reaction in which the product of one step serves as the catalyst for the next step.

catabolism Phase of metabolism involved in the degradation of nutrient molecules.

chemotaxis Cells sensing and moving toward a specific biochemical agent.

cofactor A small molecular weight substance required for the action of an enzyme. Magnesium and calcium ions are important cofactors in ATP production and coagulation.

constitutive Expressed in the resting (nonactivated) state.

cytokines Immune mediators (usually peptides) involved in signalling between cells. Factors formed by one cell that induce activity in other cells. For example, TNF and IL-1.

down regulation Decrease in cell surface receptor density (number), usually resulting from an increase in the circulating concentration of the endogenous agonist for that receptor. If a cell is down regulated, it is not as responsive to the mediator that usually stimulates the receptor on the cell. Down regulation serves to limit and control the response.

effector cell Cells involved in the activity of certain biologic responses, which produce the end-effect. For example, immune effector cells carry out the functions of the immune system.

eicosanoids Group of substances derived from arachidonic acid, including the prostaglandins, thromboxane, and leukotrienes.

endogenous Originating within the organism. Endorphin is an endogenous opioid.

enzyme A protein specialized to catalyze a specific metabolic reaction.

exogenous Originating outside the organism. Morphine sulfate is an exogenous opioid.

gluconeogenesis The biosynthesis of new carbohydrate from noncarbohydrate precursors. Occurs primarily in the liver. For example, hepatic conversion of amino acids to glucose.

glycolysis The reactions involved in breaking glucose down into molecules of pyruvate.

humoral Pertaining to the extracellular fluids, including the serum and lymph.

hydrolysis Cleavage of a molecule into two or more smaller molecules by reaction with water.

immune complexes The product of an antigen-antibody (Ag-Ab) reaction that may also contain components of the complement system.

interleukins A specific class of cytokines that signals between cells of the immune system.

in vitro Occurring outside the body. Usually refers to experimental laboratory studies.

---

*List of terms and definitions modified from Lehninger AL. Principles of biochemistry. New York: Worth Publishers, 1982 and Roitt I, Brostoff J, Male D. Immunology. 3rd ed. St. Louis: Mosby, 1993.

in vivo Occurring within the body.

leukotrienes Pharmacologically active metabolites of arachidonic acid metabolism.

ligand A molecule that binds a receptor.

major histocompatibility complex Surface antigens on body cells that play an important role in recognition of self vs. nonself and in regulating cell-to-cell interaction in the immune response.

mediator Generic term for bioactive substances that exert physiologic changes in body cells and tissues. For example, proteases, TNF, and interleukins.

metabolism Set of enzyme-catalyzed reactions.

metabolite Intermediates or end-products of enzyme-catalyzed reactions. For example, the prostaglandins are metabolites of arachidonic acid metabolism.

opsonization A process that facilitates phagocytosis through the deposition of specific substances (antibody, complement split products) on the pathogen.

oxidation A process involving the breakdown of substances, often for the production of energy. In aerobic metabolism, the oxidation of glucose yields ATP.

peptides Two or more amino acids covalently joined by peptide bonds.

prostaglandins Pharmacologically active metabolites of arachidonic acid.

protease An enzyme that catalyzes the hydrolysis of proteins.

receptor antagonist An agent that binds a receptor and prevents the normal, physiologic ligand from binding. For example, the IL-1 receptor antagonist binds the IL-1 receptor, thus preventing the IL-1 from binding its own receptor.

substrate The specific compound acted upon by an enzyme. Glucose is the substrate in glycolysis.

ureagenesis Metabolic pathway occurring in the liver that involves the formation of urea from amino (nitrogen-containing) groups.

zymogen An inactive precursor of an enzyme. For example, pepsinogen is the zymogen; pepsin is the active enzyme.

Index

A

AA. *See* Arachidonic acid
Abdominal distention, 229
Abscesses, brain, 304-305
Abuse, alcohol, 240
Acetaminophen (Tylenol), 199, 200, 211
N-Acetylcysteine, 416
Acetylsalicylic acid, 211
Acidosis
  metabolic
    with acute renal failure, 285, 287*t*
    etiology of, 408, 409*t*
  respiratory, etiology of, 408, 409*t*
  severe, action of, 109*t*
Acute lung injury, 167
  criteria for, 168, 169*t*
Acute phase response, 8
Acute Physiology and Chronic Health Evaluation (APACHE), 247
Acute renal failure, 276, 301
  classification of, 280-285
  definition of, 280-285
  etiology of, 280, 280*f*
  in children, 343
  MODS and, 294
  mortality rates from, 294, 294*t*
  pathophysiologic alterations in children and, 343-344
  prevention of, 294-298
  in sepsis, 285-290
    hemodynamic factors, 285-290
    humoral and cellular mediators, 290-293
  systemic manifestations, 285, 286*t*-288*t*
  therapeutic management of, 294-298
  in children, 344-345
Acute respiratory distress syndrome. *See also* Adult respiratory distress syndrome
  critical pathway, 188, 189*t*-192*t*
    guidelines for use, 188, 193*t*
Acute tubular necrosis, 281-283
  causes of, 282, 283*t*
  clinical course of, 284-285
  initiating phase of, 285
  ischemic, 282, 284*f*
    pathogenesis of, 282, 284*f*

Page numbers followed by *t* or *f* indicate table or figure, respectively.

Acute tubular necrosis—cont'd
  laboratory values in, 281, 282*t*, 283-284
  maintenance phase of, 285
  management and prevention of
    antiendothelin strategies for, 300-301
    future trends in, 299-301
  nephrotoxic, 282-283
    pathogenesis of, 282, 284*f*
  recovery phase of, 285
Adenosine triphosphate
  generation of during cellular metabolism, 135
  replenishment, 136-137
  synthesis of, 136, 139*f*
ADH. *See* Antidiuretic hormone
Adhesion molecules, monoclonal antibodies to, 186
Adolescents. *See also* Pediatric patients
  growth and development of, 353
Adrenergic receptors, vascular effects, 128, 129*t*
Adrenocorticotropic hormone, activity in stress state, 8, 10*t*
Adult respiratory distress syndrome, 167-195
  assessment of, 178-180
  cardiovascular support, 184-185
  clinical presentation, 178-180
  critical pathway, 188, 189*t*-192*t*
    guidelines for use, 188, 193*t*
  definition of, 167, 168, 169*t*
  diagnosis of, 168-169
  etiology of, 168
  hemodynamic parameters of, 180
  infection control and management in, 185
  investigational therapies for, 185-186
    grading of recommendations, 187, 187*t*
    quality of evidence in, 187, 187*t*
    recommendations for management with, 186-187
  laboratory findings, 178
  liver failure and, 208
  lung mechanics in, 178-180
  management of
    in future health care environment, 187-188
    protocol for, 188, 189*t*-192*t*
    therapeutic, 180-185

Adult respiratory distress syndrome—cont'd
  mechanical ventilation in, 180-184
    complications, 181
    goals, 180-181
    guidelines, 180-181
    patient considerations, 181-184
  nutritional support for, 185
  pathophysiology of, 174-178
    cascade, 176, 177*f*
  pharmacologic support for, 184
    recommendations, 187, 188*t*
  postinjury score, 408, 411*t*
  radiographic findings, 178
  research, 187-188
  signs and symptoms, 178, 179*t*
  treatment recommendations, 187, 187*t*
Aerobic metabolism, 135-136
Afterload, 386
  ventricular, 259*f*, 259-260
Aging
  effects on organ structure and function, 366-375
  immunologic theory of, 364, 365*f*
  physiology of, 361-366
  theory of, 361
Agonists, 438
Airway resistance, 170-171
Airways, causes of respiratory failure, 330
Albumin, 127
  goal, 269*t*
  serum, 155*t*
Alcohol abuse, 240
Aldactone. *See* Spironolactone
Aldomet. *See* Methyldopa
Aldosterone, activity in stress state, 8, 10*t*
Alfenta. *See* Alfentanil
Alfentanil (Alfenta), 200
ALI. *See* Acute lung injury
Alkalosis
  respiratory, etiology, 408, 409*t*
  severe, 109*t*
Alveolar dead space, 180
Alveolar macrophages, in ARDS, 175
Alveolar/pulmonary capillary blood flow, effects of gravity on, 171-172, 172*f*
American-European Consensus Conference (AECC), definitions, 167
Amobarbital (Amytal), 200

441

Amrinone, 129t, 131
  for children, 336-337, 337t
Amytal. *See* Amobarbital
Anabolic steroids, 211
Analgesics, metabolized by liver, 199, 200
Anaphylactic shock, hemodynamic parameters in, 268, 268t
Anaphylatoxins, 438
Anesthesia, immune alterations in, 31, 32t, 36
Angiotensin, action, 109t
Angiotensin II, renal effects, 292-293, 293t
Antacid therapy, 231
Antagonists
  calcium, 131
  definition of, 438
  histamine, 231-232
  receptor, 414-416
Antibiotics
  and gut, 225
  metabolized by liver, 199, 200
Antibodies
  circulating, 28f, 28-29
  monoclonal, 414
    production of, 414, 415f
    to WBC adhesion molecules, 186
  polyclonal, stimulation of, 414, 415f
Anticytokines, future trends, 416
Antidiuretic hormone, activity in stress state, 8, 10t
Antiendothelins, strategies for acute tubular necrosis, 300-301
Antiendotoxins, future trends, 416
Antiepileptics, metabolized by liver, 199, 200
Antigen-presenting cells, 60, 60t
Antiinflammatory drugs
  future trends, 416
  metabolized by liver, 199, 200
Antilipid mediators, 186
Antimediators, for liver dysfunction, 211
Antioxidants, 186, 300, 416-417
  future trends, 416
Antipyretic drugs, metabolized by liver, 199, 200
Antipyrine (Auralgan), 200
Antithrombin III
  for DIC, 97
  levels in DIC, 93t, 94
Anturane. *See* Sulfinpyrazone
APACHE. *See* Acute Physiology and Chronic Health Evaluation
APCs. *See* Antigen-presenting cells
Arachidonic acid
  definition of, 438
  metabolism of, 64, 65f
Arachidonic acid metabolites, 64-65, 432t
  action, 110, 111t

Arachidonic acid metabolites—cont'd
  in ARDS, 175-176
  biologic activity of, 108, 110f
  biologic targets, 65
  impact on MODS, 64-65
  physiologic role, 64, 65f
Arcuate nucleus, physiologic anatomy of, 310-311, 311t
ARDS. *See* Adult respiratory distress syndrome
ARF. *See* Acute renal failure
Arterial access for monitoring, 267
Arterial oxygen content (CaO$_2$)
  formula and normal values, 385, 385t
  interventions to increase, 396-397
Arterial oxygen delivery index (DaO$_2$I), formula and normal values, 385, 385t
Arterial oxygen saturation (SaO$_2$), goal, 269t
Arterial pH (pHa), 388-389
  formula and normal values, 388, 388t
Arteriovenous hemodialysis, continuous, 296t-297t
Arteriovenous hemofiltration, continuous, 296t-297t
Arteriovenous oxygen difference (AVDo$_2$)
  measurement of, 316, 316t
  monitoring, 316, 317f
    limitations of, 316, 317t
    nursing responsibilities, 316, 318t
Aspiration, with enteral feeding, 157-158
Aspirin. *See* Salicylic acid
Assist control, 181, 182t-183t
Ativan. *See* Lorazepam
ATN. *See* Acute tubular necrosis
ATP. *See* Adenosine triphosphate
Atrial natriuretic peptide, 299
Auralgan. *See* Antipyrine
Autocatalytic reaction, 438
Autodigestion, 242
Autoregulation
  gastrointestinal, 217
  myocardial, loss of, 265
  renal, 277-278
AVo$_2$. *See* Arteriovenous oxygen difference
Azactam. *See* Aztreonam
Azo Gantrisin. *See* Sulfisoxazole
Aztreonam (Azactam), 200

B

B cells
  normal values, 37, 40t
  surface immunoglobulins, 28f, 28-29
Bacteremia, 5
Bacteria
  commensal, 222-223
  fecal flora, composition of, 223, 223t

Bacteria—cont'd
  ileum, effects of dietary change on, 223, 223t
  pathogenic, overgrowth of, 228
  translocation of from gut, 226, 227f-230t
Bactrim. *See* Sulfamethoxazole
Balloon pumps, intraaortic, 273
Barotrauma, 181
Base excess/base deficit, 389
  formula and normal values, 388, 388t
Basolateral amygdala, physiologic anatomy of, 310-311, 311t
Basophils, 430t
  normal values, 37, 40t
Behavior, effects of aging on, 374-375
Benadryl. *See* Diphenhydramine
Bile, production of, 201
Bile reflux, 243
Biliary tract disease, 240, 241f
Bilirubin, metabolism by liver, 201
Bleeding, gastrointestinal, 228
  therapeutic management in children, 346-347
Blood cultures, enteric organisms in, 228
Blood flow
  cerebral, 305
  coronary, 265-266
    maldistribution of, 265-266
  gastrointestinal, factors that regulate, 215-217, 217f
  intraorgan, 114, 116t
  microvascular distribution, 143
  pulmonary
    causes of respiratory failure, 330
    effects of position on, 169, 170f
  regional, 113-119, 116t
Blood pressure
  normal values for children, 336, 336t
  systolic, goal, 269t
Blood transfusions, immune alterations in, 31, 32t, 35-36
Blood volume, circulating, maldistribution of, 107-134
  definition of, 9-12, 12t
  in pediatric patients, 329
Bradykinin, 57, 429t
  activity of, 20, 21t, 109t
Brain
  microabscesses in, 304-305
  physiologic anatomy of, 310-311, 311t
  postischemic reperfusion injury, 122
Breathing, work of, 184
Brevital. *See* Methohexital
Bumetanide (Bumex), 200
Bumex. *See* Bumetanide
Butazolidin. *See* Phenylbutazone

C

Cachectin, 435t
Calan. *See* Verapamil

Index

Calcium
  antagonists, 131
  excretion of by liver, 201
  increased, action of, 109t
  metabolism of, 266
Calcium-channel blocking agents, 300
CaO₂. See Arterial oxygen content
Capillary bed, structure of, 138-139, 140f
Capillary blood flow, alveolar/pulmonary, effects of gravity on, 171-172, 172f
Capoten. See Captopril
Captopril (Capoten), 200
Carbamazepine (Tegretol), 200
Carbohydrate metabolism
  alterations in, 150-151
  by liver, 199, 201
Cardiac index (CI), 260-261, 262t
  formula and normal values, 385, 385t
  goal, 269t
Cardiac monitoring, 268
Cardiac output (CO), 260-261, 262t
  determinants of, 385-396
  formula and normal values for, 385, 385t
  increased, etiology of, 408, 409t
  interventions to increase, 394-396
  in shock states, 268, 268t
Cardiac tamponade, hemodynamic parameters in, 268, 268t
Cardiogenic shock
  hemodynamic parameters in, 268, 268t
  low-flow, in children, 334-335
Cardiopulmonary failure, TPN solutions and, 159-160
Cardiopulmonary support for critically ill elderly, therapeutic goals for, 377-379, 378f
Cardiopulmonary targets, 392-393
Cardiovascular drugs
  metabolized by liver, 199, 200
  for pediatric patients, 336-337
Cardiovascular support in ARDS, 184-185
Cardiovascular system
  age-related changes in, 371t, 371-372
  anatomic and physiologic differences in pediatric patients, 333-334
  assessment of, 37, 38t
  dysfunction
    assessment in geriatric patients, 372
    criteria for elderly, 358-361, 360t, 366, 367t, 372
    criteria for pediatric patients, 327, 328t
  in pediatric patients, 333-338
  effects of TNF on, 62, 63t
  potential IIR impact and complications, 37, 38t
  role of in MODS, 406, 407f
Catabolism, 438

Catecholamines, activity in stress state, 8, 10t
Catheters
  nasogastric suction, 230, 231f
  pulmonary artery, 268
CAVH. See Continuous arteriovenous hemofiltration
CAVHD. See Continuous arteriovenous hemodialysis
CBF. See Cerebral blood flow
Cefobid. See Cefoperazone
Cefoperazone (Cefobid), 200
Cefotaxime (Claforan), 200
Ceftriaxone (Rocephin), 200
Cell-mediated immunity, 27-28
Cellular activity, excessive, associated mediators and contributing factors of, 49, 50t
Cellular bioenergetics, 135-138
Cellular mediators
  of acute renal failure, 290-293
  of inflammatory/immune response, 20-21, 22t
Cellular metabolism
  alterations in oxygen supply-demand imbalance, 144-145
  ATP generation during, 135
Central nervous system
  anatomic and physiologic differences in pediatric patients, 338
  assessment of, 37, 38t
  in pediatric patients, 338-339
  causes of respiratory failure, 330
  communication with neuroendocrine and immune systems, 310, 310f
  cytokines found in, 311, 312t
  IIR impact and complications, 37, 38t
Central nervous system depressants, 211
Central nervous system dysfunction, 304-324
  and cerebral blood flow, 305, 305f
  clinical manifestations of, 312-314
  environmental management and, 320
  etiology of, 304-312
  fever management and, 319-320
  future directions, 321-322
  pathophysiology of, 304-312
    in pediatric patients, 338
  patient monitoring and, 315-316
  patient positioning and, 316-319
  in pediatric patients, 338-340
  pharmacologic support for pediatric patients, 340
  summary, 322
  therapeutic management of, 314-321
    in pediatric patients, 338-340
Central venous pressure, 262t
  in shock states, 268, 268t
Cephalothin (Keflin), 200
Cerebellar Purkinje cells, physiologic anatomy of, 310-311, 311t

Cerebral blood flow, 305
  measurement of, 316, 316t
Cerebral ischemia, 305
  pathogenesis of
    excitatory amino acids hypothesis, 307-309, 308f
    oxygen-derived free radical and EAA interaction hypothesis, 309, 309f
    oxygen-derived free radical hypothesis, 306-307, 307f
  primary mechanisms in, 306-309
  secondary mechanisms in, 310-312
Cerebral metabolism (CMRO₂), 305
  measurement of, 316, 316t
Cerebral resuscitation, 320-321
  guidelines for, 321t
Cerebral vasculature, 119
Chemotaxis, 25, 26f
  definition of, 438
Chest wall, causes of respiratory failure and, 330
Children. See also Pediatric patients
  school-age, growth and development of, 353
Chloramphenicol, 200
Chlordiazepoxide (Librium), 200
Chlormethiazole, 200
Chlorpromazine (Thorazine), 200, 211
CI. See Cardiac index
Cimetidine (Tagamet), 200
Circulating mediators, assessment and laboratory findings, 41
Circulating volume, maldistribution of, 107-134
  clinical presentation and assessment, 122-125
  definition of, 9-12, 12t
  future therapy for, 131-132
  investigational therapies for, 131-132
  monitoring, 125-126
  pathophysiology of, 107-112
  in pediatric patients, 329
  pharmacologic therapy, 128-131
  prevention of, 126
  processes leading to, 115f
  therapeutic management of, 125-131
Circulation
  abnormalities in acute pancreatitis, 249
  portal, 196, 198f
  splanchnic, 116t, 118-119
Claforan. See Cefotaxime
Cleocin. See Clindamycin
Clindamycin (Cleocin), 200
Clofibrate (CPIB), 200
Clotting cascade, 75-79, 76t, 77f, 428t
  activity of, 20, 21t
  excessive activation of, 84-85
  extrinsic pathway, 75, 77f, 78-79
  interactions of, 79
  intrinsic pathway, 75-78, 77f, 78f
  pathophysiologic, 402, 405t

444 *Index*

Clotting factors, 75, 76*t*
  decreased, etiology of, 408, 410*t*
  sites of synthesis of, 75, 76*t*
CMRO₂. *See* Cerebral metabolism
CNS. *See* Central nervous system
CO. *See* Cardiac output
Coagulation, 56-57, 73-103, 111
  associated mediators and contributing factors, 49, 50*t*
  component synthesis and removal by liver, 201
  disseminated intravascular, 73-103; *see also* Disseminated intravascular coagulation
  with acute pancreatitis, 249
  in children, 341-342
  disorders associated with, 342
  impact of liver dysfunction on, 208, 209*f*
  homeostasis of, role of endothelium in, 51
  impact of on MODS, 56-57
  inhibitors of, 81-82
  physiologic role of, 56
Coagulation modulators, 416
Cofactors, 438
  hemostatic replacement of, 98
Collagenase, 434*t*
Colloids, 127-128
  vs crystalloids, 128, 269-270
Colorectum, 220-221
  blood supply, 220*f*, 221
  functional anatomy, 220-221
  secretory role and mucosa, 221
Coma, modified Glasgow scale for infants, 339
Commensal bacteria, 222-223
Compensatory mechanisms, failure of, 113
Complement, function of, 53
Complement cascade, 53-56, 54*f*, 428*t*
  activity of, 20, 21*t*
  in ARDS, 176
  impact of on MODS, 55-56
  physiologic role of in SIRS, 53-55, 54*f*, 55*f*
Compliance
  lung, 170
  ventricular, 256-259, 257*f*, 258*f*
Computed tomography findings in ARDS, 178
Confusion, 313
Congenital heart disease, causes of, 334
Consciousness, decreased level of, 313-314
  etiology of, 408, 409*t*
Continuous arteriovenous hemodialysis, 296*t*-297*t*
Continuous arteriovenous hemofiltration, 296*t*-297*t*

Continuous venovenous hemodialysis, 298*t*-299*t*
Continuous venovenous hemofiltration, 296*t*-297*t*
Contraceptive steroids, 211
Contractility
  myocardial, 386
  ventricular, 260-265, 261*f*
Coronary artery disease, 266
Coronary blood flow, 265-266
  maldistribution of, 265-266
Corticosteroids, anti-inflammatory and immunosuppressive effects of, 31-33, 33*f*
Cortisol activity in stress state, 8, 10*t*
Coumadin. *See* Warfarin
CPIB. *See* Clofibrate
Critically ill children, parenteral nutrient doses in, 348, 348*t*
Critically ill elderly
  cardiopulmonary support for, 377-379, 378*f*
  external defense mechanisms in, 363-364, 364*t*
  nutritional support for, 379-380
Crystalloids, 126-127
  vs colloids, 128, 269-270
Cullen's sign, 245
Cushing's triad, 338
Cvo₂. *See* Venous oxygen content
CVP. *See* Central venous pressure
CVVH. *See* Continuous venovenous hemofiltration
CVVHD. *See* Continuous venovenous hemodialysis
Cylcooxygenase inhibitors, 211
Cytokines, 21-23, 432*t*-435*t*
  activity of, 21
  CNS, 311, 312*t*
  definition of, 21, 438
  in infection, inflammation, and ischemia, 6

D

D-dimer assay, alterations of in DIC, 93*t*, 94
Dao₂I. *See* Arterial oxygen delivery index
Darvon. *See* Propoxyphene
Dead space, alveolar, 180
Dead-space ventilation, 170
Decadron. *See* Dexamethasone
Demerol. *See* Meperidine
Demographics, 357-358
Depakene. *See* Valproic acid
Depressants, 211
Dexamethasone (Decadron), 200
Dextran, 127-128
Dialysis
  intracerebral microdialysis, 316
  peritoneal, 298*t*-299*t*
  renal, 295, 296*t*-299*t*

Diarrhea, 153-157
Diazepam (Valium), 199, 200
DIC. *See* Disseminated intravascular coagulation
Dietary change, effects of on bacteria in ileum, 223, 223*t*
Diffusion, 171
Digestive tract
  histologic organization of, 215, 216*f*
  selective decontamination of, 232
Digitoxin, 200
Digoxin (Lanoxin), 130, 200
Dilantin. *See* Phenytoin
Diphenhydramine (Benadryl), 200
Disopyramide (Norpace), 200
Disorientation, 313
Disseminated intravascular coagulation, 73-103
  with acute pancreatitis, 249
  antithrombin III for, 97
  assessment parameters for, 91-92
  in children, 341-342
  clinical presentation of, 91-92
  conditions with, 84
  diagnosis of, 92-95
  disorders associated with, 342
  endothelial damage in, 82-83
  etiology of, 82-84
  fibrinolytic inhibitors for, 97
  hemostatic cofactor replacement for, 98
  heparin therapy for, 95-96
  impact of liver dysfunction on, 208, 209*f*
  investigational agents for, 97
  laboratory data and, 92-95, 93*t*
  MODS and, 87-91
  nursing interventions and, 99
  pathology of, removal of, 95
  pathophysiologic alterations in, 84-87, 86*f*, 89*f*
  replacement therapy for, 96-97
  therapeutic management of, 95-100
Distributive shock, hemodynamic parameters in, 268, 268*t*
Diuretics, 211
  for acute renal failure, 294
  metabolized by liver, 199, 200
Do₂. *See* Oxygen delivery
Dobutamine, 129*t*, 129-130, 271-272
  for children, 336-337, 337*t*
  relative potency of, 270*t*, 270-271
Dopamine, 128-131, 129*t*, 271
  for acute renal failure, 295
  for children, 336-337, 337*t*
  relative potency of, 270*t*, 270-271
Dopaminergic receptors, vascular effects of, 128, 129*t*
Drugs. *See also* specific drugs
  dosage adjustments in liver disease, 211, 212*t*
  excretion of by liver, 201

Drugs—cont'd
 hepatotoxic, 211
 metabolized by liver, 199, 200
 related pancreatitis and, 241-242
 vasoactive
  categories of, 129t
  for children, 336-337, 337t
  to increase cardiac output, 395-396
Duodenal reflux, 243
Duodenum, blood supply of, 219, 219f
Dvo$_2$I. See Venous oxygen delivery index
Dyazide. See Triamterene/HCTZ
DynaCirc. See Isradipine

E

EAAs. See Excitatory amino acids
Ebb phase, 148
ECLS. See Extracorporeal life support
Edema, myocardial, 266
Edematous states, causes of, 343
EDV. See End-diastolic volume
EEG. See Electroencephalography
EF. See Ejection fraction
Effector cells, 438
Eicosanoids
 in ARDS, 175-176
 definition of, 438
Ejection fraction, 261-262, 372
 in septic shock, 264t, 264-265
Elastase, 434t
Elderly. See also Geriatric patients
 critically ill
  cardiopulmonary support for, therapeutic goals for, 377-379, 378f
  nutritional support for, 379-380
 immune dysfunction in, 363, 363t
 inflammatory/immune response in, 363-365
  clinical presentation of, 365-366
  laboratory data in, 369, 369t
 metabolic stress response in, 362-363
 multiple organ dysfunction syndrome in, 358
 neuroendocrine response in, 361-362
 organ failure in, criteria for, 358-361, 360t, 366, 367t
 sepsis in, clinical treatment perspective for, 377
Electroencephalography abnormalities, 314
Electrolyte balance
 effects of aging on, 373
 imbalances in acute renal failure, 285, 286t-287t
Electron transport system, 136, 139f
Encephalopathy, hepatic, therapeutic management of in children, 345-346
End-diastolic volume index
 left-ventricular, in septic shock, 264t, 264-265

End-diastolic volume index—cont'd
 right-ventricular
  formula and normal values for, 385, 385t
  in septic shock, 264t, 264-265
 in septic shock, 264t, 264-265
End-systolic volume, 263-264
Endocrine activation, 8, 9f
Endocrine system, effects of TNF on, 62, 63t
Endorphins
 action of, 109t
 activity in stress state, 8, 10t
Endoscopic ulcerations or erosions, 229
Endothelial cells, mediators produced by, 20-21, 22t
Endothelial damage
 associated mediators and contributing factors, 49, 50t
 in DIC, 82-83
 in maldistribution of circulating volume, 111-112
 in MODS, 11f, 12-13
Endothelin, 53
 renal effects of, 292-293, 293t
 role of in injury, 53
 role of in oxygen supply-demand imbalance, 144
 role of in SIRS, 53
Endothelium, 49-52
 anatomy of, 49, 51f
 factors impairing, 13, 52
 functions of, 51
  factors impairing, 52
 hemostatic control mechanisms and, 82
 impact of on MODS, 51-52
 neutrophil adhesion and, 48, 48f
 normal hemostatic mechanisms and, 74
 role of in homeostasis of coagulation, 51
 role of in SIRS, 49-51, 51f
Endothelium-derived relaxant factor, action of, 109t
Endotoxin
 -mediated factors affecting renal blood flow, 292-293, 293t
 -mediated renal injury, 290-291, 292f
 renal effects and, 292-293, 293t
 role of in SIRS, 48-49
 in sepsis, 266-267
Energy substrates
 metabolism of
  aerobic, 135-136
  anaerobic, 137-138
 normal oxidation of, 135-136
Enteral nutrition, 153-158, 232-233
 advantages of, 153
 complications of, 153-158
 decision tree for, 153, 156f
 formulas for, 158
 monitoring of, 160, 160t

Enteral nutrition—cont'd
 vs parenteral support, 153
 tube obstruction and, 157
Enteric organisms in blood cultures, 228
Environmental management in CNS dysfunction, 320
Enzymes
 definition of, 438
 plasma cascades, 20, 21t, 428t-429t
 proteolytic, 59-60
  in ARDS, 176
Eosinophils, normal values for, 37, 40t
Epinephrine, 129t, 130, 272
 action of, 109t
 activity of in stress state, 8, 10t
 for children, 336-337, 337t
 relative potency of, 270t, 270-271
 site of action of, 109t
Epithelial cells of gut barrier, 221
Erosions, endoscopic, 229
Erythromycin, 200
Erythromycin estolate, 211
ESF. See End-systolic volume
ESV. See End-systolic volume
Ethical considerations, 381, 418
Excitatory amino acids
 hypothesis for cerebral ischemia and, 307-309, 308f
 oxygen-derived free radical interactions and, 309, 309f
Exogenous surfactant, 186
Extracorporeal life support, 337-338
Extracorporeal membrane oxygenation, 186

F

Factor X, direct activation of, 83
Factor XII, intrinsic reactions and, 76, 78f
Family support, 353-354
Fat, metabolism of by liver, 201
FDPs. See Fibrin/fibrinogen degradation products
Fecal bacterial flora, composition of, 223, 223t
Feeding tube obstruction, 157
 suggestions to prevent, 157
Fenoprofen (Nalfon), 200
Fentanyl (Sufenta), 200
Fever, 312-313
 etiology of, 408, 409t
 management of, 319-320
Fibrin, formation of, 75
Fibrin/fibrinogen degradation products, 80, 81f
 alterations in DIC and, 93, 93t
 increased, etiology of, 408, 410t
Fibrinogen, levels in DIC and, 93, 93t
Fibrinolysis, 56-57, 79, 80f, 429t
 activity of, 20, 21t
 impact of on MODS, 56-57

Fibrinolysis—cont'd
  physiologic role of, 56
Fibrinolytic inhibitors, 81-82, 97
Fibrinolytic system, 79-82, 80f, 81f
  clearance of, 80-81
  hemostatic control mechanisms of, 80-82
Flagyl. See Metronidazole
Flow phase, 148
Fluid administration to increase cardiac output, 394-395
Fluid balance, effects of aging on, 373
Fluid resuscitation, 126-128
  requirements in neonates and children in shock, 336, 336t
Flumazenil (Mazicon), 200
Formulas
  disease- or organ-specific, 159-160
  enteral, 158
Frank-Starling mechanism, 269
Free radicals, oxygen-derived, 58, 435t
  action of, 110, 111t
  EAA interactions and, 309, 309f
  effects of, 122
  hypothesis for cerebral ischemia and, 306-307, 307f
  production of
    in infection, inflammation, and ischemia, 6
    iron-dependent reactions in, 416-417, 417f
    in ischemia and reperfusion injury, 204, 206f
    by xanthine oxidase pathway, 119-120, 121f
Furosemide (Lasix), 200

G

Gallstones, 240, 241f
Gas exchange, pulmonary, effects of position on, 169, 170f
Gas transport in lung, 172-173, 174f
Gastric acid, 222
Gastric mucosal pH, 230, 390
  formula and normal values for, 388, 388t
  targets and, 393-394
Gastric output, elevated, 228-229
Gastric tonometry, 230, 231f
Gastrointestinal system, 215-237
  aging and, 369-371
  anatomy of, 215-221
  assessment of, 37, 39t
  bleeding, 228
    in children, 346-347
  blood flow in, 116t, 118-119
    factors that regulate, 215-217, 217f
  effects of TNF on, 62, 63t
  etiologic role in MODS, 226-227
  external barriers and, 23, 23t

Gastrointestinal system—cont'd
  failure of
    criteria for geriatric patients, 358-361, 360t, 366, 367t
    criteria for pediatric patients, 327, 328t
  gut barrier, 221
  gut defenses, 221-223, 226-227
  gut immunity, 222
  IIR impact and complications and, 37, 39t
  ischemia/reperfusion injury
    prevention of, 233
    surgical drainage of, 231
    therapeutic management of, 231-234
  morphology, 215, 216f
  motility and, 221-222
    impairment of, 225
  natural defenses of, 23, 23t
  oxygen countercurrent exchange mechanism and, 218, 218f
  pathophysiology of, 223-227, 224f
  physiology of, 215-221
  role of in MODS, 406, 407f
  vascular physiology of, 215-218, 216f, 217f
    escape, 217
    redistribution, 217-218
Genitourinary system
  assessment and IIR impact and complications, 37, 39t
  natural defenses and external barriers of, 23, 23t
Geriatric patients
  demographics of, 357-358
  immune response to illness in, 364, 365f
  multiple organ dysfunction syndrome in, 357-383
  statistics about, 357-358
  stress response in, 361-362, 362f
Glasgow coma scale modified for infants, 339
Global oxygen debt, 388-390
Global perfusion, 265
Glomerular filtration, 276-277
Glucagon, 131
  activity of in stress state, 8, 10t
Gluconeogenesis, 438
Glutamine, 160, 233
Glycolysis, 438
Granulocytes, normal WBC values of, 37, 40t
Gravity, effects of on alveolar/pulmonary capillary blood flow, 171-172, 172f
Grey Turner's sign, 245
Grief, parental, 354
Growth factors, 299-300
Growth hormone
  activity of in stress state, 8, 10t
  therapy and, 160

Gut
  age-related changes in, 369-370, 370t
  antibiotic administration and, 225
  bacterial translocation from, 226, 227f-230f
  defenses of, 221-223, 226-227
  immunity, 222
  oxygen supply-demand imbalance in, 143-144
  responses of in MODS, 234, 234t
  as target organ, 223-226, 226f
Gut barrier, 221
Gut failure, assessment and clinical presentation of, 227-230
Gut ischemia/reperfusion, 204, 225
  mucosal, 223-225

H

Hageman factor, 56f, 56-57, 433t
  renal effects of, 292-293, 293t
Hct. See Hematocrit
Heart. See also Cardiac
  blood flow of, 114, 116t
Heart disease, causes of, 334
Heart rate, limits of in pediatric patients, 333, 333t
Hematocrit, goal, 269t
Hematologic failure
  in acute renal failure, 285, 288t
  criteria for
    in elderly, 358-361, 360t, 366, 367t
    in pediatric patients, 327, 328t
  in pediatric patients, 340-342
Hematopoietic system, effects of TNF on, 62, 63t
Hemodialysis
  continuous arteriovenous, 296t-297t
  continuous venovenous, 298t-299t
  intermittent, 296t-297t
Hemodynamics
  alterations in
    with myocardial dysfunction, 255
    in septic shock, 264t, 264-265
    in shock, 268, 268t
  calculated variables, 260, 262t
  components and regulation of, 255, 255f
  renal, 278, 279f
Hemofiltration
  continuous arteriovenous, 296t-297t
  continuous venovenous, 296t-297t
  intermittent, 296t-297t
Hemoglobin goal, 269t
Hemorrhage
  in DIC, 87, 88f
  immune alterations in, 31, 32t, 34-35, 35f
Hemostasis
  definition of, 74
  fibrinolytic control mechanisms and, 80-82

Hemostasis—cont'd
  normal mechanisms of, 74-82
  restoration of, 95-98
Hemostatic cofactor replacement, 98
Heparin therapy for DIC, 95-96
Hepatic dysfunction, 196-214
  antimediator therapy for, 211
  assessment of, 206-207
  clinical markers for, 206
  clinical presentation of, 206-207
  criteria for, 358-361, 360t
  impact of on DIC, 208, 209f
  in MODS, 406, 407f
  nutritional support for, 210
  pathophysiologic alterations in pediatric patients and, 345
  in pediatric patients, 345-347
  therapeutic management of, 208-211
    effects of aging on, 368-369
    in pediatric patients, 345-347
Hepatic encephalopathy, therapeutic management of in children, 345-346
Hepatic venous oxygen saturation, targets and, 394
Hepatocellular dysfunction, 202f, 202-203
Hepatocyte function, Kupffer cell-mediated alteration of, 204, 205f
Hepatotoxic agents, 210-211
Hetastarch, 128
Hexobarbital, 200
HFV. *See* High-frequency ventilation
Hg. *See* Hemoglobin
High-frequency ventilation, 181, 182t-183t
Hippocampus, 313, 314f
  information flow in, 313, 315f
  physiologic anatomy of, 310-311, 311t
Histamine, 433t
  action of, 109t
  antagonists, 231-232
  in ARDS, 176
  site of action of, 109t
Hormones. *See also specific hormones*
  excretion of by liver, 201
  neuroendocrine, activity of in stress state, 8, 10t
Humoral immunity, 28f, 28-29
  definition of, 438
Humoral mediators of acute renal failure, 290-293
Hydrolysis, 438
Hypercarbia, action of, 109t
Hyperemia, 113
Hyperglycemia, etiology of, 408, 410t
Hyperkalemia with acute renal failure, 286t
Hypermagnesemia with acute renal failure, 287t

Hyperphosphatemia with acute renal failure, 286t
Hypertonic saline, 127
Hyperventilation, 319
Hypnotic drugs metabolized by liver, 199, 200
Hypocalcemia with acute renal failure, 286t
Hypoglycemia
  etiology of, 408, 410t
  therapeutic management of in children, 346
Hypoperfusion of liver, 203-204
Hypotension
  definition of, 5
  etiology of, 408, 409t
  renal response to, 278, 279f
Hypothalamus
  control of neuroendocrine response by, 8, 9f
  physiologic anatomy of, 310-311, 311t
Hypothermia, etiology of, 408, 409t
Hypovolemic shock
  hemodynamic parameters in, 268, 268t
  low-flow, in children, 334
Hypoxemia, etiology of, 408, 410t
Hypoxia, action of, 109t

I

IABPs. *See* Intraaortic balloon pumps
Ibuprofen (Motrin), 200, 416-417
ICP. *See* Intracranial pressure
IHD. *See* Intermittent hemodialysis
IHF. *See* Intermittent hemofiltration
IIR. *See* Inflammatory/immune response
IL-1. *See* Interleukin-1
Ileum, bacteria in, effects of dietary change on, 223, 223t
Ileus, 153, 228
Immune complexes, 111-112
  cellular interactions and, 111-112
  definition of, 438
Immune dysfunction
  age-related changes and, 363, 363t
  risk factors for, 20
Immune response. *See also* Inflammatory/immune response
  abnormalities of, 31-36
    clinical conditions with, 31, 32t
  assessment and laboratory findings and, 41
Immune system
  assessment and laboratory findings of, 37-41
  communication with CNS and neuroendocrine systems, 310, 310f
  failure of, criteria for in elderly, 366, 367t
Immunity
  cell-mediated, 27-28
  gut, 222

Immunity—cont'd
  humoral, 28f, 28-29
  definition of, 438
Immunoglobulins
  circulating, 28f, 28-29
  surface, 28f, 28-29
Immunologic theory of aging, 364, 365f
Immunosuppression, 31
  corticosteroid effects and, 31-33, 33f
  after hemorrhage, 34-35, 35f
Immunotherapy, 233
Inderal. *See* Propranolol
Indocin. *See* Indomethacin
Indomethacin (Indocin), 200, 211
Infants. *See also* Pediatric patients
  growth and development of, 352
  modified Glasgow coma scale for, 339
Infection
  with acute renal failure, 285, 288t
  control and management of
    in ARDS, 185
    in geriatric patients, 377
    in pediatric patients, 349
  definition of, 5
  effects of aging on, 369-371
  vs inflammation, 6-7
  mediators produced in, 6
  in pediatric patients, 348-349
  SIRS and, 46-47, 47f
  source identification, 377
Inflammation
  vs infection, 6-7
  malignant intravascular, 6-7
  mechanisms of, 23-26, 24f
  in SIRS, 47-48, 48f
  pathophysiologic cascade and, 402, 405t
  prevention and early identification of stimuli and, 413
  release of vasoactive mediators with, 108-111
  systemic, role of gut in, 225-226, 226f
Inflammatory/immune response, 9-12, 11f, 19-45
  assessment of, 36-41
  blunted, in elderly, 365-366
  cellular mediators and, 20-21, 22t
  in children, 329
  circulating mediators and, 41
  clinical presentation of, 365-366
  components of, 20-23
  in elderly, 363-365, 365f
  external barriers and, 23, 23t
  external defense mechanisms in critically ill elderly patients, 363-364, 364t
  immunologic responsiveness, assessment and laboratory findings, 41
  laboratory findings and, 36-41
  levels of host defense in, 23-31
  natural defenses and, 23, 23t

448 *Index*

Inflammatory/immune response—cont'd
  natural defenses and—cont'd
    assessment of, 37, 38*t*-39*t*
    nonspecific, 23-26
    specific, 26-31
    summary, 31
    systems assessment and, 37, 38*t*-39*t*
  triggers of, 4
Inflammatory mediators, 6, 427-435
  cellular components of, 430*t*-431*t*
  in cerebral ischemia, 310-312
  role of in MODS, 46-72
INH. *See* Isoniazid
Injury. *See also* Ischemia/reperfusion injury
  acute lung, 167
    criteria for, 168, 169*t*
    release of vasoactive mediators with, 108-111
    role of endothelin in, 53
    role of NO in, 52-53
Inotropic therapy, 270-272
  agents to increase cardiac output and, 395
  combined with vasodilator therapy, 273
  goal of, 270-271
Insult, response to, 361-365
Integument, natural defenses and external barriers of, 23, 23*t*
Interferon-γ, 433*t*
  cellular source and CNS effects of, 311, 312*t*
Interleukin-1, 62-63, 433*t*
  action of, 110, 111*t*
  in ARDS, 175
  cellular source and CNS effects of, 311, 312*t*
  impact of on MODS, 63
  physiologic role of, 62-63
  role of in SIRS, 48-49
Interleukin-2, 434*t*
  cellular source and CNS effects of, 311, 312*t*
Interleukin-6, 64, 434*t*
  cellular source and CNS effects of, 311, 312*t*
  impact of on MODS, 64
  physiologic role of, 64
Interleukins, 438
Intermittent hemodialysis, 296*t*-297*t*
Intermittent hemofiltration, 296*t*-297*t*
Intermittent mandatory ventilation, synchronized, 181, 182*t*-183*t*
Intestinal villus
  impaired, 226, 230*f*
  normal, 226, 228*f*, 229*f*
Intestines. *See* Gut; Large intestine; Small intestine
Intraaortic balloon pumps, 273, 337
Intracerebral microdialysis, 316

Intracranial pressure, control of in pediatric patients, 339-340
Intraluminal oxygenation, 233-234
Intrapulmonary shunts, 172, 180
Intrarenal disease, causes of in children, 343
Intravascular inflammation, malignant, 6-7
Inverse ratio ventilation, 181, 182*t*-183*t*
Investigational therapies, 412-418
  for ARDS, 185-186
    recommendations for management with, 186-187, 187*t*
  for DIC, 97
  to increase arterial oxygen content, 397
  for maldistribution of circulating volume, 131-132
  for metabolic support, 160
  summary of, 417-418
Iron
  dependent reaction of in oxygen-free radical production, 416-417, 417*f*
  liver storage of, 201
IRV. *See* Inverse ratio ventilation
Ischemia/reperfusion injury, 11*f*, 13, 14*f*
  cerebral, 305
    pathogenesis of, 306-309, 310-312
  free radical formation in, 204, 206*f*
  gastrointestinal, prevention of, 233
  of gut, 225
  in liver, 204
  mediators produced in, 6
  mucosal, 223-225
  myocardial, in childhood, 334
  in oxygen supply-demand imbalance, 144
  postischemic, 119-122
  renal, 290, 291*f*, 343
  splanchnic, causes and effects of, 223, 224*f*
  toxic oxygen metabolite formation in, 13, 14*f*
Ischemic acute tubular necrosis, 282, 284*f*
  causes of, 282, 283*t*
  pathogenesis of, 282, 284*f*
Ischemic heart disease, neonatal, 334
Ischemic neurologic deficit, reversible, 306
Ischemic penumbra, 305
Ischemic threshold, 305*f*, 305-306
Isoniazid (INH), 200
Isoproterenol, 129*t*, 130
  for children, 336-337, 337*t*
  relative potency of, 270*t*, 270-271
Isradipine (DynaCirc), 200

K

Kallikrein/kinin cascade, 429*t*
  activity of, 20, 21*t*
  impact of on MODS, 57

Kallikrein/kinin cascade—cont'd
  physiologic role of, 57
Keflin. *See* Cephalothin
Ketoconazole, 186
Kidney, 276-303. *See also under* Renal
  elimination of metabolic waste products of, 279
  physiology of, 276-280
  response of to hypotension, 278, 279*f*
Krebs cycle, 136, 137*f*
Kupffer cells, activity of, 204, 205*f*

L

Labetalol (Trandate or Normodyne), 200
Lactate
  formula and normal values of, 388, 388*t*
  increased, etiology of, 408, 409*t*
  serum, 389-390
Lanoxin. *See* Digoxin
Large intestine
  blood supply of, 220, 220*f*
  histologic organization of, 215, 216*f*
Lasix. *See* Furosemide
Left-ventricular ejection fraction, 264*t*, 264-265
Left-ventricular end-diastolic volume index, 264*t*, 264-265
Left-ventricular end-systolic volume, 264
Left-ventricular stroke work index, 262*t*
  formula and normal values of, 385, 385*t*
Leukocytosis, etiology of, 408, 409*t*
Leukopenia, etiology of, 408, 409*t*
Leukotrienes, 432*t*, 439
Levarterenol, relative potency of, 270*t*, 270-271
Level of consciousness, decreased, 313-314
  etiology of, 408, 409*t*
Librium. *See* Chlordiazepoxide
Lidocaine, 200
Ligands, 439
Lipids
  abnormalities of, and pancreatitis, 240-241
  mediators produced in infection, inflammation, and ischemia, 6
  metabolism of, 151
    by liver, 199
Liver. *See also* Hepatic
  aging, 368-369
  anatomy of, 196-199, 197*f*, 200
    in pediatric patients, 345
  bile production by, 201
  blood supply of, 196, 197*f*
  cell types in, 196-199
  drugs metabolized by, 199, 200
  function of, 197-199, 201-203
    drugs that compromise, 211
    metabolic, 199, 201

Liver—cont'd
  function of—cont'd
    secretory/excretory, 201
    vascular/immune, 197-199, 201
  hypermetabolism of, 201-203
  physiology of, 197-199
    in pediatric patients, 345
  postischemic reperfusion injury and, 122
  as storage reservoir, 201
  tissue perfusion and, 208-210
Liver damage
  contributing factors to, 204-205
  drugs capable of causing, 211
  mechanisms of, 203-205
Liver disease
  in children, 342
  drug dosage adjustments for, 211, 212t
  drugs that should be used with caution in, 211
  drugs that worsen, 211
Liver failure, 211
  complications of in children, 347
  criteria for
    in elderly, 366, 367t
    in pediatric patients, 327, 328t
  developmental stages of, 345t, 345-346
  impact of on ARDS, 208
  impact of on MODS, 207-208
  TPN solutions and, 159
Liver function studies in children, 346
Lopressor. *See* Metoprolol
Lorazepam (Ativan), 200
Lorcainide, 200
Low-flow shock in children
  cardiogenic, 334-335
  hypovolemic, 334
Luminal. *See* Phenobarbital
Lung. *See also* Pulmonary
  blood flow of, 116t, 116-118
  diffusion and, 171
  gas transport in, 172-173, 174f
  physiology of, 169
  surface tension of, 170
Lung compliance, 170
Lung injury, acute, 167
  criteria for, 168, 169t
Lung mechanics, 170-171
  alterations of in ARDS, 178-180
Lung perfusion, 171
LVEDVI. *See* Left-ventricular end-diastolic volume index
LVEF. *See* Left-ventricular ejection fraction
LVESV. *See* Left-ventricular end-systolic volume
LVSWI. *See* Left-ventricular stroke work index
Lymphocytes, 430t
  assessment and laboratory findings of, 37-41

Lymphocytes—cont'd
  mediators produced by, 20-21, 22t
  normal values for, 37, 40t
Lymphoid tissue, 26-31
  assessment of, 41
  primary, 29
  secondary, 29-31

M

Macrophages, 60-61, 430t
  alveolar, in ARDS, 175
  impact of on MODS, 61
  mediators produced by, 20-21, 22t, 60, 108, 111t
  physiologic role of, 60-61
  T cell interactions requiring MHC Class II surface antigens and, 29, 30f
  tissue and, 60, 60t
Magnesium, increased, action of, 109t
Maintenance fluids, pediatric requirements for, 336, 336t
Major histocompatibility complex
  Class II surface antigens, macrophage/T cell interaction requiring, 29, 30f
  definition of, 439
Maldistribution of circulating volume, 107-134
  assessment of, 122-125
  clinical presentation of, 122-125
  definition of, 9-12, 12t
  future therapy for, 131-132
  investigational therapies for, 131-132
  monitoring of, 125-126
  pathophysiology of, 107-112
  in pediatric patients, 329
  pharmacologic therapy for, 128-131
  prevention of, 126
  processes leading to, 115f
  therapeutic management of, 125-131
Maldistributive shock in children, 335
Malignant intravascular inflammation, 6-7
Malnutrition, immune alterations in, 31, 32t, 36
MAP. *See* Mean arterial pressure
Mast cells, 67, 430t
  impact of on MODS, 67
  mediators produced by, 20-21, 22t
  physiologic role of, 67
Mathematical coupling of Do_2 and Vo_2, 393
Mazicon. *See* Flumazenil
MDF. *See* Myocardial depressant factor
Mean arterial pressure, 262t
  goal for, 269t
  in shock states, 268, 268t
Mechanical support for myocardial dysfunction, 273
  in children, 337-338

Mechanical ventilation
  in ARDS, 180-184
  complications of, 181
  goals for, 180-181
  guidelines for, 180-181
  to increase arterial oxygen content, 396-397
  patient considerations for, 181-184
  patient repositioning for, 184
Mediators. *See also specific mediators*
  antilipid, 186
  cellular
    of acute renal failure, 290-293
    of inflammatory/immune response, 20-21, 22t
  circulating, assessment and laboratory findings of, 41
  definition of, 439
  humoral, of acute renal failure, 290-293
  inflammatory, 6, 427-435
    cellular components of, 430t-431t
    in cerebral ischemia, 310-312
    role of in MODS, 46-72
  intercellular, 21-23
  monoclonal antibodies to, 414
  pathophysiologic derangements associated with, 49, 50f
  receptors, monoclonal antibodies to, 414
  release of, 1-103
    by endothelial cells, 20-21, 22t
    in infection, inflammation, and ischemia, 6
    in ischemia/reperfusion injury, 6
    by macrophages, 60, 108, 111t
    by neutrophils, 58, 108, 111t
    in sepsis, 266-267
  vasoactive, 108, 109t
    release of, 108-111
Meperidine (Demerol), 200, 211
Metabolic acidosis
  with acute renal failure, 285, 287t
  etiology of, 408, 409t
Metabolic requirements, assessment of, 152-160
Metabolic response
  in elderly, 362-363
  pathophysiology of, 148-152, 150f
Metabolic support, 152-160
  benefits of, 152
  enteral route of, 153-158
  investigational therapies for, 160
  methods of, 153
  monitoring of, 160
  parenteral route for, 158-160
    vs enteral, 153
  principles of, 152
Metabolic waste products, elimination of, 279
Metabolism
  alterations in, 148-163

450 *Index*

Metabolism—cont'd
  in acute pancreatitis, 249
  consequences of, 152
  definition of, 9-12, 12*t*
  investigational therapies for, 160
  in pediatric patients, 329
  arachidonic acid, 64, 65*f*
  bilirubin, 201
  calcium, 266
  carbohydrate
    alterations in, 150-151
    in liver, 199, 201
  cellular
    alterations in, 144-145
    ATP generation during, 135
  cerebral, 305
    measurement of, 316, 316*t*
  definition of, 439
  energy substrate
    aerobic, 135-136
    anaerobic, 137-138
  failure of, criteria for elderly, 366, 367*t*
  fat, in liver, 201
  lipid
    alterations in, 151
    in liver, 199
  neuroendocrine effects on, 148, 149*f*
  protein
    alterations in, 151-152
    in liver, 199, 201
Methadone, 200
Methohexital (Brevital), 200
Methotrexate, 211
Methyldopa (Aldomet), 200, 211
Metoprolol (Lopressor), 200
Metronidazole (Flagyl), 200
MgCL$_2$-ATP, 300
MHC. *See* Major histocompatibility complex
Microabscesses, brain, 304-305
Microcirculation, capillary bed structure of, 138-139, 140*f*
Microdialysis, intracerebral, 316
Microdialysis probe, 316, 318*f*
Microorganisms, opsonization and phagocytosis of, 25, 27*f*, 53, 55*f*
Microvascular blood flow, distribution of, 143
Microvascular permeability, associated mediators of and contributing factors to, 49, 50*t*
Microvascular thrombi, associated mediators of and contributing factors to, 49, 50*t*
Midazolam (Versed), 200
Minipress. *See* Prazosin
Mitochondria, morphology of, 135-136, 138*f*
MODS. *See* Multiple organ dysfunction syndrome
MOF. *See* Multiple organ failure

Monitoring
  arterial access for, 267
  AVDo$_2$, 316, 317*f*
    limitations of, 316, 317*t*
    nursing responsibilities for, 316, 318*t*
  cardiac, 268
  in CNS dysfunction, 315-316
  in maldistribution of circulating volume, 125-126
  oxygen consumption and, 398
  oxygen delivery and, 398
  with parenteral nutrition, 160, 160*t*
  in septic shock, 267-268
  venous access for, 268
Monoclonal antibodies, 414
  clinical trials and, 414
  development of, 414
  production of, 414, 415*f*
  to WBC adhesion molecules, 186
Monocytes, 430*t*
  normal values for, 37, 40*t*
Mononuclear cells, normal values for, 37, 40*t*
Mononuclear phagocytic system, 60-61
  impact of on MODS, 61
  physiologic role of, 60-61
Morphine, 200, 211
Motrin. *See* Ibuprofen
Mucosal pH, gastric, 230, 390
  formula and normal values for, 388, 388*t*
  targets and, 393-394
Multiple organ dysfunction, 4
Multiple organ failure, 4
  postinjury score, 408, 411*t*
Muscles of ventilation, 169
Myocardial contractility, 386
Myocardial depressant factor, 266
Myocardial depression, 181
  associated mediators and contributing factors to, 49, 50*t*
Myocardial dysfunction, 252-275
  assessment of
    in geriatric patients, 372
    in pediatric patients, 335-336
  clinical presentation of, 253-265
  criteria for
    in elderly, 358-361, 360*t*, 366, 367*t*
    in pediatric patients, 327, 328*t*
  etiology of, 265-267
  historical perspective on, 252-253
  overview of, 253-255
  pathophysiology of, 253-265
  in pediatric patients, 334-335
  in pediatric patients, 333-338
  pharmacologic support for
    in pediatric patients, 336-337
  vasodilators and, 272-273
  therapeutic management of, 268-273
  in pediatric patients, 335-338
Myocardial edema, 266

Myocardial ischemia in childhood, 334
Myocardium
  blood flow in, 114-116, 116*t*
  postischemic reperfusion injury and, 120-122
Mysoline. *See* Primidone

N

Nafcil. *See* Nafcillin
Nafcillin (Nafcil), 200
Nalfon. *See* Fenoprofen
Naloxone, 131
Naprosyn. *See* Naproxen
Naproxen (Naprosyn), 200
Nasogastric suction catheter, 230, 231*f*
Natural killer cells, normal values for, 37, 40*t*
Nembutal. *See* Pentobarbital
Neonates. *See also* Pediatric patients
  causes of ischemic heart disease in, 334
  fluid resuscitation requirements in, 336, 336*t*
Nephron, 276, 277*f*
Nephrotoxic acute tubular necrosis, 282-283
  causes of, 282, 283*t*
  pathogenesis of, 282, 284*f*
Nephrotoxins
  in children, 343
  sepsis and, 293-294
Nervous system
  central
    assessment of, 37, 38*t*, 338-339
    dysfunction of, 304-324, 338
    effects of TNF on, 62, 63*t*
  peripheral, causes of respiratory failure and, 330
  sympathetic
    activation of, 8-10
    responsiveness and, 266
Neuroendocrine hormones, activity of in stress state, 8, 10*t*
Neuroendocrine response
  in elderly, 361-362
  hypothalamic control of, 8, 9*f*
Neuroendocrine system
  activation of, 8-9, 11*f*, 112
  communication of with CNS and immune systems, 310, 310*f*
  effects of on metabolism, 148, 149*f*
Neurogenic shock, hemodynamic parameters in, 268, 268*t*
Neurologic failure, criteria for
  in elderly, 358-361, 360*t*, 366, 367*t*
  in pediatric patients, 327, 328*t*
Neurologic system
  aging and, 374-375
  role in MODS in, 407*f*, 408
Neutrophils, 57-58, 431*t*
  in ARDS, 175
  assessment of, 37

Neutrophils—cont'd
  endothelial adhesion and, 48, 48f
  impact of on MODS, 58
  margination and transmigration of, 24-25, 25f
  maturational diagrams of, 37, 40f
  mediators produced by, 20-21, 22t, 58, 108, 111t
  normal values for, 37, 40t
  physiologic role of, 57-58
Nifedipine (Procardia), 200
Nitrazepam, 200
Nitric oxide, 52-53, 434t
  inhaled, 186
  renal effects of, 292-293, 293t
  role of in injury, 52-53
  role of in oxygen supply-demand imbalance, 144
  role of in SIRS, 52-53
Nitroglycerin for children, 336-337, 337t
Nitroprusside, 129t, 131, 273
  for children, 336-337, 337t
NK cells. See Natural killer cells
NO. See Nitric oxide
No-reflow phenomenon, 321
Norepinephrine, 129t, 130, 272
  action of, 109t
  activity of in stress state, 8, 10t
  for children, 336-337, 337t
  relative potency of, 270t, 270-271
  renal effects of, 292-293, 293t
  site of action of, 109t
Normodyne. See Labetalol
Norpace. See Disopyramide
Nursing
  interventions for DIC, 99
  responsibilities in AVDo$_2$ monitoring, 316, 318t
Nutrition
  effects of aging on, 369-371
  enteral, 153-158, 232-233
    monitoring of, 160, 160t
  parenteral, 158-160
    doses of in critically ill children, 348, 348t
    monitoring of, 160, 160t
  total parenteral, 158
    complications of, 159
    disease- or organ-specific formulas for, 159-160
Nutritional assessment
  comprehensive, 154
  for pediatric patients, 347
Nutritional support
  for acute renal failure, 295-298
  for ARDS, 185
  for critically ill elderly, 379-380
  goals of, 412, 413
  interventions and, 413
  for liver dysfunction, 210
  for pediatric patients, 347-348

Nutritional support—cont'd
  for pediatric patients—cont'd
    age-related factors and, 347
    daily needs and, 347, 348t
    therapeutic management of, 347-348
  provision of, 412

O

Obstructive shock, hemodynamic parameters in, 268, 268t
OER. See Oxygen extraction ratio
Opsonization
  definition of, 439
  of microorganisms, 25, 27f, 53, 55f
Organ dysfunction and failure. See also Multiple organ dysfunction; *specific organs*
  clinical presentation and assessment of, 122-125
  criteria for in elderly, 358-361, 360t, 366, 367t
  effects of degenerative process on, 358, 359f
Organ interactions, 7
Organ support, individual, 412
  in geriatric patients, 380-381
  goals and interventions of, 413
Organ viability, maintenance of, 98-100
Orinase. See Tolbutamide
Oxazepam (Serax), 200
Oxidation, 439
  of energy substrates, 135-136
  xanthine, 119-120, 121f
Oxygen, reactive species, 435t
Oxygen consumption (Vo$_2$), 140-141, 387-388
  delivery-dependent, 390, 391f
  delivery-independent, 390, 391f
  evaluation of, 384-401
  formula and normal values for, 388t, 388-389
  goal of, 269t
  indications of for monitoring, 398
  management of, 384-401
    targets related to, 392-394
  mathematical coupling and, 393
  practical considerations in, 397-398
  supply-dependent, 140-141, 141f
  therapeutic interventions for, 394-397
Oxygen consumption index (Vo$_2$I), formula and normal values for, 388, 388t
Oxygen content
  arterial, interventions to increase, 396-397
  determinants of, 386
Oxygen countercurrent exchange, mechanism of, 218, 218f
Oxygen debt, 141, 142f
  clinical evaluation of, 388-390
  global and regional, 388-390

Oxygen debt—cont'd
  pathophysiology of, 388, 389f
  repayment of, 141, 142f
  tissue and, 141
Oxygen delivery (Do$_2$), 138-140
  clinical evaluation of, 385-390
  evaluation and management of, 384-401
  goal of, 269t
  indications of for monitoring, 398
  management targets related to, 392-394
  mathematical coupling and, 393
  oxygen consumption and, 390, 391f
  practical considerations in, 397-398
  therapeutic interventions for, 394-397
  variables in, 385, 385t
Oxygen demand
  conditions that increase, 142
  decrease of, 412
Oxygen-derived free radicals, 58, 435t
  action of, 110, 111t
  EAA interactions of, 309, 309f
  effects of, 122
  hypothesis for cerebral ischemia, 306-307, 307f
  production of
    in infection, inflammation, and ischemia, 6
    iron-dependent reactions in, 416-417, 417f
    in ischemia and reperfusion injury, 204, 206f
    by xanthine oxidase pathway, 119-120, 121f
Oxygen extraction, 138-140
Oxygen extraction ratio (OER), formula and normal values for, 388, 388t
Oxygen metabolites, toxic, 58-59, 435t
  formation of in ischemia/reperfusion injury, 13, 14f
  production of in infection, inflammation, and ischemia, 6
Oxygen saturation
  arterial, goal of, 269t
  effects on oxyhemoglobin dissociation curve and, 386, 387f
  venous
    decreased, 408, 410t
    formula and normal values for, 388, 388t
    hepatic, targets and, 394
    increased, 408, 410t
Oxygen supply and demand balance
  in geriatric patients, 377-379
  relationships, 141-142
  restoration of, 411-412
  goals and interventions of, 413
Oxygen supply and demand imbalance, 135-147
  cellular metabolism alterations in, 144-145

452 *Index*

Oxygen supply and demand imbalance—cont'd
  definition of, 9-12, 12*t*
  gut example and, 143-144
  ischemia/reperfusion injury in, 144
  pathophysiology of, 142-145
  in pediatric patients, 329
  roles of nitric oxide and endothelin in, 144
Oxygen toxicity, 181
Oxygen transport, 138-141
Oxygen utilization, 138-141
  variables for, 388, 388*t*
Oxygenation
  effects of aging on, 366-368
  extracorporeal membrane and, 186
  intraluminal, 233-234
Oxyhemoglobin dissociation curve, 173, 174*f*, 386, 387*f*

P

PAF. *See* Platelet-activating factor
Pain management
  age-related factors in, 349-350
  in pediatric patients, 349-352
    assessment of, 350
    effects of growth and development on, 350, 351*f*
    therapeutic management of, 350-352
Pancreas
  aging and, 371
  anatomy of, 238-240, 239*f*
  endocrine function of, 238-240, 240*t*
    effects of aging on, 371
  exocrine function of, 240, 240*t*
    effects of aging on, 371
  physiology of, 238-240, 239*f*
  role of in MODS, 406, 407*f*
  secretions of, 240, 240*t*
  suppression of, 249-250
Pancreatic duct obstruction, 243
Pancreatitis
  acute, 238-251
    assessment of, 243-248
    causes of, 242
    clinical presentation of, 243-248
    complications of, 248
    diagnosis of, 247-248
    etiology of, 240-242
    idiopathic and drug-related causes of, 241-242
    laboratory findings in, 245-246
    metabolic complications of, 249
    modified Glasgow criteria for, 247
    multisystem involvement in, 248-249
    pathogenesis hypotheses, 242-243
    pathophysiology of, 243, 244*f*
    physical assessment of, 243-245
    progression of, 248
    radiologic studies of, 246-247
    Ranson's criteria for, 247
Pancreatitis—cont'd
  acute—cont'd
    Ranson's risk factors for, 247
    risk factors for, 247
    surgical intervention for, 250
    therapeutic management of, 249-250
  alcoholic, 240
PAOP. *See* Pulmonary artery occlusion pressure
Paralysis, peripheral vascular, 113
Parenchyma, causes of respiratory failure and, 330
Parental grief, 354
Parental needs, 353
Parenteral nutrition, 158-160
  advantages of, 158
  complications of, 158-159
  decision tree for, 153, 156*f*
  disease- or organ-specific formulas for, 159-160
  doses of in critically ill children, 348, 348*t*
  vs enteral support, 153
  monitoring for, 160, 160*t*
  total, 158
    complications of, 159
    disease- or organ-specific formulas for, 159-160
Partial pressure of oxygen in venous blood (PvO_2)
  effects of on oxyhemoglobin dissociation curve, 386, 387*f*
  formula and normal values for, 388, 388*t*
Partial thromboplastin time, alterations in DIC and, 93, 93*t*
Patient monitoring. *See* Monitoring
Patient positioning. *See* Positioning
PCV. *See* Pressure control ventilation
PCWP. *See* Pulmonary capillary wedge pressure
Pediatric patients
  cardiovascular dysfunction in, 333-338
  central nervous system dysfunction in, 338-340
  critically ill, parenteral nutrient doses in, 348, 348*t*
  daily nutrient needs for, 347, 348*t*
  family support for, 353-354
  fluid resuscitation requirements in, 336, 336*t*
  growth and development of, 352-353
  heart rate limits in, 333, 333*t*
  hematologic system dysfunction in, 340-342
  hepatic dysfunction in, 345-347
  infection in, 348-349
  inflammatory/immune response in, 329
  maintenance fluid requirements in, 336, 336*t*
Pediatric patients—cont'd
  maldistribution of circulating blood volume in, 329
  metabolism alterations in, 329
  multiple organ dysfunction syndrome in, 327-356
    criteria for, 327, 328*t*
    events reported to trigger, 327, 328
    pathophysiology of, 329-330
  myocardial ischemia in, causes of, 334
  normal pressure values for, 336, 336*t*
  nutritional assessment in, 347
  nutritional support for, 347-348
  oxygen supply and demand imbalance in, 329
  pain management in, 349-352
    effects of growth and development on, 350, 351*f*
  positive-pressure support for, guidelines for initiating, 332
  renal system dysfunction in, 342-345
  respiratory dysfunction in, 330-333
  skin integrity and, 349
  ventilatory support for, 331-332
PEEP. *See* Positive end-expiratory pressure
Pentazocine (Talwin), 200, 211
Pentobarbital (Nembutal), 200
Pentothal sodium. *See* Thiopental
Pentoxifylline, 417
Peptides, 439
Perfusion
  abnormalities, 142-143
  cardiovascular, effects of aging on, 371-372
  global, 265
  lung, 171
  regional, targets of, 393-394
Peripheral nervous system, causes of respiratory failure and, 330
Peripheral vascular paralysis, 113
Peritoneal dialysis, 298*t*-299*t*
Permeability
  changes in, 112
  microvascular, associated mediators and contributing factors in, 49, 50*t*
PGE$_1$. *See* Prostaglandin E$_1$
pH
  arterial, 388-389
    formula and normal values for, 388, 388*t*
  gastric mucosal, 230, 390
    formula and normal values for, 388, 388*t*
  targets of, 393-394
Phagocytes
  migration of from blood to tissue, 25, 26*f*
  mononuclear system of, 60-61
Phagocytosis of microorganisms, 25, 27*f*

Pharmacologic support
  for ARDS, 184
    recommendations for, 187, 188t
  for CNS dysfunction in pediatric patients, 340
  for myocardial dysfunction, 272-273
  for myocardial dysfunction in children, 336-337, 337t
Pharmacologic therapy. *See also specific drugs*
  for maldistribution of circulating volume, 128-131
Phenobarbital (Luminal), 200
Phenylbutazone (Butazolidin), 200, 211
Phenylephrine, 129t, 131, 272
  relative potency of, 270t, 270-271
Phenytoin (Dilantin), 199, 200
Pindolol (Visken), 200
Pineal gland, physiologic anatomy of, 310-311, 311t
Plasma cascades, 20, 428t-429t. *See also specific cascades*
  activity of, 20, 21t
Platelet-activating factor, 66, 434t
  action of, 110, 111t
  in ARDS, 176
  impact of on MODS, 66
  physiologic role of, 66
  renal effects of, 292-293, 293t
Platelets, 66, 431t
  aggregation of, 75
  in ARDS, 176
  count alterations in DIC, 93, 93t
  decreased, etiology of, 408, 410t
  impact of on MODS, 66
  mediators produced by, 20-21, 22t
  physiologic role of, 66
  plug formation and, 74
  release reaction and, 74-75
  role of in fibrin formation, 75
  shape change of, 74
Pleurae, causes of respiratory failure and, 330
Pneumonia, aspiration, 157-158
Polyclonal antibodies, stimulation of, 414, 415f
Portal circulation, 196, 198f
Positioning
  arterial oxygen content and, 397
  in CNS dysfunction, 316-319
  for mechanical ventilation, 184
  pulmonary blood flow and, 169, 170f
  pulmonary gas exchange and, 169, 170f
Positive end-expiratory pressure, 181, 182t-183t
Positive-pressure support, for pediatric patients, guidelines for initiating, 332
Postinjury ARDS score, 408, 411t
Postinjury MOF score, 408, 411t

Postischemic reperfusion injury, 119-122
  effects of, 120
Postischemic xanthine oxidation, 119-120
Postrenal disease, causes of in children, 343
Potassium, increased, action of, 109t
Prazosin (Minipress), 200
Prealbumin, 155t
Prednisolone, 200
Prednisone, 211
Preload, 385-386
  ventricular, 255-256, 256f
Prerenal disease, causes of in children, 343
Prerenal failure, 281
  hemodynamic classification of, 281, 281t
  laboratory values and, 281, 282t
Preschoolers. *See also* Pediatric patients
  growth and development of, 352-353
Pressure control ventilation, 181, 182t-183t
Pressure support ventilation, 181, 182t-183t
Primidone (Mysoline), 200
Procainamide (Pronestyl), 200
Procardia. *See* Nifedipine
Pronestyl. *See* Procainamide
Propoxyphene (Darvon), 200
Propranolol (Inderal), 200
Prostacyclin
  action of, 109t
  renal effects of, 292-293, 293t
  site of action of, 109t
Prostaglandin E_1, 185-186
  for children, 336-337, 337t
Prostaglandin E_2, 432t
  renal effects of, 292-293, 293t
Prostaglandin $F_{2\alpha}$, action of, 109t
Prostaglandin I_2, 432t
Prostaglandins, 439
Proteases, 434t
  action of, 110, 111t
  definition of, 439
Proteins
  metabolism of, 151-152
    in liver, 199, 201
  retinol-binding, 155t
  visceral, 153, 155t
Proteolytic activation, direct, 84
Proteolytic enzymes, 59-60
  in ARDS, 176
  impact of on MODS, 59-60
  physiologic role of, 59
Prothrombin time, alterations of in DIC, 93, 93t
Protocol management in ARDS, 188
PSV. *See* Pressure support ventilation
Psychosocial considerations, 418
Pulmonary artery catheter, 268

Pulmonary artery occlusion pressure, formula and normal values for, 385, 385t
Pulmonary blood flow
  causes of respiratory failure and, 330
  effects of position on, 169, 170f
Pulmonary capillary blood flow, effects of gravity on, 171-172, 172f
Pulmonary capillary wedge pressure, 262t
  goal of, 269t
  in acute lung injury, 169t
  in adult respiratory distress syndrome, 169t
  in shock states, 268, 268t
Pulmonary damage
  with acute pancreatitis, 248-249
  structural, 181
Pulmonary gas exchange, effects of position on, 169, 170f
Pulmonary system
  age-related changes in, 366, 368t
  assessment of, 37, 38t
  effects of TNF on, 62, 63t
  failure, criteria for in elderly, 358-361, 360t, 366, 367t
  IIR impact on and complications of, 37, 38t
  role of in MODS, 406, 407f
Pulmonary vascular resistance, 262t
Pulmonary vascular resistance index, 262t
  formula and normal values for, 385, 385t
Pulmonary vasculature, 116t, 116-118
Purkinje cells, cerebellar, physiologic anatomy of, 310-311, 311t
$P\overline{v}o_2$. *See* Venous oxygen partial pressure
PVR. *See* Pulmonary vascular resistance

Q

Quinidine, 199, 200

R

Radicals. *See* Oxygen-derived free radicals
Ranitidine (Zantac), 200
RAP. *See* Right atrial pressure
Raphe nucleus, physiologic anatomy of, 310-311, 311t
Reactive oxygen species, 435t
Receptors
  adrenergic, vascular effects of, 128, 129t
  agonists, 438
  antagonists, 414-416, 439
  dopaminergic, vascular effects of, 128, 129t
  mediator, monoclonal antibodies to, 414

Red blood cell administration to increase arterial oxygen content, 396
Reflux
  bile, 243
  duodenal, 243
Regional blood flow, 113-119, 116t
Regional oxygen debt, 388-390
Regional perfusion targets, 393-394
Regulation, effects of aging on, 374-375
Renal blood flow, 116t, 119
  endotoxin-mediated factors affecting, 292-293, 293t
Renal cell injury
  endotoxin-mediated, 290-291, 292f
  pathophysiology of, 285-289, 289f
Renal dialysis, 295, 296t-299t
Renal disease, primary, causes of in children, 343
Renal failure
  acute, 276, 301
    classification of, 280-285
    definition of, 280-285
    etiology of, 280, 280f, 343
    MODS and, 294
    mortality rates of, 294, 294t
    pathophysiologic alterations in children and, 343-344
    prevention of, 294-298
    in sepsis, 285-290, 290-293
    systemic manifestations, 285, 286t-288t
    therapeutic management of, 294-298, 344-345
  criteria for
    in elderly, 358-361, 360t, 366, 367t
    in pediatric patients, 327, 328t
  fixed, causes of in children, 343
  in pediatric patients, 342-345
  TPN solutions and, 159
Renal function
  alterations in
    with acute pancreatitis, 249
    age-related, 373, 373t
  overview of, 279-280
Renal ischemia/reperfusion injury, 290, 291f
  causes of in children, 343
Renal replacement therapy, 295, 296t-299t
Renal system
  aging, 373
  anatomic and physiologic differences of in children, 343
  effects of TNF on, 62, 63t
  hemodynamic control and, 278, 279f
  obstruction of in children, 343
  role of in MODS, 407f, 408
  vasculature of, 116t, 119, 276, 277f
Renal ultrafiltration, 295, 296t-297t
Renin-angiotensin cascade, 278, 278f

Reperfusion injury. See Ischemia/reperfusion injury
Replacement therapy
  for DIC, 96-97
  renal, 295, 296t-299t
  volume, for children, 336
Repositioning, for mechanical ventilation, 184
Research
  on ARDS, 187-188
  areas of, 160
Respiration, chemical control of, 169
Respiratory acidosis, etiology of, 408, 409t
Respiratory alkalosis, etiology of, 408, 409t
Respiratory dysfunction in pediatric patients, 330-333
  anatomic classification of, 330
  assessment of, 331-332
  criteria for, 327, 328t
  interventions for, 332-333
  pathophysiologic alterations and, 331
  therapeutic management of, 331-333
Respiratory system
  aging, 366-368
  anatomic and physiologic differences of in pediatric patients, 330-331
  natural defenses and external barriers of, 23, 23t
  neuronal control of, 169
Response to insult in geriatric patients, 361-365
Restoril. See Temazepam
Resuscitation
  cerebral, 320-321
  fluid, 126-128
Retinol-binding protein, 155t
Retrovir. See Zidovudine
Reversible ischemic neurologic deficit, 306
Rifadin. See Rifampin
Rifampin (Rifadin), 200
Right atrial pressure, formula and normal values for, 385, 385t
Right-ventricular ejection fraction, 264t, 264-265
Right-ventricular end-diastolic volume index, 264t, 264-265
  formula and normal values for, 385, 385t
Right-ventricular end-systolic volume, 264
Right-ventricular stroke work index, 262t
  formula and normal values for, 385, 385t
RIND. See Reversible ischemic neurologic deficit
Rocephin. See Ceftriaxone
RVEDVI. See Right-ventricular end-diastolic volume index

RVEF. See Right-ventricular ejection fraction
RVESV. See Right-ventricular end-systolic volume
RVSWI. See Right-ventricular stroke work index

S

Salicylic acid (Aspirin), 200
Saline, hypertonic, 127
Sao$_2$. See Arterial oxygen saturation
SBP. See Systolic blood pressure
School-age children. See also Pediatric patients
  growth and development of, 353
SDD. See Selective decontamination of digestive tract
Sedative/hypnotic drugs metabolized by liver, 199, 200
Seizures, 314
Selective decontamination of digestive tract, 232
Sepsis
  acute renal failure in, 285-290
    humoral and cellular mediators and, 290-293
  assessment of, 122
  clinical presentation of, 122, 124t
  clinical signs and symptoms of, 123
  definition of, 5
  hyperdynamic vs hypodynamic responses in, 253-255
  impact of on ventricular compliance, 257-259
  impact of on ventricular preload, 256
  mediator activity in, 266-267
  myocardial dysfunction in, 252-275
  nephrotoxins and, 293-294
  nonbacteremic, 6-7
  severe
    clinical presentation of, 123, 124t
    definition of, 5
  SIRS and, 46-47, 47f
  survivors vs nonsurvivors of, 270
  therapeutic management of, 268-273
  in elderly, 377
Septic shock
  afterload with, 259, 259f
  clinical presentation of, 123, 124t
  definition of, 5
  hemodynamic changes in, 264t, 264-265, 268, 268t
  impact of on ventricular afterload, 259-260
  impact of on ventricular contractility, 264-265
  monitoring of, 267-268
  myocardial dysfunction in, 253
  pathogenesis of, 253, 254f
  therapeutic goals in, 268, 269t
  ventricular changes in, 261-262, 263f

Septic triad, 48-49
Septra. *See* Sulfamethoxazole
Serax. *See* Oxazepam
Serotonin, 109*t*, 435*t*
Serotonin-containing region of the brain, physiologic anatomy of, 310-311, 311*t*
Serum albumin, 155*t*
Serum lactate, 389-390
Serum transferrin, 155*t*
Shock
  in children
    cardiogenic low-flow, 334-335
    fluid resuscitation requirements in, 336, 336*t*
    hypovolemic low-flow, 334
    maldistributive, 335
  distributive, 268, 268*t*
  hemodynamic parameters in, 268, 268*t*
  in neonates, fluid resuscitation requirements for, 336, 336*t*
  neurogenic, 268, 268*t*
  obstructive, 268, 268*t*
  renal cell injury in, 285-289, 289*f*
  septic
    afterload with, 259, 259*f*
    clinical presentation of, 123, 124*t*
    definition of, 5
    hemodynamic changes in, 264*t*, 264-265, 268, 268*t*
    impact of on ventricular afterload, 259-260
    impact of on ventricular contractility, 264-265
    monitoring of, 267-268
    myocardial dysfunction in, 253
    pathogenesis of, 253, 254*f*
    therapeutic goals in, 268, 269*t*
    ventricular changes in, 261-262, 263*f*
Shunts, intrapulmonary, 172, 180
SIMV. *See* Synchronized intermittent mandatory ventilation
SIRS. *See* Systemic inflammatory response syndrome
Skin integrity in pediatric patients, 349
Small intestine, 219-220
  blood supply to, 219*f*, 220, 220*f*
  functional anatomy of, 219-220
  morphologic layers of, 226, 227*f*
  secretory role of, 220
SNS. *See* Sympathetic nervous system
Sodium nitroprusside, 273
  for children, 336-337, 337*t*
Spironolactone (Aldactone), 200
Splanchnic circulation, 116*t*, 118-119
Splanchnic ischemia, causes and effects of, 223, 224*f*
Statistics, 357-358
Steroids
  anabolic and contraceptive, 211

Steroids—cont'd
  antiinflammatory and immunosuppressive effects of, 31-33, 33*f*
Stomach, 218-219
  blood supply to, 219, 219*f*
  functional anatomy of, 218-219
  histologic organization of, 215, 216*f*
  secretory role of, 219
Stress, immune alterations in, 31-34, 32*t*
Stress response, 8
  geriatric, 361-362, 362*f*
  metabolic, in elderly, 362-363
  neuroendocrine hormone activity in, 8, 10*t*
Stress ulcers, prophylaxis of, 231-232
Stroke volume, 262*t*
Stroke work index, 262*t*, 262-263
  formula and normal values for, 385, 385*t*
  left-ventricular, 262*t*, 385, 385*t*
  right-ventricular, 262*t*, 385, 385*t*
Submucosal arteries, physiology of, 215-217, 216*f*
Substance abuse, immune alterations in, 36
Substrates
  definition of, 439
  metabolism of
    aerobic, 135-136
    anaerobic, 137-138
  normal oxidation of, 135-136
Sucralfate, 232
Suction catheters, nasogastric, 230, 231*f*
Sufenta. *See* Fentanyl
Sulfamethoxazole (Bactrim or Septra), 200
Sulfinpyrazone (Anturane), 200
Sulfisoxazole (Azo Gantrisin), 200
Sumycin. *See* Tetracycline
Surfactant, exogenous, 186
Surgery, immune alterations in, 31, 32*t*, 36
SV. *See* Stroke volume
Svo_2. *See* Venous oxygen saturation
SVR. *See* Systemic vascular resistance
SWI. *See* Stroke work index
Sympathetic nervous system
  activation of, 8-10
  responsiveness of, 266
Synchronized intermittent mandatory ventilation, 181, 182*t*-183*t*
Systemic inflammatory response syndrome, 46-49, 248
  abatement of, interventions and expected response in, 397, 399*t*
  assessment of, 122
  clinical presentation of, 122
  clinical signs and symptoms of, 123
  compensated state and, 390-391, 392*f*
    interventions and expected response to, 397, 399*t*

Systemic inflammatory response syndrome—cont'd
  decompensated state and, 391-392, 392*f*
    interventions and expected response, 397, 399*t*
  definition of, 5, 46-47, 47*f*, 359, 361*t*
  intrinsic control of, 67-68
  mechanisms of inflammation in, 47-48, 48*f*
  modulation of, future trends in, 416
  pathophysiology of, 47-49, 49*f*, 50*t*
    cascade of, 402, 405*t*
  role of complement cascade in, 53-55, 54*f*, 55*f*
  role of endothelin in, 53
  role of endothelium in, 49-51, 51*f*
  role of gut in, 225-226, 226*f*
  role of nitric oxide in, 52
  summary of, 67-68
  uncompensated state and, 391, 392*f*
    interventions and expected response to, 397, 399*t*
    manifestations of, 398
Systemic vascular resistance, 262*t*
  decreased, etiology of, 408, 409*t*
  goal for, 269*t*
  in shock states, 268, 268*t*
Systemic vascular resistance index, 262*t*
  formula and normal values for, 385, 385*t*
Systolic blood pressure, goal for, 269*t*

T

T cells
  macrophage interactions requiring MHC Class II surface antigens, 29, 30*f*
  normal values for, 37, 40*t*
Tachycardia, etiology of, 408, 409*t*
Tagamet. *See* Cimetidine
Talwin. *See* Pentazocine
Tegretol. *See* Carbamazepine
Temazepam (Restoril), 200
Terminology, 5
Tetracycline (Sumycin), 200, 211
TF. *See* Tissue factor
TGF-β. *See* Transforming growth factor-β
Thalamic nuclei, physiologic anatomy of, 310-311, 311*t*
Theo-Dur. *See* Theophylline
Theophylline (Theo-Dur), 200
Thiopental (Pentothal Sodium), 200
Thorazine. *See* Chlorpromazine
Thrombi, microvascular, associated mediators and contributing factors for, 49, 50*t*
Thrombin
  in clotting cascade, 79
  hemostatic control mechanisms for, 82

Thrombin time, alterations in DIC and, 93, 93*t*
Thrombocytopenia in children, 340-341
Thrombosis in DIC, 85-87, 86*f*
Thromboxane, 432*t*
  renal effects of, 292-293, 293*t*
Thromboxane A$_2$, 109*t*
Tissue and oxygen debt, 141
Tissue factor, release of, 83-84
Tissue hypoxia, assessment of, 178, 179*t*
Tissue macrophages, 60, 60*t*
TNF. *See* Tumor necrosis factor
Tocainide (Tonocard), 200
Toddlers. *See also* Pediatric patients
  growth and development of, 352
Tolbutamide (Orinase), 200
TOM. *See* Toxic oxygen metabolites
Tonocard. *See* Tocainide
Tonometry, gastric, 230, 231*f*
Total parenteral nutrition, 158
  complications of, 159
  disease- or organ-specific formulas for, 159-160
Toxic oxygen metabolites, 58-59, 435*t*
  impact of on MODS, 59
  physiologic role of, 58-59
  production of
    in infection, inflammation, and ischemia, 6
    in ischemia/reperfusion injury, 13, 14*f*
Toxicity, oxygen, 181
TPN. *See* Total parenteral nutrition
Trandate. *See* Labetalol
Transferrin, serum, 155*t*
Transforming growth factor-β, 66-67, 435*t*
  impact of on MODS, 66-67
  physiologic role of, 66
Transforming growth factor-β1, cellular source and CNS effects of, 311, 312*t*
Trauma
  immune alterations in, 31, 32*t*, 34
  to pancreas, 241
Triamterene/HCTZ (Dyazide), 200
TRIP nasogastric suction catheter, 230, 231*f*
Trisynaptic circuit, 313, 315*f*
Tuber cinereum, physiologic anatomy of, 310-311, 311*t*
Tubular necrosis, acute, 281-283
  causes of, 282, 283*t*
  future trends in management and prevention of, 299-301
  laboratory values in, 281, 282*t*, 283-284
Tubuloglomerular feedback, 277-278
Tumor necrosis factor, 61-62, 435*t*
  action of, 110, 111*t*
  in ARDS, 175

Tumor necrosis factor—cont'd
  biologic effects of, 62, 63*t*
  impact of on MODS, 62, 63*t*
  physiologic role of, 61-62
  renal effects of, 292-293, 293*t*
  role of in SIRS, 48-49
  in sepsis, 267
Tumor necrosis factor-α, cellular source and CNS effects of, 311, 312*t*
Tylenol. *See* Acetaminophen

U

Ulcers
  endoscopic, 229
  stress, prophylaxis and, 231-232
Ultrafiltration, renal, 295, 296*t*-297*t*
Ureagenesis, 439
Uremia, with acute renal failure, 285, 287*t*-288*t*
Urine output, decreased, 408, 409*t*
Urodilatin, 299

V

V/Q. *See* Ventilation-perfusion ratio
VADs. *See* Ventricular assist devices
Valium. *See* Diazepam
Valproic acid (Depakene), 200
Vanderbilt University Medical Center, critical pathway for ARDS and, 188, 189*t*-192*t*
  guidelines for use, 188, 193*t*
Vascular disease, causes of, 334
Vascular paralysis, peripheral, 113
Vasculature
  cerebral, 119
  pulmonary, 116*t*, 116-118
  renal, 116*t*, 119, 276, 277*f*
Vasoactive drugs
  categories of, 129*t*
  for children, 336-337, 337*t*
  to increase cardiac output, 395-396
Vasoactive mediators, 108, 109*t*
  release of with injury or inflammation, 108-111
Vasoactive substances in ARDS, 176
Vasoconstriction
  associated mediators and contributing factors to, 49, 50*t*
  normal hemostatic mechanisms of, 74
Vasodilatation
  associated mediators and contributing factors to, 49, 50*t*
  causes of, 343
Vasodilators
  for gastrointestinal involvement, 232
  for myocardial dysfunction, 272-273
Vasomotor control, 112
Vasopressin, 109*t*
Vasopressor therapy, 270-272
  goal of, 270-271
  relative potencies of, 270*t*, 270-271

Venous access for monitoring, 268
Venous admixture, 180
Venous oxygen content (Cvo$_2$) formula and normal values, 385, 385*t*
Venous oxygen delivery index (Dvo$_2$I) formula and normal values, 385, 385*t*
Venous oxygen partial pressure (Pvo$_2$)
  effects of on oxyhemoglobin dissociation curve, 386, 387*f*
  formula and normal values for, 388, 388*t*
Venous oxygen saturation (Svo$_2$)
  decreased, 408, 410*t*
  formula and normal values for, 388, 388*t*
  hepatic, targets, 394
  increased, 408, 410*t*
Venovenous hemodialysis, continuous, 298*t*-299*t*
Venovenous hemofiltration, continuous, 296*t*-297*t*
Ventilation, 169-173
  control of, 169
  dead-space, 170
  distribution of, 169, 170*f*
  effects of aging on, 366-368
  high-frequency, 181, 182*t*-183*t*
  inverse ratio, 181, 182*t*-183*t*
  mechanical
    in ARDS, 180-184
    to increase arterial oxygen content, 396-397
  muscles of, 169
  pressure control, 181, 182*t*-183*t*
  pressure support, 181, 182*t*-183*t*
  support of for pediatric patients, 331-332
  synchronized intermittent mandatory, 181, 182*t*-183*t*
  ventilator strategies for, 181, 182*t*-183*t*
Ventilation-perfusion matching, 171-172, 172*f*, 173*f*
Ventilation-perfusion mismatching, 180
Ventilation-perfusion ratio (V/Q), three-zoned model of, 171-172, 172*f*
Ventilation-perfusion relationships, 172, 173*f*
Ventricular afterload, 259*f*, 259-260
  impact of disease on, 259-260
  physiologic role of, 259, 259*f*
Ventricular assist devices, 273, 337
Ventricular compliance, 256-259
  impact of disease on, 257-259
  physiologic role of, 256-257, 257*f*, 258*f*
Ventricular contractility, 260-265
  impact of disease on, 264-265
  physiologic role of, 260-264, 261*f*, 262*t*
Ventricular preload, 255-256
  definition of, 255
  impact of disease on, 256

Ventricular preload—cont'd
  physiologic role of, 255-256, 256f
Verapamil (Calan), 200
Versed. *See* Midazolam
Visceral proteins, 153, 155t
Visken. *See* Pindolol
Vitamins, liver storage of, 201
Vo$_2$. *See* Oxygen consumption
Volume, circulating, maldistribution of, 107-134
  definition of, 9-12, 12t
  in pediatric patients, 329
Volume depletion, true, 343

Volume infusion, 269-270
  goal of, 269
  response to, 269
Volume loading, 256-257, 258f
Volume overload with acute renal failure, 285, 286t
Volume replacement for children, 336

W

Warfarin (Coumadin), 200
WBCs. *See* White blood cells
White blood cells
  activation of, 120, 122f

White blood cells—cont'd
  adhesion molecules, monoclonal antibodies to, 186
  normal values for, 37, 40t

X

Xanthine oxidation, 119-120, 121f

Z

Zantac. *See* Ranitidine
Zidovudine (Retrovir), 200
Zymogen, 439

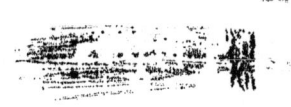